Weight Watchers®

# Dining Out Companion

PointsPlus™



Printed in U.S.A.

Weight Watchers PointsPlus

## NEW FOR 2011! 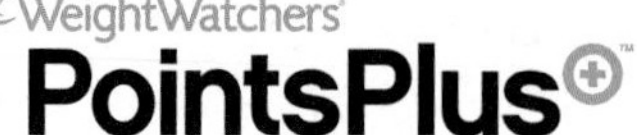


**Let 2011 be your year for enjoying the pleasures of dining out while following the Weight Watchers plan! Whether you know where you're going or haven't decided yet, this book is for you.**

### Know where you're going?

Find the menu in our extensive list of national chain restaurants beginning on page 65 and make wise choices even before you get there! Your restaurant not listed? Turn to page 9 for menu items commonly found in several types of restaurants.

### Haven't decided yet where to go?

Use the listings to find a chain or cuisine that allows you options. Or use them just to get some great ideas. That way, deciding once you get to the restaurant will be easier.

### In this book you will find:

**DINING OUT A-Z FOOD LIST:** an alphabetical ***PointsPlus***™ value guide to hundreds and hundreds of restaurant foods (Weight Watchers® Power Foods are identified by a green pyramid [▲])

**ETHNIC & REGIONAL FAVORITES:** organized by cuisine for quick and easy reference, this comprehensive listing with ***PointsPlus*** values features the most popular ethnic and regional dishes from the A-Z Food List

**RESTAURANT MENUS:** ***PointsPlus*** values for menu items from 140 national restaurant chains

### *A note about restaurant offerings:*

Since most of the restaurants listed in this book have locations in different parts of the country, keep in mind that a restaurant chain's offerings may vary by location. And all items featured in each restaurant's menu listings and photos may not be available at every location.

### *A note about PointsPlus values:*

The ***PointsPlus*** values for all of the foods in this book were calculated by Weight Watchers International, Inc. using the most current nutrition information provided by the participating restaurants at the time of the book's publication. However, since restaurants may revise their menus, recipes, or serving sizes throughout the year, feel free to ask for nutrition information or to check the restaurant's website for updated information, and use your ***PointsPlus*** Calculator to check ***PointsPlus*** values.

> It is important to know that certain foods, especially sugar-free ones, may contain sugar alcohols, which can reduce total ***PointsPlus*** values of the food. These ingredients – and also regular alcohol – are not typically included on food labels or in the nutrition information supplied by participating restaurants, so as a result, you might notice discrepancies with the ***PointsPlus*** values you see in the lists in this book and the values you calculate with your ***PointsPlus*** Calculator. For the most accurate ***PointsPlus*** values for sugar-free foods and foods containing alcohol, you can feel confident using this book, your Program materials, or if you are a subscriber to eTools, the database on WeightWatchers.com.

# CONTENTS

# CONTENTS

# Dining Out A-Z Food List

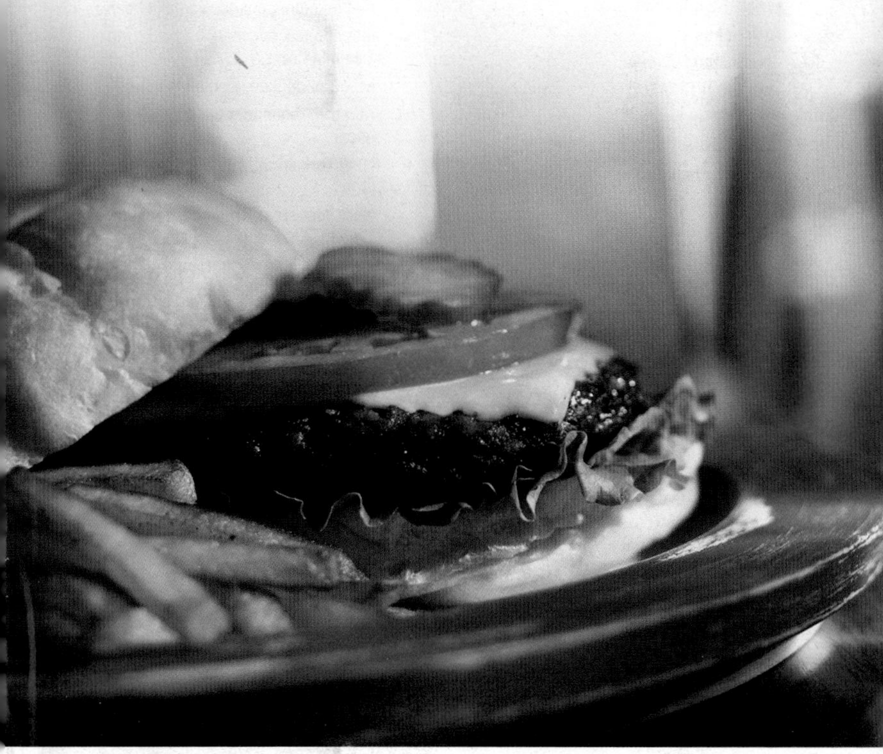

| ▲ Power Foods | PointsPlus™ value |
|---|---|
| **A** | |
| **Almond float,** 1 cup | 3 |
| **Ambrosia,** 1/2 cup | 2 |
| **Apple** | |
| baked, 1 large (7 oz) | 9 |
| caramel, 1 large (8 oz) | 13 |
| **Apple brown Betty,** 1 cup | 6 |
| **Apple crisp,** 3/4 cup | 11 |
| **Apple fritter,** restaurant-type, 1 (4 oz) | 12 |
| **Apple kuchen,** 1 piece (4 oz) | 12 |
| **Apple streusel,** 1/2 cup | 5 |
| **Arroz con pollo,** 3 oz chicken with 1 1/2 cups rice | 15 |
| **Artichokes** | |
| marinated, 1/2 cup | 4 |
| stuffed, 1 (7 3/4 oz) | 15 |
| **B** | |
| **Baba au rhum,** 1 (3 oz) | 10 |
| **Baba ganosh,** 1/4 cup | 3 |
| **Bacon** | |
| Canadian-style, cooked, 1 slice (1 oz) | 1 |
| cooked, crisp, 1 slice | 1 |
| cooked, crisp, 3 slices | 4 |
| **Bacon bits,** imitation, 1 tsp | 0 |
| **Bagel** | |
| any type, 1 mini (2 1/2" diameter) | 2 |
| any type, 1 small or 1/2 large (2 oz) | 4 |
| with cream cheese and lox, 1 large (4 3/4 oz) | 14 |
| **Baked Alaska,** 2" wedge or 1/12 of 9" cake | 6 |
| **Baklava,** 1 piece (1 1/4 oz) | 7 |
| **Banana bread,** with or without nuts, 1 slice (2 1/2 oz) | 6 |
| **Banana split,** 3 scoops (1 1/2 cups) ice cream, 1 banana, 3 Tbsp syrup, and 1/2 cup whipped cream | 21 |
| **Bananas Foster,** 1 (9 oz) | 18 |
| ▲ **Beans,** garbanzo (chick peas), cooked or canned, 1/2 cup | 3 |
| **Beans,** baked | |
| 1/2 cup | 8 |
| fast-food, 1 serving (6 oz) | 5 |
| **Beans, black, with rice,** 1 cup | 6 |
| **Beans, red, with rice,** 1 cup | 7 |
| ▲ **Beans, refried,** 1/2 cup | 4 |
| **Beans and franks,** 1 cup | 13 |
| **Bear claw,** restaurant-type, 1 (4 oz) | 11 |
| **Beef** | |
| brisket, cooked, 3 oz | 9 |
| filet mignon, cooked, 1 small (4 oz) | 10 |
| ▲ filet mignon, trimmed, cooked, 1 small (4 oz) | 6 |
| KC strip, cooked, 1 small (4 oz) | 7 |
| ▲ KC strip, trimmed, cooked, 1 small (4 oz) | 6 |
| New York steak, cooked, 1 small (4 oz) | 8 |
| ▲ New York steak, trimmed, cooked, 1 small (4 oz) | 5 |
| shortribs, lean and fat, cooked, 3 oz | 11 |
| shortribs, trimmed, cooked, 3 oz | 6 |
| ▲ steak, lean, cooked (round or loin cuts other than those listed here with all visible fat trimmed), 1 small (4 oz) | 5 |
| steak, regular, cooked, 1 small (4 oz) | 10 |
| strip sirloin, cooked, 1 small (4 oz) | 7 |
| ▲ strip sirloin, trimmed, cooked, 1 small (4 oz) | 5 |
| T-bone steak, cooked, 1 small (4 oz) | 9 |
| T-bone steak, trimmed, cooked, 1 small (4 oz) | 7 |
| **Beef, corned,** cooked, 3 oz | 6 |
| **Beef, ground** | |
| 75% lean/25% fat (regular), cooked, 1 patty (3 oz) | 5 |
| 80% lean/20% fat, cooked, 1 patty (3 oz) | 5 |

| ▲ Power Foods | *PointsPlus*™ value |
|---|---|
| 85% lean/15% fat, cooked, 1 patty (3 oz) | 5 |
| 90% lean/10% fat, cooked, 1 patty (3 oz) | 4 |
| ▲ 95% lean/5% fat, cooked, 1 patty (3 oz) | 3 |
| **Beef, orange-ginger,** 1 cup | 15 |
| **Beef, sweet and sour,** 1 cup | 13 |
| **Beef and broccoli,** 1 cup | 4 |
| **Beef bourguignon,** 1 cup | 15 |
| **Beef goulash,** 1 cup | 9 |
| **Beef masala,** 1 cup | 6 |
| **Beef stir-fry,** with garlic or black bean sauce, 1 cup | 8 |
| **Beef Stroganoff with noodles,** 1 cup stroganoff with 1 cup of noodles | 17 |
| **Beef Wellington,** 1 slice (3 1/2" x 2 1/2" x 1 1/2") | 14 |
| **Beer** | |
| light, 1 can or bottle (12 fl oz) | 3 |
| non-alcoholic, 1 can or bottle (12 fl oz) | 2 |
| regular, 1 can or bottle (12 fl oz) | 5 |
| **Beignet,** 1 (3/4 oz) | 2 |
| **Bellini,** 1 (6 fl oz) | 6 |
| **Benny cake,** 1 piece (2" x 3") | 4 |
| ▲ **Berries, mixed,** 1 cup | 0 |
| **Bhuna gosht,** 1 cup | 9 |
| **Bialy,** 1 (3 oz) | 7 |
| **Biryani** | |
| chicken, 1 cup | 11 |
| lamb, 1 cup | 15 |
| **Biscotti** | |
| chocolate, 8 mini, 2 small, or 1 regular (1 oz) | 4 |
| plain or fat-free, 8 mini, 2 small, or 1 regular (1 oz) | 3 |
| **Biscuit** | |
| cheese, 1 (2" diameter) | 6 |
| with egg and bacon, fast food, 1 | 13 |

| ▲ Power Foods | *PointsPlus*™ value |
|---|---|
| with egg and ham, fast food, 1 | 12 |
| with egg and sausage, fast food, 1 | 15 |
| with egg and steak, fast food, 1 | 11 |
| with egg, cheese, and bacon, fast food, 1 | 12 |
| with egg, fast food, 1 | 9 |
| with ham, fast food, 1 | 11 |
| with steak, fast food, 1 | 13 |
| **Bistec de palomilla (Cuban fried steak),** 1 steak (6 oz) | 11 |
| **Black Russian,** 1 (3 fl oz) | 8 |
| **Blanquette of veal,** 1 cup | 6 |
| **Blintz, cheese,** 1 (4 1/2 oz) | 6 |
| **Bloody Mary,** 1 (5 fl oz) | 4 |
| **Borscht,** without sour cream, 1 cup | 4 |
| **Boston brown bread,** 1 slice (3 3/4" x 1/2") | 3 |
| **Bouillabaisse,** 2 cups | 9 |
| **Bourbon,** 1 fl oz | 3 |
| **Brandy Alexander,** 1 (3 fl oz) | 9 |
| **Brandy,** 1 jigger (1 1/2 fl oz) | 4 |
| **Bread** | |
| any type other than those listed here (white, wheat, rye, Italian, French, pumpernickel), 1 slice (1 oz) | 2 |
| challah, 1 slice (5" x 3" x 3/4") | 3 |
| chapati, 1 piece (5" diameter) | 3 |
| enjera, 1 (9" diameter) | 2 |
| naan, 1 piece (7" x 8" diameter) | 5 |
| **Bread, garlic,** 1 slice (1 1/2 oz) | 6 |
| **Breadstick** | |
| any type, 2 long (7 1/2" x 1/2" or 3/4 oz) | 2 |
| any type, 4 short (5" x 1/2" or 3/4 oz) | 2 |
| soft, 1 (1 1/3 oz) | 3 |
| **Brioche,** 1 slice (1 oz) | 3 |
| **Broccoli rice casserole,** 1 cup | 5 |
| **Broccoli stir-fry,** 1 cup | 4 |
| **Brownie** | |
| 1 (2" square) | 6 |

*Brownie (cont'd)*

| ▲ Power Foods | PointsPlus™ value |
|---|---|
| fast food, 1 (2" square) | 7 |
| walnut, restaurant-type, 1 (4 1/2 oz) | 15 |
| **Bruschetta,** 1 slice (3 oz) | 3 |
| **Bubble and squeak,** 1 cup | 5 |
| **Buffalo wings,** cooked, 3 (4 1/2 oz) | 9 |
| **Bulgogi (beef stir-fry),** 1 cup | 5 |
| **Burgoo,** 1 cup | 5 |
| **Burrito** | |
| bean, 1 small (6") | 7 |
| bean, 1 large (8") | 10 |
| bean and cheese, fast food, 2 pieces (6 1/2 oz) | 10 |
| bean and chili peppers, fast food, 2 pieces (7 oz) | 11 |
| bean and meat, fast food, 2 pieces (8 oz) | 14 |
| bean, cheese, and chili peppers, fast food, 2 pieces (12 oz) | 18 |
| bean, fast food, 1 (5 oz) | 9 |
| beans, cheese, and beef, fast food, 2 pieces (7 oz) | 9 |
| beef and cheese, 1 small (6") | 8 |
| beef and cheese, 1 large (8") | 7 |
| beef and chili peppers, fast food, 2 pieces (7 oz) | 11 |
| beef, cheese, and chili peppers, fast food, 2 pieces (10 3/4 oz) | 17 |
| beef, fast food, 2 pieces (7 3/4 oz) | 14 |
| chicken and cheese, 1 small (6") | 6 |
| chicken and cheese, 1 large (8") | 8 |
| fruit, fast food, 1 small (2 1/2 oz) | 6 |
| vegetable, 1 small (made with a 6" tortilla) | 6 |
| vegetable, 1 large (made with a 10" tortilla) | 12 |
| **Butter,** regular, 1 tsp | 1 |
| **Butter chicken,** 1 cup | 9 |

## C

| ▲ Power Foods | PointsPlus™ value |
|---|---|
| **Cabbage,** stuffed, 2 (2" x 2 1/2") | 7 |
| **Cake** | |
| angel food, 1/16 of a 10" tube | 3 |
| Boston cream pie, 1/6 of the pie (3 1/4 oz) | 6 |
| carrot, with cream cheese icing, 1/12 of a 9" layer cake, or 3" square | 18 |
| coffee, 3" square, or 1/12 of a 9" tube | 9 |
| fruitcake, 2 1/2" x 1 3/4" x 1/2" or 2 oz | 6 |
| honey, 5" x 3" x 1" | 9 |
| pineapple upside-down, 1/8 of a 10" skillet cake | 13 |
| pound, 1 slice (5" x 3" x 1") | 9 |
| strawberry shortcake, 1/12 of a 9" cake or 1 filled individual shortcake | 8 |
| with icing, 1/12 of a 9" layer cake or 3" square | 14 |
| **Calamari** | |
| fried, 1/2 cup | 11 |
| ▲ grilled, 1/2 cup | 1 |
| **Calzone, ham and cheese,** 1 (5 1/4" x 6") | 15 |
| **Cannelloni** | |
| cheese, with meat sauce, 2 shells with 1/2 cup sauce | 22 |
| cheese, with tomato sauce, 2 shells with 1/2 cup sauce | 14 |
| meat, with cream sauce, 2 shells with 1/2 cup sauce | 19 |
| meat, with tomato sauce, 2 shells with 1/2 cup sauce | 15 |
| spinach and cheese, with cream sauce, 2 shells with 1/2 cup sauce | 17 |
| spinach and cheese, with tomato sauce, 2 shells with 1/2 cup sauce | 14 |
| **Cannoli,** 1 (3 1/2" long) | 10 |
| **Caponata (eggplant appetizer),** 1 cup | 5 |

| ▲ Power Foods | *PointsPlus*™ value |
|---|---|
| **Cappuccino** | |
| ▲ made with fat-free milk, 1 small (8 fl oz) | 1 |
| ▲ made with fat-free milk, 1 tall (12 fl oz) | 2 |
| ▲ made with fat-free milk, 1 grande (16 fl oz) | 2 |
| made with low-fat milk, 1 small (8 fl oz) | 2 |
| made with low-fat milk, 1 tall (12 fl oz) | 3 |
| made with low-fat milk, 1 grande (16 fl oz) | 3 |
| made with whole milk, 1 small (8 fl oz) | 2 |
| made with whole milk, 1 tall (12 fl oz) | 3 |
| made with whole milk, 1 grande (16 fl oz) | 4 |
| **Carne asada,** 4 oz | 10 |
| **Carne guisado (Cuban beef stew),** 1 cup | 7 |
| **Carnitas,** 1 cup | 9 |
| **Carrots and parsnips,** 1 cup | 6 |
| **Cashew chicken,** 6 1/4 oz | 7 |
| **Cassoulet,** 1 cup | 12 |
| **Cavatelli with sausage and broccoli,** 1 cup | 6 |
| **Caviar,** any type, 1 oz | 2 |
| **Ceviche,** 1/2 cup | 2 |
| **Chalupa (pork and bean dish),** 1 cup | 7 |
| **Champagne,** 1 small glass (4 fl oz) | 3 |
| ▲ **Chana dal,** 1 cup | 5 |
| **Channa masala,** 1 cup | 9 |
| **Char shiu bao (roast pork bun),** 1 (2 oz) | 5 |
| **Cheese, cottage,** regular (4%), 1 cup | 6 |
| **Cheese, hard or semisoft, dairy or soy,** regular, 1" cube, 1/4 cup shredded, or 3 Tbsp grated (1 oz) | 3 |

| ▲ Power Foods | *PointsPlus*™ value |
|---|---|
| **Cheese fries,** restaurant-type, 8 1/2 oz | 18 |
| **Cheeseburger** | |
| double, fast food, 1 | 12 |
| double, with bacon, fast food, 1 | 21 |
| large, double, with condiments and vegetables, fast food, 1 | 19 |
| large, fast food, 1 | 15 |
| large, with bacon and condiments, fast food, 1 | 15 |
| large, with condiments and vegetables, fast food, 1 | 12 |
| on bun, fast food, 1 small | 8 |
| on bun, plain, without mayonnaise, lettuce, and tomato, 1 (6 1/2 oz) | 12 |
| small, with condiments and vegetables, fast food, 1 | 10 |
| triple, plain, fast food, 1 | 21 |
| **Cheesecake** | |
| any type, fast food, 3 1/2 oz | 9 |
| with fruit topping, 1/16 of the 10" cake | 12 |
| without fruit topping, 1/16 of the 10" cake | 11 |
| **Cherries, maraschino,** 1 | 0 |
| **Chicken, blackened,** 1 breast (3 oz) | 7 |
| **Chicken, long rice,** 1 cup | 5 |
| **Chicken, nugget-style** | |
| fried, 6 pieces (2 1/2 oz) | 8 |
| fried, fast food, 6 pieces | 9 |
| **Chicken, sesame,** 1 cup | 10 |
| **Chicken, sweet and sour,** 1 cup | 11 |
| **Chicken a la king,** 1 cup | 13 |
| **Chicken adobo,** 1 thigh (4 oz) | 6 |
| **Chicken and broccoli,** 1 cup | 3 |
| **Chicken and dumplings,** cooked, with skin, 3 oz chicken with 2 dumplings | 9 |
| **Chicken and meatball fricassee,** 2 cups | 10 |

| ▲ Power Foods | *PointsPlus*™ value |
|---|---|
| **Chicken asopao,** 10 oz | 9 |
| **Chicken breast fillet,** grilled, 1 (3 oz) | 3 |
| **Chicken breast on bun,** grilled, 1 (6 oz) | 11 |
| **Chicken breast** | |
| barbecued, with skin and bone, 1 (4 1/2 oz) | 7 |
| cooked, with skin and bone, 1 (4 1/2 oz) | 5 |
| five spice, with skin and bone, 1 (4 1/2 oz) | 7 |
| fried, with skin and bone, 1 (4 1/2 oz) | 11 |
| **Chicken cacciatore,** 1 half-breast or 1 thigh and leg (6 1/2 oz) | 11 |
| **Chicken Caesar wrap,** restaurant-type, 1 (10 oz) | 16 |
| **Chicken cordon bleu,** 1 piece (6 3/4 oz) | 10 |
| **Chicken drumstick** | |
| barbecued, with skin and bone, 1 (1 1/2 oz) | 3 |
| cooked, with skin and bone, 1 (1 1/2 oz) | 2 |
| fried, with skin and bone, 1 (1 1/2 oz) | 5 |
| fried, with skin, fast food, 1 (2 oz) | 5 |
| **Chicken hekka,** 1 cup | 7 |
| **Chicken in the pot,** without skin, 2 cups | 12 |
| **Chicken jalfrezi,** 1 cup | 6 |
| **Chicken Kiev,** 1 piece (4" x 8") | 18 |
| **Chicken leg** | |
| five spice, 1 leg, thigh, and drumstick, with skin and bone (4 1/2 oz) | 9 |
| roasted, with skin and bone, 1 leg (3 1/4 oz) | 4 |
| **Chicken marsala,** without bone, with sauce, 4 oz | 14 |
| **Chicken molé,** 1 cup | 9 |
| **Chicken paprika,** 1 breast or thigh with 1/2 cup sauce | 8 |

| ▲ Power Foods | *PointsPlus*™ value |
|---|---|
| **Chicken parmigiana** | |
| with sauce, 5 oz with 1/2 cup sauce | 11 |
| without sauce, 5 1/2 oz | 8 |
| **Chicken pilaf (kotta pilafi)** | |
| 1 cup | 8 |
| 1 breast with 1 cup pilaf | 12 |
| **Chicken stir-fry, with garlic or black bean sauce,** 1 cup | 8 |
| **Chicken tenders,** restaurant-type, 3 oz | 5 |
| **Chicken tetrazzini,** 1 1/2 cups | 15 |
| **Chicken thigh** | |
| barbecued, with skin and bone, 1 (3 oz) | 6 |
| cooked, with skin and bone, 1 (3 oz) | 4 |
| fried, with skin and bone, 1 (3 oz) | 8 |
| fried, with skin, fast food, 1 (3 1/2 oz) | 8 |
| **Chicken tikka,** 4 oz | 5 |
| **Chicken wing** | |
| cooked, with skin and bone, 1 (1 1/4 oz) | 3 |
| fried, with skin, fast food, 1 (2 oz) | 6 |
| **Chicken with cashews,** 1 cup | 11 |
| **Chile beef (neua pad prik),** 1 cup | 7 |
| **Chili cheese dog,** restaurant-type, 1 (5 oz) | 10 |
| **Chili con carne** | |
| fast food, 1 cup | 7 |
| with or without beans, 1 cup | 9 |
| **Chili con queso,** 1/4 cup | 6 |
| **Chili dog on roll,** 1 (8 1/2 oz) | 11 |
| **Chili fish (macher jhol),** 1 fillet (6 oz) | 13 |
| **Chili rellenos, beef and cheese,** without sauce, 2 (7 1/2 oz) | 19 |
| **Chimichanga** | |
| beef, 1 (3" x 3 1/2") | 12 |
| beef and cheese, fast food, 1 (6 1/2 oz) | 12 |
| beef and red chili peppers, fast food, 1 (6 3/4 oz) | 11 |

| ▲ Power Foods | *PointsPlus*™ value |
|---|---|
| beef, cheese, and red chili peppers, fast food, 1 (6 1/2 oz) | 10 |
| beef, fast food, 1 (6 oz) | 12 |
| chicken, 1 (3" x 3 1/2") | 10 |
| **Chocolate mousse,** 1 cup | 15 |
| **Cholent,** 1 cup | 5 |
| **Chop suey** | |
| beef, 1 cup | 5 |
| chicken, 1 cup | 4 |
| pork, 1 cup | 5 |
| vegetable, 1 cup | 5 |
| **Chow fun, beef, chicken, pork, or shrimp,** 1 cup | 9 |
| **Chow mein** | |
| beef, 1 cup | 5 |
| chicken, 1 cup | 4 |
| chicken subgum, 1 cup | 4 |
| pork, 1 cup | 5 |
| **Chruscik,** 1 (1/4 oz) | 1 |
| **Chuleta,** 1 pork chop (6 oz) | 12 |
| **Cinnamon bun,** 1 large (4 oz) | 7 |
| **Cioppino,** 2 cups | 13 |
| **Clams** | |
| baked, 6 (2 1/2 oz) | 7 |
| breaded and fried, 20 (6 1/2 oz) | 10 |
| breaded and fried, fast food, 3/4 cup | 12 |
| fried, 1 cup | 11 |
| **Cobbler, fruit,** any type, 1 cup | 13 |
| **Coconut rice** | |
| Indian, 1 cup | 6 |
| Thai, 1 cup | 10 |
| **Coconut shrimp,** 4 jumbo (7 1/4 oz) | 17 |
| **Coffee, black,** without sugar, 1 cup | 0 |
| **Cognac,** 1 jigger (1 1/2 fl oz) | 4 |
| **Colcannon,** 1 cup | 8 |
| **Coleslaw,** fast food, 3/4 cup | 4 |
| **Conch fritters,** 2 (1 3/4 oz) | 3 |

| ▲ Power Foods | *PointsPlus*™ value |
|---|---|
| **Cookies** | |
| amaretti, 1 (1" diameter) | 3 |
| butter, 1 small | 1 |
| Chinese almond, 2 (1 oz) | 4 |
| chocolate chip, 1 medium (2 1/4" diameter) | 1 |
| fortune, 1 (1/2 oz) | 2 |
| kringla, 2 (1 1/2 oz) | 4 |
| lace, 1 | 1 |
| Mexican wedding, 2 (1 1/2" wide each) | 2 |
| rainbow, 1 (1" x 2") | 3 |
| rugalach, 1 (2 1/2" x 1 1/4") | 3 |
| sesame seed, 2 (2" long) | 4 |
| white macadamia, restaurant-type, 1 (1 3/4 oz) | 7 |
| **Coq au vin,** 2 cups | 12 |
| **Coquilles St. Jacques,** 2 shells (13 1/2 oz) | 9 |
| **Corn** | |
| cream-style, 1 cup | 5 |
| ▲ kernels, 1 cup | 4 |
| ▲ on the cob, 1 ear (up to 7" long) | 2 |
| ▲ on the cob, 1 ear (8" long) | 4 |
| on the cob, with butter, fast food, 1 ear (5 oz) | 4 |
| **Corn cake, sweet,** 1/2 cup | 10 |
| **Corn casserole,** 1/2 cup | 10 |
| **Corn dog** | |
| 1 (2 3/4 oz) | 6 |
| fast food, 1 (6 oz) | 12 |
| **Cornbread dressing,** 1 cup | 9 |
| **Cornbread** | |
| 2" square | 3 |
| Mexican, 1/12 of a 10" round or 3 1/3 oz | 8 |
| **Cornish hen,** cooked, with skin, 1/2 (4 1/2 oz) | 9 |
| **Cosmopolitan,** 1 (3 1/2 fl oz) | 6 |

| ▲ Power Foods | *PointsPlus™* value |
|---|---|
| **Couscous,** regular, cooked, 1 cup | 4 |
| **Crab, deviled,** 1/2 cup | 4 |
| **Crab cakes** | |
| 2 (2 1/4 oz each or 3" round) | 5 |
| fast food, 1 (2 oz) | 4 |
| **Crab puffs,** 6 (1 1/2" rounds) | 5 |
| **Crab Rangoon,** 1 large (4 1/2") or 5 mini | 5 |
| **Crackers** | |
| lavash, 1/4 of the 10" cracker | 7 |
| oyster, 20 or 1/2 cup | 3 |
| saltines, 4 | 1 |
| saltines, 6 | 2 |
| **Cream, sour,** regular, 1 Tbsp | 1 |
| **Cream puff,** 1 (2 oz) | 9 |
| **Creamed chipped beef, chicken, or turkey,** 1 cup | 12 |
| **Crème brûlée,** 3/4 cup | 12 |
| **Crème caramel,** 1 cup | 8 |
| **Crème de menthe,** 1 jigger (1 1/2 fl oz) | 6 |
| **Crème fraiche,** 2 Tbsp | 3 |
| **Creole** | |
| chicken, without rice, 1 cup | 7 |
| shrimp, without rice, 1 cup | 5 |
| **Crêpes** | |
| chicken, 2 (10 oz) | 12 |
| plain, 1 (6" diameter) | 2 |
| seafood, 1 (11 oz) | 12 |
| Suzette, 2 (4 3/4 oz) | 11 |
| **Croissant** | |
| apple, 1 medium (2 oz) | 4 |
| butter, 1 medium (2 oz) | 6 |
| cheese, 1 medium (2 oz) | 6 |
| chocolate-filled, 1 (3 3/4 oz) | 7 |
| plain, 1 (1 3/4 oz) | 6 |
| with egg and cheese, fast food, 1 (4 1/2 oz) | 10 |
| with egg, cheese, and bacon, fast food, 1 (4 1/2 oz) | 11 |

| ▲ Power Foods | *PointsPlus™* value |
|---|---|
| with egg, cheese, and ham, fast food, 1 (5 1/4 oz) | 13 |
| with egg, cheese, and sausage, fast food, 1 (5 3/4 oz) | 14 |
| **Croquettes** | |
| beef, 2 (2 1/2 oz each) | 10 |
| chicken, 2 (2 1/2 oz each) | 9 |
| **Croutons** | |
| packaged, regular, 1/2 cup | 3 |
| plain, 1 cup | 3 |
| seasoned, 1 cup | 5 |
| **Cruller** | |
| 1 (2 oz) | 6 |
| French, glazed, 1 (3" diameter) | 5 |
| glazed, 1 (4" diameter) | 7 |
| glazed, 1 long (approximately 5 1/4" x 2 1/2" x 1 1/2" high) | 9 |
| **Crumpet,** 1 (3" diameter) | 4 |
| **Curry** | |
| beef, 1 cup | 11 |
| Bengali fish, 1 fillet (4 1/2 oz) and 1 cup vegetables | 11 |
| chicken, 1 cup | 10 |
| egg, 1 cup | 2 |
| fish, African, 1/2 cup | 6 |
| green chicken (gaeng kheow wan gai), 1 cup | 8 |
| Japanese, 1 cup | 5 |
| lamb, 1 cup | 11 |
| shrimp, African, 1/2 cup | 7 |
| **Curry goat,** 4 oz | 6 |
| **Custard,** 1 cup | 9 |

## D

| ▲ Power Foods | *PointsPlus™* value |
|---|---|
| **Daiquiri,** 3 fl oz | 4 |
| **Danish pastry** | |
| cheese, cinnamon, or fruit, 1 (4 1/4" diameter) | 7 |
| fast food, 1 (3 oz) | 10 |
| nut, 1 (4 1/4" diameter) | 8 |

| ▲ Power Foods | *PointsPlus*™ value |
|---|---|
| **Date-nut bread,** 1 (5" x 1/2") | 7 |
| **Dhansak,** 1 cup | 7 |
| **Dim sum** | |
| bean curd roll with shrimp and vegetables, 1 (3 1/2 oz) | 3 |
| bean curd roll with vegetables, 1 (2 1/2 oz) | 2 |
| sesame seed balls, 1 (3" x 3") | 7 |
| **Dip** | |
| any type other than those listed here, 2 Tbsp | 2 |
| artichoke, baked, 1/4 oz | 6 |
| Mexican 7-layer, 1/2 cup | 4 |
| spinach, 1/4 cup | 5 |
| spinach artichoke, restaurant-type, 2 oz | 3 |
| **Dolma,** 4 (3 1/4 oz) | 5 |
| **Donair,** 4 oz meat with onion, tomato, and 2 Tbsp sauce | 16 |
| **Doro wat,** 1 cup | 7 |
| **Doughnut** | |
| cake-type, with icing, 1 (2 oz) | 7 |
| cake-type, without icing, 1 (2 oz) | 6 |
| with crème filling, 1 (3 1/2" x 2 1/2" oval) | 9 |
| yeast, glazed, 1 (4" diameter) | 7 |
| yeast, with jelly filling, 1 (3 1/2" x 2 1/2" oval) | 8 |
| **Doughnut holes, yeast,** glazed, 2 (1 oz) | 3 |
| **Dressing, salad** | |
| ginger, 2 Tbsp | 2 |
| creamy, regular, 2 Tbsp | 4 |
| Italian-type other than creamy Italian, regular, 2 Tbsp | 2 |
| **Duck,** domestic, cooked, with skin, 1/4 duck (5 oz) | 13 |
| **Duck a l'orange,** 1/4 duck with 2 Tbsp sauce | 15 |

| ▲ Power Foods | *PointsPlus*™ value |
|---|---|
| **Duck with fruit sauce,** 1/4 of the duck with skin and 1/2 cup sauce | 16 |
| **Dumpling** | |
| beef or pork, fried, 4 (6 1/2 oz) | 7 |
| beef or pork, steamed, 4 (5 3/4 oz) | 7 |
| chicken, fried, 4 (6 1/2 oz) | 5 |
| chicken, steamed, 4 (5 3/4 oz) | 5 |
| kroppkakor (potato), boiled, 1 (2" wide) | 3 |
| kroppkakor (potato), fried, 1 (2" wide) | 4 |
| potato, 6 (1" diameter) | 3 |
| shrimp, fried, 4 (6 1/2 oz) | 5 |
| shrimp, steamed, 4 (5 3/4 oz) | 5 |
| vegetarian, fried, 4 (3 1/2" x 2" wide) | 4 |
| vegetarian, steamed, 4 (3 1/2" x 2" wide) | 4 |

## E

| ▲ Power Foods | *PointsPlus*™ value |
|---|---|
| **Eclair,** 1 (5 1/4 oz) | 11 |
| ▲ **Edamame, in pods,** 1 cup | 2 |
| **Egg** | |
| deviled, 2 stuffed halves | 4 |
| fried, 1 large | 2 |
| ▲ poached, 1 large | 2 |
| scrambled, 2 or 1/2 cup | 5 |
| **Egg foo yung** | |
| beef, 1 (3" diameter) | 4 |
| chicken, 1 (3" diameter) | 4 |
| pork, 1 (3" diameter) | 5 |
| shrimp, 1 (3" diameter) | 4 |
| **Egg roll** | |
| beef, 1 (4 1/2" long) | 6 |
| chicken, 1 (4 1/2" long) | 5 |
| pork, 1 (4 1/2" long) | 6 |
| shrimp, 1 (4 1/2" long) | 4 |
| **Eggplant,** breaded and fried, 2 slices (3" diameter) | 3 |

| ▲ Power Foods | *PointsPlus*™ value |
|---|---|
| **Eggplant parmigiana** | |
| with sauce, 3" by 4" serving with 1/2 cup Italian tomato sauce | 14 |
| without sauce, 1 piece (3" x 4") | 11 |
| **Eggs Benedict,** 2 English muffin halves with 2 eggs and 1/4 cup Hollandaise sauce | 17 |
| **Empanadas,** 2 (3" diameter) | 6 |
| **Enchilada de camarones,** 1 cup | 5 |
| **Enchiladas** | |
| beef, 2 (10 1/2 oz) | 13 |
| cheese, 2 (8 1/2 oz) | 12 |
| cheese and beef, fast food, 1 (6 3/4 oz) | 9 |
| cheese, fast food, 1 (5 3/4 oz) | 9 |
| chicken, 2 (10 1/2 oz) | 11 |
| pork, 2 (10 1/2 oz) | 13 |
| sour cream, 1 (5 1/2 oz) | 9 |
| **Enchirito, with cheese, beef, and beans,** fast food, 1 (6 3/4 oz) | 9 |
| **Escargots,** 6 snails with 2 Tbsp butter | 6 |
| **Etouffee, shrimp,** 1 cup | 10 |

## F

| ▲ Power Foods | *PointsPlus*™ value |
|---|---|
| **Fadge,** 1 piece (3 1/4 oz) | 2 |
| **Fajitas** | |
| beef, 2 (9 oz) | 13 |
| chicken, 2 (8 1/2 oz) | 10 |
| pork, 2 (10 1/2 oz) | 14 |
| shrimp, 2 (9 oz) | 10 |
| vegetarian, 1 (5 1/2 oz) | 6 |
| **Falafel** | |
| in pita, 1 large pita with 4 falafel patties | 13 |
| patties, 4 (2" diameter each) | 8 |
| **Fattoush,** 2 cups | 7 |
| **Fettuccine Alfredo,** 1 cup | 17 |
| **Fish** | |
| ▲ bass, striped, cooked, 1 fillet (6 oz) | 5 |
| ▲ bluefish, cooked, 1 fillet (6 oz) | 6 |
| ▲ catfish, cooked, 1 fillet (6 oz) | 6 |
| ▲ cod, cooked, 1 fillet (3 oz) | 2 |
| ▲ flounder, cooked, 1 fillet (6 oz) | 4 |
| ▲ grouper, cooked, 1 fillet (6 oz) | 4 |
| ▲ haddock, cooked, 1 fillet (6 oz) | 4 |
| ▲ halibut, cooked, 1 fillet or steak (6 oz) | 5 |
| lox, 1 oz | 1 |
| ▲ mahimahi (dolphinfish), cooked, 1 fillet (6 oz) | 4 |
| salmon, cooked, 1 fillet or steak (6 oz) | 9 |
| ▲ snapper, cooked, 1 fillet (6 oz) | 5 |
| ▲ swordfish, cooked, 1 fillet or steak (6 oz) | 6 |
| ▲ tilapia, cooked, 1 fillet (3 oz) | 2 |
| ▲ trout, cooked, 1 fillet (6 oz) | 8 |
| ▲ trout, rainbow, cooked, 1 fillet (6 oz) | 6 |
| tuna, canned in oil, drained, 1/2 cup (4 oz) | 5 |
| ▲ tuna, canned in water, drained, 1/2 cup (4 oz) | 3 |
| ▲ tuna, cooked, 1 fillet or steak (6 oz) | 5 |
| ▲ whitefish, cooked, 1 fillet (5 1/2 oz) | 6 |
| **Fish,** baked stuffed, 6 3/4 oz | 9 |
| **Fish,** blackened, 1 fillet (6 oz) | 12 |
| **Fish,** fried, breaded with flour, 1 fillet (6 oz) | 13 |
| **Fish amandine,** 1 fillet (6 oz) | 13 |
| **Fish and brewis,** 1 cup | 14 |
| **Fish and chips,** 5 oz fish fillet with 20 chips (French fries) | 17 |
| **Fish fillet** | |
| battered or breaded, fried, fast food, 1 fillet (3 oz) | 6 |
| grilled, with garlic butter, 1 fillet (3 3/4 oz) | 3 |
| grilled, with lemon pepper, 1 fillet (3 3/4 oz) | 2 |
| **Fish Veronique,** 1 fillet (6 oz) | 12 |
| **Flan,** 3/4 cup | 9 |

| ▲ Power Foods | *PointsPlus™* value |
|---|---|
| **Flauta** | |
| beef, 1 (6" x 1 1/4") | 12 |
| chicken, 1 (6" x 1 1/4") | 11 |
| pork, 1 (6" x 1 1/4") | 11 |
| **Focaccia bread,** 1/4 of the 10" diameter | 7 |
| **Fondue, cheese,** 1/2 cup fondue with 2 oz bread | 12 |
| **Frankfurter on roll** | |
| chili, fast food, 1 (4 oz) | 8 |
| plain, 1 (4 oz) | 9 |
| plain, fast food, 1 (3 1/2 oz) | 7 |
| **French fries** | |
| 20 (4 1/2" long or 5 1/2 oz) | 11 |
| fast food, 1 small serving | 7 |
| fast food, 1 medium serving | 11 |
| fast food, 1 extra large serving | 14 |
| **French toast sticks,** fast food, 5 pieces (5 oz) | 13 |
| **French toast** | |
| 2 slices (4 1/2 oz) | 8 |
| with butter, fast food, 2 slices (4 3/4 oz) | 10 |
| **Frijoles, with cheese,** fast food, 1 cup | 5 |
| **Fritters** | |
| corn, 3 (2 1/2" x 2" each) | 6 |
| vegetable, 1 cup | 12 |
| **Frog legs,** fried, 2 (1 oz) | 4 |
| **Fromage frais (soft cheese with fruit),** 1 oz | 3 |
| **Fruit compote,** 1/2 cup | 4 |
| **Fruit cup,** restaurant-type, 1 small (6 oz) | 1 |
| **Fudge,** with or without nuts, 1 piece (1" x 2" or 1 oz) | 3 |

## G

| ▲ Power Foods | *PointsPlus™* value |
|---|---|
| **Gefilte fish,** 1 piece (1 1/2 oz) | 1 |
| **Gelatin, fruit-flavored,** prepared, 1/2 cup | 2 |
| **General Tso's chicken,** 1 cup | 17 |
| **Gin,** 1 jigger (1 1/2 fl oz) | 4 |
| **Gin and tonic,** 1 (6 fl oz) | 5 |
| **Gin gimlet,** 1 (2 1/2 fl oz) | 4 |
| **Ginger chicken,** 1 cup | 8 |
| **Ginger fish,** 1 cup | 9 |
| **Gingerbread,** 1 piece (3" square) | 11 |
| **Gnocchi** | |
| cheese, 1 cup | 12 |
| potato, 1 cup | 5 |
| spinach, 1 cup | 13 |
| **Goat masala,** 1 cup | 6 |
| **Gordita, beef,** 1 (3" diameter) | 11 |
| **Gosht shaha korma,** 1 cup | 15 |
| **Gravy** | |
| brown, 1/4 cup | 3 |
| cream, 1/4 cup | 4 |
| giblet, 1/4 cup | 2 |
| sausage, 1/4 cup | 4 |
| **Green rice,** 1 cup | 7 |
| ▲ **Greens, beet, chard, collard, dandelion, kale, mustard, turnip,** cooked or uncooked, 1 cup | 0 |
| **Guacamole,** 1/4 cup | 2 |
| **Gumbo** | |
| chicken, 1 cup | 7 |
| seafood, 1 cup | 6 |
| **Gyoza,** 3 (1 3/4 oz) | 3 |
| **Gyro,** 1 (11 oz) | 16 |

## H

| ▲ Power Foods | *PointsPlus™* value |
|---|---|
| **Ham,** glazed, with pineapple, 4 oz ham with 1/2 pineapple slice | 7 |
| **Hamantaschen,** 1 piece (3" diameter) | 3 |
| **Hamburger on bun** | |
| double patty, plain, fast food, 1 (6 oz) | 14 |
| double patty, with condiments, fast food, 1 (7 1/2 oz) | 15 |
| large, plain, fast food, 1 (4 3/4 oz) | 11 |

*Hamburger on bun (cont'd)*

| ▲ Power Foods | *PointsPlus™* value |
|---|---|
| large, with condiments, fast food, 1 (7 3/4 oz) | 13 |
| plain (without mayonnaise, lettuce, and tomato), 3 oz cooked hamburger on 1 1/2 oz bun | 10 |
| small, fast food, 1 (3 oz) | 7 |
| small, with condiments, fast food, 1 (4 oz) | 7 |
| triple patty, with condiments, fast food, 1 (9 oz) | 18 |
| **Haroset,** 1/4 cup | 1 |
| **Haupia (coconut pudding),** 2" square | 3 |
| **Herring** | |
| chopped, 1/4 cup | 4 |
| pickled, 1/2 cup | 3 |
| **Hibachi** | |
| chicken, 1 cup | 8 |
| shrimp, 1 cup | 6 |
| steak, 1 cup | 10 |
| vegetable, 1 cup | 5 |
| **Highball** | |
| made with sweetened mixer, 1 (6 fl oz) | 7 |
| made with unsweetened mixer, 1 (6 fl oz) | 4 |
| **Honeybun,** glazed, 1 (4" x 3" oval) | 7 |
| **Hot chocolate,** with or without whipped topping, 1 cup | 8 |
| **Hot cross buns,** 1 (2 1/4 oz) | 6 |
| **Hot dog on roll** | |
| chili, fast food, 1 (4 oz) | 8 |
| plain, 1 (4 oz) | 9 |
| plain, fast food, 1 (3 1/2 oz) | 7 |
| **Huevos rancheros,** 2 eggs on 2 tortillas | 16 |
| **Huli huli chicken** | |
| breast (with skin and bone), 1 (7 1/4 oz) | 13 |
| thigh (with skin and bone), 1 (3 oz) | 5 |
| drumstick (with skin and bone), 1 (2 oz) | 3 |

| ▲ Power Foods | *PointsPlus™* value |
|---|---|
| **Hummus,** 1/4 cup | 4 |
| **Hunan beef,** 1 cup | 10 |
| **Hungarian goulash,** 1 cup | 9 |
| **Hush puppies** | |
| 2 (2 1/4 oz) | 5 |
| fast food, 5 pieces (2 3/4 oz) | 7 |

## I

| | |
|---|---|
| **Ice cream** | |
| premium, 1 scoop or 1/2 cup | 8 |
| regular, 1 scoop or 1/2 cup | 4 |
| **Ice cream,** fried, 1/2 cup | 12 |
| **Ice cream cone only** | |
| cake or wafer-type, 1 large (1 oz) | 3 |
| plain or sugar, 1 small | 1 |
| **Ice cream soda,** 12 fl oz | 11 |
| **Ice cream sundae** | |
| 1 large (6 1/2 oz) | 13 |
| 1 scoop (1/2 cup) ice cream with syrup, nuts, and whipped topping | 9 |
| caramel, fast food, 1 (5 1/2 oz) | 8 |
| hot fudge, fast food, 1 (5 1/2 oz) | 8 |
| strawberry, fast food, 1 (5 1/2 oz) | 7 |
| **Ices** | |
| fruit, 1/2 cup | 4 |
| Italian, restaurant-type, 1/2 cup | 2 |
| **Imperial roll,** 1 (4 1/2" long) | 5 |
| **Irish coffee,** 6 fl oz with 2 Tbsp whipped cream | 6 |
| **Irish soda bread,** 1/12 of a 8" round loaf | 8 |
| **Italian casserole (ground beef, pasta and cheese over rolls),** 1/8 of the 10" round casserole | 15 |

## J

| | |
|---|---|
| **Jalapeño bread,** 1 slice (1 1/2 oz) | 3 |
| **Jalapeño poppers,** 1 (1 1/2 oz) | 4 |
| **Jam, regular or reduced-sugar,** 1 Tbsp | 1 |

| ▲ Power Foods | *PointsPlus™* value |
|---|---|
| **Jamaican rice and peas,** 1 cup | 8 |
| **Jambalaya, chicken or fish, with rice,** 1 1/2 cups | 11 |
| **JapChae, beef, chicken, or pork,** 1 cup | 8 |
| **Jelly,** 1 Tbsp | 1 |
| **Jerk chicken breast, without skin,** 1 large breast (5 3/4 oz) | 5 |
| **Johnny cake,** 1 piece (2 1/2" square) | 5 |
| **Juice cocktail, cranberry, regular,** 1/2 cup | 2 |

## K

| ▲ Power Foods | *PointsPlus™* value |
|---|---|
| **Kabobs** | |
| beef, 2 skewers (4 1/2 oz) | 8 |
| chicken, 2 skewers (4 1/2 oz) | 5 |
| fish, 2 skewers (4 1/2 oz) | 5 |
| lamb, 2 skewers (4 1/2 oz) | 8 |
| **Kahlua,** 1 jigger (1 1/2 fl oz) | 6 |
| **Kahlua pig,** 3 oz | 4 |
| **Kasha varnishkes,** 1 cup | 7 |
| **Kashmiri (lamb meatballs),** 6 (3 1/2 oz) | 11 |
| **Kataifi,** 1 piece (2" long) | 7 |
| **Katsu** | |
| ahi, 2 slices (4 1/2" x 1/2" x 3/4" thick) | 6 |
| chicken, 2 slices (4 1/2" x 1/2" x 3/4" thick) | 6 |
| pork, 2 slices (4 1/2" x 1/2" x 3/4" thick) | 7 |
| **Ketchup,** 1 Tbsp | 0 |
| **Khal bi,** 4 oz | 8 |
| **Kheer,** 1/2 cup | 7 |
| **Kho-phat (Thai fried rice),** 1 cup | 9 |
| **Kibbe,** baked, 3 pieces (1 1/2" squares) | 3 |
| **Kielbasa,** 1 oz | 2 |
| ▲ **Kim chee,** 1/2 cup | 0 |
| **King ranch chicken casserole,** 1 cup | 9 |
| **Kishke,** 1 small piece (3/4 oz) | 2 |
| **Knish, potato,** 1 (3 1/2" square) | 7 |
| **Kofta (vegetable balls without sauce),** 2 (3 oz) | 6 |
| **Kofta, malai (vegetable balls in cream sauce),** 2 kofta with 1/2 cup sauce | 10 |
| **Kolache** | |
| fruit-filled, 1 (3" diameter) | 5 |
| without filling, 1 (3" diameter) | 4 |
| **Korean barbecue beef,** 4 oz | 7 |
| **Korean barbecue chicken thighs,** 1 (5 oz) | 12 |
| **Korean barbecue short ribs,** 4 oz | 8 |
| **Korma** | |
| chicken, 1 cup | 15 |
| lamb, 1 cup | 16 |
| vegetable, 1 cup | 12 |
| **Kreplach** | |
| boiled, 2 pieces (4" x 3" x 3" each) | 6 |
| fried, 2 pieces (4" x 3" x 3" each) | 8 |
| **Kugel** | |
| lukschen, with fruit, 1 piece (3" x 3 1/4") | 9 |
| lukschen, without fruit, 1 piece (3" x 3 1/4") | 6 |
| potato, 1 piece (3" x 3 1/4") | 5 |
| **Kung pao** | |
| beef, 1 cup | 12 |
| chicken, 1 cup | 9 |
| pork, 1 cup | 11 |
| shrimp, 1 cup | 10 |

## L

| ▲ Power Foods | *PointsPlus™* value |
|---|---|
| ▲ **Lamb, chop, baby or regular,** trimmed, cooked, 1 slice (3 oz) | 3 |
| **Lamb masala,** 1 cup | 7 |
| **Lasagna** | |
| cheese, with tomato sauce, 1 piece (10 oz) | 9 |
| chicken, 1 cup | 7 |

Lasagna (cont'd)

| ▲ Power Foods | *PointsPlus*™ value |
|---|---|
| vegetable, 1 cup | 8 |
| vegetarian, with cheese, 1 piece (10 oz) | 12 |
| vegetarian, with cheese and spinach, 1 piece (10 1/2 oz) | 10 |
| with meat, 4" x 2 1/2" or 1 cup | 7 |
| with meat sauce, 1 cup | 7 |
| **Latte** | |
| ▲ made with fat-free milk, 1 small (8 fl oz) | 2 |
| ▲ made with fat-free milk, 1 tall (12 fl oz) | 3 |
| ▲ made with fat-free milk, 1 grande (16 fl oz) | 4 |
| made with low-fat milk, 1 small (8 fl oz) | 3 |
| made with low-fat milk, 1 tall (12 fl oz) | 4 |
| made with low-fat milk, 1 grande (16 fl oz) | 5 |
| made with whole milk, 1 small (8 fl oz) | 3 |
| made with whole milk, 1 tall (12 fl oz) | 5 |
| made with whole milk, 1 grande (16 fl oz) | 7 |
| **Lau lau (pork and fish in taro or spinach leaves),** 1 (7 1/2 oz) | 8 |
| **Lechon asado (roast pork),** 3 oz | 4 |
| **Lemon grass chicken,** 1 cup | 9 |
| **Lemonade,** 1 cup | 3 |
| **Lettuce wrap** | |
| beef, 2 (5" long by 3" wide each) | 5 |
| chicken, 2 (5" long by 3" wide each) | 4 |
| **Limeade,** 1 cup | 3 |
| **Linguine with red clam sauce,** 1 cup linguine with 1/2 cup sauce | 8 |
| **Linguine with white clam sauce,** 1 cup linguine with 1/2 cup sauce | 10 |
| **Liqueur, any type,** 1 jigger (1 1/2 fl oz) | 6 |
| **Liquor (brandy, gin, rum, scotch, tequila, vodka, whiskey),** 1 jigger (1 1/2 fl oz) | 4 |

| ▲ Power Foods | *PointsPlus*™ value |
|---|---|
| **Liver, chopped,** 1/4 cup | 5 |
| **Liver with bacon,** 2 slices (4 oz) with 2 slices bacon | 11 |
| **Liver with onions,** 2 slices (4 oz) with 1/2 cup onions | 8 |
| **Lo mein** | |
| beef, 1 cup | 10 |
| chicken, 1 cup | 9 |
| pork, 1 cup | 9 |
| shrimp, 1 cup | 9 |
| vegetable, 1 cup | 8 |
| **Lobster Cantonese,** 1 cup | 9 |
| **Lobster Newburg,** 1 cup | 14 |
| **Lobster thermidor,** 1 cup | 14 |
| **Lomi lomi salmon,** 1/2 cup | 2 |
| **Long Island iced tea,** 1 (5 fl oz) | 8 |
| **Lumpia (Filipino spring roll),** 4 1/2" x 1" x 1 1/2" | 6 |

## M

| | |
|---|---|
| **Macaroni and cheese** | |
| 1 cup | 10 |
| Bahamian, 1 cup | 9 |
| **Malasadas (Portuguese doughnuts),** 1 (3" x 2" puff) | 3 |
| **Manapua with char shiu filling,** 1 (3 1/4 oz) | 6 |
| **Mandelbrot,** 1 slice (3" x 2" x 1/2") | 5 |
| **Mango lassi,** 1 cup | 3 |
| **Manhattan,** 1 (2 fl oz) | 5 |
| **Manicotti** | |
| with meat sauce, 2 shells with 1/2 cup sauce | 16 |
| with tomato sauce, 2 shells with 1/2 cup sauce | 13 |
| **Margarine, regular,** 1 tsp | 1 |
| **Margarita,** 1 (4 fl oz) | 9 |
| **Martini** | |
| 1 (2 1/2 fl oz) | 6 |
| chocolate, 1 (2 1/2 fl oz) | 8 |
| sour apple, 1 (2 1/2 fl oz) | 8 |

| ▲ Power Foods | PointsPlus™ value |
|---|---|
| **Masala dosa** | |
| without filling, 1 (5 1/4 oz) | 12 |
| with filling, 1 (7 3/4 oz) | 13 |
| **Massaman beef curry,** 1 cup | 21 |
| **Matzo brie,** 1/4 of the 10" round or 1 cup | 5 |
| **Matzo, all varieties,** 1 board (1 oz) | 3 |
| **Mayonnaise, regular,** 1 tsp | 1 |
| **Meat loaf,** 1 slice (5/8" thick) | 6 |
| **Meatballs, with sauce,** 2 meatballs and 1/2 cup Italian tomato sauce | 13 |
| **Meatballs, without sauce,** 1 (1 1/4" each) | 10 |
| **Menudo (beef tripe and hominy stew),** 1 cup | 7 |
| **Mexican coffee,** 6 fl oz with 2 Tbsp whipped cream | 6 |
| **Milk shake, any flavor,** fast food | |
| 1 medium (12 fl oz) | 12 |
| 1 large (16 fl oz) | 16 |
| **Mimosa,** 1 (6 fl oz) | 4 |
| **Mirin,** 1 fl oz | 1 |
| **Mochi** | |
| 1 piece (1 1/4 oz) | 2 |
| butter, 1 piece (2 3/4 oz) | 7 |
| **Mojito,** 1 (12 fl oz) | 7 |
| **Molé poblano,** 1/4 cup | 5 |
| **Mongolian beef,** 1 cup | 8 |
| **Moo goo gai pan,** 1 cup | 7 |
| **Moo shoo** | |
| chicken, 1/2 cup with 2 pancakes | 8 |
| pork, 1/2 cup with 2 pancakes | 9 |
| tofu, 1/2 cup with 2 pancakes | 8 |
| **Moussaka,** 1 piece (3" x 4") | 12 |
| **Muffin** | |
| any type other than those listed here, 1 large (3" diameter) | 8 |
| any type, fast food, 1 (4 1/4 oz) | 11 |
| banana walnut, restaurant-type, 1 (5 oz) | 15 |
| blueberry, reduced-fat, restaurant-type, 1 (5 oz) | 11 |
| corn, restaurant-type, 1 (5 oz) | 13 |
| cranberry orange, restaurant-type, 1 (5 oz) | 12 |
| mini, any type, 1 (1 1/4" diameter or 1/2 oz) | 1 |
| pumpkin, restaurant-type, 1 (5 oz) | 12 |
| **Muffin, English** | |
| any type, regular, 1 (2 oz) | 3 |
| with butter, fast food, 1 (2 1/4 oz) | 5 |
| with cheese and sausage, fast food, 1 (4 oz) | 11 |
| with egg, cheese, and Canadian bacon, fast food, 1 (4 3/4 oz) | 8 |
| with egg, cheese, and sausage, fast food, 1 (5 3/4 oz) | 13 |
| **Muffuletta,** 1 (11 1/4 oz) | 22 |
| **Mun doo** | |
| fried, 4 (6 1/2 oz) | 5 |
| steamed, 4 (5 3/4 oz) | 5 |
| **Mung dal,** 1 cup | 6 |
| **Mushrooms,** marinated, 1/2 cup | 3 |
| **Mushrooms,** stuffed, 4 (2 3/4 oz) | 4 |
| **Mussels mariniere,** 4 mussels with 3 Tbsp sauce | 5 |

## N

| ▲ Power Foods | PointsPlus™ value |
|---|---|
| **Nachos** | |
| beef, 4 (8 1/2 oz) | 14 |
| cheese, 3 (3 oz) | 9 |
| cheese and bean, 4 (6 1/2 oz) | 10 |
| chicken, 4 (8 1/2 oz) | 13 |
| with cheese and jalapeño peppers, fast food, 7 1/4 oz | 17 |
| with cheese sauce, 2 3/4 oz | 6 |
| with cheese, beans, ground beef, and peppers, fast food, 6-8 nachos (9 oz) | 16 |
| with cheese, fast food, 4 oz | 9 |

Nachos (cont'd)

| ▲ Power Foods | *PointsPlus*™ value |
|---|---|
| with cinnamon and sugar, fast food, 6-8 nachos (3 3/4 oz) | 17 |
| **Napoleon,** 1 piece (4 1/2" x 2" x 1 1/2") | 15 |
| **Nebeyaki udon,** 2 cups | 7 |
| **Noodles** | |
| drunken, 1 cup | 6 |
| fried, 1 cup | 8 |
| ramen, fresh, cooked, 1 cup | 5 |
| soba, cooked, with sauce, 1 cup | 12 |
| **Nuoc cham,** 1 Tbsp | 0 |

## O

| ▲ Power Foods | *PointsPlus*™ value |
|---|---|
| **Okonmiyaki, without sauce and mayonnaise (Japanese style pizza),** 1 (8" diameter) | 9 |
| **Okra,** fried, 1 cup | 10 |
| **Old fashioned,** 1 (2 fl oz) | 6 |
| **Olives,** 10 small or 6 large (1 oz) | 1 |
| **Omelet** | |
| cheese, 2-egg, 1 | 8 |
| ham and cheese, 2-egg, 1 | 9 |
| ham and cheese, restaurant-type, 1 (9 1/2 oz) | 15 |
| herb or plain, 2-egg, 1 | 6 |
| vegetable, 2-egg, 1 | 8 |
| vegetable, restaurant-type, 1 (11 3/4 oz) | 15 |
| **Onion, blooming,** 1/4 of a 16" diameter onion | 6 |
| **Onion rings** | |
| fast food, 8-9 rings | 8 |
| fried, 4 (3 oz) | 7 |
| **Orange chicken,** 1 cup | 14 |
| **Osso bucco,** 6 oz veal with 1/4 cup sauce | 12 |
| **Oyster pie,** 1/8 of a 9" pie | 10 |
| **Oyster po' boy,** 1 (8 3/4 oz) | 19 |
| **Oysters** | |
| battered or breaded, and fried, fast food, 6 (5 oz) | 10 |
| fried, 10 (5 1/4 oz) | 8 |
| **Oysters Rockefeller,** 4 (2 oz) | 3 |

## P

| ▲ Power Foods | *PointsPlus*™ value |
|---|---|
| **Pad si-iew (stir-fried beef with noodles),** 1 cup | 7 |
| **Pad Thai (rice noodles with chicken and shrimp),** 1 cup | 10 |
| **Paella,** 1 cup | 9 |
| **Pajun (Korean green onion and shrimp pancake),** 1 (6-8" diameter) | 9 |
| **Pakora, vegetable,** 1 (2" x 3" or 1 3/4 oz) | 4 |
| **Palak paneer,** 1 cup | 15 |
| **Palak vada (vegetable dumpling)** | |
| fried, 1 (2 1/2" x 1 1/2") | 5 |
| steamed, 1 (2 1/2" x 1 1/2") | 3 |
| **Pan Cubano,** 1 (6 1/2" x 3") | 10 |
| **Panang curry** | |
| with beef, 1 cup | 14 |
| with chicken, 1 cup | 13 |
| with pork, 1 cup | 15 |
| **Pancakes** | |
| buttermilk, restaurant-type, 2 (6 oz) | 14 |
| Chinese, 1 (1 oz) | 2 |
| potato, 1 (3 1/4 oz) | 2 |
| prepared from scratch, 1 (4" diameter) | 3 |
| scallion, 1 (2 1/4 oz) | 7 |
| with butter and syrup, fast food, 1 serving (8 oz) | 14 |
| without butter and syrup, fast food, 1 serving (5 1/4 oz) | 11 |
| **Pancit canton (sauteed egg noodles),** 1 cup | 6 |
| **Paneer** | |
| fried, 1 cup | 1 |
| jalfrezi, 1 cup | 6 |
| **Panettone,** 1/12 of a 9" tube or 1 1/2 oz | 7 |
| **Panini** | |
| chicken, 1 (8 oz) | 13 |
| ham and cheese, 1 (7 1/2 oz) | 13 |

| ▲ Power Foods | *PointsPlus*™ value |
|---|---|
| turkey, restaurant-type, 1 (10 1/2 oz) | 19 |
| vegetable, 1 (13 oz) | 12 |
| **Paprikash,** 1 1/2 cups chicken mixture with 1/2 cup sauce | 10 |
| **Paratha,** 4" triangle | 4 |
| **Pasta e fagioli,** 1 cup | 6 |
| **Pasta primavera with cream sauce,** 1 cup pasta with 3/4 cup sauce | 14 |
| **Pasta primavera with marinara sauce,** 1 cup pasta with 3/4 cup sauce | 7 |
| **Pasta with garlic and oil,** 1 cup | 8 |
| **Pastelitos de carne (Cuban meat pastry),** 1 (1" x 2" diameter) | 9 |
| **Pastitsio,** 1 piece (3 1/4" x 3") | 14 |
| **Pâté, liver, beef,** 1 slice (4 1/4" x 1 1/2" x 1/2") | 3 |
| **Peach melba,** 1/2 cup ice cream with 2 peach halves and raspberry sauce | 9 |
| **Peanuts, shelled,** 40 (1 oz) | 5 |
| **Pear,** poached, 1 pear with 2 Tbsp whipped cream | 7 |
| **Peas, Bahamian style, with rice,** 1 cup | 9 |
| **Peking duck,** 2 oz duck with 1 piece duck skin and 3 pancakes | 11 |
| **Penne a la vodka,** 1 cup pasta with 1/2 cup sauce | 9 |
| **Pepper steak** | |
| 6 oz | 14 |
| Chinese, 1 cup | 5 |
| ▲ **Peppers, sweet, cooked or canned,** 1 cup | 0 |
| **Peppers, stuffed, with beef and rice,** 1 (7 3/4 oz) | 9 |
| **Pesarattu,** 1/2 of an 8" diameter | 8 |
| **Petit fours,** 2 (1 3/4" x 1 1/2" x 1" each) | 6 |
| **Petite marmite,** 2 cups | 8 |
| ▲ **Pickle, unsweetened,** 1 large or 1 cup | 0 |
| ▲ **Pico de gallo,** 1/2 cup | 0 |

| ▲ Power Foods | *PointsPlus*™ value |
|---|---|
| **Pie** | |
| chiffon, cream, or custard, with fruit, 1/8 of a 9" one-crust pie | 11 |
| chiffon, cream, or custard, without fruit, 1/8 of a 9" one-crust pie | 10 |
| fruit, fast food, 1 (3 1/2 oz) | 9 |
| fruit, one-crust, 1/8 of a 9" pie | 8 |
| fruit, two-crust, 1/8 of a 9" pie | 11 |
| meringue, 1/8 of a 9"one-crust pie | 12 |
| mincemeat, with meat, 1/8 of a 9" two-crust pie | 13 |
| mincemeat, without meat, 1/8 of a 9" two-crust pie | 16 |
| pecan, 1/8 of a 9" one-crust pie | 14 |
| pumpkin, 1/8 of a 9" one-crust pie | 11 |
| rhubarb, 1/8 of a 9" two-crust pie | 13 |
| **Pierogies** | |
| cabbage, 2 (2 1/2 oz) | 8 |
| cheese, 2 (2 1/2 oz) | 8 |
| meat, 2 (2 1/2 oz) | 9 |
| potato, 2 (2 1/2 oz) | 8 |
| **Pigs in blankets,** 2 (1 oz) | 7 |
| **Piña colada,** 1 (6 fl oz) | 8 |
| **Pineapple,** canned, crushed, sliced, or chunks, in heavy syrup, 1 cup | 6 |
| **Pizza,** fast food, single serving, cheese, 1 (8 1/2 oz) | 15 |
| **Pizza,** restaurant-type, cheese, thin crust | |
| 1 small slice (1/8 of a 12" or 1/12 of a 16" pie) | 5 |
| 1 large slice (1/8 of a 16" to 18" pie) | 7 |
| **Pizza,** restaurant-type, one-meat topping, deep dish | |
| 1 small slice (1/8 of a 12" or 1/12 of a 16" pie) | 8 |
| 1 large slice (1/8 of a 16" to 18" pie) | 13 |
| **Pizza,** restaurant-type, one-meat topping, thin crust | |
| 1 small slice (1/8 of a 12" or 1/12 of a 16" pie) | 5 |

*Pizza (cont'd)*

| ▲ Power Foods | *PointsPlus*™ value |
|---|---|
| 1 large slice (1/8 of a 16" to 18" pie) | 8 |
| **Plantain,** fried, 1 cup | 5 |
| **Plátanos maduros (fried sweet plantains),** 1 cup | 5 |
| ▲ **Poi,** 1/2 cup (4 oz) | 4 |
| **Poke** | |
| ahi, 1/2 cup | 2 |
| tako, 1/2 cup | 2 |
| **Popcorn** | |
| buttered, popped, 3 cups | 6 |
| movie, without butter, 3 cups | 4 |
| **Popover,** 2 (3" diameter or 1 1/2 oz each) | 4 |
| **Pork,** barbecue, 1 cup | 9 |
| **Pork, Chinese roast,** 1 cup | 6 |
| **Pork, sweet and sour,** 1 cup | 13 |
| **Pork and broccoli,** 1 cup | 4 |
| **Pork hash, Hawaiian,** 4 (5 3/4 oz) | 7 |
| **Pork stir-fry, with garlic or black bean sauce,** 1 cup | 9 |
| **Pork with cashews,** 1 cup | 12 |
| **Portuguese sweet bread,** 1/8 loaf (3 oz) | 7 |
| **Pot pie** | |
| any type, fast food, 1 (14 oz) | 22 |
| chicken, homemade, 8 1/2 oz | 12 |
| **Pot sticker (filled wontons)** | |
| vegetarian, fried, 4 (3 1/2" x 2" each) | 4 |
| vegetarian, steamed, 4 (3 1/2" x 2" each) | 4 |
| **Potato,** baked | |
| ▲ plain, 1 small (3 oz) | 2 |
| ▲ plain, 1 large (7 oz) | 4 |
| with cheese sauce and bacon, fast food, 1 (10 1/2 oz) | 13 |
| with cheese sauce and chili, fast food, 1 (14 oz) | 13 |
| with cheese sauce, fast food, 1 (10 1/2 oz) | 13 |
| with sour cream and chives, 1 (5 1/2 oz) | 5 |

| ▲ Power Foods | *PointsPlus*™ value |
|---|---|
| with sour cream and chives, fast food, 1 (10 3/4 oz) | 11 |
| with vegetables and cheese, fast food, 1 (13 oz) | 11 |
| **Potato,** baked, stuffed | |
| with bacon and cheese, 1 (9 1/2 oz) | 13 |
| with cheese, 1 (5 1/2 oz) | 5 |
| with vegetables and cheese, 1 (13 1/2 oz) | 12 |
| **Potato, sweet** | |
| ▲ 1 large (5" long), 7 oz cooked or 1 cup cooked | 4 |
| ▲ baked, 1 medium (2" diameter, 5" long) | 3 |
| **Potato, white or red** | |
| ▲ 1 small (2" diameter) or 3 oz | 2 |
| ▲ 1 large (5" long), or 7 oz cooked | 4 |
| ▲ 1 cup cooked | 3 |
| **Potato latkes,** 2 (3 1/2 diameter) | 7 |
| **Potato skins, with cheese, bacon and sour cream,** 1 (7 oz) | 10 |
| **Potatoes, hash brown** | |
| 1 cup | 8 |
| fast food, 1/2 cup | 4 |
| **Potatoes,** mashed | |
| 1/2 cup | 3 |
| fast food, 1/3 cup | 2 |
| garlic, 1/2 cup | 5 |
| **Potatoes,** scalloped, 1/2 cup | 5 |
| **Potatoes au gratin,** 1 cup | 14 |
| **Potatoes O'Brien,** 1 cup | 4 |
| **Poutine,** 20 French fries with 2 oz cheese and 1/2 cup sauce | 19 |
| **Praline,** 1 (2 1/2" diameter or 1 1/2 oz) | 6 |
| **Preserves,** 1 Tbsp | 1 |
| **Pretzels** | |
| sticks, 45 (3/4 oz) | 2 |
| twists, 7 regular or 15 small (3/4 oz) | 2 |
| **Profiterole,** 1 small (1 oz) | 3 |
| **Pudding** | |
| any type and flavor other than those listed here, 1 cup | 8 |

| ▲ Power Foods | *PointsPlus*™ value |
|---|---|
| banana, 1 cup | 9 |
| **Pudding, bread,** 1 cup | 16 |
| **Pudding, corn,** 1 cup | 7 |
| **Pudding, Indian,** 1 cup | 8 |
| **Pudding, plum,** 5 oz | 11 |
| **Pudding, rice,** 1 cup | 10 |
| **Pudding, tapioca** | |
| 1 cup | 6 |
| Thai, 1/2 cup | 4 |
| **Pumpkin bread,** 1 slice (3/4" thick) | 8 |
| **Puris,** 1 (4" diameter) | 3 |

## Q

| | |
|---|---|
| **Quenelles,** 8 (2 1/2" x 1 1/2" x 3/4") | 12 |
| **Quesadilla** | |
| beef, 1/2 of 6" diameter | 7 |
| cheese, 1/2 of 6" diameter | 6 |
| chicken, 1/2 of 6" diameter | 7 |
| vegetable, 1/2 of 6" diameter | 7 |
| **Quiche, vegetable,** 1/8 of a 9" pie | 9 |
| **Quiche Lorraine,** 1/8 of a 9" pie | 11 |

## R

| | |
|---|---|
| ▲ **Radishes,** 1 cup | 0 |
| **Raita,** 1/2 cup | 2 |
| **Rajmah,** 1 cup | 8 |
| **Ratatouille,** 1 cup | 5 |
| **Ravioli** | |
| cheese, with tomato sauce, 15 oz | 19 |
| cheese, without sauce, 8 3/4 oz | 16 |
| meat, with tomato sauce, 8 pieces or 1 cup with 1/2 cup sauce | 17 |
| meat, without sauce, 8 pieces or 1 cup | 14 |
| **Red snapper Veracruz,** 6 oz cooked fillet with 3/4 cup sauce | 12 |
| ▲ **Rice, brown,** cooked, 1 cup | 5 |
| **Rice, Cuban,** 1 cup | 6 |
| **Rice, dirty,** 1 cup | 11 |

| ▲ Power Foods | *PointsPlus*™ value |
|---|---|
| **Rice,** fried | |
| plain, 1 cup | 10 |
| with beef, 1 cup | 10 |
| with chicken, 1 cup | 10 |
| with pork, 1 cup | 10 |
| with shrimp, 1 cup | 9 |
| **Rice, Spanish,** 1 cup | 7 |
| **Rice, white,** cooked, 1 cup | 5 |
| ▲ **Rice, wild,** cooked, 1 cup | 4 |
| **Rice, with pigeon peas (arroz con gandules),** 1 cup | 8 |
| **Rice pilaf,** 1 cup | 7 |
| **Risotto,** 1/2 cup | 6 |
| **Rocky mountain oysters,** 2 slices (2 oz) | 10 |
| **Rogan josh,** 1 cup | 11 |
| **Roll** | |
| dinner, 1 (2 oz) | 5 |
| French, 1 (1 1/4 oz) | 3 |
| kaiser, restaurant-type, 1 (2 oz) | 4 |
| **Ropa vieja,** 1 cup | 9 |
| **Rum,** 1 jigger (1 1/2 fl oz) | 4 |

## S

| | |
|---|---|
| **Saag gosht,** 1 cup | 7 |
| **Saag paneer,** 1 cup | 8 |
| **Sachertorte,** 1/16 of a 9" cake | 9 |
| **Saganaki,** 1 piece (1" x 2" x 1/2" thick) | 6 |
| **Saimin,** 1 cup | 5 |
| **Sakatini,** 1 (3 fl oz) | 7 |
| **Sake,** 1/2 cup | 5 |
| **Salad** | |
| Caesar, 3 cups | 7 |
| Caesar, with grilled chicken, restaurant-type, 6 1/2 oz | 8 |
| carrot and raisin, 1/2 cup | 8 |
| chef's, fast food, 1 (11 1/2 oz) | 6 |
| chef's, with dressing, 4 cups | 8 |
| chef's, without dressing, 4 cups | 6 |

Salad (cont'd)

| ▲ Power Foods | PointsPlus™ value |
|---|---|
| chicken, 1/2 cup | 6 |
| chicken, Oriental, 2 cups | 8 |
| cobb (without dressing), 3 cups | 11 |
| conch, 1 cup | 3 |
| egg, 1/2 cup | 8 |
| garden, restaurant-type, 1 (6 oz) | 3 |
| Greek, with dressing, restaurant-type, 3 cups | 10 |
| Greek, without dressing, restaurant-type, 3 cups | 3 |
| green papaya, with pork and shrimp, 1 cup | 4 |
| green papaya, without meat, 1 cup | 2 |
| grilled chicken, without dressing, fast food, 1 (12 1/4 oz) | 5 |
| lobster, 1/2 cup | 4 |
| macaroni, 1/2 cup | 7 |
| ▲ mixed greens, 1 cup | 0 |
| Niçoise, with dressing, 4 cups | 20 |
| Niçoise, without dressing, 4 cups | 9 |
| pasta, 1/2 cup | 4 |
| potato, 1/2 cup | 8 |
| potato, German, 1/2 cup | 2 |
| potato, hot, with ham, 1 cup | 8 |
| seaweed, 1/2 cup | 1 |
| shrimp, 1/2 cup | 3 |
| ▲ side, without dressing, fast food, 1 (3 oz) | 0 |
| southwestern grilled chicken, restaurant-type, 1 (13 1/4 oz) | 7 |
| spinach, with dressing, 2 cups | 7 |
| taco, fast food, 1 1/2 cups | 7 |
| taco, with chili con carne, fast food, 1 1/2 cups | 7 |
| taco, with shell, without dressing, fast food, 1 | 18 |
| taco, without shell and dressing, fast food, 1 | 10 |
| Thai beef , 1 cup | 15 |
| Thai chicken, 1 cup | 12 |

| ▲ Power Foods | PointsPlus™ value |
|---|---|
| Thai seafood, 2 cups | 11 |
| three-bean, 1/2 cup | 5 |
| tomato and mozzarella, without dressing, 2 large tomato slices with 2 oz cheese | 5 |
| tuna, 1/2 cup | 8 |
| turkey cobb, restaurant-type, 1 (11 1/4 oz) | 10 |
| vegetable, with cheese and egg, without dressing, fast food, 1 1/2 cups | 3 |
| vegetable, with chicken, without dressing, fast food, 1 1/2 cups | 2 |
| vegetable, with shrimp, without dressing, fast food, 1 1/2 cups | 3 |
| vegetable, with turkey, ham and cheese, without dressing, fast food, 1 1/2 cups | 7 |
| Waldorf, 1/2 cup | 6 |
| yogurt and cucumber, 1/2 cup | 1 |
| **Salisbury steak,** 6 oz | 12 |
| **Salsa** | |
| ▲ black bean and corn, 1/2 cup | 2 |
| ▲ fat-free, 2 Tbsp | 0 |
| ▲ fat-free, 1/2 cup | 0 |
| peach, 2 Tbsp | 0 |
| pineapple, 2 Tbsp | 0 |
| **Samosa,** 1 (2 1/2" x 2 1/2" x 3" triangle) | 3 |
| **Sandwich** | |
| beef, roast, open-faced, with gravy, 1 (6 oz) | 9 |
| BLT, restaurant-type, 1 (9 1/4 oz) | 18 |
| cheese, grilled, restaurant-type, 1 (4 oz) | 14 |
| chicken fillet with cheese, fast food, 1 (8 oz) | 17 |
| chicken fillet, plain, fast food, 1 (6 1/2 oz) | 14 |
| chicken salad on regular bread, 1 (5 1/4 oz) | 10 |
| chicken, fried, fast food, 1 (7 1/4 oz) | 12 |

| ▲ Power Foods | *PointsPlus*™ value |
| --- | --- |
| chicken, grilled, fast food, 1 (6 3/4 oz) | 10 |
| club, 1 (8 3/4 oz) | 17 |
| croque monsieur, 1 (6 1/2 oz) | 12 |
| Cuban, 1/2 (6 1/2" x 3" x 4") | 12 |
| egg and cheese, fast food, 1 (5 1/4 oz) | 9 |
| egg salad , 1 (6 oz) | 12 |
| fish and cheese, fried, fast food, 1 (6 1/2 oz) | 14 |
| fish, with tartar sauce, fast food, 1 (5 1/2 oz) | 12 |
| grinder, 1 (2 3/4 oz) | 6 |
| ham and cheese, 1 (4 oz) | 10 |
| ham and cheese, fast food, 1 (5 1/4 oz) | 9 |
| ham and cheese, grilled, restaurant-type, grilled, 1 (5 1/4 oz) | 15 |
| ham, egg, and cheese, fast food, 1 (5 oz) | 9 |
| hero, 1 (11 1/4 oz) | 6 |
| hoagie, 1 (2 3/4 oz) | 6 |
| lobster roll, 1 (4 1/4 oz) | 6 |
| lobster salad, 1 (4 1/2 oz) | 8 |
| Monte Cristo, 1 (3 3/4 oz) | 7 |
| peanut butter and jelly, 1 (3 1/4 oz) | 9 |
| peanut butter and jelly, restaurant-type, 1 (4 1/4 oz) | 11 |
| Philly cheese steak, 1 (9 oz) | 14 |
| poor boy, 1 (2 3/4 oz) | 6 |
| Reuben, 1 (8 oz) | 18 |
| roast beef, 1 (7 1/2 oz) | 9 |
| roast beef with cheese, fast food, 1 (6 1/4 oz) | 12 |
| roast beef, fast food, 1 (5 3/4 oz) | 11 |
| roast beef, plain, fast food, 1 (5 oz) | 9 |
| shrimp salad, 1 (4 1/2 oz) | 8 |
| steak, fast food, 1 (7 oz) | 12 |
| submarine, 1 (2 3/4 oz) | 6 |

| ▲ Power Foods | *PointsPlus*™ value |
| --- | --- |
| submarine, with cold cuts, fast food, 1 (8 oz) | 12 |
| submarine, with roast beef, fast food, 1 (7 1/2 oz) | 11 |
| submarine, with tuna salad, fast food, 1 (9 oz) | 16 |
| tuna melt, 1 (5 3/4 oz) | 10 |
| tuna salad, 1 (6 1/4 oz) | 11 |
| turkey, 1 (4 oz) | 7 |
| **Sangria,** 1 (4 fl oz) | 3 |
| **Sashimi** | |
| ▲ any type except mackerel and salmon, 4 pieces (2 oz) | 1 |
| mackerel, 4 pieces (2 oz) | 4 |
| salmon, 4 pieces (2 oz) | 2 |
| **Satay** | |
| beef, with peanut sauce, 2 skewers with 1/4 cup sauce | 12 |
| beef, without peanut sauce, 2 skewers (3 oz) | 5 |
| chicken, with peanut sauce, 2 skewers with 1/4 cup sauce | 12 |
| chicken, without peanut sauce, 2 skewers (3 oz) | 3 |
| **Sauce** | |
| Alfredo, 1/2 cup | 10 |
| barbecue, 1 Tbsp | 0 |
| barbecue, 1/4 cup | 1 |
| béarnaise, 1/4 cup | 8 |
| Bolognese meat , 1/2 cup | 6 |
| brown, Chinese, 1/4 cup | 1 |
| cheese, 1/4 cup | 2 |
| clam, red, 1/2 cup | 3 |
| clam, white, 1/2 cup | 5 |
| curry, Hawaiian-style, 1/4 cup | 5 |
| duck, 1 Tbsp | 1 |
| hoisin, 1 tsp | 0 |
| hollandaise, 1/4 cup | 8 |
| horseradish, 1 Tbsp | 0 |

*Sauce (cont'd)*

| ▲ Power Foods | *PointsPlus*™ value |
|---|---|
| hot, 1 tsp | 0 |
| kung pao, 2 Tbsp | 2 |
| marinara, 1/2 cup | 3 |
| meat, 1/2 cup | 5 |
| mornay, 1/4 cup | 4 |
| oyster, 1 tsp | 1 |
| peanut satay, 1 Tbsp | 1 |
| peanut, spicy, 2 Tbsp | 4 |
| pepper, 1 tsp | 0 |
| pesto, 2 Tbsp | 4 |
| plum, 1 Tbsp | 2 |
| puttanesca, 1/2 cup | 12 |
| remoulade, 2 Tbsp | 4 |
| shoyu, 1 Tbsp | 0 |
| sofrito, 1/4 cup | 4 |
| soy, 1 Tbsp | 0 |
| Spanish, 1/2 cup | 3 |
| steak, 1 Tbsp | 0 |
| taco, 1 Tbsp | 0 |
| tamari, 1 Tbsp | 0 |
| tartar, 1 Tbsp | 2 |
| teriyaki, 1 Tbsp | 0 |
| ▲ tomato, Italian, 1/2 cup | 3 |
| tzatziki, 1/2 cup | 2 |
| Vietnamese spring roll dipping, 2 Tbsp | 0 |
| **Sauerbraten,** 3 oz beef with 2 Tbsp gravy | 6 |
| **Sausage biscuit,** fast food, 1 (4 1/2 oz) | 13 |
| **Sausage in brioche,** 1 slice (2" thick) | 16 |
| **Sausage patty,** restaurant-type, 1 patty (1 1/2 oz) | 4 |
| **Sausage, chorizo,** 1 link (5 1/2" long or 3 1/2 oz) | 12 |
| **Scallops,** fried | |
| 20 small (3 1/2 oz) | 6 |
| breaded, fast food, 4 pieces (5 oz) | 11 |
| **Schaum torte** | |
| with whipped cream, 1/10 of a 10" pan | 9 |

| ▲ Power Foods | *PointsPlus*™ value |
|---|---|
| without whipped cream, 1/10 of a 10" pan | 4 |
| **Schnapps,** any flavor, 1 jigger (1 1/2 fl oz) | 6 |
| **Scone** | |
| 1 small (1 1/2 oz) | 4 |
| 1 regular (2 1/2 oz) | 7 |
| blueberry, restaurant-type, 1 (4 1/2 oz) | 12 |
| chocolate, cinnamon, or raspberry, restaurant-type, 1 (4 1/2 oz) | 13 |
| cranberry or orange, restaurant-type, 1 (4 1/2 oz) | 11 |
| **Scotch,** 1 jigger (1 1/2 fl oz) | 4 |
| **Scrapple,** 1 slice (4 1/2" x 3/4" x 3/8" thick or 2 oz) | 3 |
| **Screwdriver,** 1 (6 fl oz) | 5 |
| **Seafood cakes (haw mok thalay),** 3/4 cup | 9 |
| **Seeds** | |
| sunflower, 1 tsp | 0 |
| sunflower, 1 Tbsp | 1 |
| **Seitan,** 2 slices (2 oz) | 2 |
| **Sesame noodles,** 1 cup | 7 |
| **Shabu shabu,** 4 oz beef, 2 oz tofu, and 1 1/2 cups vegetables | 10 |
| **Shawarma, chicken** | |
| 1/2 cup | 7 |
| without skin and bone, 1 thigh (2 oz) | 5 |
| **Shellfish** | |
| conch, cracked, 1 (6" long x 3") | 10 |
| ▲ crab meat, cooked, 1/2 cup (2 oz) | 1 |
| ▲ crab, Alaska king, cooked, 1 leg (4 3/4 oz) | 3 |
| ▲ lobster, steamed, 1 1/4 pound-lobster or 4 1/2 oz lobster meat | 3 |
| ▲ oyster, cooked, 6 medium (2 oz) | 1 |
| ▲ scallops, cooked, 10 small or 4 large (2 oz) | 2 |
| ▲ shrimp, canned, 1/2 cup | 2 |

| ▲ Power Foods | *PointsPlus*™ value |
|---|---|
| **Shepherd's pie,** 1 cup | 10 |
| **Sherbet,** 1/2 cup | 3 |
| **Sherry, dry or sweet,** 1/2 cup | 6 |
| **Shish kabob,** 2 small skewers (4 3/4 oz) | 8 |
| **Shoyu chicken,** 1 thigh (3 oz) | 6 |
| **Shrimp** | |
| barbecued, 4 large shrimp with 1/4 cup sauce | 11 |
| breaded and fried, fast food, 6-8 shrimp (5 3/4 oz) | 12 |
| broiled, stuffed, 6 large (6 oz) | 18 |
| fried, 10 (5 oz) | 9 |
| fried, stuffed, 6 large (9 1/2 oz) | 11 |
| sweet and sour, 1 cup | 11 |
| **Shrimp and broccoli,** 1 cup | 3 |
| **Shrimp Cantonese,** 1 cup | 9 |
| **Shrimp po' boy,** 1 (8 3/4 oz) | 20 |
| **Shrimp puffs,** 6 (2 oz) | 5 |
| **Shrimp remoulade,** 6 small shrimp with 1/4 cup remoulade sauce | 9 |
| **Shrimp scampi,** 9 medium (3 1/2 oz) | 10 |
| **Shrimp stir-fry, with garlic or black bean sauce,** 1 cup | 7 |
| **Shrimp toast,** 1 piece (1 oz) | 3 |
| **Shumai,** fried or steamed, 2 (2" diameter) | 3 |
| **Singapore sling,** 1 (6 fl oz) | 6 |
| **Sloppy Joe,** 1 (6 oz) | 9 |
| **Smoothie,** 1 cup | 4 |
| **Soft drink** | |
| club soda, 1 can or bottle (12 fl oz) | 0 |
| diet, any flavor, 1 can or bottle (12 fl oz) | 0 |
| seltzer, plain or flavored, unsweetened, 1 can or bottle (12 fl oz) | 0 |
| sweetened with sugar, any flavor, 1 can or bottle (12 fl oz) | 4 |
| tonic water, 1 bottle (11 fl oz) | 3 |

| ▲ Power Foods | *PointsPlus*™ value |
|---|---|
| **Sopaipillas,** 2 (1 oz) | 3 |
| **Sorbet,** any flavor, 1 scoop or 1/2 cup | 2 |
| **Soufflé** | |
| cheese, 1 cup | 5 |
| fruit, 1/2 cup | 4 |
| **Soup** | |
| asparagus crab, 1 cup | 2 |
| avgolemono, 1 cup | 4 |
| black bean, 1 cup | 2 |
| broccoli cheese, 1 cup | 7 |
| cabbage, 1 cup | 2 |
| Cheddar cheese, 1 cup | 10 |
| cherry, 1 cup | 8 |
| chicken enchilada, 1 cup | 6 |
| chicken noodle, 1 cup | 3 |
| chicken, with matzo balls, 1 cup soup with 2 (1 1/2") matzo balls | 3 |
| chicken, with tortilla strips and shredded cheese, 1 cup | 5 |
| ▲ chicken, without matzo balls (broth only), 1 cup | 0 |
| clam chowder, Manhattan, 1 cup | 5 |
| cream of broccoli, 1 cup | 7 |
| cream of mushroom, 1 cup | 9 |
| cream of potato, 1 cup | 3 |
| cream of tomato, 1 cup | 5 |
| egg drop, 1 cup | 1 |
| French onion au gratin, 1 cup | 8 |
| French onion, restaurant-type, 1 cup | 7 |
| gazpacho, 1 cup | 4 |
| hot and sour, 1 cup | 3 |
| hot and spicy chicken, 1 cup | 4 |
| Italian wedding, 1 cup | 5 |
| knefla, 1 cup | 7 |
| lentil, 1 cup | 4 |
| lobster bisque, 1 cup | 4 |
| minestrone, 1 cup | 5 |
| miso, 1 cup | 2 |
| mulligatawny, 1 cup | 7 |

*Soup (cont'd)*

| ▲ Power Foods | *PointsPlus*™ value |
|---|---|
| oxtail, 1 cup | 2 |
| pigeon pea and dumpling, 1 1/2 cups | 9 |
| Portuguese bean, 1 cup | 6 |
| pozole, 1 cup | 5 |
| Scotch broth, 1 cup | 6 |
| shark fin, 1 cup | 3 |
| split pea, 1 cup | 4 |
| Thai chicken coconut, 1 cup | 10 |
| tomato, 1 cup | 3 |
| tortilla, 1 cup | 7 |
| turtle, 1 cup | 3 |
| vegetable, 1 cup | 3 |
| vichyssoise, 1 cup | 3 |
| wonton, 1 cup with 4 wontons | 5 |
| yogurt and cucumber, 1 cup | 3 |
| ▲ **Soursop (guanabana),** 1/2 cup pulp | 0 |
| **Souse, chicken,** 1 leg and 1 thigh with skin (4 1/2 oz) | 8 |
| **Souvlaki, chicken** | |
| 1 large or 2 small skewers (4 1/2 oz) | 5 |
| in pita bread, 1 (6 1/2 oz) | 8 |
| **Souvlaki, lamb** | |
| 1 large or 2 small skewers (4 3/4 oz) | 8 |
| in pita bread, 1 (6 1/2 oz) | 9 |
| **Spaetzle,** 1/2 cup | 6 |
| **Spaghetti bolognese,** 1 cup spaghetti with 1/2 cup sauce | 12 |
| **Spaghetti carbonara,** 1 cup | 13 |
| **Spaghetti with marinara sauce,** 1 cup spaghetti with 1/2 cup sauce | 8 |
| **Spaghetti with meat sauce,** 1 cup spaghetti with 1/2 cup sauce | 11 |
| **Spaghetti with tomato sauce and meatballs,** 1 cup spaghetti with 1/2 cup sauce and 2 meatballs | 18 |
| **Spanakopita,** 1 (3" square) or 1 cup | 9 |
| **Spareribs,** barbecued | |
| 4 (4" long) | 9 |
| 6 (6 1/4 oz) | 13 |
| Chinese, 2 (4" long) | 4 |

| ▲ Power Foods | *PointsPlus*™ value |
|---|---|
| **Spoon bread,** 1/2 cup | 5 |
| **Spring roll** | |
| beef or pork, 1 (4 1/2" long) | 6 |
| chicken, 1 (4 1/2" long) | 5 |
| shrimp, 1 (4 1/2" long) | 4 |
| Thai, 1 (4" long) | 5 |
| Vietnamese, fresh, 1 (1 (3/4 oz) | 2 |
| Vietnamese, fried, 1 (4" long) | 5 |
| **Sprinkles,** any type, 1 Tbsp | 0 |
| ▲ **Sprouts, alfalfa or bean,** 1 cup | 0 |
| **Spumoni,** 1/2 cup | 7 |
| **Squid,** fried, 3 oz | 4 |
| **Steak,** blackened, 6 oz | 17 |
| **Steak, chicken fried** | |
| with cream gravy, 6 oz with 1/4 cup cream gravy | 18 |
| without gravy, 6 oz | 14 |
| **Steak au poivre,** 6 oz steak with 1 Tbsp sauce | 13 |
| **Stew** | |
| bean and lentil (dal maharani), 1 cup | 6 |
| beef, 1 cup | 7 |
| Brunswick, 1 1/2 cups | 7 |
| Irish brown, 1 cup | 8 |
| lamb, 1 cup | 6 |
| **Sticky rice with mango,** 1 cup sliced mangoes with 1/2 cup sticky rice | 11 |
| **Stir-fried vegetables** | |
| with beef, 1 cup | 4 |
| with chicken, 1 cup | 3 |
| with oil or sauce, 1 cup | 4 |
| with pork, 1 cup | 4 |
| **Stromboli,** 1 slice (1" thick or 2 oz) | 5 |
| **Strudel,** any type, 1 piece (6 oz) | 12 |
| **Stuffing,** 1/2 cup | 5 |
| ▲ **Succotash,** cooked, 1 cup | 6 |
| **Suimono,** 1 cup | 2 |
| **Sukiyaki with sauce,** 2 cups with 1/4 cup sauce | 15 |
| **Summer squash casserole,** 1 cup | 9 |

| ▲ Power Foods | *PointsPlus™* value |
|---|---|
| **Sunomono,** 1/2 cup | 0 |
| **Sushi** | |
| Alaskan roll, 2 pieces (1" high x 1 3/4" diameter) | 3 |
| California roll, 4 large pieces (1" high x 1 3/4" diameter or 1 oz each) | 4 |
| cone, 1 | 3 |
| inari, 1 | 3 |
| kappa maki (cucumber roll), 4 medium pieces (1 1/2" diameter x 3/4" thick) | 3 |
| kappa maki (cucumber roll), 6 small pieces (1" diameter x 1" thick) | 3 |
| maki (vegetables and rice rolled with seaweed), 4 medium pieces (1 1/2" diameter x 3/4" thick) | 3 |
| maki (vegetables and rice rolled with seaweed), 6 small pieces (1" diameter x 1" thick) | 3 |
| nigiri (sliced uncooked fish over rice), 4 medium pieces (2" long x 3/4" wide | 3 |
| nigiri (sliced uncooked fish over rice), 6 small pieces (1" long x 1" wide) | 3 |
| nigiri uni (sea urchin), 4 medium pieces (2" long x 3/4" wide) | 3 |
| nigiri, albacore (white tuna), 4 medium pieces (2" long x 3/4" wide) | 3 |
| nigiri, amaebi (sweet shrimp), 4 medium pieces (2" long x 3/4" wide) | 3 |
| nigiri, conch, 4 medium pieces (2" long x 3/4" wide) | 3 |
| nigiri, ebi (cooked shrimp), 4 medium pieces (2" long x 3/4" wide) | 3 |
| nigiri, hamachi (yellow tail), 4 medium pieces (2" long x 3/4" wide) | 3 |
| nigiri, hirame (fluke), 4 medium pieces (2" long x 3/4" wide) | 3 |
| nigiri, hokigai (surf clam), 4 medium pieces (2" long x 3/4" wide) | 3 |

| ▲ Power Foods | *PointsPlus™* value |
|---|---|
| nigiri, ikura (salmon roe), 4 medium pieces (2" long x 3/4" wide) | 3 |
| nigiri, kani (crab), 4 medium pieces (2" long x 3/4" wide) | 3 |
| nigiri, maguro (tuna), 4 medium pieces (2" long x 3/4" wide) | 3 |
| nigiri, masago (smelt roe), 4 medium pieces (2" long x 3/4" wide) | 3 |
| nigiri, saba (mackerel), 4 medium pieces (2" long x 3/4" wide) | 3 |
| nigiri, sake (fresh salmon), 4 medium pieces (2" long x 3/4" wide) | 3 |
| nigiri, smoked salmon, 4 medium pieces (2" long x 3/4" wide) | 3 |
| nigiri, suzuki (sea bass), 4 medium pieces (2" long x 3/4" wide) | 3 |
| nigiri, suzume, 4 medium pieces (2" long x 3/4" wide) | 3 |
| nigiri, tai (red snapper), 4 medium pieces (2" long x 3/4" wide) | 3 |
| nigiri, tairagai (scallops), 4 medium pieces (2" long x 3/4" wide) | 3 |
| nigiri, tako (octopus), 4 medium pieces (2" long x 3/4" wide) | 3 |
| nigiri, tobiko (flying fish roe), 4 medium pieces (2" long x 3/4" wide) | 3 |
| nigiri, unagi (fresh water eel), 4 medium pieces (2" long x 3/4" wide) | 3 |
| nigri, ika (squid), 4 medium pieces (2" long x 3/4" wide) | 3 |
| nori maki (uncooked fish and rice rolled with seaweed), 4 medium pieces (1 1/2" diameter x 3/4" thick) | 3 |
| nori maki (uncooked fish and rice rolled with seaweed), 6 small pieces (1" diameter x 1" thick) | 3 |
| Philadelphia roll, 2 large pieces (1" high x 1 3/4" diameter) | 3 |
| rainbow roll, 4 medium pieces (1 1/2" diameter x 3/4" thick) | 3 |
| rainbow roll, 6 small pieces (1" diameter x 1" thick) | 3 |

Sushi (cont'd)

| ▲ Power Foods | PointsPlus™ value |
|---|---|
| spider roll, 6 pieces (2" diameter x 1" thick) | 10 |
| tamago-yaki (omelet roll), 2 pieces (3/4" wide) | 3 |
| tempura roll, shrimp, 6 pieces (1 1/2" diameter x 1" thick) | 10 |
| tempura roll, vegetable, 6 pieces (1 1/2" diameter x 1" thick) | 5 |
| tuna roll, 4 medium pieces (1 1/2" diameter x 3/4" thick) | 3 |
| tuna roll, 6 small pieces (1" diameter x 1" thick) | 3 |
| tuna roll, spicy, 6 pieces (2" diameter x 1" thick) | 7 |
| unagi maki, 4 medium pieces (1 1/2" diameter x 3/4" thick) | 3 |
| unagi maki, 6 small pieces (1" diameter x 1" thick) | 3 |
| uni maki, 4 medium pieces (1 1/2" diameter x 3/4" thick) | 3 |
| uni maki, 6 small pieces (1" diameter x 1" thick) | 3 |
| yellow tail roll, 4 medium pieces (1 1/2" diameter x 3/4" thick) | 3 |
| yellow tail roll, 6 small pieces (1" diameter x 1" thick) | 3 |
| **Swedish meatballs,** 6 (1" diameter) | 10 |
| **Sweet potato pie,** 1/8 of a 9" pie | 11 |
| **Sweet potatoes,** candied, 1/2 cup | 5 |
| **Sweet roll,** 1 large (4 oz) | 6 |
| **Syrup, pancake,** regular, 1 Tbsp | 1 |
| **Szechuan pork hotpot,** 1 cup | 6 |

## T

| ▲ Power Foods | PointsPlus™ value |
|---|---|
| **Tabouli,** 1/2 cup | 6 |
| **Taco** | |
| beef, 1 (3 1/2 oz) | 6 |
| breakfast, 1 (3 1/2 oz) | 5 |
| chicken, 1 (3 1/2 oz) | 5 |
| fish, 1 (4 1/4 oz) | 5 |
| hard, fast food, 1 (3 oz) | 4 |
| pork, 1 (3 1/2 oz) | 5 |
| soft, fast food, 1 (3 1/2 oz) | 4 |
| **Tamale,** 2 (9 1/2 oz) | 10 |
| **Tamale pie,** 1 cup | 12 |
| **Tandoori chicken** | |
| breast, without skin, 1 piece (4 1/2 oz) | 4 |
| thigh, without skin, 1 piece (3 oz) | 4 |
| **Tandoori fish,** 3/4 cup | 5 |
| **Tandoori shrimp,** 3/4 cup | 3 |
| **Taquitos** | |
| beef, 1 (5 1/2" x 1 1/2") | 5 |
| chicken, 1 (5 1/2" x 1 1/2") | 3 |
| **Tarte aux fruits** | |
| 1/8 of a 9" tart | 11 |
| individual, 1 (4") | 15 |
| **Tea,** decaffeinated or regular, unsweetened, 1 cup | 0 |
| **Tempura** | |
| shrimp, 4 jumbo (3 3/4 oz) | 13 |
| vegetable, 1 cup | 8 |
| **Teppan yaki (mixed grill of beef, chicken, shrimp and vegetables),** 1 1/2 cups | 12 |
| **Tequila,** 1 jigger (1 1/2 fl oz) | 4 |
| **Teriyaki** | |
| beef, 2 slices (4 oz) | 7 |
| chicken, 2 slices (4 oz) | 6 |
| fish other than salmon, 4 oz | 6 |
| salmon, 4 oz | 7 |
| tofu, 1 cup | 4 |
| **Thai chicken with basil,** without skin and bone, 1 breast (3 oz) | 5 |
| **Thai coffee or tea,** 1 cup | 9 |
| **Thai crisp noodles,** 1 cup | 9 |
| **Thai grilled beef (nuea nam tok),** 1/2 cup on lettuce leaves | 6 |
| **Tirami-su** | |
| 2 1/4" square | 10 |
| restaurant-type, 1 slice (4 3/4 oz) | 12 |

| ▲ Power Foods | *PointsPlus™* value |
|---|---|
| **Tofu,** fried, agadashi, 1 1/2" x 2" | 7 |
| **Tom Collins,** 1 (6 fl oz) | 4 |
| **Tom yum kung,** 1 cup | 2 |
| **Tomatoes,** fried green, 2 slices (1 1/2" thick) | 5 |
| ▲ **Tomatoes,** fresh or canned, 1 small, medium, or large or 1 cup | 0 |
| **Tonkatsu** | |
| beef, 3/4 cup | 7 |
| chicken, 3/4 cup | 7 |
| pork, 3/4 cup | 9 |
| **Topping** | |
| butterscotch, 2 Tbsp | 3 |
| caramel, regular or fat-free, 2 Tbsp | 3 |
| fudge, regular, 1 Tbsp | 2 |
| nuts in syrup, 2 Tbsp | 5 |
| whipped, dairy or nondairy, light or fat-free, aerosol or frozen, 2 Tbsp | 0 |
| whipped, dairy or nondairy, light or fat-free, aerosol or frozen, 1/3 cup | 1 |
| **Tortellini** | |
| cheese, without sauce, 2/3 cup | 4 |
| meat, without sauce, 2/3 cup | 4 |
| **Tortiere (Canadian meat pie),** 1/8 of a 9" pie | 10 |
| **Tostada** | |
| beef, 1 (8 1/4 oz) | 11 |
| chicken, 1 (8 1/4 oz) | 10 |
| with beans and cheese, fast food, 1 (5 oz) | 6 |
| with beans, beef, and cheese, fast food, 1 (8 oz) | 9 |
| with beef and cheese, fast food, 1 (5 3/4 oz) | 8 |
| with guacamole, fast food, 2 (9 1/4 oz) | 10 |
| **Trifle,** 1 cup | 6 |
| **Tuna noodle casserole,** 1 cup | 10 |
| **Turkey, ground,** regular, cooked, 1 patty (3 oz) | 5 |
| **Turkey tetrazzini,** 1 1/2 cups | 15 |

| ▲ Power Foods | *PointsPlus™* value |
|---|---|
| **Turnover** | |
| fruit, any type, 1 (3" x 1 1/2") | 6 |
| fruit, any type, fast food, 1 (4 oz) | 9 |
| **Twice-cooked pork,** 1 cup | 10 |
| **Tzimmes, vegetable,** 3/4 cup | 4 |

## U

| | |
|---|---|
| ▲ **Urad dal (split matpe beans without skin),** 1 cup | 5 |

## V

| | |
|---|---|
| **Veal, breast,** cooked, 3 oz | 6 |
| **Veal cutlet,** breaded and fried, 4 oz | 9 |
| **Veal marsala,** 4 oz veal with sauce | 12 |
| **Veal parmigiana** | |
| with sauce, 5 oz with 1/2 cup tomato sauce | 13 |
| without sauce, 5 1/2 oz | 10 |
| **Veal piccata,** 2 slices (4 oz) | 10 |
| **Veal scaloppine,** 2 pieces (4 1/2 oz) | 9 |
| **Veal with peppers,** 5 oz | 11 |
| **Vegetable pulao,** 1 cup | 4 |
| **Vegetables** | |
| creamed (except cream-style corn), 1 cup | 2 |
| fried, 1 cup | 4 |
| sauteed, 1 cup | 7 |
| **Vegetables, Chinese** | |
| with beef, 1 cup | 7 |
| with chicken, 1 cup | 5 |
| with peas, prepared with oil, 1 cup | 5 |
| with pork, 1 cup | 7 |
| with shrimp, 1 cup | 5 |
| with tofu, 1 cup | 4 |
| **Vegetarian burger,** restaurant-type, 1 (7 1/4 oz) | 12 |
| **Vietnamese beef balls (Thit bo vien),** 6 (1 1/2 oz) | 2 |
| **Vietnamese chicken curry,** 1 cup | 9 |

| ▲ Power Foods | *PointsPlus*™ value |
|---|---|
| **Vindaloo** | |
| chicken, 1 cup | 9 |
| lamb, 1 cup | 16 |
| pork, 1 cup | 10 |
| **Vitello tonnato,** 2 slices veal (4 oz) with 1/2 cup sauce | 16 |
| **Vodka gimlet,** 1 (2 fl oz) | 1 |
| **Vodka,** 1 jigger (1 1/2 fl oz) | 4 |

## W

| ▲ Power Foods | *PointsPlus*™ value |
|---|---|
| **Whiskey,** 1 jigger (1 1/2 fl oz) | 4 |
| **Whiskey sour,** 1 (4 fl oz) | 6 |
| **White Russian,** 1 (3 fl oz) | 8 |
| **Wiener schnitzel,** 1 slice (3 oz) | 10 |
| **Wine** | |
| any type other than those listed here, 1 small glass (4 fl oz) | 4 |
| dessert, dry, 2 fl oz | 3 |
| dessert, sweet, 2 fl oz | 3 |
| light, 1 small glass (4 fl oz) | 2 |
| non-alcoholic, 1 small glass (4 fl oz) | 0 |
| **Wine cooler,** 1 (8 fl oz) | 4 |
| **Wine spritzer,** 1 (8 fl oz) | 4 |
| **Wontons** | |
| boiled, 6 (6 oz) | 6 |
| fried, 6 (4 oz) | 12 |

## Y

| ▲ Power Foods | *PointsPlus*™ value |
|---|---|
| **Yaki-soba** | |
| beef, 1/2 cup noodles with 1/2 cup beef and vegetables | 5 |
| chicken, 1/2 cup noodles with 1/2 cup chicken and vegetables | 5 |
| pork, 1/2 cup noodles with 1/2 cup pork and vegetables | 5 |
| **Yakitori,** 1 skewer (7 1/2 oz) | 6 |
| **Yogurt,** low-fat, flavored (vanilla, lemon, coffee), sweetened with sugar, 1 cup | 6 |
| **Yogurt,** frozen | |
| fat-free, sweetened with sugar, 1 scoop or 1/2 cup | 3 |
| low-fat, 1 scoop or 1/2 cup | 3 |
| **Yorkshire pudding,** 1 piece (4" square) | 7 |
| **Yosenabe,** 2 cups | 5 |

## Z

| ▲ Power Foods | *PointsPlus*™ value |
|---|---|
| **Zabaglione,** 1/2 cup | 4 |
| **Zeppole,** 1 (4" diameter) | 7 |
| **Ziti,** baked | |
| with meat, 1 cup | 10 |
| without meat, 1 cup | 7 |
| **Zuppa di pesce,** 2 cups | 11 |
| **Zuppa Inglese,** 6 1/2 oz | 9 |

# Ethnic & Regional Favorites

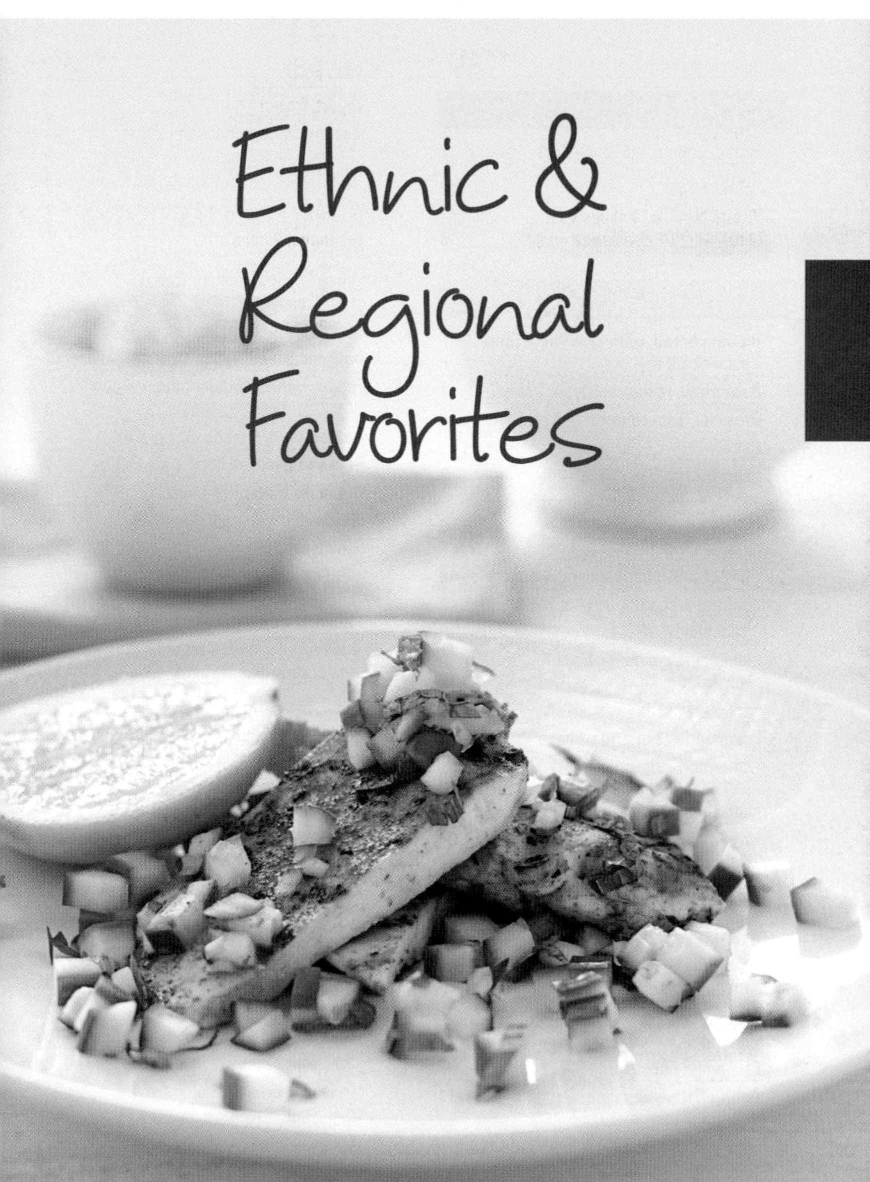

| ▲ Power Foods | *PointsPlus™* value |
|---|---|

## AFRICAN

| | |
|---|---|
| **Bread,** enjera, 1 (9" diameter) | 2 |
| **Curry** | |
| fish, African, 1/2 cup | 6 |
| shrimp, African, 1/2 cup | 7 |

## AMERICAN, BAKERY

| | |
|---|---|
| **Banana bread, with or without nuts,** 1 slice (2 1/2 oz) | 6 |
| **Bear claw,** restaurant-type, 1 (4 oz) | 11 |
| **Brownie,** 1 (2" square) | 6 |
| **Cake** | |
| angel food, 1/16 of a 10" tube | 3 |
| Boston cream pie, 1/6 of the pie (3 1/4 oz) | 6 |
| carrot, with cream cheese icing, 1/12 of a 9" layer cake, or 3" square | 18 |
| coffee, 3" square, or 1/12 of a 9" tube | 9 |
| fruitcake, 2 1/2" x 1 3/4" x 1/2" or 2 oz | 6 |
| pineapple upside-down, 1/8 of a 10" skillet cake | 13 |
| pound, 1 slice (5" x 3" x 1") | 9 |
| sponge, 1/12 of a 16 oz cake | 3 |
| strawberry shortcake, 1/12 of a 9" cake or 1 filled individual shortcake | 8 |
| white, without frosting, 1/12 of the 9" diameter | 7 |
| with icing, 1/12 of a 9" layer cake or 3" square | 14 |
| **Cheesecake** | |
| with fruit topping, 1/16 of the 10" cake | 12 |
| without fruit topping, 1/16 of the 10" cake | 11 |
| **Cinnamon bun,** 1 large (4 oz) | 7 |
| **Cobbler, fruit,** any type, 1 cup | 13 |
| **Cookies** | |
| butter, 1 small | 1 |
| chocolate chip, 1 medium (2 1/4" diameter) | 1 |
| lace, 1 | 1 |
| rainbow, 1 (1" x 2") | 3 |
| white macadamia, restaurant-type, 1 (1 3/4 oz) | 7 |
| **Danish pastry** | |
| cheese, cinnamon, or fruit, 1 (4 1/4" diameter) | 7 |
| nut, 1 (4 1/4" diameter) | 8 |
| **Date-nut bread,** 1 (5" x 1/2") | 7 |
| **Fudge,** with or without nuts, 1 piece (1" x 2" or 1 oz) | 3 |
| **Gingerbread,** 1 piece (3" square) | 11 |
| **Honeybun,** glazed, 1 (4" x 3" oval) | 7 |
| **Hot cross buns,** 1 (2 1/4 oz) | 6 |
| **Muffin** | |
| any type other than those listed here, 1 large (3" diameter) | 8 |
| banana walnut, restaurant-type, 1 (5 oz) | 15 |
| blueberry, reduced-fat, restaurant-type, 1 (5 oz) | 11 |
| corn, restaurant-type, 1 (5 oz) | 13 |
| cranberry orange, restaurant-type, 1 (5 oz) | 12 |
| mini, any type, 1 (1 1/4" diameter or 1/2 oz) | 1 |
| oat bran, 1 (2 oz) | 4 |
| pumpkin, restaurant-type, 1 (5 oz) | 12 |
| wheat bran, toaster-type with raisins, 1 (1 1/4 oz) | 3 |
| **Pie** | |
| chiffon, cream, or custard, with fruit, 1/8 of a 9" one-crust pie | 11 |
| chiffon, cream, or custard, without fruit, 1/8 of a 9" one-crust pie | 10 |
| fruit, one-crust, 1/8 of a 9" pie | 8 |
| fruit, two-crust, 1/8 of a 9" pie | 11 |
| individual, 1 (5" x 3 3/4") | 11 |
| key lime, 1/8 of a 9" one-crust pie | 14 |
| meringue, 1/8 of a 9"one-crust pie | 12 |

| ▲ Power Foods | *PointsPlus*™ value |
|---|---|
| mincemeat, with meat, 1/8 of a 9" two-crust pie | 13 |
| mincemeat, without meat, 1/8 of a 9" two-crust pie | 16 |
| pecan, 1/8 of a 9" one-crust pie | 14 |
| pumpkin, 1/8 of a 9" one-crust pie | 11 |
| rhubarb, 1/8 of a 9" two-crust pie | 13 |
| **Pumpkin bread,** 1 slice (3/4" thick) | 8 |
| **Sweet roll,** 1 large (4 oz) | 6 |
| **Turnover, fruit,** any type, 1 (3" x 1 1/2") | 6 |

## AMERICAN, BAR/PUB

| ▲ Power Foods | *PointsPlus*™ value |
|---|---|
| **Beer** | |
| light, 1 can or bottle (12 fl oz) | 3 |
| non-alcoholic, 1 can or bottle (12 fl oz) | 2 |
| **Bellini,** 1 (6 fl oz) | 6 |
| **Black Russian,** 1 (3 fl oz) | 8 |
| **Bloody Mary,** 1 (5 fl oz) | 4 |
| **Bourbon,** 1 fl oz | 3 |
| **Brandy,** 1 jigger (1 1/2 fl oz) | 4 |
| **Brandy Alexander,** 1 (3 fl oz) | 9 |
| **Buffalo wings,** cooked, 3 (4 1/2 oz) | 9 |
| **Champagne,** 1 small glass (4 fl oz) | 3 |
| **Cheese fries,** restaurant-type, 8 1/2 oz | 18 |
| **Cheeseburger, on bun, plain, without mayonnaise, lettuce, and tomato,** 1 (6 1/2 oz) | 12 |
| **Cherries, maraschino,** 1 | 0 |
| **Chili dog on roll,** 1 (8 1/2 oz) | 11 |
| **Cognac,** 1 jigger (1 1/2 fl oz) | 4 |
| **Cosmopolitan,** 1 (3 1/2 fl oz) | 6 |
| **Crème de menthe,** 1 jigger (1 1/2 fl oz) | 6 |
| **Daiquiri,** 3 fl oz | 4 |
| **Fish,** fried, breaded with flour, 1 fillet (6 oz) | 13 |
| **Gin,** 1 jigger (1 1/2 fl oz) | 4 |
| **Gin and tonic,** 1 (6 fl oz) | 5 |
| **Gin gimlet,** 1 (2 1/2 fl oz) | 4 |
| **Hamburger on bun, plain (without mayonnaise, lettuce, and tomato),** 3 oz cooked hamburger on 1 1/2 oz bun | 10 |
| **Highball** | |
| made with sweetened mixer, 1 (6 fl oz) | 7 |
| made with unsweetened mixer, 1 (6 fl oz) | 4 |
| **Hot dog on roll,** plain, 1 (4 oz) | 9 |
| **Juice cocktail, cranberry,** regular, 1/2 cup | 2 |
| **Kahlua,** 1 jigger (1 1/2 fl oz) | 6 |
| **Liqueur,** any type, 1 jigger (1 1/2 fl oz) | 6 |
| **Liquor (brandy, gin, rum, scotch, tequila, vodka, whiskey),** 1 jigger (1 1/2 fl oz) | 4 |
| **Long Island iced tea,** 1 (5 fl oz) | 8 |
| **Manhattan,** 1 (2 fl oz) | 5 |
| **Margarita,** 1 (4 fl oz) | 9 |
| **Martini** | |
| 1 (2 1/2 fl oz) | 6 |
| chocolate, 1 (2 1/2 fl oz) | 8 |
| sour apple, 1 (2 1/2 fl oz) | 8 |
| **Mimosa,** 1 (6 fl oz) | 4 |
| **Mojito,** 1 (12 fl oz) | 7 |
| **Old fashioned,** 1 (2 fl oz) | 6 |
| **Peanuts,** shelled, 40 (1 oz) | 5 |
| **Piña colada,** 1 (6 fl oz) | 8 |
| **Potato skins, with cheese, bacon and sour cream,** 1 (7 oz) | 10 |
| **Pretzels** | |
| sticks, 45 (3/4 oz) | 2 |
| twists, 7 regular or 15 small (3/4 oz) | 2 |
| **Rum,** 1 jigger (1 1/2 fl oz) | 4 |
| **Sandwich, Philly cheese steak,** 1 (9 oz) | 14 |

American, Bar/Pub (cont'd)

| ▲ Power Foods | PointsPlus™ value |
|---|---|
| **Sauce, tartar,** 1 Tbsp | 2 |
| **Scotch,** 1 jigger (1 1/2 fl oz) | 4 |
| **Screwdriver,** 1 (6 fl oz) | 5 |
| **Singapore sling,** 1 (6 fl oz) | 6 |
| **Sloppy Joe,** 1 (6 oz) | 9 |
| **Soft drink** | |
| club soda, 1 can or bottle (12 fl oz) | 0 |
| tonic water, 1 bottle (11 fl oz) | 3 |
| **Tequila,** 1 jigger (1 1/2 fl oz) | 4 |
| **Tom Collins,** 1 (6 fl oz) | 4 |
| **Vodka,** 1 jigger (1 1/2 fl oz) | 4 |
| **Vodka gimlet,** 1 (2 fl oz) | 1 |
| **Whiskey,** 1 jigger (1 1/2 fl oz) | 4 |
| **Whiskey sour,** 1 (4 fl oz) | 6 |
| **White Russian,** 1 (3 fl oz) | 8 |
| **Wine** | |
| any type other than those listed here, 1 small glass (4 fl oz) | 4 |
| dessert, dry, 2 fl oz | 3 |
| dessert, sweet, 2 fl oz | 3 |
| light, 1 small glass (4 fl oz) | 2 |
| non-alcoholic, 1 small glass (4 fl oz) | 0 |
| **Wine spritzer,** 1 (8 fl oz) | 4 |

## AMERICAN, BARBECUE

| ▲ Power Foods | PointsPlus™ value |
|---|---|
| **Beans,** baked, 1/2 cup | 8 |
| **Beef** | |
| brisket, cooked, 3 oz | 9 |
| shortribs, lean and fat, cooked, 3 oz | 11 |
| shortribs, trimmed, cooked, 3 oz | 6 |
| **Chicken breast, barbecued, with skin and bone,** 1 (4 1/2 oz) | 7 |
| **Chicken breast fillet,** grilled, 1 (3 oz) | 3 |
| **Chicken drumstick,** barbecued, with skin and bone, 1 (1 1/2 oz) | 3 |
| **Chicken thigh,** barbecued, with skin and bone, 1 (3 oz) | 6 |
| **Corn** | |
| ▲ on the cob, 1 ear (up to 7" long) | 2 |
| ▲ on the cob, 1 ear (8" long) | 4 |
| **Cornbread,** 2" square | 3 |
| **Kabobs** | |
| beef, 2 skewers (4 1/2 oz) | 8 |
| chicken, 2 skewers (4 1/2 oz) | 5 |
| **Lemonade,** 1 cup | 3 |
| **Limeade,** 1 cup | 3 |
| ▲ **Pickle,** unsweetened, 1 large or 1 cup | 0 |
| **Pork,** barbecue, 1 cup | 9 |
| **Sauce** | |
| barbecue, 1 Tbsp | 0 |
| barbecue, 1/4 cup | 1 |
| **Shrimp,** barbecued, 4 large shrimp with 1/4 cup sauce | 11 |
| **Spareribs,** barbecued | |
| 4 (4" long) | 9 |
| 6 (6 1/4 oz) | 13 |
| **Wine cooler,** 1 (8 fl oz) | 4 |

## AMERICAN, CAJUN

| Item | PointsPlus™ value |
|---|---|
| **Bananas Foster,** 1 (9 oz) | 18 |
| **Beans, red, and rice,** 1 cup | 7 |
| **Beignet,** 1 (3/4 oz) | 2 |
| **Chicken,** blackened, 1 breast (3 oz) | 7 |
| **Creole** | |
| chicken, without rice, 1 cup | 7 |
| shrimp, without rice, 1 cup | 5 |
| **Etouffee, shrimp,** 1 cup | 10 |
| **Fish,** blackened, 1 fillet (6 oz) | 12 |
| **Green rice,** 1 cup | 7 |
| **Gumbo** | |
| chicken, 1 cup | 7 |
| seafood, 1 cup | 6 |
| **Jambalaya, chicken or fish, with rice,** 1 1/2 cups | 11 |
| **Muffuletta,** 1 (11 1/4 oz) | 22 |

| ▲ Power Foods | *PointsPlus*™ value |
|---|---|
| **Oyster pie,** 1/8 of a 9" pie | 10 |
| **Oyster po' boy,** 1 (8 3/4 oz) | 19 |
| **Praline,** 1 (2 1/2" diameter or 1 1/2 oz) | 6 |
| **Rice, dirty,** 1 cup | 11 |
| **Sandwich, poor boy,** 1 (2 3/4 oz) | 6 |
| **Sauce, remoulade,** 2 Tbsp | 4 |
| **Shrimp po' boy,** 1 (8 3/4 oz) | 20 |
| **Shrimp remoulade,** 6 small shrimp with 1/4 cup remoulade sauce | 9 |
| **Soup, turtle,** 1 cup | 3 |
| **Steak,** blackened, 6 oz | 17 |

## AMERICAN, DINER

| ▲ Power Foods | *PointsPlus*™ value |
|---|---|
| **Apple,** baked, 1 large (7 oz) | 9 |
| **Bacon** | |
| cooked, crisp, 1 slice | 1 |
| cooked, crisp, 3 slices | 4 |
| **Brownie, walnut,** restaurant-type, 1 (4 1/2 oz) | 15 |
| **Crackers** | |
| oyster, 20 or 1/2 cup | 3 |
| saltines, 4 | 1 |
| saltines, 6 | 2 |
| **Egg** | |
| fried, 1 large | 2 |
| ▲ poached, 1 large | 2 |
| scrambled, 2 or 1/2 cup | 5 |
| **Fish** | |
| ▲ cod, cooked, 1 fillet (3 oz) | 2 |
| ▲ grouper, cooked, 1 fillet (6 oz) | 4 |
| ▲ haddock, cooked, 1 fillet (6 oz) | 4 |
| ▲ halibut, cooked, 1 fillet or steak (6 oz) | 5 |
| tuna, canned in oil, drained, 1/2 cup (4 oz) | 5 |
| ▲ tuna, canned in water, drained, 1/2 cup (4 oz) | 3 |
| **French fries,** 20 (4 1/2" long or 5 1/2 oz) | 11 |
| **Fruit cup,** restaurant-type, 1 small (6 oz) | 1 |
| **Hot chocolate, with or without whipped topping,** 1 cup | 8 |
| **Jam, regular or reduced-sugar,** 1 Tbsp | 1 |
| **Jelly,** 1 Tbsp | 1 |
| **Muffin, English, any type, regular,** 1 (2 oz) | 3 |
| **Omelet** | |
| cheese, 2-egg, 1 | 8 |
| ham and cheese, 2-egg, 1 | 9 |
| herb or plain, 2-egg, 1 | 6 |
| vegetable, 2-egg, 1 | 8 |
| **Onion rings,** fried, 4 (3 oz) | 7 |
| **Pancakes** | |
| buttermilk, restaurant-type, 2 (6 oz) | 14 |
| prepared from scratch, 1 (4" diameter) | 3 |
| **Potatoes, hash brown,** 1 cup | 8 |
| **Preserves,** 1 Tbsp | 1 |
| **Pudding, any type and flavor other than those listed here,** 1 cup | 8 |
| banana, 1 cup | 9 |
| **Pudding, rice,** 1 cup | 10 |
| **Pudding, tapioca,** 1 cup | 6 |
| **Salad** | |
| chef's, with dressing, 4 cups | 8 |
| chef's, without dressing, 4 cups | 6 |
| chicken, 1/2 cup | 6 |
| egg, 1/2 cup | 8 |
| garden, restaurant-type, 1 (6 oz) | 3 |
| macaroni, 1/2 cup | 7 |
| potato, 1/2 cup | 8 |
| shrimp, 1/2 cup | 3 |
| tuna, 1/2 cup | 8 |
| **Sandwich** | |
| BLT, restaurant-type, 1 (9 1/4 oz) | 18 |
| cheese, grilled, restaurant-type, 1 (4 oz) | 14 |

*American, Diner, Sandwich (cont'd)*

| ▲ Power Foods | PointsPlus™ value |
|---|---|
| ham and cheese, grilled, restaurant-type, grilled, 1 (5 1/4 oz) | 15 |
| Reuben, 1 (8 oz) | 18 |
| roast beef, 1 (7 1/2 oz) | 9 |
| shrimp salad, 1 (4 1/2 oz) | 8 |
| tuna melt, 1 (5 3/4 oz) | 10 |
| tuna salad, 1 (6 1/4 oz) | 11 |
| turkey, 1 (4 oz) | 7 |
| **Soft drink** | |
| diet, any flavor, 1 can or bottle (12 fl oz) | 0 |
| sweetened with sugar, any flavor, 1 can or bottle (12 fl oz) | 4 |
| **Soup** | |
| broccoli cheese, 1 cup | 7 |
| Cheddar cheese, 1 cup | 10 |
| chicken noodle, 1 cup | 3 |
| cream of broccoli, 1 cup | 7 |
| cream of tomato, 1 cup | 5 |
| tomato, 1 cup | 3 |
| vegetable, 1 cup | 3 |
| **Syrup, pancake,** regular, 1 Tbsp | 1 |

## AMERICAN, FAST FOOD BURGER JOINT

| ▲ Power Foods | PointsPlus™ value |
|---|---|
| **Cheeseburger** | |
| double, 1 | 12 |
| double, with bacon, 1 | 21 |
| large, double, with condiments and vegetables, 1 | 19 |
| large, 1 | 15 |
| large, with bacon and condiments, 1 | 15 |
| large, with condiments and vegetables, 1 | 12 |
| on bun, 1 small | 8 |
| small, with condiments and vegetables, 1 | 10 |
| triple, plain, 1 | 21 |
| **Chicken, nugget-style,** fried, 6 pieces | 9 |
| **Chili con carne,** 1 cup | 7 |
| **French fries** | |
| 1 small serving | 7 |
| 1 medium serving | 11 |
| 1 extra large serving | 14 |
| **Hamburger on bun** | |
| double patty, plain, 1 (6 oz) | 14 |
| double patty, with condiments, 1 (7 1/2 oz) | 15 |
| large, plain, 1 (4 3/4 oz) | 11 |
| large, with condiments, 1 (7 3/4 oz) | 13 |
| small, 1 (3 oz) | 7 |
| small, with condiments, 1 (4 oz) | 7 |
| triple patty, with condiments, 1 (9 oz) | 18 |
| **Ice cream sundae** | |
| caramel, 1 (5 1/2 oz) | 8 |
| hot fudge, 1 (5 1/2 oz) | 8 |
| strawberry, 1 (5 1/2 oz) | 7 |
| **Milk shake, any flavor** | |
| 1 medium (12 fl oz) | 12 |
| 1 large (16 fl oz) | 16 |
| **Onion rings,** 8-9 rings | 8 |
| **Pie, fruit,** 1 (3 1/2 oz) | 9 |
| **Potato,** baked | |
| with cheese sauce and bacon, 1 (10 1/2 oz) | 13 |
| with cheese sauce and chili, 1 (14 oz) | 13 |
| with cheese sauce, 1 (10 1/2 oz) | 13 |
| with sour cream and chives, 1 (10 3/4 oz) | 11 |
| with vegetables and cheese, 1 (13 oz) | 11 |
| **Sandwich** | |
| chicken fillet with cheese, 1 (8 oz) | 17 |
| chicken fillet, plain, 1 (6 1/2 oz) | 14 |
| chicken, fried, 1 (7 1/4 oz) | 12 |

| ▲ Power Foods | *PointsPlus*™ value |
|---|---|
| chicken, grilled, 1 (6 3/4 oz) | 10 |
| fish and cheese, fried, 1 (6 1/2 oz) | 14 |
| fish, with tartar sauce, 1 (5 1/2 oz) | 12 |

## AMERICAN, ICE CREAM SHOP

| ▲ Power Foods | *PointsPlus*™ value |
|---|---|
| **Banana split,** 3 scoops (1 1/2 cups) ice cream, 1 banana, 3 Tbsp syrup, and 1/2 cup whipped cream | 21 |
| **Ice cream** | |
| premium, 1 scoop or 1/2 cup | 8 |
| regular, 1 scoop or 1/2 cup | 4 |
| **Ice cream cone only** | |
| cake or wafer-type, 1 large (1 oz) | 3 |
| plain or sugar, 1 small | 1 |
| **Ice cream soda,** 12 fl oz | 11 |
| **Ice cream sundae** | |
| 1 scoop (1/2 cup) ice cream with syrup, nuts, and whipped topping | 9 |
| 1 large (6 1/2 oz) | 13 |
| **Sherbet,** 1/2 cup | 3 |
| **Sprinkles, any type,** 1 Tbsp | 0 |
| **Topping** | |
| butterscotch, 2 Tbsp | 3 |
| caramel, regular or fat-free, 2 Tbsp | 3 |
| fudge, regular, 1 Tbsp | 2 |
| nuts in syrup, 2 Tbsp | 5 |
| whipped, dairy or nondairy, light or fat-free, aerosol or frozen, 2 Tbsp | 0 |
| whipped, dairy or nondairy, light or fat-free, aerosol or frozen, 1/3 cup | 1 |

## AMERICAN, SALAD BAR

| ▲ Power Foods | *PointsPlus*™ value |
|---|---|
| **Bacon bits,** imitation, 1 tsp | 0 |
| ▲ **Beans, garbanzo (chick peas),** cooked or canned, 1/2 cup | 3 |
| **Beets** | |
| ▲ canned, 1 cup | 0 |
| pickled, 1/2 cup | 2 |
| **Cheese, cottage, regular (4%),** 1 cup | 6 |
| **Cheese, hard or semisoft, dairy or soy, regular,** 1" cube, 1/4 cup shredded, or 3 Tbsp grated (1 oz) | 3 |
| ▲ **Corn, kernels,** 1 cup | 4 |
| **Croutons, packaged, regular,** 1/2 cup | 3 |
| **Dressing, salad, creamy, regular,** 2 Tbsp | 4 |
| **Dressing, salad, Italian-type other than creamy Italian, regular,** 2 Tbsp | 2 |
| **Gelatin, fruit-flavored,** prepared, 1/2 cup | 2 |
| **Olives,** 10 small or 6 large (1 oz) | 1 |
| ▲ **Peppers,** sweet, cooked or canned, 1 cup | 0 |
| **Pineapple** | |
| canned, crushed, sliced, or chunks, in heavy syrup, 1 cup | 6 |
| canned, crushed, sliced, or chunks, in juice, 1 cup | 0 |
| ▲ **Radishes,** 1 cup | 0 |
| **Salad** | |
| carrot and raisin, 1/2 cup | 8 |
| pasta, 1/2 cup | 4 |
| three-bean, 1/2 cup | 5 |
| **Seeds** | |
| sunflower, 1 tsp | 0 |
| sunflower, 1 Tbsp | 1 |
| ▲ **Sprouts, alfalfa or bean,** 1 cup | 0 |
| ▲ **Tomatoes, fresh or canned,** 1 small, medium, or large or 1 cup | 0 |
| **Yogurt** | |
| low-fat, flavored (vanilla, lemon, coffee), sweetened with sugar, 1 cup | 6 |
| low-fat, fruit-flavored, sweetened with sugar, 1 cup | 7 |

▲ Power Foods — *PointsPlus*™ value

## AMERICAN, SEAFOOD

|  | PointsPlus™ value |
|---|---|
| **Coconut shrimp,** 4 jumbo (7 1/4 oz) | 17 |
| **Crab cakes,** 2 (2 1/4 oz each or 3" round) | 5 |
| **Crab puffs,** 6 (1 1/2" rounds) | 5 |
| **Fish** | |
| ▲ bass, striped, cooked, 1 fillet (6 oz) | 5 |
| ▲ bluefish, cooked, 1 fillet (6 oz) | 6 |
| ▲ flounder, cooked, 1 fillet (6 oz) | 4 |
| ▲ mahimahi (dolphinfish), cooked, 1 fillet (6 oz) | 4 |
| salmon, cooked, 1 fillet or steak (6 oz) | 9 |
| ▲ snapper, cooked, 1 fillet (6 oz) | 5 |
| ▲ swordfish, cooked, 1 fillet or steak (6 oz) | 6 |
| ▲ tilapia, cooked, 1 fillet (3 oz) | 2 |
| ▲ trout, cooked, 1 fillet (6 oz) | 8 |
| ▲ trout, rainbow, cooked, 1 fillet (6 oz) | 6 |
| ▲ tuna, cooked, 1 fillet or steak (6 oz) | 5 |
| **Fish,** baked stuffed, 6 3/4 oz | 9 |
| **Fish,** fried, without flour, 1 fillet (6 oz) | 14 |
| **Lobster Newburg,** 1 cup | 14 |
| **Lobster thermidor,** 1 cup | 14 |
| **Oysters,** fried, 10 (5 1/4 oz) | 8 |
| **Scallops,** fried, 20 small (3 1/2 oz) | 6 |
| **Shellfish** | |
| ▲ crab meat, cooked, 1/2 cup (2 oz) | 1 |
| ▲ crab, Alaska king, cooked, 1 leg (4 3/4 oz) | 3 |
| ▲ lobster, steamed, 1 1/4 pound-lobster or 4 1/2 oz lobster meat | 3 |
| ▲ oyster, cooked, 6 medium (2 oz) | 1 |
| ▲ scallops, cooked, 10 small or 4 large (2 oz) | 2 |
| ▲ shrimp, canned, 1/2 cup | 2 |
| **Shrimp** | |
| broiled, stuffed, 6 large (6 oz) | 18 |
| fried, 10 (5 oz) | 9 |
| fried, stuffed, 6 large (9 1/2 oz) | 11 |
| **Shrimp puffs,** 6 (2 oz) | 5 |
| **Soup** | |
| clam chowder, Manhattan, 1 cup | 5 |
| lobster bisque, 1 cup | 4 |
| **Squid,** fried, 3 oz | 4 |

## AMERICAN, SOUTHERN/SOUL

|  | PointsPlus™ value |
|---|---|
| **Apple brown Betty,** 1 cup | 6 |
| **Biscuit,** 1 small (2" diameter) or 1/2 large | 3 |
| **Chicken and dumplings,** cooked, with skin, 3 oz chicken with 2 dumplings | 9 |
| **Chicken breast,** fried, with skin and bone, 1 (4 1/2 oz) | 11 |
| **Chicken drumstick,** fried, with skin and bone, 1 (1 1/2 oz) | 5 |
| **Chicken thigh,** fried, with skin and bone, 1 (3 oz) | 8 |
| **Corn,** cream-style, 1 cup | 5 |
| **Cornbread dressing,** 1 cup | 9 |
| ▲ **Fish, catfish,** cooked, 1 fillet (6 oz) | 6 |
| **Fritters, corn,** 3 (2 1/2" x 2" each) | 6 |
| **Gravy** | |
| brown, 1/4 cup | 3 |
| cream, 1/4 cup | 4 |
| giblet, 1/4 cup | 2 |
| sausage, 1/4 cup | 4 |
| ▲ **Greens (beet, chard, collard, dandelion, kale, mustard, turnip),** cooked or uncooked, 1 cup | 0 |
| **Hush puppies,** 2 (2 1/4 oz) | 5 |
| **Macaroni and cheese,** 1 cup | 10 |
| **Okra,** fried, 1 cup | 10 |
| **Pot pie, chicken,** homemade, 8 1/2 oz | 12 |

| ▲ Power Foods | *PointsPlus*™ value |
|---|---|
| **Sauce** | |
| hot, 1 tsp | 0 |
| pepper, 1 tsp | 0 |
| **Soup, split pea,** 1 cup | 4 |
| **Spoon bread,** 1/2 cup | 5 |
| **Steak, chicken fried** | |
| with cream gravy, 6 oz with 1/4 cup cream gravy | 18 |
| without gravy, 6 oz | 14 |
| **Stew, beef,** 1 cup | 7 |
| **Brunswick,** 1 1/2 cups | 7 |
| **Stuffing,** 1/2 cup | 5 |
| ▲ **Succotash,** cooked, 1 cup | 6 |
| **Sweet potato pie,** 1/8 of a 9" pie | 11 |
| **Tomatoes, fried green,** 2 slices (1 1/2" thick) | 5 |

## AMERICAN, STEAKHOUSE

| ▲ Power Foods | *PointsPlus*™ value |
|---|---|
| **Beef** | |
| filet mignon, cooked, 1 small (4 oz) | 10 |
| ▲ filet mignon, trimmed, cooked, 1 small (4 oz) | 6 |
| KC strip, cooked, 1 small (4 oz) | 7 |
| ▲ KC strip, trimmed, cooked, 1 small (4 oz) | 6 |
| New York steak, cooked, 1 small (4 oz) | 8 |
| ▲ New York steak, trimmed, cooked, 1 small (4 oz) | 5 |
| ▲ steak, lean, cooked (with all visible fat trimmed), 1 small (4 oz) | 5 |
| steak, regular, cooked, 1 small (4 oz) | 10 |
| strip sirloin, cooked, 1 small (4 oz) | 7 |
| ▲ strip sirloin, trimmed, cooked, 1 small (4 oz) | 5 |
| T-bone steak, cooked, 1 small (4 oz) | 9 |
| T-bone steak, trimmed, cooked, 1 small (4 oz) | 7 |
| **Breadstick** | |
| any type, 2 long (7 1/2 x 1/2" or 3/4 oz) | 2 |
| any type, 4 short (5 x 1/2" or 3/4 oz) | 2 |
| **Cream, sour,** regular, 1 Tbsp | 1 |
| **Croutons** | |
| plain, 1 cup | 3 |
| seasoned, 1 cup | 5 |
| ▲ **Lamb, chop, baby or regular,** trimmed cooked, 1 slice (3 oz) | 3 |
| **Onion,** blooming, 1/4 of a 16" diameter onion | 6 |
| **Pepper steak,** 6 oz | 14 |
| **Potato,** baked | |
| ▲ plain, 1 small (3 oz) | 2 |
| ▲ plain, 1 large (7 oz) | 5 |
| with sour cream and chives, 1 (5 1/2 oz) | 5 |
| **Potato,** baked, stuffed | |
| with bacon and cheese, 1 (9 1/2 oz) | 13 |
| with cheese, 1 (5 1/2 oz) | 5 |
| with vegetables and cheese, 1 (13 1/2 oz) | 12 |
| **Potatoes,** mashed | |
| garlic, 1/2 cup | 5 |
| 1/2 cup | 3 |
| **Potatoes,** scalloped, 1/2 cup | 5 |
| **Roll, dinner,** 1 (2 oz) | 5 |
| **Salad** | |
| cobb (without dressing), 3 cups | 11 |
| ▲ mixed greens, 1 cup | 0 |
| spinach, with dressing, 2 cups | 7 |
| **Salisbury steak,** 6 oz | 12 |
| **Sauce** | |
| horseradish, 1 Tbsp | 0 |
| steak, 1 Tbsp | 0 |

▲ Power Foods — *PointsPlus*™ value

## CANADIAN

|  | *PointsPlus*™ value |
|---|---|
| **Bacon, Canadian-style,** cooked, 1 slice (1 oz) | 1 |
| **Donair,** 4 oz meat with onion, tomato, and 2 Tbsp sauce | 16 |
| **Fish and brewis,** 1 cup | 14 |
| **Poutine,** 20 French fries with 2 oz cheese and 1/2 cup sauce | 19 |
| **Sauce, donair,** 2 Tbsp | 2 |
| **Tortiere (Canadian meat pie),** 1/8 of a 9" pie | 10 |

## CARIBBEAN

|  | *PointsPlus*™ value |
|---|---|
| **Beans, black, with rice,** 1 cup | 6 |
| **Benny cake,** 1 piece (2" x 3") | 4 |
| **Bistec de palomilla (Cuban fried steak),** 1 steak (6 oz) | 11 |
| **Carne guisado (Cuban beef stew),** 1 cup | 7 |
| **Chicken asopao,** 10 oz | 9 |
| **Chuleta,** 1 pork chop (6 oz) | 12 |
| **Conch fritters,** 2 (1 3/4 oz) | 3 |
| **Curry goat,** 4 oz | 6 |
| **Jamaican rice and peas,** 1 cup | 8 |
| **Jerk chicken breast,** without skin, 1 large breast (5 3/4 oz) | 5 |
| **Johnny cake,** 1 piece (2 1/2" square) | 5 |
| **Lechon asado (roast pork),** 3 oz | 4 |
| **Macaroni and cheese, Bahamian,** 1 cup | 9 |
| **Pan Cubano,** 1 (6 1/2" x 3") | 10 |
| **Pastelitos de carne (Cuban meat pastry),** 1 (1" x 2" diameter) | 9 |
| **Peas, Bahamian style, with rice,** 1 cup | 9 |
| **Plantain,** fried, 1 cup | 5 |
| **Plátanos maduros (fried sweet plantains),** 1 cup | 5 |
| **Rice, Cuban,** 1 cup | 6 |
| **Ropa vieja,** 1 cup | 9 |
| **Salad, conch,** 1 cup | 3 |
| **Sandwich, Cuban,** 1/2 (6 1/2" x 3" x 4") | 12 |
| **Shellfish, conch,** cracked, 1 (6" long x 3") | 10 |
| **Soup, pigeon pea and dumpling,** 1 1/2 cups | 9 |
| ▲ **Soursop (guanabana),** 1/2 cup pulp | 0 |
| **Sweetsop (sugar apple),** 1/2 (2 7/8" diameter) or 1/2 cup | 0 |

## CHINESE/CANTONESE

|  | *PointsPlus*™ value |
|---|---|
| **Almond float,** 1 | 3 |
| **Beef and broccoli,** 1 cup | 4 |
| **Beef stir-fry, with garlic or black bean sauce,** 1 cup | 8 |
| **Beef, orange-ginger,** 1 cup | 15 |
| **Beef, sweet and sour,** 1 cup | 13 |
| **Broccoli stir-fry,** 1 cup | 4 |
| **Bubble tea (milk tea),** 1 cup | 2 |
| **Char shiu bao (roast pork bun),** 1 (2 oz) | 5 |
| **Chicken and broccoli,** 1 cup | 3 |
| **Chicken breast, five spice, with skin and bone,** 1 (4 1/2 oz) | 7 |
| **Chicken leg, five spice,** 1 leg, thigh, and drumstick, with skin and bone (4 1/2 oz) | 9 |
| **Chicken stir-fry, with garlic or black bean sauce,** 1 cup | 8 |
| **Chicken with cashews,** 1 cup | 11 |
| **Chicken, long rice,** 1 cup | 5 |
| **Chicken, sesame,** 1 cup | 10 |
| **Chicken, sweet and sour,** 1 cup | 11 |
| **Chop suey** | |
| beef, 1 cup | 5 |
| chicken, 1 cup | 4 |
| pork, 1 cup | 5 |
| vegetable, 1 cup | 5 |

| ▲ Power Foods | *PointsPlus™* value |
|---|---|
| **Chow fun, beef, chicken, pork, or shrimp,** 1 cup | 9 |
| **Chow mein** | |
| beef, 1 cup | 5 |
| chicken, 1 cup | 4 |
| chicken subgum, 1 cup | 4 |
| pork, 1 cup | 5 |
| **Cookies** | |
| Chinese almond, 2 (1 oz) | 4 |
| fortune, 1 (1/2 oz) | 2 |
| **Crab Rangoon,** 1 large (4 1/2") or 5 mini | 5 |
| **Dim sum** | |
| bean curd roll with vegetables, 1 (2 1/2 oz) | 2 |
| sesame seed balls, 1 (3" x 3") | 7 |
| bean curd roll with shrimp and vegetables, 1 (3 1/2 oz) | 3 |
| **Dumpling** | |
| beef or pork, fried, 4 (6 1/2 oz) | 7 |
| beef or pork, steamed, 4 (5 3/4 oz) | 7 |
| chicken, fried, 4 (6 1/2 oz) | 5 |
| chicken, steamed, 4 (5 3/4 oz) | 5 |
| shrimp, fried, 4 (6 1/2 oz) | 5 |
| shrimp, steamed, 4 (5 3/4 oz) | 5 |
| vegetarian, fried, 4 (3 1/2" x 2" wide) | 4 |
| vegetarian, steamed, 4 (3 1/2" x 2" wide) | 4 |
| **Egg foo yung** | |
| beef, 1 (3" diameter) | 4 |
| chicken, 1 (3" diameter) | 4 |
| pork, 1 (3" diameter) | 5 |
| shrimp, 1 (3" diameter) | 4 |
| **Egg roll** | |
| beef, 1 (4 1/2" long) | 6 |
| chicken, 1 (4 1/2" long) | 5 |
| pork, 1 (4 1/2" long) | 6 |
| shrimp, 1 (4 1/2" long) | 4 |
| **General Tso's chicken,** 1 cup | 17 |

| ▲ Power Foods | *PointsPlus™* value |
|---|---|
| **Ginger fish,** 1 cup | 9 |
| **Gyoza,** 3 (1 3/4 oz) | 3 |
| **Hunan beef,** 1 cup | 10 |
| **Kung pao** | |
| beef, 1 cup | 12 |
| chicken, 1 cup | 9 |
| pork, 1 cup | 11 |
| shrimp, 1 cup | 10 |
| **Lettuce wrap** | |
| beef, 2 (5" long by 3" wide each) | 5 |
| chicken, 2 (5" long by 3" wide each) | 4 |
| **Lo mein** | |
| beef, 1 cup | 10 |
| chicken, 1 cup | 9 |
| pork, 1 cup | 9 |
| shrimp, 1 cup | 9 |
| vegetable, 1 cup | 8 |
| **Lobster Cantonese,** 1 cup | 9 |
| **Mongolian beef,** 1 cup | 8 |
| **Moo goo gai pan,** 1 cup | 7 |
| **Moo shoo** | |
| chicken, 1/2 cup with 2 pancakes | 8 |
| pork, 1/2 cup with 2 pancakes | 9 |
| tofu, 1/2 cup with 2 pancakes | 8 |
| **Noodles,** fried, 1 cup | 8 |
| **Orange chicken,** 1 cup | 14 |
| **Pancakes** | |
| Chinese, 1 (1 oz) | 2 |
| scallion, 1 (2 1/4 oz) | 7 |
| **Peking duck,** 2 oz duck with 1 piece duck skin and 3 pancakes | 11 |
| **Pepper steak, Chinese,** 1 cup | 5 |
| **Pork and broccoli,** 1 cup | 4 |
| **Pork stir-fry, with garlic or black bean sauce,** 1 cup | 9 |
| **Pork with cashews,** 1 cup | 12 |
| **Pork, Chinese roast,** 1 cup | 6 |
| **Pork, sweet and sour,** 1 cup | 13 |

*Chinese/Cantonese (cont'd)*

| ▲ Power Foods | PointsPlus™ value |
|---|---|
| **Pot sticker (filled wontons)** | |
| vegetarian, fried, 4 (3 1/2" x 2" each) | 4 |
| vegetarian, steamed, 4 (3 1/2" x 2" each) | 4 |
| **Rice,** fried | |
| plain, 1 cup | 10 |
| with beef, 1 cup | 10 |
| with chicken, 1 cup | 10 |
| with pork, 1 cup | 10 |
| with shrimp, 1 cup | 9 |
| **Rice, white,** cooked, 1 cup | 5 |
| **Salad, chicken, Oriental,** 2 cups | 8 |
| **Sauce** | |
| Asian stir-fry, 1 Tbsp | 1 |
| brown, Chinese, 1/4 cup | 1 |
| duck, 1 Tbsp | 1 |
| hoisin, 1 tsp | 0 |
| kung pao, 2 Tbsp | 2 |
| oyster, 1 tsp | 1 |
| plum, 1 Tbsp | 2 |
| soy , 1 Tbsp | 0 |
| **Shrimp, sweet and sour,** 1 cup | 11 |
| **Shrimp and broccoli,** 1 cup | 3 |
| **Shrimp Cantonese,** 1 cup | 9 |
| **Shrimp stir-fry, with garlic or black bean sauce,** 1 cup | 7 |
| **Shrimp toast,** 1 piece (1 oz) | 3 |
| **Shumai,** fried or steamed, 2 (2" diameter) | 3 |
| **Soup** | |
| egg drop, 1 cup | 1 |
| shark fin, 1 cup | 3 |
| wonton, 1 cup with 4 wontons | 5 |
| **Spareribs, barbecued, Chinese,** 2 (4" long) | 4 |
| **Spring roll** | |
| beef or pork, 1 (4 1/2" long) | 6 |
| chicken, 1 (4 1/2" long) | 5 |
| shrimp, 1 (4 1/2" long) | 4 |

| ▲ Power Foods | PointsPlus™ value |
|---|---|
| **Stir-fried vegetables** | |
| with beef, 1 cup | 4 |
| with chicken, 1 cup | 3 |
| with oil or sauce, 1 cup | 4 |
| with pork, 1 cup | 4 |
| **Szechuan pork hotpot,** 1 cup | 6 |
| **Twice-cooked pork,** 1 cup | 10 |
| **Vegetables, Chinese** | |
| with beef, 1 cup | 7 |
| with chicken, 1 cup | 5 |
| with peas, prepared with oil, 1 cup | 5 |
| with pork, 1 cup | 7 |
| with shrimp, 1 cup | 5 |
| with tofu, 1 cup | 4 |

## EASTERN EUROPEAN

| | |
|---|---|
| **Beef Stroganoff with noodles,** 1 cup stroganoff with 1 cup of noodles | 17 |
| **Caviar, any type,** 1 oz | 2 |
| **Chicken Kiev,** 1 piece (4" x 8") | 18 |
| **Kielbasa,** 1 oz | 2 |
| **Kolache** | |
| fruit-filled, 1 (3" diameter) | 5 |
| without filling, 1 (3" diameter) | 4 |
| **Paprikash,** 1 1/2 cups chicken mixture with 1/2 cup sauce | 10 |
| **Pierogies** | |
| cabbage, 2 (2 1/2 oz) | 8 |
| cheese, 2 (2 1/2 oz) | 8 |
| meat, 2 (2 1/2 oz) | 9 |
| potato, 2 (2 1/2 oz) | 8 |
| **Soup, cabbage,** 1 cup | 2 |

## ENGLISH/IRISH

| | |
|---|---|
| **Beef Wellington,** 1 slice (3 1/2" x 2 1/2" x 1 1/2") | 14 |
| **Beef, corned,** cooked, 3 oz | 6 |
| **Bubble and squeak,** 1 cup | 5 |

| ▲ Power Foods | *PointsPlus*™ value |
|---|---|
| **Burgoo,** 1 cup | 5 |
| **Carrots and parsnips,** 1 cup | 6 |
| **Colcannon,** 1 cup | 8 |
| **Cream, clotted (English double devon cream),** 2 Tbsp | 4 |
| **Crumpet,** 1 (3" diameter) | 4 |
| **Fadge,** 1 piece (3 1/4 oz) | 2 |
| **Fish and chips,** 5 oz fish fillet with 20 chips (French fries) | 17 |
| **Irish coffee,** 6 fl oz with 2 Tbsp whipped cream | 6 |
| **Irish soda bread,** 1/12 of a 8" round loaf | 8 |
| **Popover,** 2 (3" diameter or 1 1/2 oz each) | 4 |
| **Pudding, bread,** 1 cup | 16 |
| **Pudding, plum,** 5 oz | 11 |
| **Scone** | |
| blueberry, restaurant-type, 1 (4 1/2 oz) | 12 |
| chocolate, cinnamon, or raspberry, restaurant-type, 1 (4 1/2 oz) | 13 |
| cranberry or orange, restaurant-type, 1 (4 1/2 oz) | 11 |
| 1 small (1 1/2 oz) | 4 |
| 1 regular (2 1/2 oz) | 7 |
| **Shepherd's pie,** 1 cup | 10 |
| **Stew** | |
| Irish brown, 1 cup | 8 |
| lamb, 1 cup | 6 |
| **Trifle,** 1 cup | 6 |
| **Yorkshire pudding,** 1 piece (4" square) | 7 |

## FRENCH

| ▲ Power Foods | *PointsPlus*™ value |
|---|---|
| **Baba au rhum,** 1 (3 oz) | 10 |
| **Beef bourguignon,** 1 cup | 15 |
| **Blanquette of veal,** 1 cup | 6 |
| **Bouillabaisse,** 2 cups | 9 |
| **Brioche,** 1 slice (1 oz) | 3 |
| **Cassoulet,** 1 cup | 12 |
| **Chicken cordon bleu,** 1 piece (6 3/4 oz) | 10 |
| **Chocolate mousse,** 1 cup | 15 |
| **Coq au vin,** 2 cups | 12 |
| **Coquilles St. Jacques,** 2 shells (13 1/2 oz) | 9 |
| **Cream puff,** 1 (2 oz) | 9 |
| **Crème brûlée,** 3/4 cup | 12 |
| **Crème caramel,** 1 cup | 8 |
| **Crème fraiche,** 2 Tbsp | 3 |
| **Crêpes** | |
| chicken, 2 (10 oz) | 12 |
| plain, 1 (6" diameter) | 2 |
| seafood, 1 (11 oz) | 12 |
| Suzette, 2 (4 3/4 oz) | 11 |
| **Croissant** | |
| apple, 1 medium (2 oz) | 4 |
| butter, 1 medium (2 oz) | 6 |
| cheese, 1 medium (2 oz) | 6 |
| chocolate-filled, 1 (3 3/4 oz) | 7 |
| plain, 1 (1 3/4 oz) | 6 |
| **Croquettes** | |
| beef, 2 (2 1/2 oz each) | 10 |
| chicken, 2 (2 1/2 oz each) | 9 |
| **Cruller, French,** glazed, 1 (3" diameter) | 5 |
| **Duck a l'orange,** 1/4 duck with 2 Tbsp sauce | 15 |
| **Eclair,** 1 (5 1/4 oz) | 11 |
| **Escargots,** 6 snails with 2 Tbsp butter | 6 |
| **Fish amandine,** 1 fillet (6 oz) | 13 |
| **Fish Veronique,** 1 fillet (6 oz) | 12 |
| **Fondue, cheese,** 1/2 cup fondue with 2 oz bread | 12 |
| **Frog legs,** fried, 2 (1 oz) | 4 |
| **Fromage frais (soft cheese with fruit),** 1 oz | 3 |

*French (cont'd)*

| ▲ Power Foods | *PointsPlus™* value |
|---|---|
| **Mussels mariniere,** 4 mussels with 3 Tbsp sauce | 5 |
| **Napoleon,** 1 piece (4 1/2" x 2" x 1 1/2") | 15 |
| **Oysters Rockefeller,** 4 (2 oz) | 3 |
| **Pâté, liver, beef,** 1 slice (4 1/4" x 1 1/2" x 1/2") | 3 |
| **Peach melba,** 1/2 cup ice cream with 2 peach halves and raspberry sauce | 9 |
| **Petit fours,** 2 (1 3/4" x 1 1/2" x 1" each) | 6 |
| **Petite marmite,** 2 cups | 8 |
| **Potatoes au gratin,** 1 cup | 14 |
| **Profiterole,** 1 small (1 oz) | 3 |
| **Quenelles,** 8 (2 1/2" x 1 1/2" x 3/4") | 12 |
| **Quiche, vegetable,** 1/8 of a 9" pie | 9 |
| **Quiche Lorraine,** 1/8 of a 9" pie | 11 |
| **Ratatouille,** 1 cup | 5 |
| **Roll, French,** 1 (1 1/4 oz) | 3 |
| **Salad Niçoise** | |
| with dressing, 4 cups | 20 |
| without dressing, 4 cups | 9 |
| **Sandwich, croque monsieur,** 1 (6 1/2 oz) | 12 |
| **Sauce** | |
| béarnaise, 1/4 cup | 8 |
| hollandaise, 1/4 cup | 8 |
| mornay, 1/4 cup | 4 |
| **Sausage in brioche,** 1 slice (2" thick) | 16 |
| **Sorbet, any flavor,** 1 scoop or 1/2 cup | 2 |
| **Soufflé** | |
| cheese, 1 cup | 5 |
| fruit, 1/2 cup | 4 |
| **Soup** | |
| cherry, 1 cup | 8 |
| French onion au gratin, 1 cup | 8 |
| French onion, restaurant-type, 1 cup | 7 |
| vichyssoise, 1 cup | 3 |
| **Steak au poivre,** 6 oz steak with 1 Tbsp sauce | 13 |
| **Tarte aux fruits** | |
| individual, 1 (4") | 15 |
| 1/8 of a 9" tart | 11 |

## GERMAN

| ▲ Power Foods | *PointsPlus™* value |
|---|---|
| **Apple fritter,** restaurant-type, 1 (4 oz) | 12 |
| **Apple kuchen,** 1 piece (4 oz) | 12 |
| **Apple streusel,** 1/2 cup | 5 |
| **Beer, regular,** 1 can or bottle (12 fl oz) | 5 |
| **Dumpling, potato,** 6 (1" diameter) | 3 |
| **Luncheon meat, bratwurst,** cooked, 2 oz | 5 |
| **Pancakes, potato,** 1 (3 1/4 oz) | 2 |
| **Peppers,** stuffed, with beef and rice, 1 (7 3/4 oz) | 9 |
| **Sachertorte,** 1/16 of a 9" cake | 9 |
| **Salad, potato, German,** 1/2 cup | 2 |
| **Sauerbraten,** 3 oz beef with 2 Tbsp gravy | 6 |
| ▲ **Sauerkraut,** 1 cup | 0 |
| **Schaum torte** | |
| with whipped cream, 1/10 of a 10" pan | 9 |
| without whipped cream, 1/10 of a 10" pan | 4 |
| **Schnapps, any flavor,** 1 jigger (1 1/2 fl oz) | 6 |
| **Spaetzle,** 1/2 cup | 6 |
| **Strudel, any type,** 1 piece (6 oz) | 12 |
| **Wiener schnitzel,** 1 slice (3 oz) | 10 |

## GREEK

| ▲ Power Foods | *PointsPlus™* value |
|---|---|
| **Baklava,** 1 piece (1 1/4 oz) | 7 |
| **Dolma,** 4 (3 1/4 oz) | 5 |
| **Gyro,** 1 (11 oz) | 16 |

| ▲ Power Foods | *PointsPlus™* value |
|---|---|
| **Kataifi,** 1 piece (2" long) | 7 |
| **Moussaka,** 1 piece (3" x 4") | 12 |
| **Pastitsio,** 1 piece (3 1/4" x 3") | 14 |
| **Saganaki,** 1 piece (1" x 2" x 1/2" thick) | 6 |
| **Salad** | |
| Greek, with dressing, restaurant-type, 3 cups | 10 |
| Greek, without dressing, restaurant-type, 3 cups | 3 |
| yogurt and cucumber, 1/2 cup | 1 |
| **Sauce, tzatziki,** 1/2 cup | 2 |
| **Soup** | |
| avgolemono, 1 cup | 4 |
| yogurt and cucumber, 1 cup | 3 |
| **Souvlaki, chicken** | |
| in pita bread, 1 (6 1/2 oz) | 8 |
| 1 large or 2 small skewers (4 1/2 oz) | 5 |
| **Souvlaki, lamb** | |
| in pita bread, 1 (6 1/2 oz) | 9 |
| 1 large or 2 small skewers (4 3/4 oz) | 8 |
| **Spanakopita,** 1 (3" square) or 1 cup | 9 |

## HAWAIIAN

| | |
|---|---|
| **Chicken hekka,** 1 cup | 7 |
| **Haupia (coconut pudding),** 2" square | 3 |
| **Huli huli chicken** | |
| drumstick (with skin and bone), 1 (2 oz) | 3 |
| breast (with skin and bone), 1 (7 1/4 oz) | 13 |
| thigh (with skin and bone), 1 (3 oz) | 5 |
| **Kahlua pig,** 3 oz | 4 |
| **Lau lau (pork and fish in taro or spinach leaves),** 1 (7 1/2 oz) | 8 |
| **Manapua with char shiu filling,** 1 (3 1/4 oz) | 6 |
| **Mochi, butter** | |
| 1 piece (2 3/4 oz) | 7 |
| 1 piece (1 1/4 oz) | 2 |
| **Mun doo** | |
| fried, 4 (6 1/2 oz) | 5 |
| steamed, 4 (5 3/4 oz) | 5 |
| ▲ **Poi,** 1/2 cup (4 oz) | 4 |
| **Pork hash,** 4 (5 3/4 oz) | 7 |
| **Salad, green papaya, without meat,** 1 cup | 2 |
| **Sauce, curry, Hawaiian-style,** 1/4 cup | 5 |
| **Soup, oxtail, Hawaiian-style,** 1 cup | 7 |

## INDIAN

| | |
|---|---|
| **Beef masala,** 1 cup | 6 |
| **Bhuna gosht,** 1 cup | 9 |
| **Biryani** | |
| chicken, 1 cup | 11 |
| lamb, 1 cup | 15 |
| **Bread** | |
| chapati, 1 piece (5" diameter) | 3 |
| naan, 1 piece (7" x 8" diameter) | 5 |
| **Butter chicken,** 1 cup | 9 |
| **Cashew chicken,** 6 1/4 oz | 7 |
| ▲ **Chana dal,** 1 cup | 5 |
| **Channa masala,** 1 cup | 9 |
| **Chicken jalfrezi,** 1 cup | 6 |
| **Chicken paprika,** 1 breast or thigh with 1/2 cup sauce | 8 |
| **Chicken tikka,** 4 oz | 5 |
| **Chili fish (macher jhol),** 1 fillet (6 oz) | 13 |
| **Coconut rice, Indian,** 1 cup | 6 |
| **Curry** | |
| beef, 1 cup | 11 |
| Bengali fish, 1 fillet (4 1/2 oz) and 1 cup vegetables | 11 |
| chicken, 1 cup | 10 |
| egg, 1 cup | 2 |
| lamb, 1 cup | 11 |

*Indian (cont'd)*

| ▲ Power Foods | *PointsPlus™* value |
|---|---|
| **Dhansak,** 1 cup | 7 |
| **Fritters, vegetable,** 1 cup | 12 |
| **Goat masala,** 1 cup | 6 |
| **Gosht shaha korma,** 1 cup | 15 |
| **Kashmiri (lamb meatballs),** 6 (3 1/2 oz) | 11 |
| **Kheer,** 1/2 cup | 7 |
| **Kofta (vegetable balls without sauce),** 2 (3 oz) | 6 |
| **Kofta, malai (vegetable balls in cream sauce),** 2 kofta with 1/2 cup sauce | 10 |
| **Korma** | |
| chicken, 1 cup | 15 |
| lamb, 1 cup | 16 |
| vegetable, 1 cup | 12 |
| **Lamb masala,** 1 cup | 7 |
| **Mango lassi,** 1 cup | 3 |
| **Masala dosa** | |
| with filling, 1 (7 3/4 oz) | 13 |
| without filling, 1 (5 1/4 oz) | 12 |
| **Mung dal,** 1 cup | 6 |
| **Mutter paneer,** 1 cup | 13 |
| **Pakora, vegetable,** 1 (2" x 3" or 1 3/4 oz) | 4 |
| **Palak paneer,** 1 cup | 15 |
| **Palak vada (vegetable dumpling)** | |
| fried, 1 (2 1/2" x 1 1/2") | 5 |
| steamed, 1 (2 1/2" x 1 1/2") | 3 |
| **Paneer** | |
| fried, 1 cup | 1 |
| jalfrezi, 1 cup | 6 |
| **Paratha,** 4" triangle | 4 |
| **Pesarattu,** 1/2 of an 8" diameter | 8 |
| **Puris,** 1 (4" diameter) | 3 |
| **Raita,** 1/2 cup | 2 |
| **Rajmah,** 1 cup | 8 |
| **Rogan josh,** 1 cup | 11 |

| ▲ Power Foods | *PointsPlus™* value |
|---|---|
| **Saag gosht,** 1 cup | 7 |
| **Saag paneer,** 1 cup | 8 |
| **Samosa,** 1 (2 1/2" x 2 1/2" x 3" triangle) | 3 |
| **Soup, mulligatawny,** 1 cup | 7 |
| **Stew, bean and lentil (dal maharani),** 1 cup | 6 |
| **Tandoori chicken** | |
| breast, without skin, 1 piece (4 1/2 oz) | 4 |
| thigh, without skin, 1 piece (3 oz) | 4 |
| **Tandoori fish,** 3/4 cup | 5 |
| **Tandoori shrimp,** 3/4 cup | 3 |
| ▲ **Urad dal (split matpe beans without skin),** 1 cup | 5 |
| **Vegetable pulao,** 1 cup | 4 |
| **Vindaloo** | |
| chicken, 1 cup | 9 |
| lamb, 1 cup | 16 |
| pork, 1 cup | 10 |

## ITALIAN, RESTAURANT

| Food | Value |
|---|---|
| **Artichokes** | |
| marinated, 1/2 cup | 4 |
| stuffed, 1 (7 3/4 oz) | 15 |
| **Biscotti** | |
| chocolate, 8 mini, 2 small, or 1 regular (1 oz) | 4 |
| plain or fat-free, 8 mini, 2 small, or 1 regular (1 oz) | 3 |
| cheese, 1 (2" diameter) | 6 |
| **Bread, garlic,** 1 slice (1 1/2 oz) | 6 |
| **Bruschetta,** 1 slice (3 oz) | 3 |
| **Calamari** | |
| fried, 1/2 cup | 11 |
| ▲ grilled, 1/2 cup | 1 |

| ▲ Power Foods | *PointsPlus*™ value |
|---|---|
| **Calzone, ham and cheese,** 1 (5 1/4" x 6") | 15 |
| **Cannelloni** | |
| cheese, with meat sauce, 2 shells with 1/2 cup sauce | 22 |
| cheese, with tomato sauce, 2 shells with 1/2 cup sauce | 14 |
| meat, with cream sauce, 2 shells with 1/2 cup sauce | 19 |
| meat, with tomato sauce, 2 shells with 1/2 cup sauce | 15 |
| spinach and cheese, with cream sauce, 2 shells with 1/2 cup sauce | 17 |
| spinach and cheese, with tomato sauce, 2 shells with 1/2 cup sauce | 14 |
| **Cannoli,** 1 (3 1/2" long) | 10 |
| **Caponata (eggplant appetizer),** 1 cup | 5 |
| **Cappuccino** | |
| ▲ made with fat-free milk, 1 small (8 fl oz) | 1 |
| ▲ made with fat-free milk, 1 tall (12 fl oz) | 2 |
| ▲ made with fat-free milk, 1 grande (16 fl oz) | 2 |
| made with low-fat milk, 1 small (8 fl oz) | 2 |
| made with low-fat milk, 1 tall (12 fl oz) | 3 |
| made with low-fat milk, 1 grande (16 fl oz) | 3 |
| made with whole milk, 1 small (8 fl oz) | 2 |
| made with whole milk, 1 tall (12 fl oz) | 3 |
| made with whole milk, 1 grande (16 fl oz) | 4 |
| **Cavatelli with sausage and broccoli,** 1 cup | 6 |
| **Cheese, mozzarella,** fried, 2 slices (2 3/4" x 1" x 1/2" each) | 10 |

| ▲ Power Foods | *PointsPlus*™ value |
|---|---|
| **Chicken cacciatore,** 1 half-breast or 1 thigh and leg (6 1/2 oz) | 11 |
| **Chicken marsala, without bone, with sauce,** 4 oz | 14 |
| **Chicken parmigiana** | |
| with sauce, 5 oz with 1/2 cup sauce | 11 |
| without sauce, 5 1/2 oz | 8 |
| **Chicken tetrazzini,** 1 1/2 cups | 15 |
| **Cioppino,** 2 cups | 13 |
| **Clams** | |
| baked, 6 (2 1/2 oz) | 7 |
| breaded and fried, 20 (6 1/2 oz) | 10 |
| breaded and fried, fast food, 3/4 cup | 12 |
| fried, 1 cup | 11 |
| **Cookies** | |
| amaretti, 1 (1" diameter) | 3 |
| sesame seed, 2 (2" long) | 4 |
| **Eggplant parmigiana** | |
| with sauce, 3" by 4" serving with 1/2 cup Italian tomato sauce | 14 |
| without sauce, 1 piece (3" x 4") | 11 |
| **Fettuccine Alfredo,** 1 cup | 17 |
| **Focaccia bread,** 1/4 of the 10" diameter | 7 |
| **Gnocchi** | |
| cheese, 1 cup | 12 |
| potato, 1 cup | 5 |
| spinach, 1 cup | 13 |
| **Ices,** Italian, restaurant-type, 1/2 cup | 2 |
| **Italian casserole (ground beef, pasta and cheese over rolls),** 1/8 of the 10" round casserole | 15 |
| **Lasagna** | |
| cheese, with tomato sauce, 1 piece (10 oz) | 9 |
| chicken, 1 cup | 7 |
| vegetable, 1 cup | 8 |
| vegetarian, with cheese, 1 piece (10 oz) | 12 |

*Italian Restaurant, Lasagna (cont'd)*

| ▲ Power Foods | *PointsPlus*™ value |
|---|---|
| vegetarian, with cheese and spinach, 1 piece (10 1/2 oz) | 10 |
| with meat, 4" x 2 1/2" or 1 cup | 7 |
| with meat sauce, 1 cup | 7 |
| **Latte** | |
| ▲ made with fat-free milk, 1 small (8 fl oz) | 2 |
| ▲ made with fat-free milk, 1 tall (12 fl oz) | 3 |
| ▲ made with fat-free milk, 1 grande (16 fl oz) | 4 |
| made with low-fat milk, 1 small (8 fl oz) | 3 |
| made with low-fat milk, 1 tall (12 fl oz) | 4 |
| made with low-fat milk, 1 grande (16 fl oz) | 5 |
| made with whole milk, 1 small (8 fl oz) | 3 |
| made with whole milk, 1 tall (12 fl oz) | 5 |
| made with whole milk, 1 grande (16 fl oz) | 7 |
| **Linguine with red clam sauce,** 1 cup linguine with 1/2 cup sauce | 8 |
| **Linguine with white clam sauce,** 1 cup linguine with 1/2 cup sauce | 10 |
| **Manicotti** | |
| with meat sauce, 2 shells with 1/2 cup sauce | 16 |
| with tomato sauce, 2 shells with 1/2 cup sauce | 13 |
| **Meatballs, with sauce,** 2 meatballs and 1/2 cup Italian tomato sauce | 13 |
| **Mushrooms,** marinated, 1/2 cup | 3 |
| **Osso bucco,** 6 oz veal with 1/4 cup sauce | 12 |
| **Panettone,** 1/12 of a 9" tube or 1 1/2 oz | 7 |

| ▲ Power Foods | *PointsPlus*™ value |
|---|---|
| **Panini** | |
| chicken, 1 (8 oz) | 13 |
| ham and cheese, 1 (7 1/2 oz) | 13 |
| vegetable, 1 (13 oz) | 12 |
| **Pasta e fagioli,** 1 cup | 6 |
| **Pasta primavera with cream sauce,** 1 cup pasta with 3/4 cup sauce | 14 |
| **Pasta primavera with marinara sauce,** 1 cup pasta with 3/4 cup sauce | 7 |
| **Pasta with garlic and oil,** 1 cup | 8 |
| **Penne a la vodka,** 1 cup pasta with 1/2 cup sauce | 9 |
| **Ravioli** | |
| cheese, with tomato sauce, 15 oz | 19 |
| cheese, without sauce, 8 3/4 oz | 16 |
| meat, with tomato sauce, 8 pieces or 1 cup with 1/2 cup sauce | 17 |
| meat, without sauce, 8 pieces or 1 cup | 14 |
| **Risotto,** 1/2 cup | 6 |
| **Salad** | |
| Caesar, 3 cups | 7 |
| Caesar, with grilled chicken, restaurant-type, 6 1/2 oz | 8 |
| tomato and mozzarella, without dressing, 2 large tomato slices with 2 oz cheese | 5 |
| **Sauce** | |
| Alfredo, 1/2 cup | 10 |
| Bolognese meat , 1/2 cup | 6 |
| clam, red, 1/2 cup | 3 |
| clam, white, 1/2 cup | 5 |
| marinara, 1/2 cup | 3 |
| meat, 1/2 cup | 5 |
| pesto, 2 Tbsp | 4 |
| puttanesca, 1/2 cup | 12 |
| ▲ tomato, Italian, 1/2 cup | 3 |

| ▲ Power Foods | *PointsPlus™* value |
|---|---|
| **Shrimp scampi,** 9 medium (3 1/2 oz) | 10 |
| **Soup** | |
| Italian wedding, 1 cup | 5 |
| lentil, 1 cup | 4 |
| minestrone, 1 cup | 5 |
| **Spaghetti bolognese,** 1 cup spaghetti with 1/2 cup sauce | 12 |
| **Spaghetti carbonara,** 1 cup | 13 |
| **Spaghetti with marinara sauce,** 1 cup spaghetti with 1/2 cup sauce | 8 |
| **Spaghetti with meat sauce,** 1 cup spaghetti with 1/2 cup sauce | 11 |
| **Spaghetti with tomato sauce and meatballs,** 1 cup spaghetti with 1/2 cup sauce and 2 meatballs | 18 |
| **Spumoni,** 1/2 cup | 7 |
| **Stromboli,** 1 slice (1" thick or 2 oz) | 5 |
| **Tirami-su,** restaurant-type, 1 slice (4 3/4 oz) | 12 |
| **Tortellini** | |
| cheese, without sauce, 2/3 cup | 4 |
| meat, without sauce, 2/3 cup | 4 |
| **Tortoni,** 2 1/2 oz | 7 |
| **Turkey tetrazzini,** 1 1/2 cups | 15 |
| **Veal marsala,** 4 oz veal with sauce | 12 |
| **Veal parmigiana** | |
| with sauce, 5 oz with 1/2 cup tomato sauce | 13 |
| without sauce, 5 1/2 oz | 10 |
| **Veal piccata,** 2 slices (4 oz) | 10 |
| **Veal scaloppine,** 2 pieces (4 1/2 oz) | 9 |
| **Veal with peppers,** 5 oz | 11 |
| **Vitello tonnato,** 2 slices veal (4 oz) with 1/2 cup sauce | 16 |
| **Zabaglione,** 1/2 cup | 4 |
| **Zeppole,** 1 (4" diameter) | 7 |
| **Ziti,** baked | |
| with meat, 1 cup | 10 |
| without meat, 1 cup | 7 |
| **Zuppa di pesce,** 2 cups | 11 |
| **Zuppa Inglese,** 6 1/2 oz | 9 |

## ITALIAN, PIZZERIA

| ▲ Power Foods | *PointsPlus™* value |
|---|---|
| **Pizza,** restaurant-type, cheese, thin crust | |
| 1 small slice (1/8 of a 12" or 1/12 of a 16" pie) | 5 |
| 1 large slice (1/8 of a 16" to 18" pie) | 7 |
| **Pizza,** restaurant-type, one-meat topping, deep dish | |
| 1 small slice (1/8 of a 12" or 1/12 of a 16" pie) | 8 |
| 1 large slice (1/8 of a 16" to 18" pie) | 13 |
| **Pizza,** restaurant-type, one-meat topping, thin crust | |
| 1 small slice (1/8 of a 12" or 1/12 of a 16" pie) | 5 |
| 1 large slice (1/8 of a 16" to 18" pie) | 8 |

## JAPANESE

| ▲ Power Foods | *PointsPlus™* value |
|---|---|
| **Curry, Japanese,** 1 cup | 5 |
| **Dressing, salad, ginger,** 2 Tbsp | 2 |
| ▲ **Edamame, in pods,** 1 cup | 2 |
| **Hibachi** | |
| chicken, 1 cup | 8 |
| shrimp, 1 cup | 6 |
| steak, 1 cup | 10 |
| vegetable, 1 cup | 5 |
| **Katsu** | |
| ahi, 2 slices (4 1/2" x 1/2" x 3/4" thick) | 6 |
| chicken, 2 slices (4 1/2" x 1/2" x 3/4" thick) | 6 |
| pork, 2 slices (4 1/2" x 1/2" x 3/4" thick) | 7 |
| **Lomi lomi salmon,** 1/2 cup | 2 |
| **Mirin,** 1 fl oz | 1 |
| **Nebeyaki udon,** 2 cups | 7 |

*Japanese (cont'd)*

| ▲ Power Foods | *PointsPlus*™ value |
|---|---|
| **Noodles** | |
| ramen, fresh, cooked, 1 cup | 5 |
| soba, cooked, with sauce, 1 cup | 12 |
| **Okonmiyaki, without sauce and mayonnaise (Japanese style pizza),** 1 (8" diameter) | 9 |
| **Poke** | |
| ahi, 1/2 cup | 2 |
| tako, 1/2 cup | 2 |
| **Saimin,** 1 cup | 5 |
| **Sakatini,** 1 (3 fl oz) | 7 |
| **Sake,** 1/2 cup | 5 |
| **Salad, seaweed,** 1/2 cup | 1 |
| **Sashimi** | |
| ▲ any type except mackerel and salmon, 4 pieces (2 oz) | 1 |
| mackerel, 4 pieces (2 oz) | 4 |
| salmon, 4 pieces (2 oz) | 2 |
| **Sauce** | |
| shoyu, 1 Tbsp | 0 |
| tamari, 1 Tbsp | 0 |
| teriyaki, 1 Tbsp | 0 |
| teriyaki, 1/4 cup | 2 |
| **Shabu shabu,** 4 oz beef, 2 oz tofu, and 1-1/2 cups vegetables | 10 |
| **Shoyu chicken,** 1 thigh (3 oz) | 6 |
| **Soup, miso,** 1 cup | 2 |
| **Suimono,** 1 cup | 2 |
| **Sukiyaki with sauce,** 2 cups with 1/4 cup sauce | 15 |
| **Sunomono,** 1/2 cup | 0 |
| **Sushi** | |
| Alaskan roll, 2 pieces (1" high x 1 3/4" diameter) | 3 |
| California roll, 4 large pieces (1" high x 1 3/4" diameter or 1 oz each) | 4 |
| cone, 1 | 3 |

| ▲ Power Foods | *PointsPlus*™ value |
|---|---|
| inari, 1 | 3 |
| kappa maki (cucumber roll), 4 medium pieces (1 1/2" diameter x 3/4" thick) | 3 |
| kappa maki (cucumber roll), 6 small pieces (1" diameter x 1" thick) | 3 |
| maki (vegetables and rice rolled with seaweed), 4 medium pieces (1 1/2" diameter x 3/4" thick) | 3 |
| maki (vegetables and rice rolled with seaweed), 6 small pieces (1" diameter x 1" thick) | 3 |
| nigiri (sliced uncooked fish over rice), 4 medium pieces (2" long x 3/4" wide) | 3 |
| nigiri (sliced uncooked fish over rice), 6 small pieces (1" long x 1" wide) | 3 |
| nigiri uni (sea urchin), 4 medium pieces (2" long x 3/4" wide) | 3 |
| nigiri, albacore (white tuna), 4 medium pieces (2" long x 3/4" wide) | 3 |
| nigiri, amaebi (sweet shrimp), 4 medium pieces (2" long x 3/4" wide) | 3 |
| nigiri, conch, 4 medium pieces (2" long x 3/4" wide) | 3 |
| nigiri, ebi (cooked shrimp), 4 medium pieces (2" long x 3/4" wide) | 3 |
| nigiri, hamachi (yellow tail), 4 medium pieces (2" long x 3/4" wide) | 3 |
| nigiri, hirame (fluke), 4 medium pieces (2" long x 3/4" wide) | 3 |
| nigiri, hokigai (surf clam), 4 medium pieces (2" long x 3/4" wide) | 3 |
| nigiri, ikura (salmon roe), 4 medium pieces (2" long x 3/4" wide) | 3 |
| nigiri, kani (crab), 4 medium pieces (2" long x 3/4" wide) | 3 |
| nigiri, maguro (tuna), 4 medium pieces (2" long x 3/4" wide) | 3 |

| ▲ Power Foods | *PointsPlus*™ value |
|---|---|
| nigiri, masago (smelt roe), 4 medium pieces (2" long x 3/4" wide) | 3 |
| nigiri, saba (mackerel), 4 medium pieces (2" long x 3/4" wide) | 3 |
| nigiri, sake (fresh salmon), 4 medium pieces (2" long x 3/4" wide) | 3 |
| nigiri, smoked salmon, 4 medium pieces (2" long x 3/4" wide) | 3 |
| nigiri, suzuki (sea bass), 4 medium pieces (2" long x 3/4" wide) | 3 |
| nigiri, suzume, 4 medium pieces (2" long x 3/4" wide) | 3 |
| nigiri, tai (red snapper), 4 medium pieces (2" long x 3/4" wide) | 3 |
| nigiri, tairagai (scallops), 4 medium pieces (2" long x 3/4" wide) | 3 |
| nigiri, tako (octopus), 4 medium pieces (2" long x 3/4" wide) | 3 |
| nigiri, tobiko (flying fish roe), 4 medium pieces (2" long x 3/4" wide) | 3 |
| nigiri, unagi (fresh water eel), 4 medium pieces (2" long x 3/4" wide) | 3 |
| nigri, ika (squid), 4 medium pieces (2" long x 3/4" wide) | 3 |
| nori maki (uncooked fish and rice rolled with seaweed), 4 medium pieces (1 1/2" diameter x 3/4" thick) | 3 |
| nori maki (uncooked fish and rice rolled with seaweed), 6 small pieces (1" diameter x 1" thick) | 3 |
| Philadelphia roll, 2 large pieces (1" high x 1 3/4" diameter) | 3 |
| rainbow roll, 4 medium pieces (1 1/2" diameter x 3/4" thick) | 3 |
| rainbow roll, 6 small pieces (1" diameter x 1" thick) | 3 |
| spider roll, 6 pieces (2" diameter x 1" thick) | 10 |
| tamago-yaki (omelet roll), 2 pieces (3/4" wide) | 3 |

| ▲ Power Foods | *PointsPlus*™ value |
|---|---|
| tempura roll, shrimp, 6 pieces (1 1/2" diameter x 1" thick) | 10 |
| tempura roll, vegetable, 6 pieces (1 1/2" diameter x 1" thick) | 5 |
| tuna roll, 4 medium pieces (1 1/2" diameter x 3/4" thick) | 3 |
| tuna roll, 6 small pieces (1" diameter x 1" thick) | 3 |
| tuna roll, spicy, 6 pieces (2" diameter x 1" thick) | 7 |
| unagi maki, 4 medium pieces (1 1/2" diameter x 3/4" thick) | 3 |
| unagi maki, 6 small pieces (1" diameter x 1" thick) | 3 |
| uni maki, 4 medium pieces (1 1/2" diameter x 3/4" thick) | 3 |
| uni maki, 6 small pieces (1" diameter x 1" thick) | 3 |
| yellow tail roll, 4 medium pieces (1 1/2" diameter x 3/4" thick) | 3 |
| yellow tail roll, 6 small pieces (1" diameter x 1" thick) | 3 |
| **Tempura** | |
| shrimp, 4 jumbo (3 3/4 oz) | 13 |
| vegetable, 1 cup | 8 |
| **Teppan yaki (mixed grill of beef, chicken, shrimp and vegetables),** 1 1/2 cups | 12 |
| **Teriyaki** | |
| beef, 2 slices (4 oz) | 7 |
| chicken, 2 slices (4 oz) | 6 |
| fish other than salmon, 4 oz | 6 |
| salmon, 4 oz | 7 |
| tofu, 1 cup | 4 |
| **Tofu,** fried, agadashi, 1 1/2" x 2" | 7 |
| **Tonkatsu** | |
| beef, 3/4 cup | 7 |
| chicken, 3/4 cup | 7 |
| pork, 3/4 cup | 9 |

*Japanese (cont'd)*

| ▲ Power Foods | PointsPlus™ value |
|---|---|
| **Yaki-soba** | |
| beef, 1/2 cup noodles with 1/2 cup beef and vegetables | 5 |
| chicken, 1/2 cup noodles with 1/2 cup chicken and vegetables | 5 |
| pork, 1/2 cup noodles with 1/2 cup pork and vegetables | 5 |
| **Yakitori,** 1 skewer (7 1/2 oz) | 6 |
| **Yosenabe,** 2 cups | 5 |

## JEWISH

| ▲ Power Foods | PointsPlus™ value |
|---|---|
| **Bagel** | |
| any type, 1 mini (2 1/2" diameter) | 2 |
| any type, 1 small or 1/2 large (2 oz) | 4 |
| with cream cheese and lox, 1 large (4 3/4 oz) | 14 |
| **Bialy,** 1 (3 oz) | 7 |
| **Blintz, cheese,** 1 (4 1/2 oz) | 6 |
| **Borscht, without sour cream,** 1 cup | 4 |
| **Bread, challah,** 1 slice (5" x 3" x 3/4") | 3 |
| **Cabbage,** stuffed, 2 (2" x 2 1/2") | 7 |
| **Cake, honey,** 5" x 3" x 1" | 9 |
| **Chicken and meatball fricassee,** 2 cups | 10 |
| **Chicken in the pot, without skin,** 2 cups | 12 |
| **Cholent,** 1 cup | 5 |
| **Cookies, rugalach,** 1 (2 1/2" x 1 1/4") | 3 |
| **Fish** | |
| lox, 1 oz | 1 |
| ▲ whitefish, cooked, 1 fillet (5 1/2 oz) | 6 |
| **Flanken,** 2 slices (4 oz) | 8 |
| **Fruit compote,** 1/2 cup | 4 |
| **Gefilte fish,** 1 piece (1 1/2 oz) | 1 |
| **Hamantaschen,** 1 piece (3" diameter) | 3 |
| **Haroset,** 1/4 cup | 1 |
| **Herring** | |
| chopped, 1/4 cup | 4 |
| pickled, 1/2 cup | 3 |
| **Kasha varnishkes,** 1 cup | 7 |
| **Kishke,** 1 small piece (3/4 oz) | 2 |
| **Knish, potato,** 1 (3 1/2" square) | 7 |
| **Kreplach** | |
| boiled, 2 pieces (4" x 3" x 3" each) | 6 |
| fried, 2 pieces (4" x 3" x 3" each) | 8 |
| **Kugel** | |
| lukschen, with fruit, 1 piece (3" x 3 1/4") | 9 |
| lukschen, without fruit, 1 piece (3" x 3 1/4") | 6 |
| potato, 1 piece (3" x 3 1/4") | 5 |
| **Liver,** chopped, 1/4 cup | 5 |
| **Mandelbrot,** 1 slice (3" x 2" x 1/2") | 5 |
| **Matzo, all varieties,** 1 board (1 oz) | 3 |
| **Matzo brie,** 1/4 of the 10" round or 1 cup | 5 |
| **Potato latkes,** 2 (3 1/2 diameter) | 7 |
| **Soup** | |
| chicken, with matzo balls, 1 cup soup with 2 (1 1/2") matzo balls | 3 |
| ▲ chicken, without matzo balls (broth only), 1 cup | 0 |
| hot and sour, 1 cup | 3 |
| mushroom barley, 1 cup | 4 |
| **Tzimmes, vegetable,** 3/4 cup | 4 |

## KOREAN

| ▲ Power Foods | PointsPlus™ value |
|---|---|
| **Bulgogi (beef stir-fry),** 1 cup | 5 |
| **JapChae, beef, chicken, or pork,** 1 cup | 8 |
| **Khal bi,** 4 oz | 8 |
| ▲ **Kim chee,** 1/2 cup | 0 |
| **Korean barbecue beef,** 4 oz | 7 |

| ▲ Power Foods | *PointsPlus*™ value |
|---|---|
| **Korean barbecue chicken thighs,** 1 (5 oz) | 12 |
| **Korean barbecue short ribs,** 4 oz | 8 |
| **Pajun (Korean green onion and shrimp pancake),** 1 (6-8" diameter) | 9 |

## MEXICAN/TEX-MEX

| ▲ Power Foods | *PointsPlus*™ value |
|---|---|
| **Arroz con pollo,** 3 oz chicken with 1 1/2 cups rice | 15 |
| ▲ **Beans,** refried, 1/2 cup | 4 |
| **Burrito** | |
| bean, 1 small (6") | 7 |
| bean, 1 large (8") | 10 |
| bean and cheese, fast food, 2 pieces (6 1/2 oz) | 10 |
| bean and chili peppers, fast food, 2 pieces (7 oz) | 11 |
| bean and meat, fast food, 2 pieces (8 oz) | 14 |
| bean, cheese, and chili peppers, fast food, 2 pieces (12 oz) | 18 |
| bean, fast food, 1 (5 oz) | 9 |
| beans, cheese, and beef, fast food, 2 pieces (7 oz) | 9 |
| beef and cheese, 1 small (6") | 8 |
| beef and cheese, 1 large (8") | 7 |
| beef and chili peppers, fast food, 2 pieces (7 oz) | 11 |
| beef, cheese, and chili peppers, fast food, 2 pieces (10 3/4 oz) | 17 |
| beef, fast food, 2 pieces (7 3/4 oz) | 14 |
| chicken and cheese, 1 small (6") | 6 |
| chicken and cheese, 1 large (8") | 8 |
| fruit, fast food, 1 small (2 1/2 oz) | 6 |
| vegetable, 1 small (made with a 6" tortilla) | 6 |
| vegetable, 1 large (made with a 10" tortilla) | 12 |

| ▲ Power Foods | *PointsPlus*™ value |
|---|---|
| **Carne asada,** 4 oz | 10 |
| **Carnitas,** 1 cup | 9 |
| **Chalupa (pork and bean dish),** 1 cup | 7 |
| **Chicken adobo,** 1 thigh (4 oz) | 6 |
| **Chicken molé,** 1 cup | 9 |
| **Chili con carne, with or without beans,** 1 cup | 9 |
| **Chili con queso,** 1/4 cup | 6 |
| **Chili rellenos, beef and cheese, without sauce,** 2 (7 1/2 oz) | 19 |
| **Chimichanga** | |
| beef, 1 (3" x 3 1/2") | 12 |
| beef and cheese, fast food, 1 (6 1/2 oz) | 12 |
| beef and red chili peppers, fast food, 1 (6 3/4 oz) | 11 |
| beef, cheese, and red chili peppers, fast food, 1 (6 1/2 oz) | 10 |
| beef, fast food, 1 (6 oz) | 12 |
| chicken, 1 (3" x 3 1/2") | 10 |
| **Cookies, Mexican wedding,** 2 (1 1/2" wide each) | 2 |
| **Corn cake, sweet,** 1/2 cup | 10 |
| **Cornbread, Mexican,** 1/12 of a 10" round or 3 1/3 oz | 8 |
| **Dip, Mexican 7-layer,** 1/2 cup | 4 |
| **Enchilada de camarones,** 1 cup | 5 |
| **Empanadas,** 2 (3" diameter) | 6 |
| **Enchiladas** | |
| beef, 2 (10 1/2 oz) | 13 |
| cheese, 2 (8 1/2 oz) | 12 |
| cheese and beef, fast food, 1 (6 3/4 oz) | 9 |
| cheese, fast food, 1 (5 3/4 oz) | 9 |
| chicken, 2 (10 1/2 oz) | 11 |
| pork, 2 (10 1/2 oz) | 13 |
| sour cream, 1 (5 1/2 oz) | 9 |

*Mexican/Tex-Mex (cont'd)*

| ▲ Power Foods | *PointsPlus™* value |
|---|---|
| **Enchirito, with cheese, beef, and beans,** fast food, 1 (6 3/4 oz) | 9 |
| **Fajitas** | |
| beef, 2 (9 oz) | 13 |
| chicken, 2 (8 1/2 oz) | 10 |
| pork, 2 (10 1/2 oz) | 14 |
| shrimp, 2 (9 oz) | 10 |
| vegetarian, 1 (5 1/2 oz) | 6 |
| **Flauta** | |
| beef, 1 (6" x 1 1/4") | 12 |
| chicken, 1 (6" x 1 1/4") | 11 |
| pork, 1 (6" x 1 1/4") | 11 |
| **Gordita, beef,** 1 (3" diameter) | 11 |
| **Guacamole,** 1/4 cup | 2 |
| **Huevos rancheros,** 2 eggs on 2 tortillas | 16 |
| **Ice cream,** fried, 1/2 cup | 12 |
| **Jalapeño poppers,** 1 (1 1/2 oz) | 4 |
| **King ranch chicken casserole,** 1 cup | 9 |
| **Menudo (beef tripe and hominy stew),** 1 cup | 7 |
| **Mexican coffee,** 6 fl oz with 2 Tbsp whipped cream | 6 |
| **Molé poblano,** 1/4 cup | 5 |
| **Nachos** | |
| beef, 4 (8 1/2 oz) | 14 |
| cheese, 3 (3 oz) | 9 |
| cheese and bean, 4 (6 1/2 oz) | 10 |
| chicken, 4 (8 1/2 oz) | 13 |
| with cheese and jalapeño peppers, fast food, 7 1/4 oz | 17 |
| with cheese sauce, 2 3/4 oz | 6 |
| with cheese, beans, ground beef, and peppers, fast food, 6-8 nachos (9 oz) | 16 |
| with cheese, fast food, 4 oz | 9 |
| with cinnamon and sugar, fast food, 6-8 nachos (3 3/4 oz) | 17 |

| ▲ Power Foods | *PointsPlus™* value |
|---|---|
| **Picadillo,** 1 cup | 11 |
| ▲ **Pico de gallo,** 1/2 cup | 0 |
| **Quesadilla** | |
| beef, 1/2 of 6" diameter | 7 |
| cheese, 1/2 of 6" diameter | 6 |
| chicken, 1/2 of 6" diameter | 7 |
| vegetable, 1/2 of 6" diameter | 7 |
| **Rice, Spanish,** 1 cup | 7 |
| **Rice, with pigeon peas (arroz con gandules),** 1 cup | 8 |
| **Salad** | |
| taco, fast food, 1 1/2 cups | 7 |
| taco, with chili con carne, fast food, 1 1/2 cups | 7 |
| taco, with shell, without dressing, fast food, 1 | 18 |
| taco, without shell and dressing, fast food, 1 | 10 |
| **Salsa** | |
| ▲ black bean and corn, 1/2 cup | 2 |
| ▲ fat-free, 2 Tbsp | 0 |
| ▲ fat-free, 1/2 cup | 0 |
| **Sangria,** 1 (4 fl oz) | 3 |
| **Sauce** | |
| chili, green, 1/4 cup | 0 |
| chili, red, 1 Tbsp | 0 |
| sofrito, 1/4 cup | 4 |
| taco, 1 Tbsp | 0 |
| **Sausage, chorizo,** 1 link (5 1/2" long or 3 1/2 oz) | 12 |
| **Sopaipillas,** 2 (1 oz) | 3 |
| **Soup** | |
| chicken enchilada, 1 cup | 6 |
| chicken, with tortilla strips and shredded cheese, 1 cup | 5 |
| gazpacho, 1 cup | 4 |
| pozole, 1 cup | 5 |
| tortilla, 1 cup | 7 |
| **Taco** | |
| beef, 1 (3 1/2 oz) | 6 |

| Power Foods | PointsPlus™ value |
|---|---|
| breakfast, 1 (3 1/2 oz) | 5 |
| chicken, 1 (3 1/2 oz) | 5 |
| fish, 1 (4 1/4 oz) | 5 |
| hard, fast food, 1 (3 oz) | 4 |
| pork, 1 (3 1/2 oz) | 5 |
| soft, fast food, 1 (3 1/2 oz) | 4 |
| **Tamale,** 2 (9 1/2 oz) | 10 |
| **Tamale pie,** 1 cup | 12 |
| **Taquitos** | |
| beef, 1 (5 1/2" x 1 1/2") | 5 |
| chicken, 1 (5 1/2" x 1 1/2") | 3 |
| **Tostada** | |
| beef, 1 (8 1/4 oz) | 11 |
| chicken, 1 (8 1/4 oz) | 10 |
| with beans and cheese, fast food, 1 (5 oz) | 6 |
| with beans, beef, and cheese, fast food, 1 (8 oz) | 9 |
| with beef and cheese, fast food, 1 (5 3/4 oz) | 8 |
| with guacamole, fast food, 2 (9 1/4 oz) | 10 |

## MIDDLE EASTERN

| Power Foods | PointsPlus™ value |
|---|---|
| **Baba ganosh,** 1/4 cup | 3 |
| **Beef goulash,** 1 cup | 9 |
| **Candy, sesame,** 1 piece (2" x 1") | 3 |
| **Chicken pilaf (kotta pilafi),** 1 cup | 8 |
| **Chicken pilaf (kotta pilafi),** 1 breast with 1 cup pilaf | 12 |
| **Couscous, regular,** cooked, 1 cup | 4 |
| **Crackers, lavash,** 1/4 of the 10" cracker | 7 |
| **Doro wat,** 1 cup | 7 |
| **Falafel** | |
| in pita, 1 large pita with 4 falafel patties | 13 |
| patties, 4 (2" diameter each) | 8 |
| **Fattoush,** 2 cups | 7 |
| **Hummus,** 1/4 cup | 4 |
| **Hungarian goulash,** 1 cup | 9 |
| **Kibbe,** baked, 3 pieces (1 1/2" squares) | 3 |
| **Rice pilaf,** 1 cup | 7 |
| **Shawarma, chicken** | |
| without skin and bone, 1 thigh (2 oz) | 5 |
| 1/2 cup | 7 |
| **Shish kabob,** 2 small skewers (4 3/4 oz) | 8 |
| **Tabouli,** 1/2 cup | 6 |

## PORTUGUESE

| Power Foods | PointsPlus™ value |
|---|---|
| **Malasadas (Portuguese doughnuts),** 1 (3" x 2" puff) | 3 |
| **Portuguese sweet bread,** 1/8 loaf (3 oz) | 7 |
| **Soup, Portuguese bean,** 1 cup | 6 |

## SCANDINAVIAN

| Power Foods | PointsPlus™ value |
|---|---|
| **Bread, lefse,** 1 (8-10" diameter) | 6 |
| **Chruscik,** 1 (1/4 oz) | 1 |
| **Cookies, kringla,** 2 (1 1/2 oz) | 4 |
| **Dumpling** | |
| kroppkakor (potato), boiled, 1 (2" wide) | 3 |
| kroppkakor (potato), fried, 1 (2" wide) | 4 |
| **Fish, salmon,** smoked, 1 oz | 1 |
| **Soup, knefla,** 1 cup | 7 |

## SOUTHEAST ASIA

| Power Foods | PointsPlus™ value |
|---|---|
| **Lumpia (Filipino spring roll),** 4 1/2" x 1" x 1 1/2" | 6 |
| **Pancit canton (sauteed egg noodles),** 1 cup | 6 |

| ▲ Power Foods | *PointsPlus™* value |
|---|---|

## SPANISH

| | |
|---|---|
| **Ceviche,** 1/2 cup | 2 |
| **Flan,** 3/4 cup | 9 |
| **Paella,** 1 cup | 9 |
| **Red snapper Veracruz,** 6 oz cooked fillet with 3/4 cup sauce | 12 |
| **Salad, green papaya, with pork and shrimp,** 1 cup | 4 |
| **Sauce, Spanish,** 1/2 cup | 3 |
| **Soup, black bean,** 1 cup | 2 |

## THAI

| | |
|---|---|
| **Chile beef (neua pad prik),** 1 cup | 7 |
| **Coconut rice, Thai,** 1 cup | 10 |
| **Curry, green chicken (gaeng kheow wan gai),** 1 cup | 8 |
| **Ginger chicken,** 1 cup | 8 |
| **Kho-phat (Thai fried rice),** 1 cup | 9 |
| **Massaman beef curry,** 1 cup | 21 |
| **Nam Prik,** 1 Tbsp | 1 |
| **Noodles, drunken,** 1 cup | 6 |
| **Pad si-iew (stir-fried beef with noodles),** 1 cup | 7 |
| **Pad Thai (rice noodles with chicken and shrimp),** 1 cup | 10 |
| **Panang curry** | |
| with beef, 1 cup | 14 |
| with chicken, 1 cup | 13 |
| with pork, 1 cup | 15 |
| **Pudding, tapioca, Thai,** 1/2 cup | 4 |
| **Salad** | |
| Thai beef , 1 cup | 15 |
| Thai chicken, 1 cup | 12 |
| Thai seafood, 2 cups | 11 |
| **Satay** | |
| beef, with peanut sauce, 2 skewers with 1/4 cup sauce | 12 |
| beef, without peanut sauce, 2 skewers (3 oz) | 5 |
| chicken, with peanut sauce, 2 skewers with 1/4 cup sauce | 12 |
| chicken, without peanut sauce, 2 skewers (3 oz) | 3 |
| **Sauce** | |
| peanut satay, 1 Tbsp | 1 |
| peanut, spicy, 2 Tbsp | 4 |
| **Seafood cakes (haw mok thalay),** 3/4 cup | 9 |
| **Sesame noodles,** 1 cup | 7 |
| **Soup** | |
| hot and spicy chicken, 1 cup | 4 |
| Thai chicken coconut, 1 cup | 10 |
| **Spring roll, Thai,** 1 (4" long) | 5 |
| **Sticky rice with mango,** 1 cup sliced mangoes with 1/2 cup sticky rice | 11 |
| **Thai chicken with basil, without skin and bone,** 1 breast (3 oz) | 5 |
| **Thai coffee or tea,** 1 cup | 9 |
| **Thai crisp noodles,** 1 cup | 9 |
| **Thai grilled beef (nuea nam tok),** 1/2 cup on lettuce leaves | 6 |
| **Tom yum kung,** 1 cup | 2 |

▲ Power Foods — *PointsPlus*™ value

## VIETNAMESE

| Food | *PointsPlus*™ value |
|---|---|
| **Imperial roll,** 1 (4 1/2" long) | 5 |
| **Lemon grass chicken,** 1 cup | 9 |
| **Nuoc cham,** 1 Tbsp | 0 |
| **Sauce, Vietnamese spring roll dipping,** 2 Tbsp | 0 |
| **Soup, asparagus crab,** 1 cup | 2 |
| **Spring roll** | |
| Vietnamese, fresh, 1 (1 (3/4 oz) | 2 |
| Vietnamese, fried, 1 (4" long) | 5 |
| **Vietnamese beef balls (Thit bo vien),** 6 (1 1/2 oz) | 2 |
| **Vietnamese chicken curry,** 1 cup | 9 |

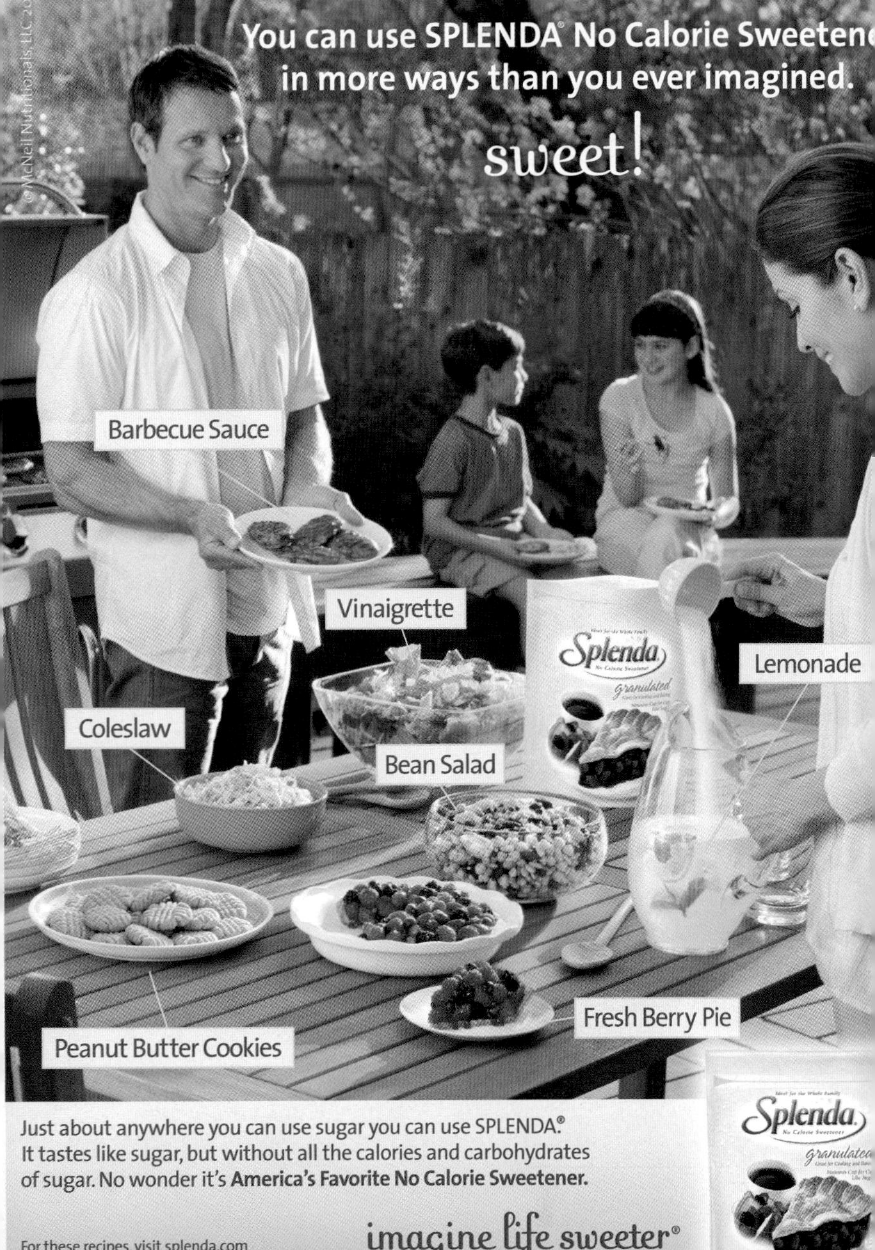

© McNeil Nutritionals, LLC 2010
You can use SPLENDA® No Calorie Sweetene
in more ways than you ever imagined.
sweet!
Barbecue Sauce
Vinaigrette
Lemonade
Coleslaw
Bean Salad
Fresh Berry Pie
Peanut Butter Cookies
Splenda
No Calorie Sweetener
Granulated

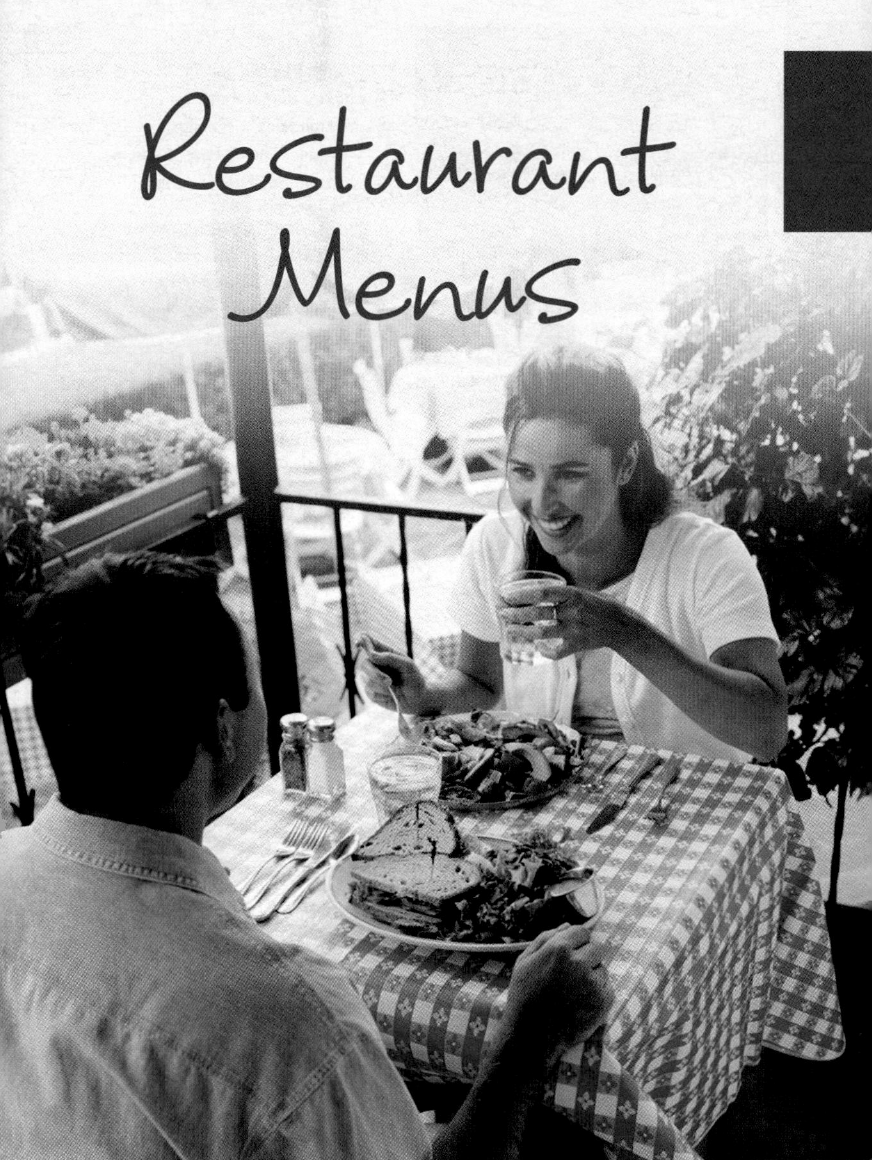

# Restaurant Menus

# A&W® ALL AMERICAN FOOD®

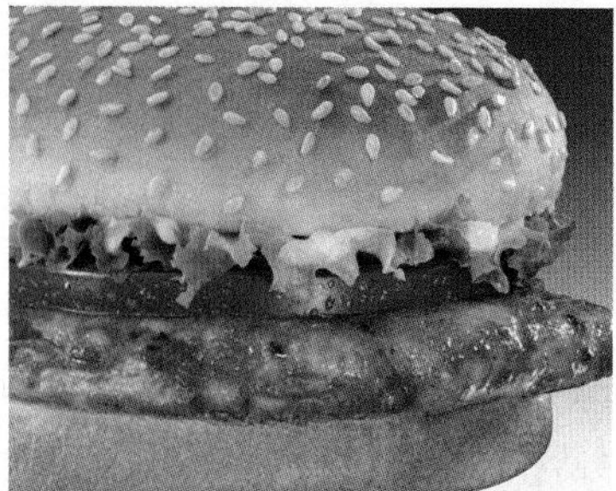

| ▲ Power Foods | *PointsPlus™* value |
|---|---|
| **SANDWICHES & STRIPS** | |
| **Cheeseburger,** 1 | 11 |
| **Chicken Strips,** 3 pieces | 13 |
| **Crispy Chicken Sandwich,** 1 | 14 |
| **Grilled Chicken Sandwich,** 1 | 10 |
| **Hamburger,** 1 | 10 |
| **Original Bacon Cheeseburger,** 1 | 14 |
| **Original Bacon Double Cheeseburger,** 1 | 20 |
| **Original Double Cheeseburger,** 1 | 18 |
| **Papa Burger®,** 1 | 18 |
| **Papa Single Burger,** 1 | 12 |
| **HOT DOGS** | |
| **Coney (Chili) Dog,** 1 | 9 |
| **Coney Chili/Cheese Dog,** 1 | 10 |
| **Hot Dog (plain),** 1 | 8 |
| **SIDES** | |
| **Breaded Onion Rings,** 1 regular | 9 |
| **Cheese Curds,** 1 serving | 16 |
| **Cheese Fries,** 1 serving | 10 |
| **Chili Fries,** 1 serving | 10 |
| **Chili/Cheese Fries,** 1 serving | 10 |

| ▲ Power Foods | *PointsPlus™* value |
|---|---|
| **Corn Dog Nuggets®,** 1 small (5 pieces) | 5 |
| **Extra Burger Patty,** 1 | 5 |
| **Large Fries,** 1 serving | 11 |
| **Regular French Fries,** 1 serving | 8 |
| **Small/Kids Fries,** 1 serving | 5 |
| **DIPPING SAUCES** | |
| **BBQ,** 1 serving | 1 |
| **Honey Mustard,** 1 serving | 3 |
| **Ranch,** 1 serving | 5 |
| **Sweet & Sour,** 1 serving | 1 |
| **ROOT BEER & FLOATS** | |
| **A&W® Root Beer,** 1 small | 6 |
| **A&W® Root Beer Float,** 1 small | 9 |
| **A&W® Root Beer Freeze,** 1 medium | 15 |
| **Diet A&W® Root Beer,** 1 small | 0 |
| **Diet A&W® Root Beer Float,** 1 small | 5 |
| **SWEETS & TREATS** | |
| **Caramel Sundae,** 1 | 9 |
| **Chocolate Milkshake,** 1 small | 19 |
| **Chocolate Sundae,** 1 | 9 |
| **Hot Fudge Sundae,** 1 | 9 |
| **M&M's® Polar Swirl®,** 1 | 19 |
| **Oreo® Polar Swirl®,** 1 | 19 |
| **Reese's® Polar Swirl®,** 1 | 20 |
| **Strawberry Milkshake,** 1 small | 18 |
| **Strawberry Sundae,** 1 | 8 |
| **Vanilla Cone,** 1 | 7 |
| **Vanilla Milkshake,** 1 small | 20 |

| ▲ Power Foods | PointsPlus™ value |
|---|---|
| **BURGERS** | |
| **1/4 lb. Black Angus Burger,** 1 | 11 |
| **1/4 lb. Black Angus Cheese,** 1 | 12 |
| **1/4 lb. Black Angus Bacon Cheese,** 1 | 14 |
| **1/4 lb. Black Angus Mushroom 'n Swiss,** 1 | 12 |
| **1/4 lb. Black Angus Deluxe,** 1 | 12 |
| **1/2 lb. Black Angus Burger,** 1 | 16 |
| **1/2 lb. Black Angus Cheese,** 1 | 19 |
| **1/2 lb. Black Angus Deluxe,** 1 | 19 |
| **Black Angus Hamburger,** 1 | 7 |
| **Black Angus Double Burger,** 1 | 10 |
| **Black Angus Ranch Burger,** 1 | 13 |
| **Black Angus Cheeseburger,** 1 | 8 |
| **Black Angus Double Cheeseburger,** 1 | 12 |
| **Black Angus BBQ Bacon Cheeseburger,** 1 | 10 |
| **Black Angus Bacon Double Cheeseburger,** 1 | 14 |
| **Black Angus Triple Cheeseburger,** 1 | 12 |
| **ENTRÉES** | |
| **1/4 lb. Black Angus Hot Dog,** 1 | 13 |
| **2-piece Chicken Fingers,** 1 serving | 7 |
| **Chicken Rings (5 pieces),** 1 serving | 7 |
| **Grilled Lemon Pepper Chicken Sandwich,** 1 | 9 |
| ▲ **Halibut,** 2 pieces | 6 |
| **SIDES** | |
| **Onion Rings,** 1 serving | 21 |
| **French Fry,** 1 small serving | 7 |
| **French Fry,** 1 regular serving | 10 |
| **French Fry,** 1 large serving | 32 |

| ▲ Power Foods | PointsPlus™ value |
|---|---|
| **SALADS** | |
| **Crispy Chicken Salad (without dressing or shell),** 1 | 17 |
| **Grilled Chicken Salad (without dressing),** 1 | 12 |
| **Grilled Chicken Salad without Dressing and Shell,** 1 | 7 |
| **Taco Salad,** 1 | 23 |
| **Taco Salad without Shell,** 1 | 19 |
| **Taco Salad without White Sauce and Shell,** 1 | 10 |
| **SALAD DRESSINGS** | |
| **Kens Thousand Island,** 1 packet | 5 |
| **Litehouse Blue Cheese,** 1 packet | 9 |
| **Litehouse Caesar Dressing,** 1 packet | 8 |
| **Litehouse Ginger Sesame,** 1 packet | 2 |
| **Litehouse Lite Ranch,** 1 packet | 4 |
| **Litehouse Ranch Dressing,** 1 packet | 7 |
| **CONDIMENTS & SAUCES** | |
| **Barbecue Sauce,** 1 serving | 1 |
| **Fry Sauce,** 1 serving | 2 |
| **Salsa,** 1 serving | 0 |
| **Sweet 'n Sour Sauce,** 1 serving | 1 |
| **Tartar Sauce,** 1 serving | 2 |
| **White Sauce,** 1 serving | 5 |
| **ICE CREAM** | |
| **Courtesy Cone,** 1 | 1 |
| **Ice Cream Cone,** 1 | 4 |
| **Small Vanilla Shake,** 1 | 8 |
| **Regular Vanilla Shake,** 1 | 11 |
| **Large Vanilla Shake,** 1 | 14 |

# ATLANTA BREAD

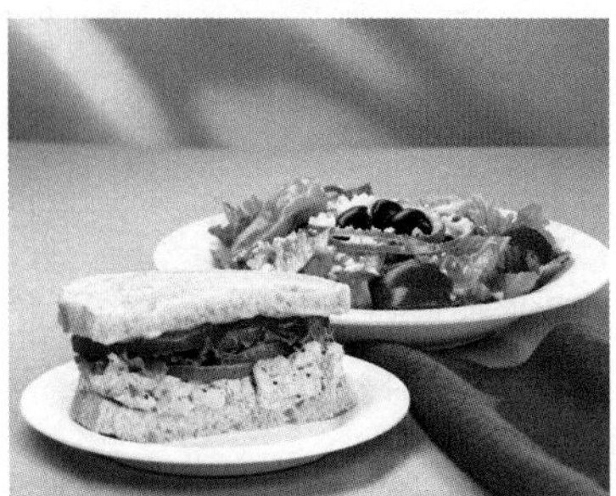

| ▲ Power Foods | *PointsPlus*™ value |
|---|---|
| **SOUP** | |
| **Baja Chicken Enchilada,** 1 1/4 cups | 9 |
| **Baked Potato Soup,** 1 1/4 cups | 6 |
| **Broccoli & Cheese,** 1 1/4 cups | 7 |
| **Chicken and Sausage Gumbo Soup,** 1 1/4 cups | 5 |
| **Chicken Peppercorn,** 1 1/4 cups | 12 |
| **Classic Chicken Noodle,** 1 1/4 cups | 3 |
| **French Onion,** 1 1/4 cups | 2 |
| **Garden Vegetable,** 1 1/4 cups | 2 |
| **Homestyle Chicken & Dumpling,** 1 1/4 cups | 11 |
| **New England Clam Chowder,** 1 1/4 cups | 5 |
| **Tomato Fennel & Dill,** 1 1/4 cups | 8 |
| **Wisconsin Cheese,** 1 1/4 cups | 8 |
| **CHILI** | |
| **Classic Beef Chili,** 1 1/4 cups | 7 |
| **Frontier Chicken Chili,** 1 1/4 cups | 7 |
| **SANDWICHES** | |
| **ABC Special Sandwich,** 1 | 20 |
| **Bella Chicken Sandwich,** 1 | 16 |
| **California Avocado Sandwich,** 1 | 25 |
| **Chicken Cordon Bleu Panini,** 1 | 18 |

| ▲ Power Foods | *PointsPlus*™ value |
|---|---|
| **Chicken Pesto Panini,** 1 | 19 |
| **Cubano Panini,** 1 | 17 |
| **Italian Veggie Panini,** 1 | 15 |
| **Kid's Grilled Cheese,** 1 | 10 |
| **Kid's Peanut Butter & Jelly,** 1 | 9 |
| **NY Hot Pastrami Sandwich,** 1 | 17 |
| **Tuna Salad on French,** 1 | 17 |
| **Turkey Club Panini,** 1 | 18 |
| **Turkey on Nine Grain,** 1 | 9 |
| **Veggie on Nine Grain,** 1 | 13 |
| **SIGNATURE SANDWICHES** | |
| **Bistro Chicken Press,** 1 | 21 |
| **Chicken Waldorf,** 1 | 12 |
| **Turkey Bacon Rustica,** 1 | 26 |
| **BAGEL SANDWICHES** | |
| **Bacon, Egg & Cheese Sandwich,** 1 | 13 |
| **Egg & Cheese Sandwich,** 1 | 12 |
| **Ham, Egg & Cheddar Cheese Sandwich,** 1 | 13 |
| **Sausage, Egg & Cheese Sandwich,** 1 | 20 |
| **PASTA** | |
| **Asiago Cream,** 1 serving | 24 |
| **Basil Pesto,** 1 serving | 28 |
| **Chicken Parmesan,** 1 serving | 23 |
| **Fettuccine Salmone,** 1 serving | 22 |
| **Kid's Penne & Cheese,** 1 serving | 12 |
| **Penne Bolognese,** 1 serving | 26 |
| **Penne Pomodoro Pasta,** 1 serving | 24 |
| **PIZZA** | |
| **BBQ Chicken,** 1/2 pizza | 8 |
| **Chicken Pesto Calzone,** 1 serving | 22 |
| **Four Cheese,** 1/2 pizza | 14 |

| ▲ Power Foods | *PointsPlus™* value |
|---|---|
| **Kid's Cheese,** 1/2 pizza | 8 |
| **Margherita,** 1/2 pizza | 13 |
| **Pepperoni,** 1/2 pizza | 9 |
| **White,** 1/2 pizza | 12 |

## SALADS

| | |
|---|---|
| **Balsamic Bleu Salad,** 1 | 9 |
| **Caesar Salad, without dressing,** 1 | 4 |
| **Chopstix Chicken Salad, without dressing,** 1 | 6 |
| **Greek Salad, without dressing,** 1 | 6 |
| **House Salad, without dressing,** 1 | 2 |
| **Salsa Fresca Salmon Salad,** 1 | 15 |

## BREADS & ROLLS

| | |
|---|---|
| **Asiago Foccacia,** 1/6 loaf | 7 |
| **Asiago Loaf,** 1 slice | 2 |
| **Asiago Strip,** 1/2 loaf | 9 |
| **Ciabatta,** 1 | 7 |
| **Cinnamon Raisin Bread,** 1 serving | 7 |
| **French Baguette,** 1 serving | 2 |
| **French Loaf,** 1 slice | 3 |
| **French Roll,** 1 | 4 |
| **Honey Wheat,** 1 serving | 4 |
| **Nine Grain,** 1 serving | 3 |
| **Panini Bread,** 1/2 loaf | 12 |
| **Pumpernickel Loaf,** 1 serving | 3 |
| **Rye Loaf,** 1 serving | 2 |
| **Sourdough Baguette,** 1 serving | 2 |
| **Sourdough Bread,** 1 serving | 3 |
| **Sourdough Soup Bowl,** 1 | 10 |

## CROISSANTS

| | |
|---|---|
| **Almond Croissant,** 1 | 17 |
| **Apple Croissant,** 1 | 11 |
| **Cheese Croissant,** 1 serving | 10 |
| **Chocolate Croissant,** 1 | 15 |

| ▲ Power Foods | *PointsPlus™* value |
|---|---|
| **French Croissant,** 1 | 9 |
| **Raspberry Cheese Croissant,** 1 | 12 |

## BREAKFAST

| | |
|---|---|
| **Belgian Waffle with Maple Syrup & Whipped Cream,** 1 serving | 14 |
| **French Toast with Maple Syrup,** 2 slices | 17 |
| **Morning Classic with Bacon,** 1 serving | 12 |
| **Morning Classic with Ham,** 1 serving | 11 |
| **Morning Classic with Sausage,** 1 serving | 18 |
| **Scrambled Eggs,** 1 serving | 5 |

## OMELETS

| | |
|---|---|
| **Florentine Omelet,** 1 serving | 13 |
| **Ham and Swiss Omelet,** 1 serving | 14 |
| **Spanish Omelet,** 1 serving | 13 |
| **Three Cheese Omelette,** 1 serving | 30 |
| **Tomato Bacon Omelet,** 1 serving | 10 |

## BAGELS

| | |
|---|---|
| **Apple Spice,** 1 | 9 |
| **Asiago Bagel,** 1 | 10 |
| **Cinnamon Crisp,** 1 | 9 |
| **Cinnamon Raisin Bagel,** 1 | 7 |
| **Everything Bagel,** 1 | 9 |
| **Plain Bagel,** 1 | 8 |
| **Poppy Seed Bagel,** 1 | 9 |
| **Sesame Seed Bagel,** 1 | 10 |
| **Wheat Bagel,** 1 | 7 |
| **Whole Grain,** 1 | 7 |

| ▲ Power Foods | *PointsPlus™* value |
|---|---|
| **CREAM CHEESE** | |
| **Chive Cream Cheese,** 1 serving | 5 |
| **Honey Raisin Walnut Cream Cheese,** 2 oz | 5 |
| **Olive Cream Cheese,** 2 oz | 5 |
| **Plain Cream Cheese,** 1 serving | 5 |
| **Raspberry Cream Cheese,** 2 oz | 3 |
| **Vegetable Cream Cheese,** 1 serving | 5 |
| **MUFFINS** | |
| **Banana Nut,** 1 | 17 |
| **Blueberry Muffin,** 1 | 9 |
| **Chocolate Chip Muffin,** 1 | 18 |
| **Low Fat Pumpkin Muffin,** 1 | 6 |
| **Lowfat Apple Muffin,** 1 | 6 |
| **Mocha Chip Muffin,** 1 | 17 |
| **Pumpkin Muffin,** 1 | 15 |
| **MUFFIN TOPS** | |
| **Banana Nut Muffin Top,** 1 top | 11 |
| **Blueberry Muffin Top,** 1 top | 7 |
| **Chocolate Chip Muffin Top,** 1 top | 11 |
| **Lowfat Pumpkin Muffin Top,** 1 top | 5 |
| **Mocha Chip Muffin Top,** 1 top | 11 |
| **COOKIES** | |
| **Chocolate Chunk Cookie,** 1 | 12 |
| **Chocolate Oatmeal & Craisin Cookie,** 1 | 11 |
| **Chocolate Toffee Cookie,** 1 | 11 |
| **Oatmeal Raisin Cookie,** 1 | 10 |
| **Peanut Butter Cookie,** 1 | 12 |
| **Shortbread Cookie,** 1 | 11 |
| **Toffee Chocolate Chunk Cookie,** 1 | 13 |
| **White Chocolate Macadamia Nut Cookie,** 1 | 13 |

| ▲ Power Foods | *PointsPlus™* value |
|---|---|
| **DANISH/SWEET ROLLS/PASTRIES** | |
| **Apple Danish,** 1 | 12 |
| **Cheese Danish,** 1 | 13 |
| **Gooey Butter Danish,** 1 | 15 |
| **Raspberry Cheese Danish,** 1 | 12 |
| **BROWNIES** | |
| **Creamy Caramel Brownie,** 1 | 13 |
| **Double Chocolate Brownie,** 1 | 13 |
| **CHEESECAKE** | |
| **Caramel Nut Cheesecake,** 1 slice | 18 |
| **Carrot Cake Cheesecake,** 1 slice | 19 |
| **Cookies and Cream Cheesecake,** 1 slice | 12 |
| **Pecan Turtle Cheesecake,** 1 slice | 17 |
| **Plain Cheesecake,** 1 slice | 16 |
| **Pumpkin Cheesecake,** 1 slice | 14 |
| **OTHER PASTRIES & SWEETS** | |
| **Bearclaw,** 1 | 14 |
| **Cinnamon Roll,** 1 | 17 |
| **Key Lime Pie,** 1 slice | 14 |
| **Pecan Roll,** 1 | 24 |
| **Sticky Bun,** 1 | 15 |

▲ Power Foods — *PointsPlus*™ value

## BREADS

| Item | PointsPlus value |
|---|---|
| **Artisan Baguette (salad size),** 1 slice | 6 |
| **Artisan Baguette (sandwich size),** 1 | 8 |
| **Artisan Honey Multigrain Baguette (salad size),** 1 piece | 6 |
| **Artisan Honey Multigrain Baguette (sandwich size),** 1 | 9 |
| **Artisan Multigrain Bread,** 1 slice | 7 |
| **Artisan Sundried Tomato Bread,** 4 oz | 7 |
| **Asiago Breadstick,** 1" slice | 5 |
| **Bacon and Cheese Mini Loaf,** 1 serving | 15 |
| **Basil Pesto Cheese Toasts,** 3 pieces | 4 |
| **Bread Bowl,** 1 | 16 |
| **Cheddar Jalapeno Breadstick,** 1 | 4 |
| **Cheese Bread,** 1 piece | 10 |
| **Ciabatta,** 1 | 5 |
| **Ciabatta (large),** 1 | 8 |
| **Cinnamon Raisin Breadstick,** 1 | 5 |
| **Country White Bread,** 1 slice | 7 |
| **Everything Breadstick,** 1 | 5 |
| **Farm House Rolls,** 1 | 8 |
| **Focaccia,** 1 | 9 |
| **Lahvash,** 1 serving | 8 |
| **Rosemary Garlic Bread Stick,** 1 | 5 |
| **Sesame Breadstick,** 1 | 5 |
| **Soft Roll,** 1 | 11 |

## BAGELS (WITHOUT SPREAD)

| Item | PointsPlus value |
|---|---|
| **Apple Cheddar Bagel,** 1 | 9 |
| **Asiago Cheese Bagel,** 1 | 9 |
| **Cinnamon Crisp Bagel,** 1 | 11 |
| **Cinnamon Raisin Bagel,** 1 | 8 |
| **Everything Bagel,** 1 | 9 |
| **Honey 9 Grain Bagel,** 1 | 10 |
| **Jalapeño Double Cheddar Bagel,** 1 | 10 |
| **Onion Dill Bagel,** 1 | 7 |

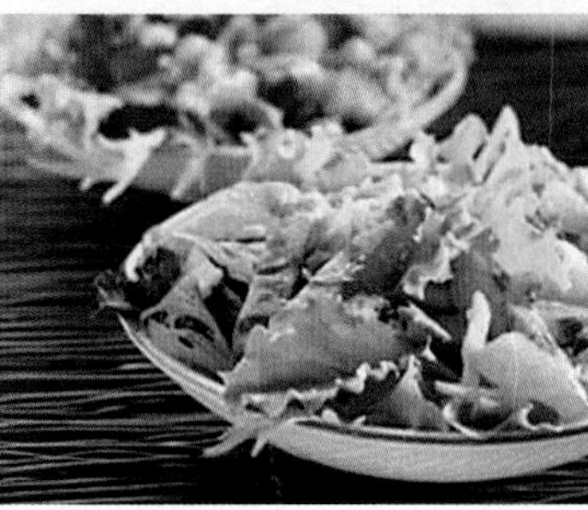

▲ Power Foods — *PointsPlus*™ value

| Item | PointsPlus value |
|---|---|
| **Plain Bagel,** 1 | 7 |
| **Poppy Seed Bagel,** 1 | 8 |
| **Sesame Seed Bagel,** 1 | 9 |

## BAGEL SPREADS

| Item | PointsPlus value |
|---|---|
| **Artichoke Aioli,** 1 serving (1 oz) | 2 |
| **Basil Pesto,** 1 serving (1 oz) | 3 |
| **Chili Dijon,** 1 serving (1 oz) | 3 |
| **Herb Bagel Spread,** 1 serving (2 oz) | 4 |
| **Herb Mayonnaise,** 1 serving (1 oz) | 3 |
| **Honey Mustard Sauce,** 1 serving (2 1/2 oz) | 5 |
| **Honey Pecan Cream Cheese,** 1 serving (2 oz) | 5 |
| **Jalapeno Mayonnaise,** 1 serving (1 oz) | 2 |
| **Lite Cream Cheese Spread,** 1 serving (2 oz) | 3 |
| **Mayonnaise,** 1 serving (1 oz) | 2 |
| **Mediterranean Spread,** 1 serving (1 oz) | 3 |
| **Mustard,** 1 tsp | 0 |
| **Plain Cream Cheese,** 1 serving (2 oz) | 5 |
| **Strawberry Cream Cheese,** 1 serving (2 oz) | 5 |
| **Sundried Tomato Cream Cheese,** 1 serving (2 oz) | 4 |

Bagel Spreads (cont'd)

| ▲ Power Foods | PointsPlus™ value |
|---|---|
| **Sun-Dried Tomato Spread,** 1 serving (1/2 oz) | 1 |
| **Vegetable Cream Cheese,** 1 serving (2 oz) | 5 |

## CROISSANTS

| ▲ Power Foods | PointsPlus™ value |
|---|---|
| **Almond Croissant,** 1 | 17 |
| **Apple Croissant,** 1 | 8 |
| **Chocolate Croissant,** 1 | 12 |
| **Ham & Cheese Croissant,** 1 | 11 |
| **Plain Croissant,** 1 | 8 |
| **Raspberry Cheese Croissant,** 1 | 9 |
| **Spinach & Cheese Croissant,** 1 | 8 |
| **Sweet Cheese Croissant,** 1 | 11 |

## BREAKFAST SANDWICHES

| ▲ Power Foods | PointsPlus™ value |
|---|---|
| **Bacon and Bagel,** 1 | 9 |
| **Bacon and Egg Melt on Ciabatta,** 1 | 13 |
| **Breakfast Quesadilla Sandwich,** 1 | 14 |
| **Egg on a Bagel Sandwich,** 1 | 9 |
| **Egg on a Bagel with Bacon Sandwich,** 1 | 11 |
| **Egg on a Bagel with Bacon & Cheese Sandwich,** 1 | 13 |
| **Egg on a Bagel with Cheese Sandwich,** 1 | 11 |
| **Mediterranean Spinach Breakfast Sandwich,** 1 | 14 |
| **Portobello, Egg and Cheddar,** 1 | 13 |
| **Prosciutto & Egg on Asiago Bagel,** 1 | 14 |
| **Sausage, Egg & Cheddar on Asiago Bagel,** 1 | 22 |
| **Smoked Salmon & Wasabi on Onion Dill Bagel,** 1 | 12 |

## OATMEAL

| ▲ Power Foods | PointsPlus™ value |
|---|---|
| **Muesli,** 1 serving | 11 |
| ▲ **Oatmeal,** 1 small | 4 |

## MUFFINS

| ▲ Power Foods | PointsPlus™ value |
|---|---|
| **Blueberry Muffin,** 1 | 13 |
| **Carrot Walnut Muffin,** 1 | 14 |
| **Corn Muffin,** 1 | 12 |
| **Cranberry Walnut Muffin,** 1 | 13 |
| **Double Chocolate Chunk Muffin,** 1 | 15 |
| **Low-fat Triple Berry Muffin,** 1 | 8 |
| **Mushroom, Gorgonzola and Red Pepper Muffin,** 1 | 13 |
| **Pumpkin Muffin,** 1 | 14 |
| **Raisin Bran Muffin,** 1 | 12 |
| **Southwest Jalapeno Muffin,** 1 | 15 |

## CAFÉ SANDWICHES

| ▲ Power Foods | PointsPlus™ value |
|---|---|
| **Arizona Chicken Sandwich,** 1 | 18 |
| **Baja Turkey Sandwich,** 1 | 16 |
| **Caprese Sandwich,** 1 | 18 |
| **Chicken Pesto Sandwich,** 1 | 17 |
| **Chicken Tarragon,** 1 | 16 |
| **Chilean Chicken Sandwich,** 1 | 19 |
| **Ham & Cheddar Sandwich (on Ciabatta),** 1 | 17 |
| **Mozzarella Chicken Sandwich,** 1 | 18 |
| **Portabello & Goat Cheese Sandwich,** 1 | 14 |
| **Prosciutto Mozzarella Sandwich,** 1 | 21 |
| **Roast Beef Caesar Sandwich,** 1 | 17 |
| **Smoked Turkey Club Sandwich,** 1 | 18 |
| **Spicy Tuna Sandwich,** 1 | 13 |
| **The Montana Sandwich,** 1 | 16 |
| **Turkey & Swiss Sandwich (on baquette),** 1 | 16 |
| **Turkey and Cranberry Chutney Sandwich,** 1 | 13 |

## HOT SANDWICHES & MELTS

| ▲ Power Foods | PointsPlus™ value |
|---|---|
| **BBQ Chicken on Farmhouse Roll,** 1 | 20 |
| **Cajun Shrimp Hot Wrap,** 1 | 17 |

| ▲ Power Foods | *PointsPlus*™ value |
|---|---|
| **Eggplant and Mozzarella Sandwich,** 1 | 17 |
| **Hot Steak Churrasco Wrap,** 1 | 15 |
| **Mayan Chicken Hot Wrap,** 1 | 15 |
| **Steak Teriyaki Hot Wrap,** 1 | 16 |
| **Steakhouse on Ciabatta,** 1 | 19 |
| **Tuna Melt,** 1 | 18 |
| **Turkey Melt,** 1 | 20 |

## WRAPS

| | |
|---|---|
| **Chicken Caesar Asiago Wrap,** 1 | 17 |
| **Chopped Turkey Cobb Wrap,** 1 | 17 |
| **Fields & Feta Wrap,** 1 | 13 |
| **Mediterranean Wrap,** 1 | 16 |
| **Southwest Tuna Wrap,** 1 | 20 |
| **Thai Peanut Chicken Wrap,** 1 | 16 |
| **Turkey Spinach Sonoma Wrap,** 1 | 14 |

## TOPPINGS

| | |
|---|---|
| **All Natural Chicken Breast,** 1 serving | 3 |
| **Bacon,** 1 serving | 2 |
| **Brie Cheese,** 1 serving | 4 |
| **Cheddar Cheese,** 2 slices | 4 |
| **Goat Cheese,** 1 serving | 3 |
| **Gorgonzola Cheese,** 1 serving | 5 |
| **Granola Topping,** 1 serving | 6 |
| **Guacamole,** 1 serving | 1 |
| ▲ **Ham,** 1 serving | 3 |
| **Mozzarella Cheese,** 1 serving | 3 |
| **Prosciutto,** 1 serving | 3 |
| **Provolone Cheese,** 1 serving | 4 |
| **Roast Beef,** 1 serving | 4 |
| **Roasted Red Pepper Hummus,** 1 serving | 2 |
| ▲ **Roasted Red Peppers,** 1 serving | 0 |
| **Sausage Patty,** 1 serving | 6 |
| **Swiss Cheese,** 1 serving | 4 |
| **Tarragon Mayonnaise Sauce,** 1 serving | 12 |

| ▲ Power Foods | *PointsPlus*™ value |
|---|---|
| **Tuna Salad Mix,** 1 serving | 4 |
| ▲ **Turkey Breast,** 1 serving | 2 |

## KIDS

| | |
|---|---|
| **All Natural Grilled Chicken Sandwich,** 1 | 12 |
| **Chicken Nuggets,** 1 serving | 5 |
| **Grilled Cheese,** 1 | 18 |
| **Kid's Buttered Penne Pasta,** 1 serving | 7 |
| **Macaroni and Cheese,** 1 kid's serving | 6 |
| **Smoked Turkey Sandwich,** 1 | 11 |

## FRESH SALADS (WITHOUT DRESSING)

| | |
|---|---|
| **Bagged Croutons,** 1 serving | 5 |
| **Caesar Asiago Salad,** 1 | 6 |
| **Caesar Asiago Salad (side),** 1 serving | 3 |
| **Chef's Salad,** 1 | 6 |
| **Chicken Pesto Salad,** 1 | 4 |
| **Garden Salad,** 1 | 2 |
| **Grilled Chicken Caesar Asiago,** 1 | 8 |
| **Mediterranean Chicken Salad,** 1 | 7 |
| **Riviera Salad,** 1 | 7 |
| **Side Garden Salad,** 1 | 1 |
| **Smoked Turkey Cobb Salad,** 1 | 8 |
| **Thai Peanut Chicken Salad,** 1 | 6 |
| **Tuna Garden Salad,** 1 | 6 |
| **Turkey Spinach Sonoma Salad,** 1 | 6 |

## HOT ENTRÉES

| | |
|---|---|
| **Cheese Tortellini Primavera,** 1 | 15 |
| **Chicken Penne Broccoli Alfredo,** 1 | 17 |
| **Meat Lasagna,** 1 | 13 |
| **Penne Marinara with Vegetables,** 1 | 9 |
| **Penne with Chicken and Fire-Roasted Pepper Sauce,** 1 | 14 |
| **Spinach and Artichoke Lasagna,** 1 | 11 |

# AU BON PAIN®

▲ Power Foods — *PointsPlus™* value

## HARVEST RICE BOWLS

| Item | PointsPlus value |
|---|---|
| **Cajun Shrimp Harvest Rice Bowl,** 1 | 13 |
| **Cajun Shrimp Harvest Rice Bowl with Brown Rice,** 1 | 14 |
| **Mayan Chicken Harvest Rice Bowl,** 1 | 13 |
| **Mayan Chicken Harvest Rice Bowl with Brown Rice,** 1 | 13 |
| **Salmon Curry Harvest Rice Bowl,** 1 | 15 |
| **Salmon Curry Harvest Rice Bowl with Brown Rice,** 1 | 16 |
| **Steak Churrasco Harvest Rice Bowl,** 1 | 14 |
| **Steak Churrasco Harvest Rice Bowl with Brown Rice,** 1 | 15 |
| **Steak Teriyaki Harvest Rice Bowl,** 1 | 15 |
| **Steak Teriyaki Harvest Rice Bowl with Brown Rice,** 1 | 15 |

## PIZZETTAS

| Item | PointsPlus value |
|---|---|
| **Spinach and Artichoke Pizzetta,** 1 | 14 |
| **Three Cheese Pizzetta,** 1 | 18 |
| **Tomato, Mozzarella, Basil Pizzetta,** 1 | 17 |

## SALADS

| Item | PointsPlus value |
|---|---|
| **Butternut Squash Salad,** 1 serving | 7 |
| **Chickpea and Tomato Cucumber Salad,** 1 | 6 |
| **Green Bean and Almond Salad,** 1 serving | 3 |
| **Green Bean and Beet Salad,** 1 | 5 |
| **Mandarin Sesame Chicken Salad,** 1 | 10 |
| **Mediterranean Tuna Salad,** 1 serving | 3 |
| **Mozzarella and Tomato,** 1 serving | 5 |
| **Mozzarella, Olives, Roasted Peppers and Tomato,** 1 serving | 5 |
| **Pear and Gorgonzola Salad,** 1 | 10 |

## SALAD DRESSINGS

| Item | PointsPlus value |
|---|---|
| **Balsamic Vinaigrette,** 2 oz | 3 |
| **Blue Cheese Dressing,** 2 oz | 9 |
| **Caesar Dressing,** 2 oz | 8 |
| **Fat Free Raspberry Vinaigrette,** 2 oz | 1 |
| **Hazelnut Vinaigrette Dressing,** 2 oz | 8 |
| **Lite Honey Mustard Dressing,** 2 oz | 5 |
| **Lite Olive Oil Vinaigrette Dressing,** 2 oz | 3 |
| **Lite Ranch Dressing,** 2 oz | 3 |
| **Sesame Ginger Dressing,** 2 oz | 7 |
| **Thai Peanut Dressing,** 2 oz | 4 |

## SOUPS

| Item | PointsPlus value |
|---|---|
| **Baked Stuffed Potato,** 1 medium (12 oz) | 9 |
| **Baked Stuffed Potato,** 1 large (16 oz) | 12 |
| **Beef Stew,** 1 medium (12 oz) | 8 |
| **Beef Stew,** 1 large (16 oz) | 11 |
| **Broccoli Cheddar,** 1 medium (12 oz) | 8 |
| **Butternut Squash and Apple Soup,** 1 medium (12 oz) | 6 |
| **Carrot Ginger Soup,** 1 medium (12 oz) | 4 |
| **Carrot Ginger Soup,** 1 large (16 oz) | 5 |
| **Chicken and Dumpling Soup,** 1 medium (12 oz) | 6 |
| **Chicken and Dumpling Soup,** 1 large (16 oz) | 7 |
| **Chicken Florentine,** 1 medium (12 oz) | 7 |
| **Chicken Gumbo Soup,** 1 medium (12 oz) | 5 |
| **Chicken Noodle Soup,** 1 medium (12 oz) | 4 |
| **Chicken Noodle Soup,** 1 large (16 oz) | 5 |
| **Chicken Vegetable Stew,** 1 medium (12 oz) | 8 |
| **Chicken Vegetable Stew,** 1 large (16 oz) | 11 |

| ▲ Power Foods | PointsPlus™ value |
|---|---|
| **Corn and Green Chili Bisque,** 1 medium (12 oz) | 7 |
| **Corn Chowder,** 1 medium (12 oz) | 10 |
| **Cream of Chicken and Wild Rice Soup,** 1 large (16 oz) | 9 |
| **Curried Rice & Lentil,** 1 medium (12 oz) | 4 |
| **French Moroccan Tomato Lentil,** 1 medium (12 oz) | 4 |
| **French Onion Soup,** 1 medium (12 oz) | 4 |
| **French Onion Soup,** 1 large (16 oz) | 4 |
| **Garden Vegetable Soup,** 1 medium (12 oz) | 2 |
| **Gazpacho,** 1 medium (12 oz) | 3 |
| **Gazpacho,** 1 large (16 oz) | 3 |
| **Harvest Pumpkin Soup,** 1 medium (12 oz) | 6 |
| **Harvest Pumpkin Soup,** 1 large (16 oz) | 9 |
| **Hearty Cabbage Soup,** 1 medium (12 oz) | 3 |
| **Italian Wedding Soup,** 1 medium (12 oz) | 4 |
| **Italian Wedding Soup,** 1 large (16 oz) | 6 |
| **Jamaican Black Bean Soup,** 1 medium (12 oz) | 5 |
| **Macaroni and Cheese,** 1 medium (12 oz) | 12 |
| **Macaroni and Cheese,** 1 large (16 oz) | 15 |
| **Mediterranean Pepper Soup,** 1 medium (12 oz) | 3 |
| **Old Fashioned Tomato Rice,** 1 medium (12 oz) | 3 |
| **Pasta e fagioli,** 1 medium (12 oz) | 6 |
| **Portuguese Kale Soup,** 1 medium (12 oz) | 3 |
| **Portuguese Kale Soup,** 1 large (16 oz) | 4 |
| **Potato Cheese Soup,** 1 medium (12 oz) | 7 |
| **Potato Leek,** 1 medium (12 oz) | 8 |
| **Red Beans, Italian Sausage & Rice,** 1 medium (12 oz) | 6 |

| ▲ Power Foods | PointsPlus™ value |
|---|---|
| **Southern Black Eyed Pea,** 1 medium (12 oz) | 4 |
| **Southwest Tortilla Soup,** 1 medium (12 oz) | 5 |
| **Southwest Vegetable,** 1 medium (12 oz) | 3 |
| **Split Pea with Ham,** 1 medium (12 oz) | 6 |
| **Thai Coconut Curry Soup,** 1 medium (12 oz) | 4 |
| **Thai Coconut Curry Soup,** 1 large | 5 |
| **Tomato Basil Bisque,** 1 medium (12 oz) | 5 |
| **Tomato Basil Bisque,** 1 large (16 oz) | 7 |
| **Tomato Cheddar Soup,** 1 medium (12 oz) | 7 |
| **Tomato Florentine Soup,** 1 medium (12 oz) | 3 |
| **Tuscan Vegetable,** 1 medium (12 oz) | 4 |
| **Vegetable Beef Barley Soup,** 1 medium (12 oz) | 4 |
| **Vegetable Beef Barley Soup,** 1 large (16 oz) | 5 |
| **Vegetarian Chili,** 1 medium (12 oz) | 5 |
| **Vegetarian Lentil,** 1 medium (12 oz) | 4 |
| **Vegetarian Minestrone,** 1 medium (12 oz) | 3 |
| **Wild Mushroom Bisque,** 1 medium (12 oz) | 5 |

## ADDITIONAL OFFERINGS

| | |
|---|---|
| **Apples, Blue Cheese and Cranberries,** 1 serving | 6 |
| **Asparagus and Almonds,** 1 serving | 2 |
| **BBQ Chicken,** 1 serving | 3 |
| **Black Bean and Corn Salad,** 1 serving | 3 |
| **Brie, Fruit and Crackers,** 1 serving | 5 |
| **Brown Rice and Hazelnut Waldorf Salad,** 1 serving | 5 |
| **Cheddar, Fruit and Crackers,** 1 serving | 5 |

*Additional Offerings (cont'd)*

| ▲ Power Foods | PointsPlus™ value |
|---|---|
| **Chickpea and Tomato Salad,** 1 serving | 2 |
| **Herb Cheese, Fruit and Crackers,** 1 serving | 5 |
| **Honey Mustard Chicken,** 1 serving | 3 |
| **Hummus and Cucumber,** 1 serving | 3 |
| **Smoked Turkey, Asparagus, Cranberry Chutney and Gorgonzola,** 1 serving | 3 |
| **Thai Beef and Peanut,** 1 serving | 3 |
| **Thai Peanut Chicken and Snow Peas,** 1 serving | 4 |

## COOKIES & DESSERTS

| ▲ Power Foods | PointsPlus™ value |
|---|---|
| **Banana Nut Pound Cake,** 1 serving | 14 |
| **Blondie,** 4 oz | 12 |
| **Blueberry Tulip,** 1 | 10 |
| **Cappuccino Pound Cake,** 1 serving | 14 |
| **Chocolate Bundt Cake,** 1 serving | 12 |
| **Chocolate Cheesecake Brownie,** 4 oz | 10 |
| **Chocolate Chip Brownie,** 4 oz | 11 |
| **Chocolate Chip Cookie,** 1 | 7 |
| **Chocolate Dipped Cranberry Almond Macaroon,** 1 | 9 |
| **Chocolate Dipped Shortbread,** 1 | 9 |
| **Chocolate Duo,** 1 serving | 5 |
| **Chocolate Pound Cake,** 1 slice | 14 |
| **Chocolate Raspberry Tulip,** 1 | 12 |
| **Confetti Cookie with M&M's,** 1 | 8 |
| **Creme de Fleur,** 1 | 13 |
| **Crumb Cake,** 1 | 13 |
| **English Toffee Cookie,** 1 | 6 |
| **Fruit Romanoff with Almonds,** 1 serving | 6 |
| **Gingerbread Man Cookie,** 1 | 9 |
| **Hazelnut Mocha Brownie,** 1 | 12 |
| **Hazelnut Crème Pastry,** 1 | 15 |
| **Hazelnut Dream Cookie,** 1 | 11 |
| **Hazelnut Fudge Cookie,** 1 | 8 |
| **Holiday Tree Cookie,** 1 | 5 |
| **Iced Cinnamon Rolls,** 1 | 11 |
| **Key Lime Sugar Cookie,** 1 | 7 |
| **Key Lime Tulip,** 1 | 12 |
| **Lemon Pound Cake,** 1 slice | 14 |
| **Mango Coconut Mousse,** 1 serving | 5 |
| **Marble Pound Cake,** 1 slice | 14 |
| **Mini Chocolate Chip Cookie,** 1 | 2 |
| **Mini Oatmeal Raisin Cookie,** 1 | 2 |
| **Mint Chocolate Pound Cake,** 1 | 15 |
| **Oatmeal Raisin Cookie,** 1 | 6 |
| **Palmier,** 1 | 12 |
| **Pecan Roll,** 1 | 18 |
| **Raspberry Mousse,** 1 serving | 4 |
| **Rocky Road Brownie,** 1 | 11 |
| **Shortbread Cookie,** 1 | 9 |
| **Tiramisu,** 1 slice | 5 |
| **White Chocolate Chunk Macadamia Nut Cookie,** 1 serving | 8 |

## SCONES

| ▲ Power Foods | PointsPlus™ value |
|---|---|
| **Cinnamon Scone,** 1 | 14 |
| **Orange Scone,** 1 | 13 |

## DANISH/SWEET ROLLS/PASTRIES

| ▲ Power Foods | PointsPlus™ value |
|---|---|
| **Cherry Danish,** 1 | 11 |
| **Lemon Danish,** 1 | 12 |

## STRUDEL

| ▲ Power Foods | PointsPlus™ value |
|---|---|
| **Apple Strudel,** 1 piece | 12 |
| **Cherry Strudel,** 1 piece | 12 |

## SNACKS

| ▲ Power Foods | PointsPlus™ value |
|---|---|
| **Assorted Nuts,** 1 serving | 6 |
| **Chocolate Covered Almonds,** 1 serving | 4 |
| **Chocolate Covered Strawberry,** 1 | 1 |
| **Chocolate Nonpareils,** 1 serving | 6 |

| ▲ Power Foods | *PointsPlus*™ value |
|---|---|
| **Dark Chocolate Cranberries,** 1 serving | 5 |
| ▲ **Fruit Cup,** 1 small | 2 |
| **Healthy Soy Mix,** 1/4 cup | 4 |
| **Jell-O,** 1 serving | 4 |
| **Kookaburra Red Licorice,** 1 serving | 4 |
| **MaJuKa Fruit Trail Mix,** 1 serving | 4 |
| **New Trail Mix,** 1 serving | 3 |
| **Tamari Almonds,** 1 serving | 5 |
| **The 19th Hole Snack Mix,** 1 serving | 4 |
| **Turkish Apricots,** 1 serving | 3 |

## COFFEE & ESPRESSO

| | |
|---|---|
| **Caffe Americano,** 1 small | 0 |
| **Caffe Latte,** 1 small | 6 |
| **Cappuccino,** 1 small | 3 |
| **Caramel Macchiato,** 1 small | 9 |
| **Chai Latte,** 1 small | 8 |
| **Iced Caffe Latte,** 1 small | 4 |
| **Iced Caramel Macchiato,** 1 small | 8 |
| **Iced Chai Latte,** 1 small | 5 |
| **Iced Decaf French Roast Coffee,** 1 large | 0 |
| **Iced French Roast Coffee,** 1 large | 0 |
| **Iced French Vanilla Coffee,** 1 large | 0 |
| **Iced Mocha Latte,** 1 small | 6 |
| **Iced Vanilla Latte,** 1 small | 7 |
| **Iced White Chocolate Latte,** 1 small | 7 |
| **Maple Spice Latte,** 1 large | 14 |
| **Mocha Latte,** 1 small | 9 |
| **Vanilla Latte,** 1 small | 9 |
| **White Chocolate Latte,** 1 small | 9 |

## SPECIALTY DRINKS

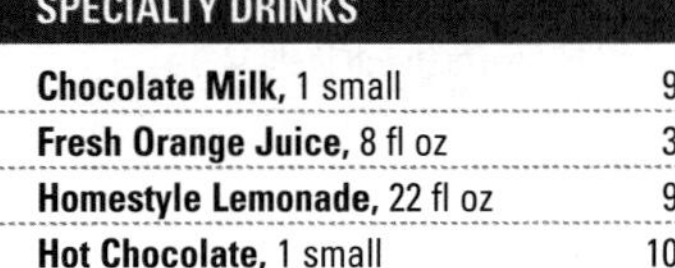

| | |
|---|---|
| **Chocolate Milk,** 1 small | 9 |
| **Fresh Orange Juice,** 8 fl oz | 3 |
| **Homestyle Lemonade,** 22 fl oz | 9 |
| **Hot Chocolate,** 1 small | 10 |

| ▲ Power Foods | *PointsPlus*™ value |
|---|---|

## ICED SPECIALTY DRINKS

| | |
|---|---|
| **Peach Iced Tea,** 1 large serving | 4 |
| **Peach Iced Tea,** 1 medium | 3 |

## BLASTS & SMOOTHIES

| | |
|---|---|
| **Banana Wildberry Smoothie,** 1 medium | 9 |
| **Caramel Blast,** 1 medium | 16 |
| **Coffee Blast,** 1 medium | 14 |
| **Coffee Blast,** 1 large | 21 |
| **Mocha Blast,** 1 medium | 14 |
| **Peach Smoothie,** 1 medium | 8 |
| **Strawberry Smoothie,** 1 medium | 8 |
| **Vanilla Blast,** 1 medium | 16 |
| **Wildberry Smoothie,** 1 medium | 10 |

## YOGURT

| | |
|---|---|
| **Blueberry Yogurt with Fruit,** 1 small | 6 |
| **Blueberry Yogurt with Granola & Fruit,** 1 small | 8 |
| **Strawberry Yogurt with Blueberries,** 1 large | 6 |
| **Strawberry Yogurt with Granola and Blueberries,** 1 large | 17 |
| **Vanilla Yogurt with Blueberries,** 1 large | 10 |
| **Vanilla Yogurt with Granola and Blueberries,** 1 large | 17 |

| ▲ Power Foods | *PointsPlus*™ value |
|---|---|
| **PRETZELS** | |
| **Almond Pretzel, with butter,** 1 | 10 |
| **Almond Pretzel, without butter,** 1 | 9 |
| **Cinnamon Sugar Pretzel, with butter,** 1 | 13 |
| **Cinnamon Sugar Pretzel, without butter,** 1 | 10 |
| **Garlic Pretzel, without butter and salt,** 1 | 8 |
| **Garlic Pretzel, without salt,** 1 | 9 |
| **Garlic Pretzel, with butter,** 1 | 9 |
| **Garlic Pretzel, without butter,** 1 | 8 |
| **Glazin' Raisin® Pretzel, with butter,** 1 | 13 |
| **Glazin' Raisin® Pretzel, without butter,** 1 | 12 |
| **Jalapeño Pretzel, with butter,** 1 | 8 |
| **Jalapeño Pretzel, without butter,** 1 | 7 |
| **Original Pretzel, without butter and salt,** 1 | 8 |
| **Original Pretzel, without salt,** 1 | 9 |
| **Original Pretzel, with butter,** 1 | 9 |
| **Original Pretzel, without butter,** 1 | 8 |
| **Pepperoni Pretzel,** 1 | 12 |
| **Pepperoni Pretzel, without butter,** 1 | 11 |
| **Sesame Pretzel, with butter,** 1 | 11 |
| **Sesame Pretzel, without butter,** 1 | 9 |
| **Sour Cream & Onion Pretzel, without butter and salt,** 1 | 8 |
| **Sour Cream & Onion Pretzel, without salt,** 1 | 9 |
| **Sour Cream & Onion Pretzel, with butter,** 1 | 9 |
| **Sour Cream & Onion Pretzel, without butter,** 1 | 8 |

| ▲ Power Foods | *PointsPlus*™ value |
|---|---|
| **PRETZEL STIX** | |
| **Cinnamon Sugar Stix, with butter,** 6 | 13 |
| **Cinnamon Sugar Stix, without butter,** 6 | 10 |
| **Original Stix, with butter,** 6 | 9 |
| **Original Stix, without butter,** 6 | 8 |
| **PRETZEL DOG** | |
| **Pretzel Dog, without butter,** 1 | 9 |
| **Pretzel Dog, with butter,** 1 | 10 |
| **DIPPING SAUCES** | |
| **Caramel Dip,** 1 1/2 oz | 3 |
| **Cheese Sauce,** 1 serving | 3 |
| **Heated Marinara Sauce,** 2 oz | 1 |
| **Hot Salsa Cheese,** 1 serving | 3 |
| **Light Cream Cheese,** 1 serving | 2 |
| **Sweet Dip,** 1 serving | 3 |
| **Sweet Mustard,** 1 1/4 oz | 2 |
| **DUTCH ICE®** | |
| **Blue Raspberry Dutch Ice®,** 14 fl oz | 4 |
| **Grape Dutch Ice®,** 14 fl oz | 5 |
| **Kiwi-Banana Dutch Ice®,** 14 fl oz | 5 |
| **Lemonade Dutch Ice®,** 14 fl oz | 8 |
| **Mocha Dutch Ice®,** 14 fl oz | 11 |
| **Orange Crème Dutch Ice®,** 14 fl oz | 7 |
| **Piña Colada Dutch Ice®,** 14 fl oz | 6 |
| **Strawberry Dutch Ice®,** 14 fl oz | 5 |
| **Strawberry Lemonade Dutch Ice®,** 14 fl oz | 9 |
| **Watermelon Dutch Ice®,** 14 fl oz | 5 |
| **Wild Cherry Dutch Ice®,** 14 fl oz | 5 |

| ▲ Power Foods | *PointsPlus*™ value |
|---|---|
| **BEVERAGES** | |
| **Blue Raspberry Dutch Smoothie,** 14 fl oz | 6 |
| **Caramel Dutch Latte™,** 14 fl oz | 10 |
| **Chocolate Dutch Shake,** 14 fl oz | 16 |
| **Coffee Dutch Latte™,** 14 fl oz | 8 |
| **Coffee Dutch Shake,** 14 fl oz | 16 |
| **Grape Dutch Smoothie,** 14 fl oz | 6 |
| **Kiwi-Banana Dutch Smoothie,** 14 fl oz | 6 |
| **Lemonade Dutch Smoothie,** 14 fl oz | 8 |
| **Mocha Dutch Latte™,** 14 fl oz | 10 |
| **Mocha Dutch Smoothie,** 14 fl oz | 9 |
| **Orange Crème Dutch Smoothie,** 14 fl oz | 7 |
| **Pina Colada Dutch Smoothie,** 14 fl oz | 7 |
| **Strawberry Dutch Shake,** 14 fl oz | 16 |
| **Strawberry Dutch Smoothie,** 14 fl oz | 7 |
| **Vanilla Dutch Shake,** 14 fl oz | 14 |
| **Wild Cherry Dutch Smoothie,** 14 fl oz | 7 |

# BACK YARD BURGERS

| ▲ Power Foods | *PointsPlus™* value |
|---|---|
| **CLASSIC BURGERS** | |
| **Back Yard Burger, 2/3 lb.,** 1 burger | 29 |
| **Back Yard American Cheeseburger, Jr.,** 1 burger | 16 |
| **Back Yard American Cheeseburger, 2/3 lb.,** 1 burger | 31 |
| **SPECIALTY BURGERS** | |
| **Back Yard Bleu Cheeseburger, Jr.,** 1 burger | 17 |
| **Back Yard Bleu Cheeseburger, 1/3 lb.,** 1 burger | 21 |
| **Back Yard Bleu Cheeseburger, 2/3 lb.,** 1 burger | 34 |
| **Back Yard Cheddar Cheeseburger, Jr.,** 1 burger | 17 |
| **Back Yard Cheddar Cheeseburger, 1/3 lb.,** 1 burger | 21 |
| **Back Yard Cheddar Cheeseburger, 2/3 lb.,** 1 burger | 35 |
| **Back Yard Pepper Jack Cheeseburger, Jr.,** 1 burger | 16 |
| **Back Yard Pepper Jack Cheeseburger,** 1/3 lb., 1 burger | 20 |
| **Back Yard Pepper Jack Cheeseburger,** 2/3 lb., 1 burger | 32 |
| **Back Yard Swiss Cheeseburger, Jr.,** 1 burger | 17 |
| **Back Yard Swiss Cheeseburger, 1/3 lb.,** 1 burger | 21 |
| **Back Yard Swiss Cheeseburger, 2/3 lb.,** 1 burger | 35 |
| **Bak-Pak Dog,** 1 | 9 |

| ▲ Power Foods | *PointsPlus™* value |
|---|---|
| **BACK YARD SPECIALTIES** | |
| **Back Yard Big Dog,** 1 serving | 13 |
| **Blackened Chicken,** 1 serving | 14 |
| **Chicken Tender Meal,** 1 meal | 34 |
| **Chili,** 1 serving | 4 |
| **Chili Cheese Big Dog,** 1 | 17 |
| **Crispy Chicken,** 1 serving | 16 |
| **Garden Veggie Burger,** 1 | 10 |
| **Grilled Chicken,** 1 serving | 9 |
| **Hawaiian Chicken,** 1 serving | 12 |
| **Kids Chicken Tender Meal,** 1 meal | 30 |
| **Tea, Sweetened,** 1 cup (20 oz) | 5 |
| **Tea, Sweetened,** 1 cup (32 oz) | 8 |
| **Tea, Unsweetened,** 1 cup | 0 |
| **CONDIMENTS** | |
| **Margarine Cup,** 1 serving | 2 |
| **Mayonnaise,** 1 packet | 3 |
| **Mayonnaise, light,** 1 packet | 1 |
| **BAKED POTATOES & FRENCH FRIES** | |
| **Seasoned Fries,** 1 large serving (9 oz) | 27 |
| **Texas Toothpicks,** 1 serving | 7 |
| **SALADS** | |
| **Fried Chicken Salad,** 1 salad | 11 |
| **Garden Fresh Salad,** 1 salad | 3 |
| **Grilled Chicken Salad,** 1 salad | 6 |
| ▲ **Side Salad,** 1 salad | 1 |

| ▲ Power Foods | *PointsPlus*™ value |
|---|---|
| **SALAD DRESSINGS** | |
| **Balsamic Vinaigrette,** 1 packet | 5 |
| **Bleu Cheese,** 1 serving | 6 |
| **Ranch, Lite,** 1 serving | 4 |
| **ICE CREAM** | |
| **Chocolate Shake,** 1 serving | 17 |
| **Ice Cream A La Carte,** 1 serving | 4 |
| **COBBLERS** | |
| **Apple Cobbler A la Mode,** 1 serving | 14 |
| **Blackberry Cobbler A La Mode,** 1 serving | 12 |
| **Cherry Cobbler A La Mode,** 1 serving | 14 |
| **Peach Cobbler A La Mode,** 1 serving | 13 |
| **Pecan Cobbler,** 1 serving | 20 |
| **Pecan Cobbler A La Mode,** 1 serving | 24 |
| **Strawberry Cobbler A La Mode,** 1 serving | 16 |
| **BEVERAGES** | |
| **Dr. Pepper, Diet,** 1 can (20 oz) | 0 |
| **Lemonade,** 1 cup (20 oz) | 14 |
| **Lemonade,** 1 cup (32 oz) | 23 |
| **Mountain Dew,** 1 can (20 oz) | 8 |
| **Mug Root Beer,** 1 can (20 oz) | 7 |
| **Pepsi,** 1 can (20 oz) | 8 |
| **Pepsi, Diet,** 1 can (20 oz) | 0 |
| **Sierra Mist,** 1 can (20 oz) | 7 |
| **Sobe Lean Cranberry Grapefruit,** 1 cup (20 oz) | 0 |
| **Tropical Fruit Punch,** 1 cup (20 oz) | 8 |

# BAJA FRESH MEXICAN GRILL

| ▲ Power Foods | *PointsPlus™* value |
|---|---|
| **BURRITOS (WITHOUT CHIPS & SOUR CREAM)** | |
| **Baja Burrito with Breaded Fish,** 1 serving | 23 |
| **Baja Burrito with Carnitas,** 1 serving | 22 |
| **Baja Burrito with Chicken,** 1 serving | 21 |
| **Baja Burrito with Mahi Mahi,** 1 serving | 21 |
| **Baja Burrito with Shrimp,** 1 serving | 20 |
| **Baja Burrito with Steak,** 1 serving | 23 |
| **Bare Burrito® with Carnitas,** 1 serving | 16 |
| **Bare Burrito® with Chicken,** 1 serving | 15 |
| **Bare Burrito® with Steak,** 1 serving | 17 |
| **Bare Burrito® with Veggie and Cheese,** 1 serving | 14 |
| **Bean and Cheese Burrito No Meat,** 1 serving | 21 |
| **Bean and Cheese Burrito with Breaded Fish,** 1 serving | 26 |
| **Bean and Cheese Burrito with Carnitas,** 1 serving | 25 |
| **Bean and Cheese Burrito with Chicken,** 1 serving | 24 |
| **Bean and Cheese Burrito with Mahi Mahi,** 1 serving | 24 |
| **Bean and Cheese Burrito with Shrimp,** 1 serving | 23 |
| **Bean and Cheese Burrito with Steak,** 1 serving | 26 |
| **Burrito "Dos Manos" with Charbroiled Chicken,** 1/2 | 19 |
| **Burrito "Dos Manos" with Charbroiled Steak,** 1/2 | 20 |
| **Burrito Mexicano with Breaded Fish,** 1 serving | 21 |
| **Burrito Mexicano with Carnitas,** 1 serving | 20 |
| **Burrito Mexicano with Chicken,** 1 serving | 19 |
| **Burrito Mexicano with Mahi Mahi,** 1 serving | 19 |
| **Burrito Mexicano with Shrimp,** 1 serving | 19 |
| **Burrito Mexicano with Steak,** 1 serving | 21 |
| **Burrito Ultimo® with Breaded Fish,** 1 serving | 24 |
| **Burrito Ultimo® with Carnitas,** 1 serving | 24 |
| **Burrito Ultimo® with Chicken,** 1 serving | 23 |
| **Burrito Ultimo® with Mahi Mahi,** 1 serving | 22 |
| **Burrito Ultimo® with Shrimp,** 1 serving | 22 |
| **Burrito Ultimo® with Steak,** 1 serving | 24 |
| **Chicken Fajita Burrito,** 1 | 23 |
| **Grilled Veggie Burrito,** 1 serving | 20 |
| **Salad Burrito Cabo Style,** 1 serving | 26 |
| **Salad Burrito Caesar Style,** 1 serving | 25 |
| **Steak Fajita Burrito,** 1 | 25 |
| **"Enchilado" Style Added to Any Burrito,** 1 serving | 17 |
| **"Enchilado" Style Added to Any Burrito "Dos Manos",** 1 serving | 17 |
| **TACOS** | |
| **Americano Soft Taco with Breaded Fish,** 1 serving | 6 |
| **Americano Soft Taco with Carnitas,** 1 serving | 6 |
| **Americano Soft Taco with Chicken,** 1 serving | 6 |
| **Americano Soft Taco with Mahi Mahi,** 1 serving | 6 |
| **Americano Soft Taco with Shrimp,** 1 serving | 6 |
| **Americano Soft Taco with Steak,** 1 serving | 7 |
| **Baja Fish Taco – Fried, with Breaded Fish,** 1 serving | 7 |
| **Grilled Mahi Mahi Taco,** 1 serving | 6 |

| ▲ Power Foods | *PointsPlus*™ value |
| --- | --- |
| **Original Baja Taco with Carnitas,** 1 serving | 6 |
| **Original Baja Taco with Chicken,** 1 serving | 5 |
| **Original Baja Taco with Shrimp,** 1 serving | 5 |
| **Original Baja Taco with Steak,** 1 serving | 6 |
| **Taco "Chilito" with Charbroiled Chicken,** 1 serving | 8 |
| **Taco "Chilito" with Charbroiled Steak,** 1 serving | 8 |

## TAQUITOS

| ▲ Power Foods | *PointsPlus*™ value |
| --- | --- |
| **Charbroiled Steak Taquitos with Beans,** 1 serving | 20 |
| **Charbroiled Steak Taquitos with Rice,** 1 serving | 20 |
| **Chicken Taquitos with Beans,** 1 serving | 20 |
| **Chicken Taquitos with Rice,** 1 serving | 20 |

## TOSTADAS

| ▲ Power Foods | *PointsPlus*™ value |
| --- | --- |
| **Tostada with Breaded Fish,** 1 serving | 30 |
| **Tostada with Charbroiled Chicken,** 1 serving | 28 |
| **Tostada with Charbroiled Fish,** 1 serving | 28 |
| **Tostada with Charbroiled Shrimp,** 1 serving | 28 |
| **Tostada with Charbroiled Steak,** 1 serving | 31 |
| **Tostada with Savory Pork Carnitas,** 1 serving | 29 |
| **Vegetarian Tostada (no meat),** 1 serving | 25 |

## FAJITAS

| ▲ Power Foods | *PointsPlus*™ value |
| --- | --- |
| **Breaded Fish Fajitas with Corn Tortillas,** 1 serving | 27 |
| **Breaded Fish Fajitas with Flour Tortillas,** 1 serving | 34 |
| **Breaded Fish Fajitas with Mixed Tortillas,** 1 serving | 32 |
| **Carnitas Fajitas with Corn Tortillas,** 1 serving | 23 |
| **Carnitas Fajitas with Flour Tortillas,** 1 serving | 31 |
| **Carnitas Fajitas with Mixed Tortillas,** 1 serving | 28 |
| **Chicken Fajitas with Corn Tortillas,** 1 serving | 21 |
| **Chicken Fajitas with Flour Tortillas,** 1 serving | 29 |
| **Chicken Fajitas with Mixed Tortillas,** 1 serving | 27 |
| **Mahi Mahi Fajitas with Corn Tortillas,** 1 serving | 21 |
| **Mahi Mahi Fajitas with Flour Tortillas,** 1 serving | 28 |
| **Mahi Mahi Fajitas with Mixed Tortillas,** 1 serving | 26 |
| **Shrimp Fajitas with Corn Tortillas,** 1 serving | 21 |
| **Shrimp Fajitas with Flour Tortillas,** 1 serving | 28 |
| **Shrimp Fajitas with Mixed Tortillas,** 1 serving | 26 |
| **Steak Fajitas with Corn Tortillas,** 1 serving | 24 |
| **Steak Fajitas with Flour Tortillas,** 1 serving | 32 |
| **Steak Fajitas with Mixed Tortillas,** 1 serving | 30 |

# BAJA FRESH MEXICAN GRILL

| ▲ Power Foods | *PointsPlus™* value |
|---|---|
| **MEXICAN FAVORITES (WITHOUT CHIPS)** | |
| **Mini Quesa-dita™ with Charbroiled Chicken,** 1 | 16 |
| **Mini Quesa-dita™ with Charbroiled Steak,** 1 | 17 |
| **Mini Quesa-dita™ with Cheese,** 1 | 15 |
| **Mini Tosta-dita™ with Charbroiled Chicken,** 1 | 14 |
| **Mini Tosta-dita™ with Charbroiled Steak,** 1 | 15 |
| **SPECIALTIES (WITHOUT CHIPS)** | |
| **Enchiladas Verdes with Charbroiled Chicken (without Sour Cream),** 1 serving | 19 |
| **Enchiladas Verdes with Cheese (without Sour Cream),** 1 serving | 21 |
| **Enchiladas with Charbroiled Chicken,** 1 serving | 19 |
| **Enchiladas with Charbroiled Steak,** 1 serving | 22 |
| **Enchiladas with Cheese,** 1 serving | 22 |
| **Vegetarian Enchiladas Verdes (without Sour Cream),** 1 serving | 18 |
| **Baja Ensalada Chicken™ (without salad dressing),** 1 serving | 7 |
| **Chicken Picado,** 1 serving | 16 |
| **Steak Picado,** 1 serving | 21 |
| **LIFESTYLE CHOICES (LIGHTER/LOW FAT)** | |
| **Baja Style Tacos - Chicken,** 1 serving | 5 |
| **Baja Style Tacos - Shrimp,** 1 serving | 5 |
| **Enchiladas Verano,** 1 serving | 14 |
| **Shrimp Ensalada,** 1 serving | 4 |
| **NACHOS** | |
| **Nachos with Breaded Fish,** 1 serving | 54 |
| **Nachos with Charbroiled Chicken,** 1 serving | 52 |
| **Nachos with Charbroiled Mahi Mahi,** 1 serving | 52 |
| **Nachos with Charbroiled Shrimp,** 1 serving | 51 |
| **Nachos with Charbroiled Steak,** 1 serving | 54 |
| **Nachos with Cheese,** 1 serving | 49 |
| **Nachos with Savory Pork Carnitas,** 1 serving | 53 |
| **TORTA** | |
| **Torta with Chips,** 1 serving | 24 |
| **Torta without Chips,** 1 serving | 16 |
| **QUESADILLA** | |
| **Quesadilla with Breaded Fish,** 1 serving | 38 |
| **Quesadilla with Charbroiled Mahi Mahi,** 1 serving | 35 |
| **Quesadilla with Charbroiled Shrimp,** 1 serving | 35 |
| **Quesadilla with Charbroiled Steak,** 1 serving | 38 |
| **Quesadilla with Charbroiled Chicken,** 1 serving | 36 |
| **Quesadilla with Cheese,** 1 serving | 33 |
| **Quesadilla with Savory Pork Carnitas,** 1 serving | 37 |
| **Vegetarian Quesadilla,** 1 serving | 34 |
| **KID'S FAVORITES** | |
| **Chicken Taquitos,** 1 serving | 16 |
| **Mini Bean & Cheese Burrito,** 1 serving | 13 |
| **Mini Bean & Cheese Burrito with Chicken,** 1 serving | 15 |
| **Mini Cheese Quesadilla,** 1 serving | 16 |
| **Mini Cheese Quesadilla with Chicken,** 1 serving | 17 |
| **Mini Nachos,** 1 serving | 18 |

# BAJA FRESH MEXICAN GRILL

▲ Power Foods — *PointsPlus™* value

## SALADS

|  | *PointsPlus™* value |
|---|---|
| **"Side-By-Side",** 1 serving | 13 |
| **Baja Ensalada® with Charbroiled Chicken,** 1 serving | 7 |
| **Baja Ensalada® with Charbroiled Shrimp,** 1 serving | 6 |
| **Baja Ensalada® with Charbroiled Steak,** 1 serving | 11 |
| **Baja Ensalada® with Savory Pork Carnitas,** 1 serving | 9 |
| **Baja Ensalada® with Charbroiled Fish (without salad dressing),** 1 serving | 9 |
| **Chile Lime Chicken Salad,** 1 serving | 15 |
| **Chipotle Glazed Charbroiled Chicken Salad,** 1 serving | 15 |
| **Fresh Mahi Mahi Ensalada Charbroiled Fish,** 1 serving | 9 |
| **Side Salad with a Side of Shrimp, Salsa Verde - no tortilla chips,** 1 serving | 5 |

## SALAD DRESSINGS

|  | *PointsPlus™* value |
|---|---|
| **Baja Dressing,** 2 oz | 9 |
| **Fat Free Salsa Verde Dressing,** 2 1/2 oz | 0 |
| **Olive Oil Vinaigrette,** 2 1/2 oz | 8 |
| **Ranch Dressing,** 2 1/2 oz | 7 |

## SOUPS

|  | *PointsPlus™* value |
|---|---|
| **Tortilla Soup (with charbroiled chicken),** 1 serving | 8 |
| **Tortilla Soup (without charbroiled chicken),** 1 serving | 7 |

## SIDE ORDERS

|  | *PointsPlus™* value |
|---|---|
| ▲ **Black Beans,** 1 serving | 7 |
| **Cebollitas,** 12 pieces | 1 |
| **Charbroiled Fish,** 6 1/2 oz | 5 |
| **Chips and Guacamole,** 1 serving | 37 |
| **Chips and Salsa Baja,** 1 serving | 20 |
| **Guacamole,** 1 serving (3 oz) | 4 |
| **Guacamole,** 1 serving (8 oz) | 11 |
| **Mini Tostada Shell,** 1 | 5 |
| **Onions, Peppers, & Chilies,** 1 serving | 2 |
| **Pico de Gallo,** 1 serving (8 oz) | 1 |
| ▲ **Pinto Beans,** 1 serving | 6 |
| **Pronto Guacamole™,** 1 serving | 15 |
| **Rice,** 1 serving | 7 |
| **Rice & Beans Plate,** 1 serving | 9 |
| **Salsa Baja,** 1 serving (8 oz) | 1 |
| **Salsa Roja,** 1 serving (8 oz) | 2 |
| **Salsa Verde,** 1 serving (8 oz) | 1 |
| **Side Breaded Fish,** 1 serving | 10 |
| **Side Carnitas,** 1 serving | 8 |
| **Side Chicken,** 1 serving | 5 |
| **Side Corn Tortilla Chips,** 1 serving (5 oz) | 19 |
| ▲ **Side Mahi Mahi,** 1 serving | 5 |
| **Side Salad,** 1 serving | 3 |
| ▲ **Side Shrimp,** 1 serving | 3 |
| **Side Steak,** 1 serving | 8 |
| **Sour Cream,** 1 serving | 2 |
| **Tostada Shell,** 1 serving | 12 |
| ▲ **Veggie Mix (grilled peppers, chilies and onions),** 1 serving | 2 |

## TORTILLAS

|  | *PointsPlus™* value |
|---|---|
| **Corn Tortilla (with oil),** 2 | 4 |
| **Corn Tortilla Strips,** 1 serving | 4 |
| **Flour Tortilla 12-13 inches,** 1 | 9 |
| **Flour Tortilla 8-inch,** 4 | 14 |
| **Flour Tortilla 8-inch,** 4 | 14 |
| **Fresh Corn Tortilla,** 5 | 10 |

## DESSERT

|  | *PointsPlus™* value |
|---|---|
| **Churros,** 1 serving | 9 |

# BASKIN-ROBBINS®

| ▲ Power Foods | *PointsPlus*™ value |
|---|---|
| **BRight Choices®** | |
| **Lemon Sorbet,** 1 small scoop (2 1/2 oz) | 2 |
| **Mango Sorbet,** 1 small scoop (2 1/2 oz) | 2 |
| **Premium Churned Light Aloha Brownie Ice Cream,** 1 small scoop (2 1/2 oz) | 4 |
| **Premium Churned Light Cappuccino Chip Ice Cream,** 1 small scoop (2 1/2 oz) | 4 |
| **Premium Churned Light Milk Chocolate Ice Cream,** 1 scoop (4 oz) | 6 |
| **Premium Churned Light Raspberry Chip Ice Cream,** 1 scoop (4 oz) | 6 |
| **Premium Churned Light Vanilla Ice Cream,** 1 scoop (4 oz) | 6 |
| **Premium Churned Reduced Fat, No Sugar Added Cabana Berry Banana,** 1 small scoop (2 1/2 oz) | 3 |
| **Premium Churned Reduced-Fat, No Sugar Added Caramel Turtle Truffle Ice Cream,** 1 small scoop (2 1/2 oz) | 4 |
| **Premium Churned Reduced-Fat, No Sugar Added Chocolate Overload Ice Cream,** 1 small scoop (2 1/2 oz) | 3 |
| **ICE CREAM** | |
| **America's Birthday Cake Ice Cream,** 1 scoop (4 oz) | 8 |
| **Apple Pie a la Mode Ice Cream,** 1 scoop (4 oz) | 7 |
| **Banana Nut Ice Cream,** 1 scoop (4 oz) | 7 |
| **Bananas 'n Strawberries Ice Cream,** 1 scoop (4 oz) | 7 |
| **Baseball Nut® Ice Cream,** 1 scoop (4 oz) | 8 |
| **Black Walnut Ice Cream,** 1 scoop (4 oz) | 8 |
| **Cherries Jubilee,** 1 scoop (4 oz) | 7 |
| **Chocolate,** 1 scoop (4 oz) | 8 |
| **Chocolate Almond Ice Cream,** 1 scoop (4 oz) | 9 |
| **Chocolate Chip,** 1 scoop (4 oz) | 8 |
| **Chocolate Chip Cookie Dough,** 1 scoop (4 oz) | 8 |
| **Chocolate Fudge,** 1 scoop (4 oz) | 8 |
| **Chocolate Mousse Royale® Ice Cream,** 1 scoop (4 oz) | 9 |
| **Chocolate Oreo® Ice Cream,** 1 scoop (4 oz) | 10 |
| **Cotton Candy Ice Cream,** 1 scoop (4 oz) | 7 |
| **French Vanilla,** 1 scoop (4 oz) | 8 |
| **Fudge Brownie Ice Cream,** 1 scoop (4 oz) | 9 |
| **German Chocolate Cake Ice Cream,** 1 scoop (4 oz) | 9 |
| **GOLD MEDAL RIBBON™,** 1 scoop (4 oz) | 7 |
| **Icing on the Cake Ice Cream,** 1 scoop (4 oz) | 8 |
| **JAMOCA®,** 1 scoop (4 oz) | 7 |
| **JAMOCA® Almond Fudge,** 1 scoop (4 oz) | 8 |
| **JAMOCA ® Oreo® Ice Cream,** 1 small scoop (2 1/2 oz) | 7 |
| **Lemon Custard Ice Cream,** 1 scoop (4 oz) | 7 |
| **Love Potion #31® Ice Cream,** 1 scoop (4 oz) | 7 |
| **Made with Snickers® Ice Cream,** 1 scoop (4 oz) | 7 |
| **Makin' Cookies Ice Cream,** 1 scoop (4 oz) | 8 |
| **Mint Chocolate Chip,** 1 scoop (4 oz) | 8 |
| **Mississippi Mud Ice Cream,** 1 scoop (4 oz) | 8 |
| **New York Cheesecake Ice Cream,** 1 scoop (4 oz) | 8 |

| ▲ Power Foods | *PointsPlus™* value |
| --- | --- |
| **Old Fashioned Butter Pecan,** 1 scoop (4 oz) | 8 |
| **Oregon Blackberry Ice Cream,** 1 scoop (4 oz) | 6 |
| **OREO® Cookies 'N Cream,** 1 scoop (4 oz) | 8 |
| **Peanut Butter 'N Chocolate,** 1 scoop (4 oz) | 9 |
| **Pink Bubblegum Ice Cream,** 1 scoop (4 oz) | 7 |
| **Pistachio Almond,** 1 scoop (4 oz) | 8 |
| **Pralines 'N Cream,** 1 scoop (4 oz) | 8 |
| **Quarterback Crunch® Ice Cream,** 1 scoop (4 oz) | 7 |
| **Reese's® Peanut Butter Cup Ice Cream,** 1 scoop (4 oz) | 9 |
| **Rock 'n Pop Swirl Sherbet,** 1 scoop (4 oz) | 5 |
| **Rocky Road,** 1 scoop (4 oz) | 8 |
| **Rum Raisin Ice Cream,** 1 scoop (4 oz) | 7 |
| **Splish Splash Sherbet,** 1 scoop (4 oz) | 4 |
| **Strawberry Cheesecake Ice Cream,** 1 scoop (4 oz) | 8 |
| **Strawberry Shortcake Ice Cream,** 1 scoop (4 oz) | 8 |
| **Tax Crunch® Ice Cream,** 1 scoop (4 oz) | 8 |
| **Tiramisu Ice Cream,** 1 scoop (4 oz) | 6 |
| **Tropical Ice,** 1 scoop (4 oz) | 4 |
| **Vanilla,** 1 scoop (4 oz) | 7 |
| **Very Berry Strawberry,** 1 scoop (4 oz) | 6 |
| **Wild 'n Reckless Sherbet,** 1 scoop (4 oz) | 4 |
| **Winter White Chocolate® Ice Cream,** 1 scoop (4 oz) | 6 |
| **WORLD CLASS® Chocolate,** 1 scoop (4 oz) | 8 |
| **York® Peppermint Pattie Ice Cream,** 1 scoop (4 oz) | 9 |

| ▲ Power Foods | *PointsPlus™* value |
| --- | --- |
| **CONES** | |
| **Cake Cone,** 1 cone | 1 |
| **Sugar Cone,** 1 cone | 1 |
| **Waffle Cone,** 1 cone | 4 |
| **FRUIT BLAST BARS** | |
| **Blue Raspberry Fruit Blast Bar,** 1 | 2 |
| **Mango Fruit Blast Bar,** 1 | 2 |
| **Strawberry Fruit Blast Bar,** 1 | 1 |
| **GRAB-N-GO** | |
| **Pralines 'n Cream Sundae Cup,** 1 | 8 |
| **Reese's® Peanut Butter Cup Sundae Cup,** 1 | 9 |
| **ICES, SHERBETS, SORBETS, FROZEN FRUIT BARS** | |
| **Daiquiri Ice,** 1 scoop (4 oz) | 4 |
| **Orange Sherbet,** 1 scoop (4 oz) | 4 |
| **Rainbow Sherbet,** 1 scoop (4 oz) | 4 |
| **SUNDAES** | |
| **Banana Royale Sundae,** 1 serving | 18 |
| **Brownie Sundae,** 1 serving | 25 |
| **Classic Banana Split,** 1 serving | 27 |
| **BEVERAGES** | |
| **Cappuccino Blast® Caramel,** 1 medium | 20 |
| **Cappuccino Blast® Mocha,** 1 small | 10 |
| **Cappuccino Blast® Nonfat,** 1 small | 6 |
| **Cappuccino Blast®, Original,** 1 small | 8 |
| **Chocolate Shake with Chocolate Ice Cream,** 1 small | 18 |

*Beverages (cont'd)*

| ▲ Power Foods | *PointsPlus*™ value |
|---|---|
| **Chocolate Shake with Premium Churned Milk Chocolate Ice Cream,** 1 medium | 17 |
| **Chocolate Shake with Vanilla Ice Cream,** 1 small | 19 |
| **Freeze with Orange Sherbet,** 1 small | 10 |
| **Ice Cream Float with Vanilla Ice Cream & Root Beer,** 1 small | 13 |
| **Mango Fruit Blast Smoothie,** 1 small | 12 |
| **Mint Chocolate Chip Shake,** 1 small | 21 |
| **Oreo® 'n Cookies Cappuccino Blast®,** 1 small | 15 |
| **Peach Passion Fruit Blast Smoothie,** 1 small | 12 |
| **Strawberry Shake with Very Berry Strawberry Ice Cream,** 1 small | 13 |
| **Vanilla Shake,** 1 small | 18 |
| **Vanilla Shake with Premium Churned Light Vanilla Ice Cream,** 1 medium | 22 |
| **Wild Mango Fruit Blast,** 1 small | 9 |

▲ Power Foods — *PointsPlus*™ value

## MEATS

| Item | PointsPlus value |
|---|---|
| **Chicken,** 1 serving (3 oz) | 3 |
| **Fajita Marinated Chicken,** 1 serving (3 oz) | 2 |
| ▲ **Lamb,** 1 serving (3 oz) | 3 |
| ▲ **NY Strip,** 1 serving (3 oz) | 2 |
| ▲ **Pork,** 1 serving (3 oz) | 3 |
| ▲ **Ribeye,** 1 serving (3 oz) | 3 |
| **Sausage,** 1 serving (3 oz) | 8 |
| ▲ **Turkey,** 1 serving (3 oz) | 3 |

## SEAFOOD

| Item | PointsPlus value |
|---|---|
| ▲ **Calamari,** 1 serving (3 oz) | 2 |
| ▲ **Cod,** 1 serving (3 oz) | 2 |
| ▲ **Crawfish,** 1 serving (3 oz) | 2 |
| ▲ **Krab (Surimi),** 1 serving (3 oz) | 2 |
| **Salmon,** 1 serving (3 oz) | 4 |
| ▲ **Scallops,** 1 serving (3 oz) | 2 |
| ▲ **Shrimp,** 1 serving (3 oz) | 1 |
| ▲ **Tuna,** 1 serving (3 oz) | 3 |

## NOODLES & RICE

| Item | PointsPlus value |
|---|---|
| **Lo Mein,** 1 serving (2 oz) | 4 |
| **Pasta,** 1 serving (2 oz) | 5 |
| **Rice,** 3/4 cup | 4 |

## SALAD FIXINGS

| Item | PointsPlus value |
|---|---|
| ▲ **Artichoke,** 1 serving | 0 |
| ▲ **Bean Sprouts,** 1 serving | 0 |
| ▲ **Beets,** 1 serving | 0 |
| **Black Olives,** 1 serving | 1 |
| ▲ **Celery,** 1 serving | 0 |
| **Cheddar Cheese,** 1 serving | 3 |
| ▲ **Cucumbers,** 1 serving | 0 |
| ▲ **Head Lettuce,** 1 serving | 0 |
| ▲ **Iceberg Lettuce,** 1 serving | 0 |
| ▲ **Lemons,** 1 wedge | 0 |
| ▲ **Limes,** 1 wedge | 0 |
| ▲ **Mushrooms,** 1 serving | 0 |
| ▲ **Pineapple,** 1 serving | 0 |
| ▲ **Romaine lettuce,** 1 serving | 0 |

## SALAD DRESSINGS

| Item | PointsPlus value |
|---|---|
| **Balsamic Vinaigrette,** 1 serving (1 oz) | 2 |
| **Blue Cheese,** 1 serving (1 oz) | 5 |
| **Caesar,** 1 serving (1 oz) | 7 |
| **Fat Free French,** 1 serving (1 oz) | 1 |
| **Greek Feta,** 1 serving (1 oz) | 2 |
| **Honey Mustard,** 1 serving (1 oz) | 5 |
| **Raspberry Vinaigrette,** 1 serving (1 oz) | 1 |

## SOUPS

| Item | PointsPlus value |
|---|---|
| **Chicken Noodle,** 1 serving (8 oz) | 2 |
| **Chicken Tortilla Soup,** 1 serving (8 oz) | 3 |
| **Clam Chowder,** 1 serving (8 oz) | 5 |
| **Country Potato,** 1 serving (8 oz) | 6 |
| **Hearty Vegetable,** 1 serving (8 oz) | 3 |
| **Hot and Sour,** 1 serving (8 oz) | 2 |
| **Mangia Mangia Mushroom,** 1 serving (8 oz) | 6 |

## VEGETABLES

| Item | PointsPlus value |
|---|---|
| ▲ **Bok choy,** 1 serving | 0 |
| ▲ **Broccoli,** 1 serving | 0 |
| ▲ **Cabbage (green),** 1 serving | 0 |
| ▲ **Cabbage (red),** 1 serving | 0 |
| ▲ **Carrots,** 1 serving | 0 |
| **Cilantro,** 1 tsp | 0 |
| ▲ **Corn (baby),** 1 serving | 0 |
| ▲ **Onions (yellow),** 1 serving | 0 |
| ▲ **Pea Pods,** 1 serving | 1 |
| ▲ **Peppers (green),** 1 serving | 0 |

*Vegetables (cont'd)*

| ▲ Power Foods | ***PointsPlus***™ value |
|---|---|
| ▲ **Peppers (red),** 1 serving | 0 |
| ▲ **Water Chestnuts,** 1 serving | 0 |

## SAUCES

| | |
|---|---|
| **Asian Black Bean,** 1 serving (1 oz) | 1 |
| **Barbeque,** 1 serving (1 oz) | 1 |
| **Chili Garlic,** 1 serving (1 oz) | 1 |
| **Fajita,** 1 serving (1 oz) | 1 |
| **Kung Pao,** 1 serving (1 oz) | 1 |
| **Lemon,** 1 serving (1 oz) | 1 |
| **Lite Soy,** 1 serving (1 oz) | 0 |
| **Mongo Marinara,** 1 serving (1 oz) | 0 |
| **Mongolian Ginger,** 1 serving (1 oz) | 1 |
| **Peanut,** 1 serving (1 oz) | 3 |
| **Sesame Oil,** 1 serving (1/2 oz) | 4 |
| **Shiitake Mushroom,** 1 serving (1 oz) | 1 |
| **Spicy Buffalo,** 1 serving (1 oz) | 1 |
| **Sweet & Sour,** 1 serving (1 oz) | 1 |
| **Sweet Orange Peel Sauce,** 1 serving (1 oz) | 2 |
| **Teriyaki,** 1 serving (1 oz) | 1 |

## TORTILLA

| | |
|---|---|
| **Tortilla,** 1 | 2 |

## LIMITED TIME OFFERINGS

| | |
|---|---|
| **Alfredo Sauce,** 1 serving (1 oz) | 1 |
| **Grated Parmesan,** 1 tsp | 0 |
| **Italian Sausage,** 1 serving (3 oz) | 8 |
| **Meatball,** 6 meatballs | 7 |
| **Tomato Bisque,** 1 serving (8 oz) | 9 |

## bd's MINI DESSERTS

| | |
|---|---|
| **Cheesecake Mini,** 1 | 6 |
| **Cookies and Cream Mini,** 1 | 6 |
| **Peanut Butter Cup Mini,** 1 | 11 |

▲ Power Foods | *PointsPlus*™ value

## CLASSIC TART SOFT SERVE

|  | *PointsPlus*™ value |
|---|---|
| **Berrylicious,** 16 fl oz | 7 |
| **Black 'n Blue,** 16 fl oz | 7 |
| **Mango Tango,** 16 fl oz | 8 |
| **Mangolada,** 16 fl oz | 8 |
| **Mondo Mango,** 16 fl oz | 7 |
| **Peach Palm,** 16 fl oz | 8 |
| **Pina Paradise,** 16 fl oz | 8 |
| **Pomegranate Berry Blue,** 16 fl oz | 6 |
| **Pomegranate Berry Red,** 16 fl oz | 6 |
| **Purely Peach,** 16 fl oz | 7 |
| **Straight-Up Strawberry,** 16 fl oz | 7 |
| **Strawberry Bananza,** 16 fl oz | 8 |
| **Strawberry Fling,** 16 fl oz | 8 |

## GOLDEN VANILLA SOFT SERVE

|  | *PointsPlus*™ value |
|---|---|
| **Berrylicious,** 16 fl oz | 7 |
| **Black 'n Blue,** 16 fl oz | 7 |
| **Mango Tango,** 16 fl oz | 9 |
| **Mangolada,** 1/2 cup | 9 |
| **Mondo Mango,** 16 fl oz | 8 |
| **Peach Palm,** 16 fl oz | 8 |
| **Pina Paradise,** 16 fl oz | 9 |
| **Pink Pineapple,** 16 fl oz | 9 |
| **Pomegranate Berry Blue,** 16 fl oz | 6 |
| **Pomegranate Berry Red,** 16 fl oz | 6 |
| **Purely Peach,** 16 fl oz | 7 |
| **Straight-Up Strawberry,** 16 fl oz | 7 |
| **Strawberry Bananza,** 16 fl oz | 8 |
| **Strawberry Fling,** 16 fl oz | 9 |

▲ Power Foods | *PointsPlus*™ value

## VANILLA BEAN HAND SCOOPED

|  | *PointsPlus*™ value |
|---|---|
| **Berrylicious,** 16 fl oz | 8 |
| **Black 'n Blue,** 16 fl oz | 8 |
| **Mango Tango,** 16 fl oz | 9 |
| **Mangolada,** 16 fl oz | 9 |
| **Mondo Mango,** 16 fl oz | 8 |
| **Peach Palm,** 16 fl oz | 9 |
| **Pina Paradise,** 16 fl oz | 9 |
| **Pink Pineapple,** 16 fl oz | 9 |
| **Pomegranate Berry Blue,** 16 fl oz | 7 |
| **Pomegranate Berry Red,** 16 fl oz | 7 |
| **Purely Peach,** 16 fl oz | 8 |
| **Straight-Up Strawberry,** 16 fl oz | 8 |
| **Strawberry Bananza,** 16 fl oz | 9 |
| **Strawberry Fling,** 16 fl oz | 9 |

# BILL MILLER BAR-B-Q

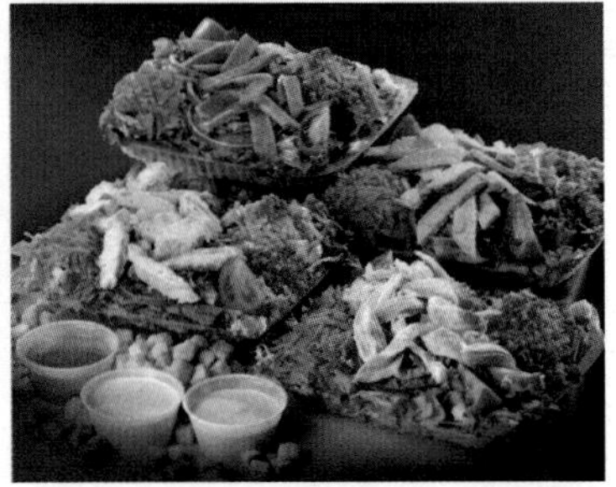

| ▲ Power Foods | *PointsPlus™* value |
|---|---|
| **SOUP & SALADS** | |
| **Bacon Bits,** 1 scoop | 1 |
| **Captain's Wafers,** 1 packet | 1 |
| **Cheddar Cheese,** 1 scoop | 1 |
| **Fat Free Ranch,** 1 packet | 1 |
| **Italian Dressing,** 1 container | 10 |
| **Ranch Dressing,** 1 container | 13 |
| **Salad De-Lite,** 1 container | 1 |
| **Thousand Island Dressing,** 1 container | 7 |
| **Vegetable Beef Soup,** 1 pint | 4 |

| ▲ Power Foods | *PointsPlus™* value |
|---|---|
| **ENTRÉES** | |
| **Bar-B-Q Chicken, Dark Meat, Skinless,** 1/4 chicken | 7 |
| ▲ **Bar-B-Q Chicken, White Meat, Skinless,** 1/4 chicken | 4 |
| ▲ **Bar-B-Q Turkey Breast,** 1 serving (3 oz) | 3 |
| **Ham,** 1 serving (3 oz) | 3 |
| **Turkey Poor Boy,** 1 | 10 |
| **SIDES** | |
| **Coleslaw,** 1 serving | 3 |
| **Fruit Salad,** 1 pint | 5 |
| ▲ **Green Beans,** 1 serving | 1 |
| **DESSERT** | |
| **Sugar Free Lemon Pie,** 1 slice | 9 |

▲ Power Foods — *PointsPlus*™ value

## SANDWICHES

| Item | *PointsPlus*™ value |
|---|---|
| **Blimpie Best,** 1 (4") | 7 |
| **Blimpie Best,** 1 (6") | 11 |
| **Blimpie Best (super stacked),** 1 (6") | 14 |
| **Blimpie Trio (super stacked),** 1 (6") | 12 |
| **BLT (super stacked),** 1 (6") | 17 |
| **BLT Sub,** 1 (6") | 9 |
| **Chicken Cheddar Bacon Ranch,** 1 (6") | 17 |
| **Chicken Teriyaki,** 1 (6") | 11 |
| **Ciabatta, Buffalo Chicken,** 1 | 15 |
| **Ciabatta, Grilled Chicken Caesar,** 1 | 16 |
| **Ciabatta, Mediterranean,** 1 | 11 |
| **Ciabatta, Roast Beef, Turkey & Cheddar,** 1 | 16 |
| **Ciabatta, Sicilian,** 1 | 17 |
| **Ciabatta, Turkey Italiano,** 1 | 12 |
| **Ciabatta, Tuscan,** 1 | 15 |
| **Ciabatta, Ultimate Club,** 1 | 13 |
| **Club,** 1 (4") | 6 |
| **Club,** 1 (6") | 10 |
| **Cuban,** 1 (6") | 10 |
| **French Dip,** 1 (6") | 10 |
| **Ham & Swiss,** 1 (4") | 6 |
| **Ham & Swiss,** 1 (6") | 10 |
| **Ham, Salami & Cheese,** 1 (6") | 11 |
| **Hot Pastrami,** 1 (6") | 11 |
| **Hot Pastrami (super stacked),** 1 (6") | 15 |
| **Meatball,** 1 (6") | 16 |
| **Philly Steak & Onion,** 1 (6") | 13 |
| **Reuben,** 1 (6") | 15 |
| **Roast Beef & Provolone,** 1 (4") | 7 |
| **Roast Beef & Provolone,** 1 (6") | 11 |
| **Roast Beef, Turkey & Cheddar,** 1 (6") | 15 |
| **Seafood,** 1 (6") | 9 |

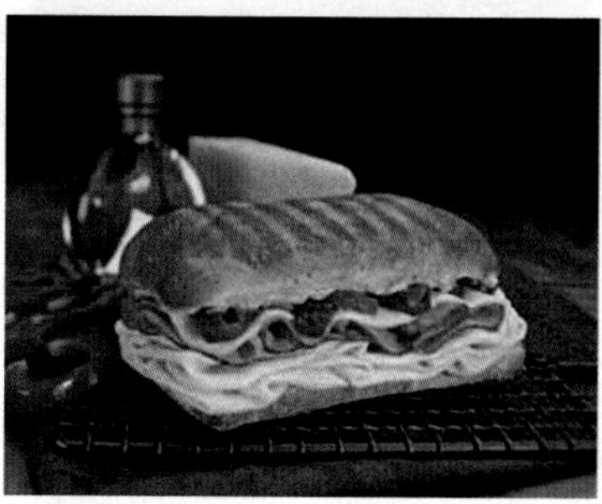

▲ Power Foods — *PointsPlus*™ value

| Item | *PointsPlus*™ value |
|---|---|
| **Special Vegetarian,** 1 (6") | 16 |
| **Tuna,** 1 (4") | 7 |
| **Tuna,** 1 (6") | 12 |
| **Turkey & Avocado,** 1 (6") | 10 |
| **Turkey & Provolone,** 1 (4") | 6 |
| **Turkey & Provolone,** 1 (6") | 10 |
| **Turkey and Bacon (super stacked),** 1 (6") | 15 |
| **Turkey and Cranberry,** 1 (6") | 9 |
| **Veggie Supreme,** 1 (6") | 15 |
| **VegiMax™ (on white roll, with cheese, lettuce, tomato & onion),** 1 (6") | 13 |

## WRAPS

| Item | *PointsPlus*™ value |
|---|---|
| **Chicken Caesar Wrap,** 1 | 16 |
| **Roast Beef & Cheddar Wrap,** 1 | 18 |
| **Southwestern Wrap,** 1 | 14 |
| **Steak & Onion Wrap,** 1 | 21 |
| **Zesty Wrap,** 1 | 15 |

## SALADS

| Item | *PointsPlus*™ value |
|---|---|
| **Antipasto Salad,** 1 serving | 6 |
| **Buffalo Chicken Salad,** 1 regular serving | 5 |

*Salads (cont'd)*

| ▲ Power Foods | *PointsPlus*™ value |
|---|---|
| **Chef Salad,** 1 serving | 4 |
| **Chicken Caesar Salad,** 1 serving | 5 |
| ▲ **Garden Salad,** 1 regular serving | 1 |
| **Northwest Potato Salad,** 1 regular serving | 7 |
| **Seafood Salad,** 1 regular serving | 3 |
| **Tuna Salad,** 1 serving | 7 |
| **Ultimate Club Salad,** 1 serving | 7 |

## SALAD DRESSINGS

| | |
|---|---|
| **Bleu Cheese Dressing,** 1 serving | 7 |
| **Buttermilk Ranch Dressing,** 1 serving | 6 |
| **Creamy Caesar Dressing,** 1 serving | 6 |
| **Creamy Italian Dressing,** 1 serving | 4 |
| **Dijon Honey Mustard Dressing,** 1 serving | 5 |
| **Fat Free Italian Dressing,** 1 serving | 1 |
| **Light Buttermilk Ranch Dressing,** 1 serving | 2 |
| **Lite Italian Dressing,** 1 serving | 0 |
| **Peppercorn Dressing,** 1 serving | 7 |
| **Thousand Island Dressing,** 1 serving | 6 |

## SOUPS

| ▲ Power Foods | *PointsPlus*™ value |
|---|---|
| **Bean with Ham Soup,** 1 serving | 3 |
| **Beef Steak & Noodle Soup,** 1 serving | 3 |
| **Beef Stew,** 1 serving | 4 |
| **Captain's Corn Chowder,** 1 serving | 5 |
| **Chicken & Dumplings Soup,** 1 serving | 4 |
| **Chicken Gumbo,** 1 serving | 2 |
| **Chicken Noodle Soup,** 1 serving | 3 |
| **Chicken Soup with White & Wild Rice,** 1 serving | 5 |
| **Cream of Broccoli with Cheese,** 1 serving | 4 |
| **Cream of Potato Soup,** 1 serving | 5 |
| **French Onion Soup,** 1 serving | 2 |
| **Grande Chili with Beans & Beef,** 1 serving | 6 |
| **Harvest Vegetable Soup,** 1 serving | 2 |
| **Italian Style Wedding Soup,** 1 serving | 4 |
| **Minestrone Soup,** 1 serving | 2 |
| **New England Clam Chowder,** 1 serving | 4 |
| **Pasta Fagioli with Sausage Soup,** 1 serving | 4 |
| **Pilgrim Turkey Vegetables with Rice Soup,** 1 serving | 3 |
| **Potato Salad,** 1 serving | 6 |
| **Seafood Gumbo,** 1 serving | 2 |
| **Split Pea with Ham Soup,** 1 serving | 3 |
| **Tomato Basil with Raviolini,** 1 serving | 3 |
| **Yankee Pot Roast Soup,** 1 serving | 2 |

## SIDES

| | |
|---|---|
| **American Cheese,** 1 serving | 3 |
| **Cole Slaw,** 1 serving | 4 |
| **Macaroni Salad,** 1 serving | 9 |
| **Mild Cheddar Cheese Shredded,** 1 serving | 3 |
| **Parmesan Cheese Shredded,** 1 serving | 2 |

## BREAKFAST ITEMS

| | |
|---|---|
| **Bacon, Egg & Cheese Biscuit,** 1 | 12 |
| **Bacon, Egg & Cheese Bluffin,** 1 | 8 |
| **Bacon, Egg & Cheese Burrito,** 1 | 15 |
| **Bacon, Egg & Cheese Croissant,** 1 | 34 |
| **Breakfast Panini,** 1 (6") | 20 |
| **Breakfast Panini,** 1 (4") | 13 |
| **Cinnamon Roll,** 1 | 12 |
| **Egg & Cheese Biscuit,** 1 | 11 |
| **Egg & Cheese Bluffin,** 1 | 7 |
| **Egg & Cheese Burrito,** 1 | 13 |

| ▲ Power Foods | *PointsPlus™* value |
|---|---|
| **Egg & Cheese Croissant,** 1 | 33 |
| **Ham, Egg & Cheese Biscuit,** 1 | 11 |
| **Ham, Egg & Cheese Bluffin,** 1 | 7 |
| **Ham, Egg & Cheese Burrito,** 1 | 15 |
| **Ham, Egg & Cheese Croissant,** 1 | 34 |
| **Plain Biscuit,** 1 | 7 |
| **Plain Bluffin,** 1 | 3 |
| **Plain Croissant,** 1 | 30 |
| **Sausage, Egg & Cheese Biscuit,** 1 | 15 |
| **Sausage, Egg & Cheese Bluffin,** 1 | 11 |
| **Sausage, Egg & Cheese Burrito,** 1 | 18 |
| **Sausage, Egg & Cheese Croissant,** 1 | 37 |

## KID'S MEALS

| | |
|---|---|
| **Ham & American Cheese,** 1 (3") | 7 |
| **Tuna,** 1 (3") | 7 |
| **Turkey,** 1 (3") | 5 |

## BREAD & WRAPS

| | |
|---|---|
| **Cheddar Jalapeno Bread,** 1 | 6 |
| **Ciabatta Bread,** 1 | 6 |
| **Honey Oat Bread,** 1 | 7 |
| **Marbled Rye Bread,** 1 | 6 |
| **Spinach Herb Wrap,** 1 (12") | 8 |
| **Traditional Wrap,** 1 (12") | 8 |
| **Wheat Roll,** 1 (6") | 5 |
| **White Roll,** 1 (6") | 6 |
| **Zesty Parmesan Roll,** 1 (6") | 6 |

## CHEESE

| | |
|---|---|
| **Cheddar Cheese,** 1 slice | 2 |
| **Pepper Jack Cheese,** 1 slice | 2 |
| **Provolone Cheese,** 1 slice | 2 |
| **Swiss Cheese,** 1 slice | 2 |

## TOPPINGS, SAUCES & DRESSINGS

| ▲ Power Foods | *PointsPlus™* value |
|---|---|
| **Deli Style Mustard,** 1 serving | 0 |
| **Guacamole,** 1 serving | 1 |
| **Honey Mustard,** 1 serving | 1 |
| ▲ **Hot Ring Peppers,** 12 pieces | 0 |
| ▲ **Jalapeno Peppers,** 18 pieces | 0 |
| ▲ **Lettuce,** 1 serving | 0 |
| **Mayonnaise,** 1 serving | 6 |
| **Oil Blend,** 1 serving | 4 |
| **Olives,** 1 serving | 1 |
| ▲ **Onion,** 3 pieces | 0 |
| **Red Hot Sauce, Original,** 1 serving | 0 |
| **Red Wine Vinegar,** 1 serving | 0 |
| ▲ **Roasted Red Peppers,** 1 serving | 0 |
| **Special Dressing,** 1 serving | 2 |
| **Spicy Brown Mustard,** 1 serving | 0 |
| ▲ **Sweet Pepper Strips,** 6 pieces | 0 |
| ▲ **Tomato,** 2 pieces | 0 |

## DESSERTS

| | |
|---|---|
| **Apple Turnover,** 1 | 9 |
| **Brownie,** 1 | 5 |
| **Cherry Turnover,** 1 | 9 |
| **Chocolate Chunk Cookie,** 1 | 5 |
| **Oatmeal Raisin Cookie,** 1 | 5 |
| **Peanut Butter Cookie,** 1 | 5 |
| **Sugar Cookie,** 1 | 9 |
| **White Chocolate Macadamia Nut Cookie,** 1 | 5 |

# BOB EVANS®

| ▲ Power Foods | *PointsPlus™* value |
|---|---|

## SALADS

| Item | *PointsPlus™* value |
|---|---|
| **Chili and Cheese Taco Salad,** 1 serving | 25 |
| **Chili and Cheese Taco Salad (Savor Size),** 1 serving | 20 |
| **Cobb Salad,** 1 salad | 13 |
| **Cobb Salad (Savor Size),** 1 salad portion | 10 |
| **Country Caesar Salad,** 1 salad | 20 |
| **Country Caesar Salad (Savor Size),** 1 salad | 15 |
| **Country Spinach Salad,** 1 salad | 11 |
| **Country Spinach Salad (Savor Size),** 1 salad | 10 |
| **Cranberry Pecan Chicken Salad,** 1 salad | 17 |
| **Cranberry Pecan Chicken Salad (Savor Size),** 1 salad | 18 |
| **Garden Salad,** 1 salad | 1 |
| **Heritage Chef Salad,** 1 salad | 10 |
| **Heritage Chef Salad (Savor Size),** 1 salad | 8 |
| **Specialty Garden Salad,** 1 salad | 3 |
| **Wildfire Fried Chicken Salad,** 1 salad | 19 |
| **Wildfire Fried Chicken Salad (Savor Size),** 1 salad | 15 |
| **Wildfire Grilled Chicken Salad,** 1 salad | 10 |
| **Wildfire Grilled Chicken Salad (Savor Size),** 1 serving | 14 |

## SALAD DRESSINGS

| Item | *PointsPlus™* value |
|---|---|
| **Avocado Ranch Dressing,** 1 side portion | 6 |
| **Bleu Cheese Dressing,** 6 Tbsp | 13 |
| **Blue Cheese Dressing,** 1 side portion | 7 |
| **Blue Cheese Dressings,** 1 dinner portion | 12 |
| **Buttermilk Ranch Dressing,** 1 dinner portion | 8 |
| **Buttermilk Ranch Dressing,** 1 side portion | 5 |
| **Caesar Dressing,** 1 dinner portion | 12 |
| **Caesar Dressing,** 1 side serving | 7 |
| **Colonial Dressing,** 1 dinner portion | 12 |
| **Colonial Dressing,** 1 side portion | 7 |
| **French Dressing,** 1 dinner portion | 12 |
| **French Dressing,** 1 side portion | 7 |
| **Honey Mustard Dressing,** 1 dinner portion | 10 |
| **Honey Mustard Dressing,** 1 side portion | 6 |
| **Hot Bacon Dressing,** 1 dinner portion | 5 |
| **Hot Bacon Dressing,** 1 side portion | 3 |
| **Lite Ranch Dressing,** 1 side portion | 3 |
| **Lite Ranch Dressing,** 1 dinner portion | 5 |
| **Raspberry Reduced Fat Dressing,** 1 dinner portion | 6 |
| **Raspberry Reduced Fat Dressing,** 1 side portion | 3 |
| **Sweet Italian Dressing,** 1 dinner portion | 7 |
| **Sweet Italian Dressing,** 1 side portion | 5 |
| **Swiss Bacon Dressing,** 1 dinner portion | 13 |
| **Thousand Island Dressing,** 1 dinner portion | 11 |
| **Vinegar & Oil Dressing,** 1 side portion | 1 |
| **Vinegar & Oil Dressing,** 1 dinner portion | 2 |
| **Wildfire Ranch Dressing,** 1 dinner portion | 7 |
| **Wildfire Ranch Dressing,** 1 side portion | 3 |

## SOUPS

| Item | *PointsPlus™* value |
|---|---|
| **Bean Soup,** 1 cup | 3 |
| **Bean Soup,** 1 bowl | 5 |

| ▲ Power Foods | PointsPlus™ value |
|---|---|
| **Cheddar Baked Potato Soup,** 1 bowl | 10 |
| **Sausage Chili,** 1 bowl | 10 |
| **Vegetable Beef Soup,** 1 cup | 3 |
| **Vegetable Beef Soup,** 1 bowl | 5 |

## APPETIZERS

| ▲ Power Foods | PointsPlus™ value |
|---|---|
| **Blue Ribbon Apple Pie,** 1 serving | 13 |
| **County Fair Cheese Bites,** 1 serving | 25 |
| **Itsy Bitsy Sandwich Trio,** 1 serving | 30 |
| **Itsy Bitsy Trio, Mini Pot Roast Sandwich (1 To Mix-&-Match),** 1 serving | 6 |
| **Itsy Bitsy Trio, Mini Pulled Pork Sandwich (1 To Mix-&-Match),** 1 serving | 7 |
| **Itsy Bitsy Trio, Mini Sausage Sandwich (1 To Mix-&-Match),** 1 serving | 8 |
| **Loaded Potato Bites,** 1 serving | 27 |
| **Wildfire Chicken Quesadilla,** 1 serving | 20 |

## DINNER ITEMS
(WITHOUT SIDE DISHES OR ROLL)

| ▲ Power Foods | PointsPlus™ value |
|---|---|
| **Chicken Salad Plate,** 1 serving | 19 |
| **Chicken Stir-Fry,** 1 serving | 16 |
| **Chicken-N-Noodles Deep-Dish (Dinner),** 1 serving | 21 |
| **Country Fried Steak (No Gravy),** 1 serving | 13 |
| **Cranberry Apple Pork Loin, A La Carte,** 1 | 14 |
| **Cranberry Apple Pork Loin, A La Carte,** 2 | 19 |
| **Garden Vegetable & Salmon Alfredo,** 1 serving | 27 |
| **Garden Vegetable Alfredo,** 1 serving | 23 |
| **Garlic Butter Salmon, Ala Carte,** 1 serving | 8 |
| **Green Pepper and Onion Pasta,** 1 serving | 14 |
| **Grilled Chicken Breast, Ala Carte,** 1 piece | 6 |
| **Italian Sausage and Pepper Pasta,** 1 serving | 21 |
| **Pot Roast Beef Stew Deep-Dish,** 1 serving | 18 |
| **Pot Roast Stroganoff,** 1 serving | 22 |
| **Potato-Crusted Flounder, A La Carte,** 1 serving | 5 |
| **Salmon Stir-Fry,** 1 serving | 19 |
| **Salmon, Ala Carte,** 1 serving | 6 |
| **Sirloin Steak, Ala Carte,** 1 serving | 11 |
| **Steak Tips & Noodles,** 1 serving | 27 |
| **Steak Tips Stir-Fry,** 1 serving | 27 |
| **Steak Tips, A La Carte,** 1 serving | 7 |
| **Turkey & Dressing,** 1 serving | 17 |
| **Vegetable Stir Fry,** 1 serving | 14 |
| **Wildfire Grilled Chicken Breast, A La Carte,** 1 serving | 6 |
| **Wildfire Salmon, Ala Carte,** 1 serving | 8 |

## SIDE DISHES

| ▲ Power Foods | PointsPlus™ value |
|---|---|
| **Baked Potato,** 1 serving | 6 |
| **Blue Cheese,** 1 serving | 3 |
| **Bread & Celery Dressing,** 1 serving | 8 |
| **Cole Slaw,** 1 serving | 6 |
| **Coleslaw,** 1 serving | 6 |
| **Cranberry Relish,** 1 serving | 2 |
| **Dill Pickle Slices,** 1 slice | 0 |
| **Fruit Cup,** 1 cup | 4 |
| **Garden Vegetables,** 1 serving | 3 |
| **Green Beans,** 1 serving | 1 |
| **Grilled Mushrooms,** 1 serving | 2 |
| **Lettuce & Tomato,** 1 serving | 0 |
| **Lettuce, Tomato & Pickle,** 1 serving | 0 |
| **Loaded Baked Potato,** 1 serving | 11 |

*Side Dishes (cont'd)*

| ▲ Power Foods | *PointsPlus*™ value |
|---|---|
| **Mashed Potatoes,** 1 serving | 4 |
| **Monterey Jack Cheese,** 1 slice | 2 |
| **Onion Petals,** 1 serving | 8 |
| **Rice Pilaf,** 1 serving | 3 |
| **Sweet Corn Griddle Cakes,** 1 serving | 11 |

## SENIORS ENTRÉES (WITHOUT SIDE DISHES OR ROLL)

| ▲ Power Foods | *PointsPlus*™ value |
|---|---|
| **Bowl Of Sausage Gravy,** 1 serving | 8 |
| **Chicken & Broccoli Alfredo,** 1 serving | 12 |
| **Chicken Parmesan,** 1 serving | 16 |
| **Chicken Parmesan with Meat Sauce,** 1 serving | 22 |
| **Chicken Stir-Fry,** 1 serving | 10 |
| **Country Fried Steak (With Gravy),** 1 serving | 15 |
| **Country Fried Steak, A La Carte,** 1 piece | 13 |
| **Cup Of Sausage Gravy,** 1 serving | 5 |
| **Fried Chicken Breast, A La Carte,** 1 piece | 7 |
| **Fried Haddock, A La Carte,** 1 piece | 10 |
| **Garden Vegetable & Chicken Alfredo,** 1 serving | 14 |
| **Garden Vegetable Alfredo,** 1 serving | 12 |
| **Garlic Butter Grilled Chicken, A La Carte,** 1 piece | 4 |
| **Green Pepper and Onion Pasta,** 1 serving | 9 |
| **Grilled Chicken Breast, A La Carte,** 1 piece | 4 |
| **Italian Sausage and Pepper Pasta,** 1 serving | 16 |
| **Meat Loaf, A La Carte,** 1 serving | 10 |
| **Open-Faced Roast Beef,** 1 serving | 11 |
| **Pot Roast Stroganoff, Savor Size,** 1 serving | 11 |
| **Slow-Roasted Chicken Pot Pie,** 1 serving | 25 |
| **Slow-Roasted Chicken-N-Noodles,** 1 serving | 5 |
| **Spaghetti with Meat Sauce, Savor Size,** 1 serving | 13 |
| **Steak Tip Stir-Fry,** 1 serving | 15 |
| **Steak Tips & Noodles,** 1 serving | 14 |
| **Turkey & Dressing,** 1 serving | 11 |
| **Turkey and Dressing, Senior,** 1 serving | 14 |
| **Turkey Sausage Breakfast,** 1 serving | 9 |
| **Vegetable Stir-Fry, with Rice,** 1 serving | 8 |

## FIT FROM THE FARM

| ▲ Power Foods | *PointsPlus*™ value |
|---|---|
| **Apple Sauce,** 1 serving | 2 |
| **Apple-Cranberry Spinach Salad with Reduced-Fat Raspberry Dressing,** 1 serving | 10 |
| **Apple-Cranberry Spinach Salad with Reduced-Fat Raspberry Dressing (Savor Size),** 1 serving | 9 |
| **Beef Vegetable Soup with Saltine Crackers,** 1 serving | 4 |
| **Blueberry-Banana French Toast,** 1 serving | 6 |
| **Blueberry-Banana Mini Fruit & Yogurt Parfait,** 1 serving | 5 |
| **Bob Evans Egg Lites with A Slice Of Tomato,** 1 serving | 1 |
| **Chicken, Spinach & Tomato Pasta (Savor Size),** 1 serving | 14 |
| **Chicken-N-Noodles with Saltine Crackers,** 1 serving | 5 |
| **Classic Bean Soup with Saltine Crackers,** 1 serving | 3 |
| **Cup Of Quaker Oatmeal with Brown Sugar & Milk,** 1 serving | 6 |
| **Diet Coca-Cola,** 1 serving | 1 |
| **Dry English Muffin with Smucker's Jelly,** 1 serving | 4 |
| **Dry Wheat Toast with Smucker's Jelly,** 1 serving | 3 |

| ▲ Power Foods | *PointsPlus™* value |
|---|---|
| **Fresh Fruit Cup,** 1 serving | 4 |
| **Fresh Fruit Dish,** 1 serving | 2 |
| **Fresh Fruit Plate with Low Fat Cottage Cheese,** 1 serving | 9 |
| **Fresh Fruit Plate with Low Fat Strawberry Yogurt,** 1 serving | 10 |
| **Fresh Garden Salad without Croutons Or Dressing,** 1 serving | 0 |
| **Fruit & Yogurt Crepe with Quaker Oatmeal,** 1 serving | 16 |
| **Grilled Chicken Breast with Plain Baked Potato & Steamed Broccoli Florets,** 1 serving | 11 |
| **Grilled Salmon Fillet with Plain Baked Potato & Steamed Broccoli Florets,** 1 serving | 12 |
| **Hot English Breakfast Tea,** 1 serving | 0 |
| **Iced Tea,** 1 serving | 0 |
| **Low-Fat Strawberry Yogurt,** 1 serving | 3 |
| ▲ **Plain Baked Potato,** 1 serving | 6 |
| **Steamed Broccoli Florets,** 1 serving | 1 |
| **Veggie Omelet with Fresh Fruit Dish & Dry Wheat Toast with Smucker's Jelly,** 1 serving | 7 |

## BREADS

| | |
|---|---|
| **Banana Nut Bread,** 1 | 6 |
| **Biscuit,** 1 | 7 |
| **Cherry Bread,** 1 | 8 |
| **Cinnamon Swirl (Frosted),** 1 | 18 |
| **Cinnamon Swirl (Unfrosted),** 1 | 15 |
| **Dinner Rolls,** 1 | 5 |
| **English Muffin,** 1 | 4 |
| **Kaiser Bun,** 1 | 5 |
| **Mini Bun,** 1 | 3 |
| **Parmesan Crusted Garlic Bread,** 1 | 5 |
| **Pumpkin Bread,** 1 | 6 |
| **Rye Bread,** 1 | 3 |
| **Rye Bread, Toasted and Buttered,** 1 | 3 |
| **Sourdough Bread,** 1 | 3 |
| **Texas Toast,** 1 | 2 |
| **Wheat Bread,** 1 | 2 |
| **Wheat Bread, Toasted and Buttered,** 1 | 3 |
| **White Bread,** 1 | 2 |
| **White Bread, Toasted and Buttered,** 1 | 3 |

## BREAKFAST

| | |
|---|---|
| **Bacon (A La Carte),** 1 serving | 1 |
| **Biscuit Sandwich,** 1 sandwich | 16 |
| **Blueberry & Banana Yogurt Parfait,** 1 serving | 5 |
| **Blueberry Banana & Yogurt Crepe,** 2 | 19 |
| **Blueberry Crepe,** 1 | 8 |
| **Blueberry Hotcake, No Topping (A La Carte),** 1 | 9 |
| **Blueberry Stuffed French Toast,** 1 serving | 16 |
| **Border Scramble Biscuit Bowl,** 1 serving | 27 |
| **Border Scramble Burrito with Bob Evans Egg Lites,** 1 serving | 17 |
| **Border Scramble Burrito with Egg,** 1 serving | 17 |
| **Border Scramble Burrito with Egg Whites,** 1 serving | 22 |
| **Border Scramble Omelet,** 1 serving | 17 |
| **Border Scramble Omelet with Bob Evans Egg Lites,** 1 serving | 11 |
| **Border Scramble Omelet with Egg Whites,** 1 serving | 11 |
| **Buttermilk Hotcake, No Topping (A La Carte),** 1 | 9 |
| **Cinnamon Hotcake, No Topping (A La Carte),** 1 | 10 |
| **Country Biscuit Breakfast,** 1 serving | 18 |
| **Eggs (A La Carte),** 1 egg | 4 |
| **Farmer's Market Omelet with Bob Evans Egg Lites,** 1 serving | 10 |

*Breakfast (cont'd)*

| ▲ Power Foods | *PointsPlus™* value |
|---|---|
| **Farmer's Market Omelet with Egg Whites,** 1 serving | 10 |
| **Farmer's Market Omelette,** 1 serving | 16 |
| **Fit From The Farm Breakfast with A Parfait,** 1 serving | 10 |
| **Fit From The Farm Breakfast with A Yogurt Crepe,** 1 serving | 15 |
| **Fit From The Farm Breakfast with Oatmeal,** 1 serving | 9 |
| **French Toast (A La Carte),** 1slice | 3 |
| **Fruit & Yogurt Plate,** 1 serving | 9 |
| **Garden Harvest Omelet,** 1 serving | 14 |
| **Garden Harvest Omelet with Bob Evans Egg Lites,** 1 serving | 8 |
| **Garden Harvest Omelet with Egg Whites,** 1 serving | 8 |
| **Grits,** 1 cup | 4 |
| **Ham & Cheddar Omelet,** 1 serving | 13 |
| **Ham & Cheddar Omelet with Bob Evans Egg Lites,** 1 serving | 7 |
| **Ham & Cheddar Omelet with Egg Whites,** 1 serving | 7 |
| **Ham & Cheese Benedict,** 1 serving | 22 |
| ▲ **Hard Boiled Egg,** 1 egg | 2 |
| ▲ **Hardcooked Egg (A La Carte),** 1 egg | 2 |
| **Meat Lover's Boburrito,** 1 serving | 21 |
| **Meat Lover's Boburrito with Bob Evans Egg Lites,** 1 serving | 16 |
| **Meat Lover's Boburrito with Egg Whites,** 1 serving | 16 |
| **Multigrain Hotcake, No Topping (A La Carte),** 1 | 10 |
| **Mush (A La Carte),** 1 serving | 4 |
| ▲ **Oatmeal,** 1 cup | 2 |
| ▲ **Omelet Shell (A La Carte),** 1 | 5 |
| ▲ **Omelet Shell, Bob Evans Egg Lites (A La Carte),** 1 serving | 2 |
| ▲ **Omelet Shell, Egg Whites (A La Carte),** 1 serving | 2 |
| **Plain Crepe,** 1 | 7 |
| **Pot Roast Hash,** 1 serving | 18 |

| ▲ Power Foods | *PointsPlus™* value |
|---|---|
| **Pumpkin Griddle Bread,** 1 serving | 31 |
| **Roasted Caramel Apple Crepe,** 1 | 8 |
| **Roasted Caramel Apple Stuffed French Toast,** 1 serving | 16 |
| **Sausage & Cheddar Omelet,** 1 serving | 15 |
| **Sausage & Cheddar Omelet with Bob Evans Egg Lites,** 1 serving | 8 |
| **Sausage & Cheddar Omelet with Egg Whites,** 1 serving | 8 |
| **Sausage Biscuit Bowl,** 1 serving | 27 |
| **Sausage Breakfast Patty (A La Carte),** 1 | 4 |
| **Sausage Country Benedict,** 1 serving | 25 |
| **Sausage Gravy,** 1 cup | 5 |
| **Sausage Link (A La Carte),** 1 | 4 |
| **Scrambled Bob Evans Egg Lites (1 Egg Equivalent) (A La Carte),** 1 serving | 1 |
| **Scrambled Bob Evans Egg Lites (2 Eggs Equivalent) (A La Carte),** 1 serving | 1 |
| **Scrambled Bob Evans Egg Lites (3 Egg Equivalent) (A La Carte),** 1 serving | 2 |
| **Scrambled Egg (1 Egg Equivalent) (A La Carte),** 1 serving | 2 |
| **Scrambled Egg (2 Egg Equivalent) (A La Carte),** 1 serving | 4 |
| **Scrambled Egg (3 Egg Equivalent) (A La Carte),** 1 serving | 6 |
| **Scrambled Egg Whites (1 Egg Equivalent) (A La Carte),** 1 serving | 1 |
| **Scrambled Egg Whites (2 Egg Equivalent) (A La Carte),** 1 serving | 1 |
| **Scrambled Egg Whites (3 Egg Equivalent) (A La Carte),** 1 serving | 2 |
| **Scrambled Eggs (2 Egg Equivalent), A La Carte,** 1 serving | 4 |

| ▲ Power Foods | PointsPlus™ value |
|---|---|
| **Scrambled Eggs (3),** 1 serving | 6 |
| **Smoked Ham,** 1 | 3 |
| **Spinach, Bacon & Tomato Biscuit Bowl,** 1 serving | 28 |
| **Stacked & Stuffed Blueberry Cream Hotcakes,** 1 serving | 41 |
| **Stacked & Stuffed Caramel Banana Pecan Hotcakes,** 1 serving | 29 |
| **Stacked & Stuffed Cinnamon Cream Hotcakes,** 1 serving | 38 |
| **Stacked & Stuffed Roasted Caramel Apple Cream Hotcakes,** 1 serving | 28 |
| **Stacked & Stuffed Strawberry Banana Cream Hotcakes,** 1 serving | 31 |
| **Strawberry Banana Crepes,** 1 | 9 |
| **Strawberry Banana Fruit & Yogurt Crepe,** 2 | 19 |
| **Strawberry Banana Mini Fruit & Yogurt Parfait,** 1 serving | 4 |
| **Strawberry Blueberry Fruit & Yogurt Crepe,** 2 | 18 |
| **Strawberry Blueberry Mini Fruit & Yogurt Parfait,** 1 serving | 4 |
| **Stuffed French Toast, No Topping,** 1 serving | 13 |
| **Sunshine Skillet,** 1 serving | 15 |
| **Sweet Cream Waffle, No Topping,** 1 serving | 10 |
| **Three Cheese Omelet,** 1 serving | 14 |
| **Three Cheese Omelet with Bob Evans Egg Lites,** 1 serving | 8 |
| **Three Cheese Omelet with Egg Whites,** 1 serving | 8 |
| **Turkey & Spinach Omelet,** 1 serving | 15 |
| **Turkey & Spinach Omelet with Bob Evans Egg Lites,** 1 serving | 9 |
| **Turkey & Spinach Omelet with Egg Whites,** 1 serving | 9 |
| **Turkey Sausage (A La Carte),** 1 serving | 2 |
| **Western Boburrito,** 1 serving | 20 |

| ▲ Power Foods | PointsPlus™ value |
|---|---|
| **Western Boburrito with Bob Evans Egg Lites,** 1 serving | 14 |
| **Western Boburrito with Egg Whites,** 1 serving | 14 |
| **Western Omelet,** 1 serving | 14 |
| **Western Omelet with Bob Evans Egg Lites,** 1 serving | 8 |
| **Western Omelet with Egg Whites,** 1 serving | 8 |

## SANDWICHES

| | |
|---|---|
| **Bacon Cheeseburger,** 1 sandwich | 16 |
| **Bob-B-Q Pulled Pork Sandwich,** 1 sandwich | 16 |
| **Bob's BLT& E,** 1 sandwich | 15 |
| **Cheeseburger,** 1 sandwich | 14 |
| **Chicken Salad Sandwich, Half,** 1 sandwich | 9 |
| **Fried Chicken Club Sandwich,** 1 sandwich | 17 |
| **Fried Chicken Sandwich,** 1 sandwich | 13 |
| **Fried Haddock Sandwich,** 1 sandwich | 21 |
| **Grilled Cheese Sandwich,** 1 sandwich | 7 |
| **Grilled Chicken Club Sandwich,** 1 sandwich | 13 |
| **Grilled Chicken Sandwich,** 1 sandwich | 9 |
| **Hamburger,** 1 sandwich | 11 |
| **Hamburger Patty, A La Carte,** 1 sandwich | 5 |
| **Knife & Fork Bob-B-Q Pulled Pork Sandwich,** 1 sandwich | 20 |
| **Knife & Fork Farmhouse Philly Sandwich,** 1 sandwich | 19 |
| **Knife & Fork Meatloaf Sandwich,** 1 sandwich | 18 |
| **Knife & Fork Pork Loin Sandwich,** 1 sandwich | 19 |

*Sandwiches (cont'd)*

| ▲ Power Foods | *PointsPlus*™ value |
|---|---|
| **Knife & Fork Turkey Sandwich,** 1 sandwich | 17 |
| **Pot Roast Sandwich,** 1 sandwich | 15 |
| **Pot Roast Sandwich, Half,** 1 sandwich | 10 |
| **Ranch Steak Burger,** 1 sandwich | 25 |
| **Turkey Bacon Melt,** 1 sandwich | 8 |
| **Turkey Bacon Melt (1/2 Combo),** 1 sandwich | 8 |

## KID'S SELECTIONS

| ▲ Power Foods | *PointsPlus*™ value |
|---|---|
| **Apple Juice,** 1 kids serving | 3 |
| **Applesauce,** 1 kids serving | 2 |
| ▲ **Broccoli Florets,** 1 kids serving | 0 |
| **Cherry Coca-Cola,** 1 kids serving | 3 |
| **Chocolate Milk 1%,** 1 kids serving | 6 |
| **Coca-Cola,** 1 kids serving | 3 |
| **Corn,** 1 kids serving | 5 |
| **Cottage Cheese,** 1 kids serving | 2 |
| **Diet Coke,** 1 kids serving | 0 |
| **Dr. Pepper,** 1 kids serving | 2 |
| **French Fries,** 1 kids serving | 9 |
| **Fresh Garden Salad,** 1 kids serving | 1 |
| **Fried Chicken Strips, Ala Carte,** 1 piece | 4 |
| **Fruit & Yogurt Dippers,** 1 kids serving | 6 |
| **Fruit Dish,** 1 kids serving | 2 |
| **Fudge Blast Sundae,** 1 kids serving | 6 |
| **Glazed Carrots,** 1 kids serving | 3 |
| **Grilled Cheese Triangles,** 1 kids serving | 8 |
| **Grilled Chicken Tender,** 1 kids serving | 1 |
| **Hi-C Fruit Punch,** 1 kids serving | 3 |
| **Home Fries,** 1 kids serving | 4 |
| **Hot Cocoa,** 1 kids serving | 7 |
| **Kids Pasta,** 1 kids serving | 5 |
| **Kids Strawberry Sundae,** 1 kids serving | 7 |
| **Lemonade,** 1 kids serving | 3 |
| **Macaroni & Cheese,** 1 kids serving | 7 |
| **Mini Cheeseburgers,** 1 kids serving | 7 |
| **Plenty-O-Pancakes,** 1 kids serving | 9 |
| **Reeses I'm Smiling Sundae,** 1 kids serving | 8 |
| **Root Beer,** 1 kids serving | 3 |
| **Smiley Face Potatoes,** 1 kids serving | 7 |
| **Spaghetti with Meat Sauce,** 1 kids serving | 12 |
| **Sprite,** 1 kids serving | 2 |
| **Strawberry Sundae,** 1 kids serving | 5 |
| **Strawberry Yogurt,** 1 kids serving | 3 |
| **Turkey Lurkey,** 1 kids serving | 4 |

## SAUCES & TOPPINGS

| ▲ Power Foods | *PointsPlus*™ value |
|---|---|
| **2% Milk, Pitcher,** 1 serving | 1 |
| **American Cheese,** 1 slice | 1 |
| **Bacon Bits,** 1 serving | 4 |
| **Beef Gravy,** 1 serving | 1 |
| **Blueberry Topping,** 1 serving | 3 |
| **Brown Sugar,** 1 serving | 3 |
| **Caramel Topping,** 1 serving | 2 |
| **Chicken Roasted Gravy,** 1 serving | 1 |
| **Chocolate Fudge Topping,** 1 serving | 2 |
| **Cocktail Sauce,** 1 serving | 1 |
| **Country Gravy,** 1 serving | 2 |
| **Cranberries,** 1 serving | 2 |
| **Cranberry Apple Topping,** 1 serving | 2 |
| **Hollandaise Sauce,** 1 serving | 1 |
| **Honey Roasted Pecans,** 1 serving | 4 |
| **Marinara Sauce,** 1 serving | 1 |
| **Pork Roasted Gravy,** 1 serving | 2 |
| **Queso Sauce,** 1 serving | 4 |
| **Raisins,** 1 serving | 2 |
| **Ranchero Picante Sauce,** 1 serving | 1 |
| **Roasted Caramel Apple Topping,** 1 serving | 2 |
| **Shredded Cheddar Cheese,** 1 serving | 3 |

| ▲ Power Foods | *PointsPlus*™ value |
|---|---|
| **Sour Cream,** 1 serving | 1 |
| **Strawberry Topping,** 1 serving | 1 |
| **Tartar Sauce,** 1 serving | 3 |
| **Whipped Topping,** 1 serving | 1 |
| **Wildfire Bbq Sauce,** 1 serving | 2 |

## CONDIMENTS

| | |
|---|---|
| **Apple Butter,** 1 packet | 1 |
| **Apple Jelly,** 1 serving | 1 |
| **Butter Cups,** 1 cup | 1 |
| **Captain Wafers Crackers,** 1 cracker | 1 |
| **Diet Blackberry Jam,** 1 packet | 0 |
| **Grape Jelly,** 1 packet | 1 |
| **Half and Half Cups,** 1 cup | 1 |
| **Honey,** 1 packet | 1 |
| ▲ **Lemon,** 1 wedge | 0 |
| **Margarine Buttery Taste Spread Cup,** 1 cup | 1 |
| **Mayonnaise,** 1 serving | 3 |
| **Non-Dairy Creamer,** 1 cup | 0 |
| **Orange Marmalade,** 1 packet | 1 |
| **Pancake Syrup,** 1 serving | 6 |
| **Saltine Crackers,** 1 cracker | 1 |
| **Strawberry Jam,** 1 packet | 1 |
| **Sugar Free Pancake Syrup,** 1 serving | 1 |

## BEVERAGES

| | |
|---|---|
| **Arnold Palmer,** 1 serving | 1 |
| **Caramel Iced Coffee,** 1 serving | 3 |
| **Caramel Mocha,** 1 serving | 7 |
| **Chamomile Hot Tea,** 1 serving | 0 |
| **Cherry Coca-Cola,** 1 serving | 4 |
| **Cherry Hot Chocolate,** 1 serving | 7 |
| **Earl Grey Hot Decaf Tea,** 1 serving | 0 |
| **English Breakfast Hot Tea,** 1 serving | 0 |
| **Green Tea,** 1 serving | 0 |
| **Hazelnut Iced Coffee,** 1 serving | 4 |

| ▲ Power Foods | *PointsPlus*™ value |
|---|---|
| **Hot Apple Cider,** 1 large | 6 |
| **Iced Coffee,** 1 serving | 1 |
| **Lemonade,** 1 regular | 2 |
| **Premium Decaf Coffee,** 1 serving | 0 |
| **Premium Regular Coffee,** 1 serving | 0 |
| **Sweet Iced Tea,** 1 serving | 2 |
| **Vanilla Iced Coffee,** 1 serving | 3 |
| **Wild Raspberry Iced Tea,** 1 serving | 2 |
| **Wild Raspberry Lemonade,** 1 serving | 5 |
| **Wild Strawberry Iced Tea,** 1 large | 2 |
| **Wild Strawberry Lemonade,** 1 serving | 6 |

## DESSERTS

| | |
|---|---|
| **Apple Dumpling Pie,** 1 serving | 16 |
| **Apple Dumpling Pie A La Mode,** 1 serving | 18 |
| **Blackberry Cobbler,** 1 serving | 16 |
| **Blackberry Cobbler A La Mode,** 1 serving | 19 |
| **Cherry Deep Dish Cobbler,** 1 serving | 19 |
| **Cherry Deep Dish Cobbler A La Mode,** 1 serving | 22 |
| **Chocolate Fudge Sundae,** 1 serving | 17 |
| **Coconut Cream Pie,** 1 serving | 14 |
| **French Silk Pie,** 1 serving | 18 |
| **Lemon Supreme Pie,** 1 serving | 18 |
| **No-Sugar-Added Apple Pie,** 1 serving | 14 |
| **No-Sugar-Added Apple Pie A La Mode,** 1 serving | 17 |
| **Peanut Butter Cup Sundae,** 1 serving | 22 |
| **Pumpkin Pie,** 1 slice | 16 |
| **Strawberry Shortcake,** 1 serving | 15 |
| **Strawberry Supreme Pie,** 1 serving | 19 |
| **Vanilla Ice Cream,** 1 serving | 3 |

# BOJANGLES'®

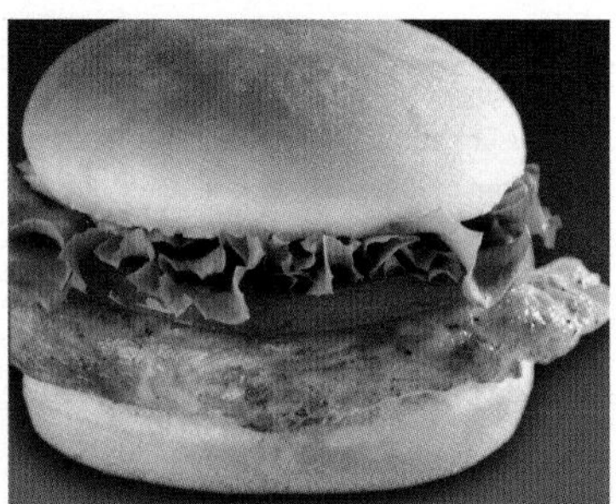

| ▲ Power Foods | *PointsPlus*™ value |
|---|---|
| **BISCUIT & BISCUIT SANDWICHES** | |
| **Bacon Biscuit,** 1 | 8 |
| **Bacon, Egg & Cheese Biscuit,** 1 | 15 |
| **Biscuit, plain,** 1 | 6 |
| **Cajun Filet Biscuit,** 1 | 12 |
| **Country Ham Biscuit,** 1 | 7 |
| **Egg Biscuit,** 1 | 11 |
| **Sausage Biscuit,** 1 | 9 |
| **Smoked Sausage Biscuit,** 1 | 10 |
| **Steak Biscuit,** 1 | 18 |
| **SANDWICHES** | |
| **Cajun Filet Sandwich, with mayonnaise,** 1 | 12 |
| **Cajun Filet Sandwich, without mayonnaise,** 1 | 9 |
| **Grilled Filet Sandwich, with mayonnaise,** 1 | 9 |
| **Grilled Filet Sandwich, without mayonnaise,** 1 | 6 |
| **CAJUN SPICED® CHICKEN** | |
| **Breast,** 1 (as served with skin) | 7 |
| **Leg,** 1 (as served with skin) | 7 |
| **Thigh,** 1 (as served with skin) | 8 |
| **Wing,** 1 (as served with skin) | 9 |

| ▲ Power Foods | *PointsPlus*™ value |
|---|---|
| **SNACKS** | |
| **Buffalo Bites®,** 1 serving | 4 |
| **Chicken Supremes,** 1 serving | 9 |
| **INDIVIDUAL FIXIN'** | |
| **Botato Rounds®,** 1 serving | 6 |
| **Cajun Pintos®,** 1 serving | 2 |
| **Dirty Rice®,** 1 serving | 5 |
| **Green Beans,** 1 serving | 0 |
| **Macaroni & Cheese,** 1 serving | 5 |
| **Marinated Cole Slaw,** 1 serving | 3 |
| **Potatoes, without gravy,** 1 serving | 2 |
| **Seasoned Fries,** 1 serving | 9 |
| **SWEET BISCUITS** | |
| **Bo Berry™ Biscuit,** 1 | 6 |
| **Cinnamon Biscuit,** 1 | 9 |

▲ Power Foods — *PointsPlus*™ value

## ENTRÉES

| Food | *PointsPlus*™ value |
|---|---|
| **1 Thigh & 1 Drumstick,** 1 serving | 8 |
| **1/2 Rotisserie Chicken,** 1 serving | 16 |
| **1/4 Rotisserie Chicken,** 1 serving | 8 |
| **1/4 White Rotisserie Chicken,** 1 serving | 8 |
| **1/4 White Rotisserie Chicken, without Skin,** 1 serving | 6 |
| **3 Piece Dark (2 Thighs & Drumstick),** 1 serving | 13 |
| **Beef Au Jus,** 1 serving | 1 |
| **Beef Brisket,** 1 serving | 8 |
| **Half Rotisserie Chicken, without Skin,** 1 serving | 8 |
| **Meatloaf,** 1 serving | 14 |
| **Pastry Top Chicken Pot Pie,** 1 serving | 21 |
| ▲ **Roasted Turkey,** 1 serving | 4 |

## SALADS

| Food | *PointsPlus*™ value |
|---|---|
| **Caesar Salad Entrée,** 1 serving | 12 |
| **Caesar Salad Entrée without Dressing,** 1 serving | 4 |
| **Caesar Side Salad,** 1 serving | 5 |
| **Caesar Side Salad without Dressing,** 1 serving | 1 |
| **Market Chopped Salad,** 1 serving | 13 |
| **Market Chopped Salad without Dressing,** 1 entrée portion | 5 |
| **Roasted Turkey,** 1 serving | 3 |
| **Rotisserie Chicken,** 1 serving | 4 |

## SALAD DRESSINGS

| Food | *PointsPlus*™ value |
|---|---|
| **Caesar Salad Dressing,** 1 serving | 10 |
| **Lite Ranch Dressing,** 1 serving | 2 |
| **Market Chopped Salad Dressing,** 1 serving | 10 |

## SANDWICHES

| Food | *PointsPlus*™ value |
|---|---|
| **Boston Chicken Carver,** 1 serving | 19 |
| **Boston Chicken Carver, with Spread and Cheese,** 1 sandwich | 19 |
| **Boston Meatloaf Carver,** 1 | 26 |
| **Boston Turkey Carver,** 1 serving | 18 |
| **Boston Turkey Carver, with Spread and Cheese,** 1 sandwich | 19 |
| **Brisket Dip Carver,** 1 sandwich | 24 |
| **Classic Chicken Salad Sandwich,** 1 sandwich | 21 |
| **Half Boston Chicken Carver,** 1 serving | 10 |
| **Half Boston Turkey Carver,** 1 serving | 9 |
| **Meatloaf Open-Faced Sandwich,** 1 sandwich | 18 |
| **Rotisserie Chicken Open-Faced Sandwich,** 1 sandwich | 8 |

## SOUPS & SIDES

| Food | *PointsPlus*™ value |
|---|---|
| **Beef Gravy,** 1 serving | 1 |
| **Chicken Noodle Soup,** 1 serving | 6 |
| **Chicken Tortilla Soup with Toppings,** 1 serving | 11 |
| **Chicken Tortilla Soup without Toppings,** 1 serving | 4 |
| **Cinnamon Apples,** 1 serving | 6 |
| **Creamed Spinach,** 1 serving | 8 |
| **Fresh Steamed Vegetables,** 1 serving | 1 |
| **Fresh Vegetable Stuffing,** 1 serving | 5 |
| **Garlic Dill New Potatoes,** 1 serving | 3 |
| **Green Beans,** 1 serving | 2 |
| **Macaroni and Cheese,** 1 serving | 7 |
| **Mashed Potatoes,** 1 serving | 7 |
| **Poultry Gravy,** 1 serving | 1 |
| **Seasonal Fresh Fruit Salad,** 1 serving | 2 |
| **Sweet Corn,** 1 serving | 5 |
| **Sweet Potato Casserole,** 1 serving | 13 |

# BOSTON MARKET®

| ▲ Power Foods | *PointsPlus™* value |
|---|---|
| **CORNBREAD & DESSERT** | |
| **Apple Gallette,** 1 serving | 12 |
| **Apple Pie,** 1 slice | 19 |
| **Chocolate Cake,** 1 serving | 16 |
| **Chocolate Chip Fudge Brownie,** 1 serving | 9 |
| **Chocolate Chunk Cookie,** 1 serving | 9 |
| **Cornbread,** 1 serving | 5 |

| ▲ Power Foods | *PointsPlus*™ value |
|---|---|

## BREAD

| | |
|---|---|
| **100% Whole Wheat,** 1 slice | 2 |
| **Apple Pie Bread,** 1 slice | 3 |
| **Austrian Pumpernickel,** 1 slice | 2 |
| **Beer Bread,** 1 slice | 2 |
| **Brioche,** 1 slice | 4 |
| **Cherry Walnut,** 1 slice | 2 |
| **Chocolate Babka,** 1 slice | 4 |
| **Chocolate Bread,** 1 slice | 3 |
| **Ciabatta,** 1 slice | 2 |
| **Cinnamon Spice,** 1 slice | 2 |
| **Cinnamon Swirl,** 1 slice | 3 |
| **Cornbread,** 1 slice | 3 |
| **Country Buttertop,** 1 slice | 3 |
| **Country Sourdough,** 1 slice | 2 |
| **Cranberry Cornbread,** 1 slice | 3 |
| **Cranberry Orange,** 1 slice | 2 |
| **Cranberry Sourdough Whole Grain,** 1 slice | 2 |
| **Dark Rye,** 1 slice | 2 |
| **Deli Rye,** 1 slice | 2 |
| **English Muffin,** 1 slice | 2 |
| **Farmer's Wheat,** 1 slice | 3 |
| **Flax Seed,** 1 slice | 2 |
| **Freedom Bread,** 1 slice | 2 |
| **French,** 1 slice | 3 |
| **French Baguette,** 1 slice | 1 |
| **French Peasant,** 1 slice | 2 |
| **Frontier Bread,** 1 slice | 2 |
| **Garlic Onion,** 1 slice | 2 |
| **Greek Olive,** 1 slice | 2 |
| **Greek Olive Ciabatta,** 1 slice | 2 |
| **Honey Challah,** 1 slice | 2 |
| **Honey Oat Bran,** 1 slice | 3 |
| **Honey Oat Bran with Cranberries,** 1 slice | 3 |
| **Honey Raisin,** 1 slice | 2 |
| **Honey Raisin Challah,** 1 slice | 2 |
| **Honey Raisin Pecan,** 1 slice | 3 |
| **Honey Stoneground Wheat,** 1 slice | 2 |
| **Honey Sunflower Whole Wheat,** 1 slice | 3 |
| **Honey Wheat,** 1 slice | 3 |
| **Honey White,** 1 slice | 2 |
| **Honey Whole Wheat,** 1 slice | 2 |
| **Irish Oat Bran,** 1 slice | 3 |
| **Irish Soda Bread,** 1 slice | 4 |
| **Jalapeno Cornbread,** 1 slice | 3 |
| **Maple Walnut,** 1 slice | 3 |
| **Marathon Multigrain,** 1 slice | 3 |
| **Marble Rye,** 1 slice | 2 |
| **Mediterranean Herb,** 1 slice | 2 |
| **Multigrain,** 1 slice | 3 |
| **Multigrain Sandwich Bread,** 1 slice | 2 |
| **Multigrain Whole Wheat,** 1 slice | 3 |
| **Norwegian Rye,** 1 slice | 2 |
| **Onion Rye,** 1 slice | 2 |
| **Panettone,** 1 slice | 3 |
| **Pecan Sourdough Whole Grain,** 1 slice | 3 |
| **Peppercorn Swiss,** 1 slice | 3 |
| **Pepperoni Bread,** 1 slice | 2 |
| **Potato Cheddar Chive,** 1 slice | 2 |
| **Potato Flake,** 1 slice | 2 |
| **Pretzel Bread,** 1 slice | 2 |
| **Pumpernickel Brick,** 1 slice | 2 |
| **Raisin Cinnamon,** 1 slice | 3 |
| **Raisin Cinnamon Walnut,** 1 slice | 3 |
| **Raisin Cinnamon Whole Wheat,** 1 slice | 3 |

Bread (cont'd)

| ▲ Power Foods | *PointsPlus™* value |
|---|---|
| **Raisin Walnut,** 1 slice | 3 |
| **Rosemary Country Bread,** 1 slice | 2 |
| **Rosemary Fougasse,** 1 slice | 2 |
| **Rosemary Garlic Ciabatta,** 1 slice | 2 |
| **Rosemary Multigrain Sandwich Bread,** 1 slice | 2 |
| **Russian Rye,** 1 slice | 2 |
| **Rustic Italian,** 1 slice | 4 |
| **Semolina,** 1 slice | 2 |
| **Sourdough,** 1 slice | 3 |
| **Sourdough Whole Grain,** 1 slice | 2 |
| **Stollen,** 1 slice | 3 |
| **Stoneground Wheat,** 1 slice | 2 |
| **Swedish Limpa Rye,** 1 slice | 3 |
| **Sweet Bellagio,** 1 slice | 2 |
| **Tomato Basil,** 1 slice | 2 |
| **Traditional Rye,** 1 slice | 2 |
| **Tuscan Herb Formaggio,** 1 slice | 2 |
| **Tuscan Rustica,** 1 slice | 2 |
| **Vanilla Egg,** 1 slice | 3 |
| **Wheat Flax Seed,** 1 slice | 2 |

## BUNS

| | |
|---|---|
| **Hamburger Bun,** 1 | 6 |
| **Hot Dog Bun,** 1 | 6 |
| **Soft Bun,** 1 | 6 |
| **Soft Onion Bun,** 1 | 6 |
| **Soft Tomato Basil Bun,** 1 | 6 |
| **Soft Wheat Bun,** 1 | 6 |

## MUFFINS

| | |
|---|---|
| **Banana Chocolate Chip Muffin,** 1 | 11 |
| **Banana Muffin,** 1 | 11 |
| **Blueberry Corn Muffin,** 1 | 12 |
| **Chocolate Muffin,** 1 | 15 |
| **Cranberry Orange Muffin,** 1 | 12 |
| **Pumpkin Muffin,** 1 | 14 |
| **Pumpkin Walnut Muffin,** 1 | 15 |
| **Raisin Bran Muffin,** 1 | 10 |
| **Zucchini Muffin,** 1 | 16 |

## COOKIES

| | |
|---|---|
| **Chocolate Chip,** 1 | 7 |
| **Chocolate Chocolate Chip,** 1 | 7 |
| **Ginger,** 1 | 6 |
| **Oatmeal Raisin,** 1 | 6 |
| **Peanut Butter,** 1 | 8 |
| **Wheat Peanut Butter,** 1 | 8 |

## DESSERT BREAD

| | |
|---|---|
| **Banana Chocolate Chip Dessert Bread,** 1 slice | 4 |
| **Banana Dessert Bread,** 1 slice | 4 |
| **Banana Walnut Dessert,** 1 slice | 4 |
| **Blueberry Corn Dessert Bread,** 1 slice | 4 |
| **Chocolate Dessert Bread,** 1 slice | 5 |
| **Cranberry Orange Dessert Bread,** 1 slice | 4 |
| **Lemon Poppyseed Dessert Bread,** 1 slice | 4 |
| **Pumpkin Chocolate Chip Dessert Bread,** 1 slice | 4 |
| **Pumpkin Dessert Bread,** 1 slice | 4 |
| **Pumpkin Walnut Dessert Bread,** 1 slice | 4 |
| **Zucchini Dessert Bread,** 1 slice | 5 |

## OTHER SWEETS

| | |
|---|---|
| **Biscotti - Almond,** 1 | 3 |
| **Biscotti - Chocolate Hazelnut,** 1 | 3 |
| **Biscotti - Lemon Anise,** 1 | 3 |
| **Brownie,** 1 | 13 |

| ▲ Power Foods | *PointsPlus*™ value |
|---|---|
| **Brownie with Walnuts,** 1 | 14 |
| **Cinnamon Bun with Cream Cheese Icing,** 1 | 13 |
| **Cinnamon Claw,** 1 | 8 |
| **Coffee Cake,** 1 serving | 9 |
| **Coffee Cake (Individual),** 1 | 10 |
| **Hot Cross Bun,** 1 | 8 |
| **Scone,** 1 | 12 |
| **Sweet Swirl,** 1 | 13 |

## OTHER ITEMS

| | |
|---|---|
| **Croutons,** 1/8 of the package (1 oz) | 2 |
| **Focaccia (without Topping),** 1/8 loaf | 4 |
| **Pizza Dough,** 1/8 of a package (2 oz) | 4 |
| **Wheat Pizza Dough,** 1/8 of a package (2 oz) | 3 |

# BRUEGGER'S®

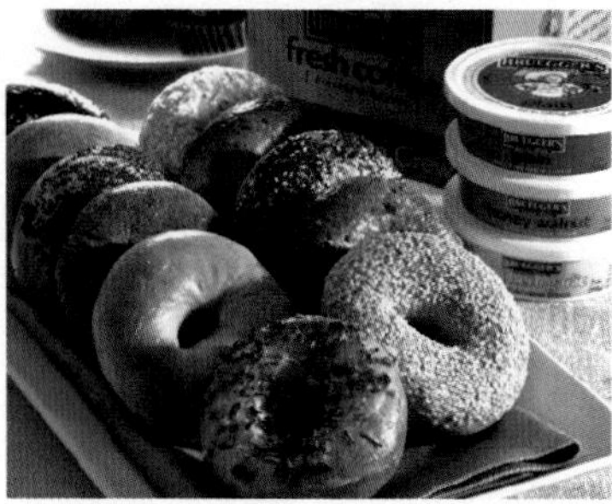

▲ Power Foods — *PointsPlus™* value

## BAGELS (WITHOUT SPREAD)

|  | PointsPlus™ value |
|---|---|
| **Asiago Parmesan Bagel,** 1 | 9 |
| **Blueberry Bagel,** 1 | 8 |
| **Chocolate Chip Bagel,** 1 | 9 |
| **Cinnamon Raisin Bagel,** 1 | 9 |
| **Cinnamon Sugar Bagel,** 1 | 9 |
| **Cranberry Orange Bagel,** 1 | 9 |
| **Everything Bagel,** 1 | 8 |
| **Fortified Multi-Grain Bagel,** 1 | 9 |
| **Garlic Bagel,** 1 | 8 |
| **Honey Grain Bagel,** 1 | 9 |
| **Jalapeño Bagel,** 1 | 8 |
| **Onion Bagel,** 1 | 8 |
| **Plain Bagel,** 1 | 8 |
| **Poppy Bagel,** 1 | 8 |
| **Pumpernickel Bagel,** 1 | 9 |
| **Rosemary Olive Oil Bagel,** 1 | 10 |
| **Sesame Bagel,** 1 | 8 |
| **Sourdough Bagel,** 1 | 8 |
| **Square Asiago Parmesan Bagel,** 1 | 9 |
| **Square Everything Bagel,** 1 | 8 |
| **Square Plain Bagel,** 1 | 9 |
| **Square Sesame Bagel,** 1 | 9 |
| **Sundried Tomato Bagel,** 1 | 8 |
| **Whole Wheat Bagel,** 1 | 11 |

▲ Power Foods — *PointsPlus™* value

## BRUEGGER'S® CREAM CHEESE & HUMMUS

|  | PointsPlus™ value |
|---|---|
| **Bacon Scallion,** 1 serving | 4 |
| **Garden Veggie,** 1 serving | 4 |
| **Honey Walnut,** 1 serving | 4 |
| **Hummus,** 1 scoop | 3 |
| **Jalapeño,** 1 serving | 4 |
| **Light Garden Veggie,** 1 serving | 2 |
| **Light Herb Garlic,** 1 serving | 3 |
| **Light Plain,** 1 serving | 2 |
| **Olive Pimento,** 1 serving | 4 |
| **Onion & Chive,** 1 serving | 4 |
| **Plain,** 1 serving | 4 |
| **Smoked Salmon,** 1 serving | 4 |
| **Strawberry,** 1 serving | 4 |

## BREAKFAST SANDWICHES

|  | PointsPlus™ value |
|---|---|
| **Egg and American Cheese Sandwich on Plain Bagel,** 1 | 14 |
| **Egg, American Cheese & Bacon on Plain Bagel,** 1 | 15 |
| **Plain Bagel with Light Cream Cheese,** 1 | 9 |
| **Smoked Salmon Sandwich on Plain Bagel,** 1 | 13 |
| **Spinach & Cheddar Omelet on Plain Bagel,** 1 | 14 |
| **Spinach & Cheddar Omelet on Plain Bagel,** 1 | 13 |

## DELI SANDWICHES

|  | PointsPlus™ value |
|---|---|
| **Garden Veggie Sandwich on A Plain Bagel,** 1 | 10 |
| **Ham Sandwich with Brown Mustard on A Plain Bagel (With Lettuce and Tomato),** 1 | 11 |
| **Turkey Sandwich on A Plain Bagel (With Lettuce, Tomato, and Mayo),** 1 | 13 |

| ▲ Power Foods | *PointsPlus*™ value |
|---|---|
| **Turkey Sandwich on Honey Wheat Bread (With Lettuce, Tomato, and Mustard),** 1 | 13 |

## SIGNATURE & CLASSIC SANDWICHES

| | |
|---|---|
| **Herby Turkey® on Sesame Bagel,** 1 | 16 |
| **Herby Turkey® Sandwich on A Plain Bagel,** 1 | 14 |
| **Leonardo Da Veggie® Asiago Softwich,** 1 | 15 |
| **Leonardo De Veggie® Sandwich on A Plain Bagel,** 1 | 13 |

## HOT PANINI

| | |
|---|---|
| **Ham & Swiss on Honey Wheat,** 1 | 16 |
| **Turkey Toscana on Hearty White,** 1 | 17 |

## SALADS

| | |
|---|---|
| **Caesar Salad with Caesar Dressing,** 1 | 7 |
| **Ceasar Chicken Salad with Caesar Dressing,** 1 | 10 |
| **Mandarin Medley Salad with Balsamic Vinaigrette,** 1 | 9 |
| **Mandarin Medley Salad with Chicken & Balsamic Vinaigrette,** 1 | 11 |
| **Sesame Salad with Asian Sesame Dressing,** 1 | 12 |
| **Sesame Salad with Chicken and Asian Sesame Dressing,** 1 | 14 |

## SOUPS

| | |
|---|---|
| **Chicken Spaetzle,** 1 cup | 4 |
| **Fire Roasted Tomato,** 1 cup | 3 |
| **White Chicken Chili,** 1 cup | 6 |

# BRUSTER'S® REAL ICE CREAM

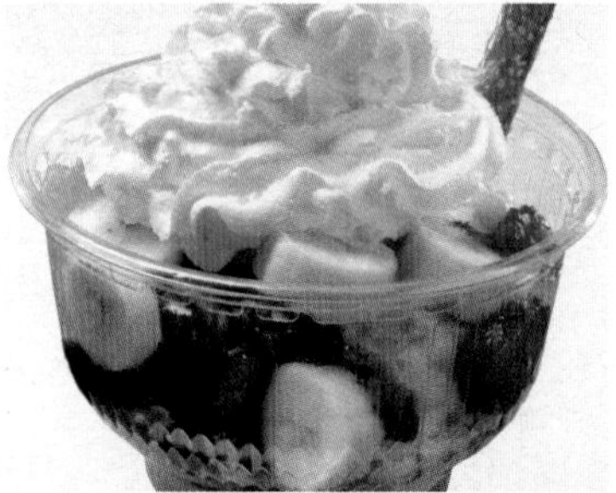

| ▲ Power Foods | *PointsPlus*™ value |
|---|---|
| **ICE CREAM** | |
| **Caramel Swirl No Sugar Added/Fat Free Ice Cream,** 1/2 cup | 3 |
| **Chocolate,** 1/2 cup | 6 |
| **Chocolate Caramel No Sugar Added/Fat Free Ice Cream,** 1/2 cup | 4 |
| **Chocolate Fudge No Sugar Added/Fat Free Ice Cream,** 1/2 cup | 4 |
| **Chocolate Ice Cream,** 1/2 cup | 6 |
| **Chocolate No Sugar Added/Fat Free Ice Cream,** 1/2 cup | 3 |
| **Chocolate Raspberry No Sugar Added/Fat Free Ice Cream,** 1/2 cup | 4 |
| **Cinnamon No Sugar Added/Fat Free Ice Cream,** 1/2 cup | 3 |
| **Coffee Caramel Swirl No Sugar Added/Fat Free Ice Cream,** 1/2 cup | 3 |
| **Coffee Caramel Swirl No Sugar Added/Fat Free Ice Cream,** 1/2 cup | 4 |
| **Coffee No Sugar Added/Fat Free Ice Cream,** 1/2 cup | 3 |

| ▲ Power Foods | *PointsPlus*™ value |
|---|---|
| **Coffee No Sugar Added/Fat Free Ice Cream,** 1/2 cup | 3 |
| **Coffee Ripple No Sugar Added/Fat Free Ice Cream,** 1/2 cup | 4 |
| **Coffee Ripple No Sugar Added/Fat Free Ice Cream,** 1/2 cup | 4 |
| **Fudge Ripple No Sugar Added/Fat Free Ice Cream,** 1/2 cup | 4 |
| **Fudge Ripple No Sugar Added/Fat Free Ice Cream,** 1/2 cup | 4 |
| **Orange Sherbet,** 1/2 cup | 6 |
| **Raspberry Swirl No Sugar Added/Fat Free Ice Cream,** 1/2 cup | 3 |
| **Strawberry Sorbet,** 1/2 cup | 6 |
| **Vanilla Ice Cream,** 1 serving | 6 |
| **Vanilla No Sugar Added/Fat Free Ice Cream,** 1/2 cup | 3 |
| **Caramel Swirl No Sugar Added/Fat Free Ice Cream,** 1/2 cup | 3 |
| **FROZEN YOGURT** | |
| **Vanilla Frozen Yogurt,** 1/2 cup | 4 |
| **Chocolate Frozen Yogurt,** 1/2 cup | 4 |
| **SHERBET & SORBET** | |
| **Orange Sherbet,** 3 1/2 oz | 6 |
| **Strawberry Sorbet,** 3 1/2 oz | 6 |

| ▲ Power Foods | *PointsPlus*™ value |
| --- | --- |

## WHOPPER® SANDWICHES

| | |
| --- | --- |
| **WHOPPER® Sandwich,** 1 | 18 |
| **WHOPPER® Sandwich (without mayonnaise),** 1 | 14 |
| **WHOPPER® Sandwich with Cheese,** 1 | 21 |
| **WHOPPER® with Cheese Sandwich (without mayonnaise),** 1 | 16 |
| **WHOPPER JR.® Sandwich,** 1 | 9 |
| **WHOPPER JR.® Sandwich (without mayonnaise),** 1 | 7 |
| **WHOPPER JR.® Sandwich with Cheese,** 1 | 10 |
| **WHOPPER JR.® Sandwich with Cheese (without mayonnaise),** 1 | 9 |
| **DOUBLE WHOPPER® Sandwich,** 1 | 25 |
| **DOUBLE WHOPPER® Sandwich (without mayonnaise),** 1 | 20 |
| **DOUBLE WHOPPER® Sandwich with Cheese,** 1 | 27 |
| **DOUBLE WHOPPER® Sandwich with Cheese (without mayonnaise),** 1 | 23 |
| **TRIPLE WHOPPER® Sandwich (with mayonnaise),** 1 | 31 |
| **TRIPLE WHOPPER® Sandwich (without mayonnaise),** 1 | 27 |
| **TRIPLE WHOPPER® Sandwich with Cheese (with mayonnaise),** 1 | 34 |
| **TRIPLE WHOPPER® Sandwich with Cheese (without mayonnaise),** 1 | 29 |
| **TEXAS WHOPPER® Sandwich,** 1 serving | 22 |
| **TEXAS DOUBLE WHOPPER® Sandwich,** 1 serving | 29 |
| **TEXAS TRIPLE WHOPPER® Sandwich,** 1 serving | 35 |

## FLAME-BROILED BURGERS

| | |
| --- | --- |
| **Hamburger,** 1 | 7 |
| **Double Hamburger,** 1 | 10 |
| **Cheeseburger,** 1 | 8 |
| **Double Cheeseburger,** 1 | 12 |

| ▲ Power Foods | *PointsPlus*™ value |
| --- | --- |
| **BK Burger Shot® 2-Pack,** 1 serving | 6 |
| **BK Burger Shot® 6-Pack,** 1 serving | 18 |
| **BK™ Double Stacker,** 1 | 15 |
| **BK™ Triple Stacker,** 1 | 20 |
| **BK™ Quad Stacker,** 1 | 25 |
| **Mushroom and Swiss Steakhouse XT™,** 1 serving | 22 |
| **Rodeo Cheeseburger,** 1 serving | 10 |
| **Sourdough Bacon Cheeseburger,** 1 serving | 21 |
| **Steakhouse Burger,** 1 | 24 |
| **Steakhouse XT™,** 1 serving | 25 |
| **3 Cheese Steakhouse XT™,** 1 serving | 28 |

## HAVE IT YOUR WAY OPTIONS

| | |
| --- | --- |
| **American Cheese,** 1 slice | 1 |
| **Bacon,** 1 strip | 0 |
| **Green Chilies,** 1/2 oz | 0 |
| **Barbecue Dipping Sauce,** 1 packet (2 Tbsp) | 1 |
| **Breakfast Syrup,** 1 packet (2 Tbsp) | 2 |
| **Buffalo Dipping Sauce,** 1 packet (2 Tbsp) | 2 |
| **Honey Mustard Dipping Sauce,** 1 packet (2 Tbsp) | 2 |
| **Ranch Dipping Sauce,** 1 packet (2 Tbsp) | 4 |
| **Strawberry or Grape Jam,** 1 packet (2 Tbsp) | 1 |
| **Sweet and Sour Dipping Sauce,** 1 packet (2 Tbsp) | 1 |
| **Zesty Onion Ring Dipping Sauce,** 1 packet (2 Tbsp) | 4 |

## CHICKEN, FISH, VEGGIE & KIDS

| | |
| --- | --- |
| **BK BIG FISH® Sandwich,** 1 | 17 |
| **BK BIG FISH® Sandwich (no tartar sauce),** 1 | 12 |
| **BK VEGGIE® Burger (no mayonnaise),** 1 | 8 |

*Chicken, Fish, Veggie & Kids (cont'd)*

| ▲ Power Foods | *PointsPlus*™ value |
|---|---|
| **BK VEGGIE® Burger (with regular mayonnaise),** 1 | 10 |
| **BK VEGGIE® Burger with Cheese,** 1 | 12 |
| **BK™ CHICKEN FRIES,** 6 pieces | 7 |
| **BK™ CHICKEN FRIES,** 9 pieces | 10 |
| **BK™ CHICKEN FRIES,** 12 pieces | 13 |
| **CHICKEN TENDERS®,** 4 pieces | 5 |
| **CHICKEN TENDERS®,** 5 pieces | 6 |
| **CHICKEN TENDERS®,** 6 pieces | 7 |
| **CHICKEN TENDERS®,** 8 pieces | 10 |
| **Kraft Macaroni and Cheese,** 1 serving | 4 |
| **Original Chicken Sandwich,** 1 | 17 |
| **Original Chicken Sandwich (without mayonnaise),** 1 | 11 |
| **Spicy CHICK'N CRISP™ Sandwich (with mayonnaise),** 1 | 12 |
| **Spicy CHICK'N CRISP™ Sandwich (without mayonnaise),** 1 | 8 |
| **Tacos (2),** 1 serving | 9 |
| **TENDERCRISP® Chicken Sandwich (with mayonnaise),** 1 | 22 |
| **TENDERCRISP® Chicken Sandwich (without mayonnaise),** 1 | 16 |
| **TENDERGRILL™ chicken sandwich (with mayonnaise),** 1 | 13 |

## SALADS, SALAD DRESSING & CROUTONS

| ▲ Power Foods | *PointsPlus*™ value |
|---|---|
| **TENDERCRISP® Chicken Garden Salad,** 1 | 11 |
| **TENDERGRILL™ Chicken Garden Salad,** 1 | 5 |
| **Garden Salad (no chicken),** 1 serving | 2 |
| **Side Salad,** 1 serving | 1 |
| **KEN'S® Creamy Caesar Dressing,** 1 packet | 6 |
| **KEN'S® Honey Mustard Dressing,** 1 packet | 8 |
| **KEN'S® Light Italian Dressing,** 1 packet | 3 |
| **KEN'S® Ranch Dressing,** 1 packet | 5 |
| **Garlic Parmesan Croutons,** 1 serving | 2 |

## SIDE ORDERS

| ▲ Power Foods | *PointsPlus*™ value |
|---|---|
| **CHEESY TOTS™ Potatoes,** 6 pieces | 6 |
| **CHEESY TOTS™ Potatoes,** 9 pieces | 9 |
| **CHEESY TOTS™ Potatoes,** 12 pieces | 12 |
| **French Fries,** 1 small serving | 9 |
| **French Fries,** 1 medium serving | 12 |
| **French Fries,** 1 large serving | 15 |
| **French Fries,** 1 value side | 6 |
| **Onion Rings,** 1 small serving | 8 |
| **Onion Rings,** 1 medium serving | 11 |
| **Onion Rings,** 1 large serving | 13 |
| **Onion Rings,** 1 value serving | 4 |
| ▲ **BK™ Fresh Apple Fries,** 1 serving | 0 |
| **Caramel Sauce,** 1 serving | 1 |

## BREAKFAST

| ▲ Power Foods | *PointsPlus*™ value |
|---|---|
| **Bacon, Egg & Cheese Biscuit,** 1 serving | 12 |
| **Biscuits (2) & Sausage Gravy Platter,** 1 serving | 19 |
| **BK Breakfast Shots 2-Pack Bacon and Cheese,** 1 serving | 8 |
| **BK Breakfast Shots 2-Pack Ham and Cheese,** 1 serving | 7 |
| **BK Breakfast Shots 2-Pack Sausage and Cheese,** 1 serving | 11 |
| **Breakfast Burrito - Bacon, Egg, Cheese, & Salsa,** 1 serving | 8 |
| **Breakfast Burrito - Potato, Egg, Cheese, & Salsa,** 1 serving | 9 |
| **Breakfast Burrito - Sausage, Egg, Cheese & Salsa,** 1 serving | 12 |
| **Cheesy Bacon BK WRAPPER™,** 1 serving | 10 |
| **CROISSAN'WICH® Bacon, Egg & Cheese,** 1 | 9 |

| ▲ Power Foods | *PointsPlus*™ value |
|---|---|
| **CROISSAN'WICH® Egg & Cheese,** 1 serving | 8 |
| **CROISSAN'WICH® Ham, Egg & Cheese,** 1 serving | 9 |
| **CROISSAN'WICH® Sausage and Cheese,** 1 | 10 |
| **CROISSAN'WICH® Sausage, Egg, & Cheese,** 1 serving | 13 |
| **DOUBLE CROISSAN'WICH™ with Bacon, Egg & Cheese,** 1 | 11 |
| **DOUBLE CROISSAN'WICH™ with Ham, Bacon, Egg, & Cheese,** 1 | 11 |
| **DOUBLE CROISSAN'WICH™ with Ham, Egg, & Cheese,** 1 | 11 |
| **DOUBLE CROISSAN'WICH™ with Ham, Sausage, Egg, & Cheese,** 1 | 15 |
| **DOUBLE CROISSAN'WICH™ with Sausage, Bacon, Egg & Cheese,** 1 | 15 |
| **DOUBLE CROISSAN'WICH™ with Sausage, Egg, & Cheese,** 1 | 18 |
| **French Toast Sticks (3 pieces),** 3 sticks | 6 |
| **French Toast Sticks (5 pieces),** 5 sticks | 10 |
| **Ham Omelet Sandwich,** 1 | 7 |
| **Ham, Egg, & Cheese Biscuit,** 1 serving | 11 |
| **Hash Browns - medium,** 1 medium serving | 14 |
| **Hash Browns - small,** 1 small serving | 11 |
| **Hash Browns - value,** 1 value serving | 7 |
| **Pancake Platter with 1 oz Breakfast Syrup,** 1 serving | 9 |
| **Pancake Platter with Sausage & 1 oz Breakfast Syrup,** 1 serving | 14 |
| **Sausage Biscuit,** 1 | 12 |
| **Sausage, Egg & Cheese Biscuit,** 1 | 15 |
| **SOURDOUGH Breakfast Sandwich with Bacon, Egg & Cheese,** 1 serving | 12 |
| **SOURDOUGH Breakfast Sandwich with Ham, Egg & Cheese,** 1 serving | 11 |
| **SOURDOUGH Breakfast Sandwich with Sausage, Egg & Cheese,** 1 serving | 15 |
| **Cini-minis (4 minis),** 1 serving | 11 |
| **Vanilla Icing (for Cini-minis),** 1 serving (2 Tbsp) | 2 |

## SHAKES, MILK & ICED COFFEE

| ▲ Power Foods | *PointsPlus*™ value |
|---|---|
| **Chocolate Milk Shake,** 1 small | 12 |
| **Chocolate Milk Shake,** 1 medium | 18 |
| **Chocolate Milk Shake,** 1 large | 26 |
| **Chocolate Milk Shake,** 1 value serving | 9 |
| **HERSHEY®'S 1% Low Fat Chocolate Milk,** 8 fl oz | 5 |
| **HERSHEY®'S Fat Free Milk,** 8 fl oz | 2 |
| **Mocha BK JOE® Iced Coffee,** 1 | 9 |
| **OREO® BK™ Sundae Shake - Chocolate,** 1 small | 18 |
| **OREO® BK™ Sundae Shake - Chocolate,** 1 medium | 26 |
| **OREO® BK™ Sundae Shake - Strawberry,** 1 small | 20 |
| **OREO® BK™ Sundae Shake - Strawberry,** 1 medium | 28 |
| **OREO® BK™ Sundae Shake - Vanilla,** 1 medium serving | 22 |
| **Strawberry Milk Shake,** 1 small | 12 |
| **Strawberry Milk Shake,** 1 medium | 17 |
| **Strawberry Milk Shake,** 1 large | 26 |
| **Strawberry Milk Shake,** 1 value serving | 9 |
| **Vanilla Milk Shake,** 1 small | 10 |
| **Vanilla Milk Shake,** 1 medium | 14 |
| **Vanilla Milk Shake,** 1 large | 21 |
| **Vanilla Milk Shake,** 1 value serving | 8 |

## DESSERTS

| ▲ Power Foods | *PointsPlus*™ value |
|---|---|
| **Dutch Apple Pie,** 1 serving | 9 |
| **HERSHEY'S® Sundae Pie,** 1 serving | 8 |

# CAMILLE'S SIDEWALK CAFÉ

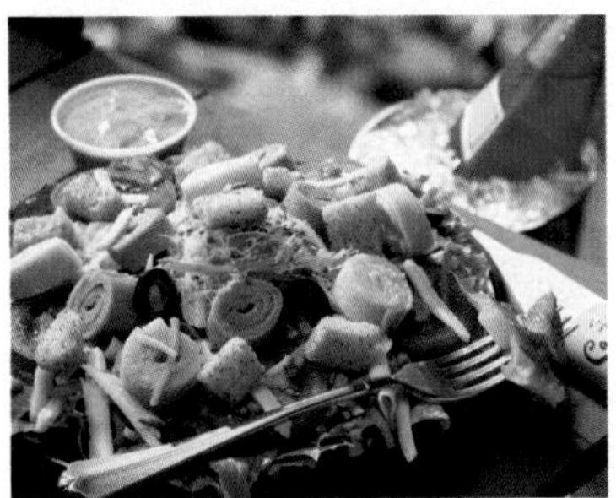

| ▲ Power Foods | *PointsPlus™* value |
|---|---|
| **WRAPS** (WITHOUT CHIPS OR SALSA) | |
| **Bangkok Thai,** 1 serving | 19 |
| **Chicken Caesar,** 1 serving | 17 |
| **Chicken California,** 1 serving | 16 |
| **Hail Caesar! Natu Wrap,** 1 serving | 19 |
| **Poblano Chicken Natu Wrap,** 1 serving | 18 |
| **Somona Veggie,** 1 serving | 16 |
| **Sonoma Veggie,** 1 serving | 16 |
| **Spicy Chicken Tender,** 1 serving | 21 |
| **Tex Mex Club,** 1 serving | 16 |
| **The Quesadilla,** 1 serving | 17 |
| **GRILLED HOT WRAPS** (WITHOUT SIDE SPRINT MIX SALAD OR RASPBERRY VINAIGRETTE) | |
| **Club Med,** 1 serving | 12 |
| **Mexican Daredevil,** 1 serving | 18 |
| **Paris Bistro,** 1 serving | 15 |
| **The Michelangelo,** 1 serving | 12 |
| **SANDWICHES** (WITHOUT BREAD, CHIPS OR SALSA) | |
| **Apple-Walnut Tuna Salad Sandwich,** 1 serving | 14 |
| **Café Chicken Salad,** 1 serving | 12 |
| **Camille's Club,** 1 serving | 12 |
| **Ham and Swiss,** 1 serving | 6 |
| **Turkey Deluxe,** 1 serving | 7 |

| ▲ Power Foods | *PointsPlus™* value |
|---|---|
| **BREAD** | |
| **Honey Wheatberry Bread,** 1 serving | 3 |
| **Marble Reuben Rye Bread,** 1 serving | 3 |
| **White Bread,** 1 serving | 3 |
| **PANINI SANDWICHES** (WITHOUT CHIPS OR SALSA) | |
| **Italian Roast Beef,** 1 serving | 16 |
| **Napa Valley Chicken,** 1 serving | 15 |
| **Turkey Habanero,** 1 serving | 15 |
| **Veganini,** 1 serving | 15 |
| **SIDES** | |
| **Camille's Salsa,** 1 serving | 0 |
| **Saltines,** 2 crackers | 1 |
| **Tri-colored Tortilla Chips,** 1 serving | 4 |
| **FLATBREAD PIZZAS** | |
| **Bangkok Thai,** 9" pizza | 21 |
| **Just a Cheese,** 9" pizza | 16 |
| **Kickin' BBQ Chicken,** 9" pizza | 18 |
| **Rustic Italian,** 9" pizza | 14 |
| **Zorba the Greek,** 1 pizza | 20 |
| **SOUPS** | |
| **Creamy Tuscan Tomato,** 1 small serving | 6 |
| **Red Chicken Chili,** 1 small serving | 4 |
| **Red Potato and Cheddar,** 1 small serving | 7 |
| **Rosemary Chicken Noodle,** 1 small serving | 2 |
| **SALADS** | |
| **Apple-Walnut Tuna Salad, without saltines & dressing,** 1 serving | 12 |
| **Bangkok Thai Salad, without saltines & dressing,** 1 serving | 7 |

| ▲ Power Foods | *PointsPlus™* value |
|---|---|
| **Caesar Salad with 2 oz Caesar Dressing - without saltines,** 1 serving | 7 |
| **Café Chicken Salad, without saltines & dressing,** 1 serving | 11 |
| **Chicken Caesar Salad with 2 oz Caesar Dressing, without saltines,** 1 serving | 8 |
| **Spring Mix Salad, tossed with raspberry vinaigrette,** 1 serving | 1 |
| **The Chef Salad, without saltines & dressing,** 1 serving | 9 |
| **The House Salad, without saltines & dressing,** 1 serving | 5 |
| **The Ultimate Salad - Chicken Salad, with 2 oz Caesar Dressing, without saltines,** 1 serving | 17 |
| **The Ultimate Salad - Tuna Salad, with 2 oz Caesar Dressing - without saltines,** 1 serving | 18 |

## SALAD DRESSINGS

| | |
|---|---|
| **Blue Cheese Dressing,** 1 serving | 8 |
| **Creamy Caesar Dressing,** 1 serving | 5 |
| **Golden Italian Dressing,** 1 serving | 7 |
| **Honey Mustard Dressing,** 1 serving | 7 |
| **Ranch Dressing,** 1 serving | 5 |
| **Raspberry Vinaigrette Kraft Free Dressing,** 1 serving | 1 |
| **Sesame Oriental Dressing,** 1 serving | 7 |
| **Tangy Tomato Bacon Kraft Signature Dressing,** 1 serving | 4 |

## BREAKFAST

| ▲ Power Foods | *PointsPlus™* value |
|---|---|
| **3 Cheese Scrambler,** 1 serving | 16 |
| **Breakfast on a Muffin with Bacon,** 1 serving | 13 |
| **Breakfast on a Muffin with Ham,** 1 serving | 12 |
| **Herb Garden,** 1 serving | 11 |
| **Original Breakfast Wrap with Bacon,** 1 serving | 15 |
| **Original Breakfast Wrap with Ham,** 1 serving | 14 |
| **Ranchero,** 1 serving | 15 |
| **Seasonal Fruit Cup,** 1 serving | 2 |
| **Swiss Scrambler,** 1 serving | 12 |
| **Vegetarian Zenergy,** 1 serving | 10 |

## KIDS MENU (WITHOUT CHIPS OR SALSA)

| | |
|---|---|
| **Banana Wrap,** 1 serving | 20 |
| **Chicken Wrapper,** 1 serving | 12 |
| **Classic PB&J,** 1 serving | 17 |
| **Grilled Cheese,** 1 serving | 16 |

## SMOOTHIES

| | |
|---|---|
| **Banana Berry,** 1 serving | 8 |
| **Banana Boat,** 1 serving | 6 |
| **Banana Split Swirl,** 1 serving | 23 |
| **Blueberries Cozumel,** 1 serving | 4 |
| **Peach Paradise,** 1 serving | 5 |
| **Strawberry Breeze,** 1 serving | 10 |
| **Strawberry Coconut,** 1 serving | 11 |

## DESSERTS

| | |
|---|---|
| **Chocolate Chunk Cookie,** 1 serving | 9 |
| **Oatmeal Raisin Cookie,** 1 serving | 5 |
| **Peanut Butter Cookie,** 1 serving | 11 |
| **White Chocolate Cherry Cookie,** 1 serving | 8 |
| **White Chocolate Macadamia Nut Cookie,** 1 serving | 10 |

# CAPTAIN D'S SEAFOOD

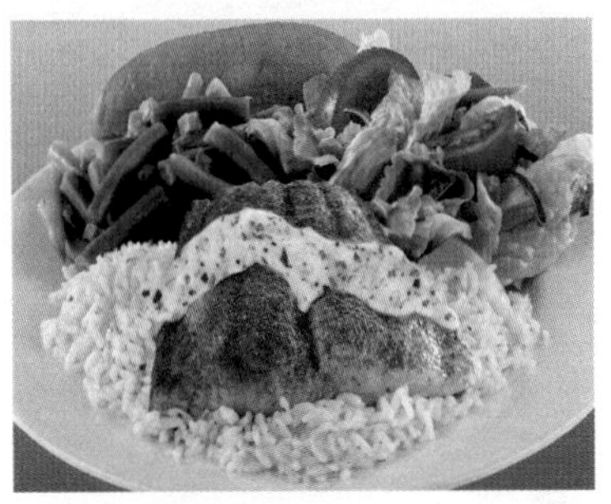

| ▲ Power Foods | *PointsPlus™* value |
|---|---|
| **APPETIZERS** | |
| **Cheese Sticks - No Sauce,** 4 pieces | 6 |
| **Jalapeno Poppers,** 5 pieces | 5 |
| **CLASSIC FISH** | |
| **Batter Dipped Fish,** 1 piece | 4 |
| **Catfish,** 1 piece | 3 |
| **Country Style Fish,** 1 piece | 6 |
| ▲ **Flounder,** 1 piece | 5 |
| **Wild Alaskan Salmon,** 1 fillet | 14 |
| **SHRIMP FAVORITES** | |
| **3 Piece Premium Shrimp,** 1 order | 2 |
| **Bite Size Shrimp,** 1/2 order | 6 |
| **Shrimp Skewers,** 1 | 19 |
| **OTHER SELECTIONS** | |
| **Breaded Chicken Tender,** 1 piece | 5 |
| **Stuffed Crab Shell,** 1 | 3 |

| ▲ Power Foods | *PointsPlus™* value |
|---|---|
| **SANDWICHES** | |
| **Chicken Ranch Sandwich (without ranch dressing),** 1 | 16 |
| **Chicken Snack Smacker (without ranch dressing),** 1 | 12 |
| **Deluxe Classic Fish Sandwich (without tartar sauce),** 1 | 16 |
| **Fish Snack Smacker (without tartar sauce),** 1 | 9 |
| **Grilled Alaskan Salmon Sandwich (without tartar sauce),** 1 | 13 |
| **SALADS** | |
| **Bite Size Shrimp Salad,** 1 | 7 |
| **Grilled Wild Alaskan Salmon Salad,** 1 | 8 |
| **Side Salad,** 1 | 1 |
| **DRESSING & SAUCES** | |
| **Blue Cheese Dressing,** 1 serving | 7 |
| **Ginger Teriyaki Sauce,** 1 serving | 2 |
| **Ranch Dressing,** 1 serving | 3 |
| **Scampi Butter Sauce,** 1 serving | 3 |
| **Sweet Chili Sauce,** 1 serving | 3 |
| **Tartar Sauce,** 2 Tbsp | 3 |
| **Thousand Island Dressing,** 1 serving | 3 |
| **SIDES** | |
| ▲ **Baked Potato - Plain,** 1 | 6 |
| **Breadstick,** 2 | 8 |
| ▲ **Broccoli,** 1 order | 0 |
| ▲ **Corn on the Cob,** 1 ear | 5 |

| ▲ Power Foods | *PointsPlus*™ value |
|---|---|
| **French Fries,** 1 serving (3 1/2 oz) | 8 |
| **Fried Okra,** 1 order | 6 |
| **Home-Style Cole Slaw,** 1 order | 4 |
| **Hush Puppies,** 4 | 11 |
| **Lemon Herb Rice,** 1 order | 4 |
| **Macaroni & Cheese,** 1 order | 4 |
| **Roasted Red Potatoes,** 1 order | 5 |
| **Southern-Style Green Beans,** 1 order | 1 |

## DESSERTS

| | |
|---|---|
| **Cheesecake with Strawberries,** 1 slice | 12 |
| **Chocolate Cake,** 1 slice | 8 |
| **Pecan Pie,** 1 slice | 13 |
| **Pineapple Cream Cheese Pie,** 1 slice | 9 |

# CARIBOU COFFEE®

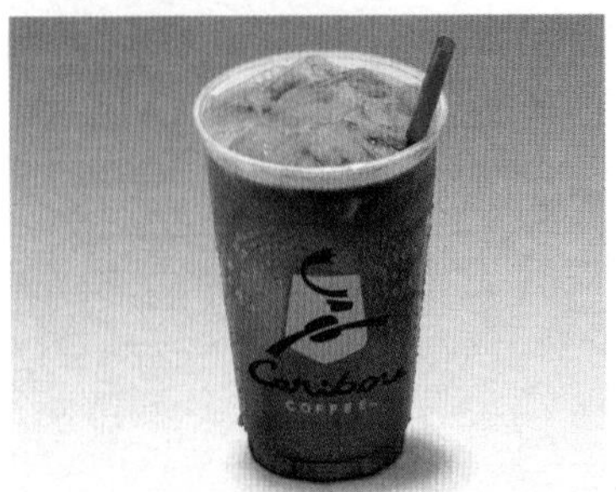


▲ Power Foods — *PointsPlus*™ value

## CLASSICS

|  | *PointsPlus*™ value |
|---|---|
| **Coffee with Steamed Milk - 2%,** 1 small | 2 |
| ▲ **Coffee with Steamed Milk - Skim,** 1 small | 1 |
| ▲ **Coffee with Steamed Milk - Soy,** 1 small | 1 |
| **Coffee, Regular or De-Caf,** 1 small | 0 |
| **Coffee, Regular or Decaf, with 2% milk,** 1 small | 2 |
| ▲ **Coffee, Regular or Decaf, with Skim Milk,** 1 small | 1 |
| ▲ **Coffee, Regular or Decaf, with Soy Milk,** 1 small | 1 |
| **Cold Press Iced Coffee, without Milk,** 1 junior | 0 |
| **Depth Charge®,** 1 small | 0 |
| **Hot Cocoa - 2%,** 1 small | 11 |
| **Hot Cocoa - Skim - No Whip,** 1 small | 6 |
| **Hot Cocoa - Skim - Whipped Cream,** 1 small | 10 |

▲ Power Foods — *PointsPlus*™ value

## ESPRESSO

|  | *PointsPlus*™ value |
|---|---|
| **Americano,** 1 small | 0 |
| **Breve,** 1 small | 10 |
| **Cappuccino - 2%,** 1 small | 1 |
| ▲ **Cappuccino - Skim Milk,** 1 small | 1 |
| ▲ **Cappuccino, with Soy Milk,** 1 small | 1 |
| **Espresso,** 1 small | 0 |
| ▲ **Latte - Skim,** 1 small | 2 |
| **Latte, with 2% Milk,** 1 small | 4 |
| ▲ **Latte, with Soy Milk,** 1 small | 3 |
| **Macchiato - skim,** 1 small | 0 |
| **Macchiato, with 2% Milk,** 1 small | 0 |
| **Macchiato, with Soy Milk,** 1 small | 0 |
| **Mocha - skim,** 1 small | 9 |
| **Mocha, with 2% Milk,** 1 small | 10 |
| **White Chocolate Mocha - Skim,** 1 small | 10 |
| **White Chocolate Mocha, with 2% Milk,** 1 small | 11 |

## COFFEE COOLERS

|  | *PointsPlus*™ value |
|---|---|
| **Caramel,** 1 junior | 10 |
| **Chocolate,** 1 junior | 11 |
| **Coffee Cooler,** 1 junior | 5 |
| **Cookies & Cream Snowdrift, with 2% Milk,** 1 junior | 13 |
| **Cookies & Cream Snowdrift™ - Skim,** 1 junior | 12 |
| **Espresso Cooler,** 1 junior | 4 |
| **Iced Americano, without Milk,** 1 junior | 0 |
| ▲ **Iced Latte - Skim,** 1 junior | 2 |

| ▲ Power Foods | *PointsPlus*™ value |
|---|---|
| **Iced Latte, with 2% Milk,** 1 junior | 3 |
| ▲ **Iced Latte, with Soy Milk,** 1 junior | 2 |
| **Iced Mocha - Skim,** 1 junior | 4 |
| **Iced Mocha, with 2% Milk,** 1 junior | 5 |
| **Iced Mocha, with Soy Milk,** 1 junior | 5 |
| **Mint Snowdrift, with 2% Milk,** 1 junior | 5 |
| **Mint Snowdrift**™, 1 junior | 10 |
| **Vanilla,** 1 junior | 11 |

## ALASKAN FRUIT SMOOTHIES

| | |
|---|---|
| **Passion Fruit Green Tea,** 1 junior | 5 |
| **Pom a Mango,** 1 junior | 6 |
| **Strawberry Banana,** 1 junior | 6 |
| **Wildberry,** 1 junior | 5 |

## NORTHERN LITE COOLERS

| | |
|---|---|
| **Caramel,** 1 junior | 5 |
| **Chocolate,** 1 junior | 6 |
| **Coffee,** 1 junior | 3 |
| **Espresso,** 1 junior | 3 |
| **Vanilla,** 1 junior | 6 |

## NORTHERN LITE LATTE

| | |
|---|---|
| ▲ **Caramel,** 1 small | 2 |
| ▲ **Vanilla,** 1 small | 2 |

## TEA

| ▲ Power Foods | *PointsPlus*™ value |
|---|---|
| **Black Tea, without Milk,** 1 small | 0 |
| **Blended Chai Tea Latte - 2% Milk,** 1 junior | 3 |
| **Blended Chai Tea Latte - Skim Milk,** 1 junior | 3 |
| **Blended Chai Tea Latte, with Soy Milk,** 1 junior | 3 |
| **Chai Tea Latte, with 2% Milk,** 1 small | 6 |
| **Chai Tea Latte, with Skim Milk,** 1 small | 4 |
| **Chai Tea Latte, with Soy Milk,** 1 small | 5 |
| **Green Tea, without Milk,** 1 small | 0 |
| **Herbal Tea, without Milk,** 1 small | 0 |
| **Iced Chai Latte - 2% Milk,** 1 junior | 3 |
| **Iced Chai Tea Latte, with Soy Milk,** 1 junior | 3 |
| **Tea (all flavors) - Iced,** 1 small | 0 |

## WILD DRINKS

| | |
|---|---|
| **Caramel Highrise**™ **- 2%,** 1 medium | 10 |
| **Hot Apple Blast®,** 1 medium | 11 |
| **Lite White Berry® (skim),** 1 medium | 12 |

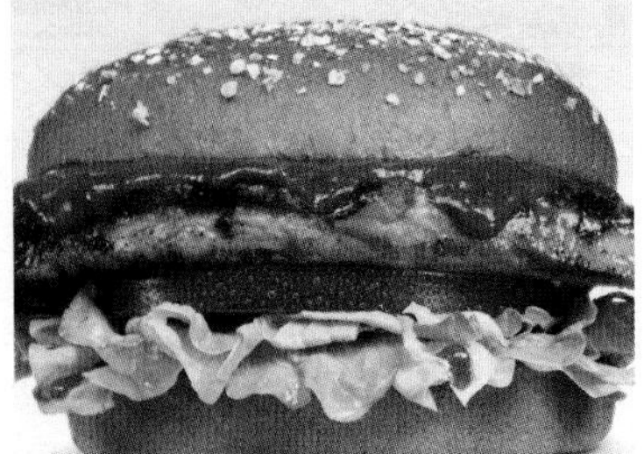

▲ Power Foods — ***PointsPlus™* value**

## CHARBROILED BURGERS

|  | PointsPlus™ value |
|---|---|
| **Big Hamburger,** 1 | 12 |
| **Chili Cheeseburger,** 1 | 22 |
| **Double Western Bacon Cheeseburger™,** 1 | 26 |
| **Famous Star® with Cheese,** 1 | 18 |
| **Jalapeno Burger™,** 1 | 19 |
| **Kid's Hamburger,** 1 | 12 |
| **Super Star® with Cheese,** 1 | 25 |
| **The Bacon Cheese Six Dollar Burger®,** 1 | 29 |
| **The Guacamole Bacon Six Dollar Burger®,** 1 | 31 |
| **The Jalapeno Six Dollar Burger™,** 1 | 28 |
| **The Low Carb Six Dollar Burger®,** 1 | 13 |
| **The Original Six Dollar Burger®,** 1 | 27 |
| **The Western Bacon Six Dollar Burger®,** 1 | 30 |
| **Western Bacon Cheeseburger®,** 1 | 19 |

## CHICKEN & OTHER CHOICES

|  | PointsPlus™ value |
|---|---|
| **Bacon Swiss Crispy Chicken Sandwich,** 1 | 19 |
| **Carl's Catch Fish Sandwich™,** 1 | 18 |
| **Charbroiled BBQ Chicken™ Sandwich,** 1 | 9 |
| **Charbroiled Chicken Club Sandwich™,** 1 | 14 |
| **Charbroiled Santa Fe Chicken Sandwich™,** 1 | 16 |
| **Chicken Breast Strips,** 5 pieces | 19 |
| **Chicken Breast Strips,** 3 pieces | 11 |
| **Spicy Chicken Sandwich,** 1 | 15 |

## SALADS

|  | PointsPlus™ value |
|---|---|
| **Charbroiled Chicken Salad (without dressing),** 1 serving | 6 |
| **Side Salad (without dressing),** 1 serving | 1 |

## SALAD DRESSINGS

|  | PointsPlus™ value |
|---|---|
| **Blue Cheese Dressing,** 1 packet (2 oz) | 9 |
| **House Dressing,** 1 packet (2 oz) | 6 |
| **Low Fat Balsamic Dressing,** 1 packet (2 oz) | 1 |
| **Thousand Island Dressing,** 1 packet (2 oz) | 7 |

## SIDES

|  | PointsPlus™ value |
|---|---|
| **Chicken Stars,** 4 pieces | 5 |
| **Chicken Stars,** 6 pieces | 7 |
| **Chicken Stars,** 9 pieces | 10 |
| **Chili Cheese Fries,** 1 serving | 33 |
| **CrissCut® Fries,** 1 serving | 11 |
| **Fish & Chips,** 1 serving | 17 |
| **Fried Zucchini,** 1 serving | 9 |
| **Natural Cut Fries,** 1 small serving | 12 |
| **Natural Cut Fries,** 1 medium serving | 16 |
| **Natural Cut Fries,** 1 large serving | 19 |
| **Natural Cut Fries,** 1 kids serving | 8 |
| **Onion Rings,** 1 serving | 12 |

| ▲ Power Foods | *PointsPlus*™ value |
|---|---|

## BREAKFAST

| | |
|---|---|
| **Bacon & Egg Burrito,** 1 | 15 |
| **Breakfast Burger,** 1 serving | 22 |
| **French Toast Dips®, without syrup,** 5 pieces | 12 |
| **Hash Brown Nuggets,** 1 serving | 9 |
| **Loaded Breakfast Burrito,** 1 serving | 22 |
| **Sourdough Breakfast Sandwich,** 1 | 12 |
| **Steak & Egg Burrito,** 1 | 18 |
| **Sunrise Croissant® Sandwich,** 1 | 15 |

## HAND-SCOOPED ICE CREAM SHAKES & MALTS™

| | |
|---|---|
| **Chocolate Malt,** 1 | 21 |
| **Chocolate Shake,** 1 | 19 |
| **OREO® Cookie Malt,** 1 | 21 |
| **OREO® Cookie Shake,** 1 | 19 |
| **Strawberry Malt,** 1 | 21 |
| **Strawberry Shake,** 1 | 19 |
| **Vanilla Malt,** 1 | 21 |
| **Vanilla Shake,** 1 | 19 |

## DESSERTS

| | |
|---|---|
| **Chocolate Chip Cookie,** 1 serving | 10 |
| **Strawberry Swirl Cheesecake,** 1 serving | 8 |
| **Chocolate Cake,** 1 serving | 8 |

# CARL'S JR.®/GREEN BURRITO®

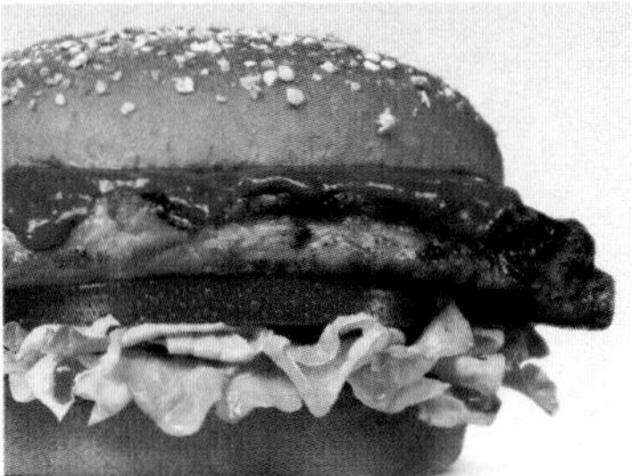

▲ Power Foods — *PointsPlus*™ value

## BURRITOS

|  | PointsPlus™ value |
|---|---|
| **Bean & Cheese Burrito,** 1 serving | 22 |
| **Bean & Cheese Burrito - Chicken,** 1 serving | 19 |
| **Bean & Cheese Burrito - Ground Beef,** 1 serving | 23 |
| **Bean & Cheese Burrito - Steak,** 1 serving | 20 |
| **Carne Asada Burrito,** 1 serving | 18 |
| **Grilled Chicken Burrito,** 1 serving | 28 |
| **The Green Burrito® - Chicken,** 1 serving | 24 |
| **The Green Burrito® - Steak,** 1 serving | 25 |

## TACOS

|  | PointsPlus™ value |
|---|---|
| **Fish Taco,** 1 serving | 8 |
| **Hard Taco - Chicken,** 1 serving | 5 |
| **Hard Taco - Ground Beef,** 1 serving | 6 |
| **Hard Taco - Steak,** 1 serving | 5 |
| **Soft Taco - Chicken,** 1 serving | 5 |
| **Soft Taco - Ground Beef,** 1 serving | 6 |

▲ Power Foods — *PointsPlus*™ value

## SPECIALTIES

|  | PointsPlus™ value |
|---|---|
| **Crisp Burritos,** 10 pieces | 48 |
| **Crisp Burritos,** 5 pieces | 24 |
| **Crisp Burritos,** 3 pieces | 14 |
| **Enchiladas - Cheese,** 2 | 13 |
| **Quesadilla - Cheese,** 1 serving | 10 |
| **Quesadilla - Chicken,** 1 serving | 13 |
| **Quesadilla - Steak,** 1 serving | 13 |
| **Super Nachos - Chicken,** 1 serving | 25 |
| **Super Nachos - Ground Beef,** 1 serving | 29 |
| **Super Nachos - Steak,** 1 serving | 26 |
| **Taco Salad - Chicken,** 1 serving | 22 |
| **Taco Salad - Ground Beef,** 1 serving | 26 |
| **Taco Salad - Steak,** 1 serving | 23 |
| **Taquitos - Chicken,** 5 | 9 |
| **Taquitos - Chicken,** 2 | 4 |

## SIDES

|  | PointsPlus™ value |
|---|---|
| **Chips,** 1 serving | 8 |
| **Chips & Cheese,** 1 serving | 19 |
| **Guacamole,** 1 serving | 2 |
| **Pinto Beans & Cheese,** 1 serving | 9 |
| **Rice,** 1 serving | 9 |
| **Sour Cream,** 1 serving | 2 |

▲ Power Foods — *PointsPlus*™ value

## ICE CREAM

|  | *PointsPlus*™ value |
|---|---|
| **Chocolate,** 1 small | 7 |
| **Chocolate,** 1 regular | 11 |
| **Chocolate,** 1 large | 16 |
| **No Fat Chocolate,** 1 small | 4 |
| **No Fat Chocolate,** 1 regular | 7 |
| **No Fat Chocolate,** 1 large | 10 |
| **No Fat Vanilla,** 1 small | 4 |
| **No Fat Vanilla,** 1 regular | 7 |
| **No Fat Vanilla,** 1 large | 10 |
| **No Sugar Added Vanilla,** 1 small | 5 |
| **No Sugar Added Vanilla,** 1 regular | 9 |
| **No Sugar Added Vanilla,** 1 large | 13 |
| **Sherbet,** 1 small | 5 |
| **Sherbet,** 1 regular | 8 |
| **Sherbet,** 1 large | 11 |
| **Vanilla,** 1 small | 7 |
| **Vanilla,** 1 regular | 12 |
| **Vanilla,** 1 large | 17 |
| **Slice of Ice Cream Cake,** 1 serving | 7 |

## ICE CREAM CONES

|  | *PointsPlus*™ value |
|---|---|
| **Cake Cone with Chocolate,** 1 kids | 4 |
| **Cake Cone with Vanilla,** 1 kids | 5 |
| **Sugar Cone with Chocolate,** 1 small | 8 |
| **Sugar Cone with Vanilla,** 1 small | 9 |
| **Waffle Cone with Chocolate,** 1 small | 9 |
| **Waffle Cone with Vanilla,** 1 small | 9 |

## CLASSIC SUNDAES

|  | *PointsPlus*™ value |
|---|---|
| **Bittersweet Fudge,** 1 regular | 19 |
| **Bittersweet Fudge,** 1 large | 25 |
| **Caramel,** 1 regular | 18 |
| **Hot Fudge,** 1 regular | 18 |
| **Hot Fudge,** 1 large | 24 |
| **No Fat Classic Sundae (Fudge),** 1 regular | 10 |

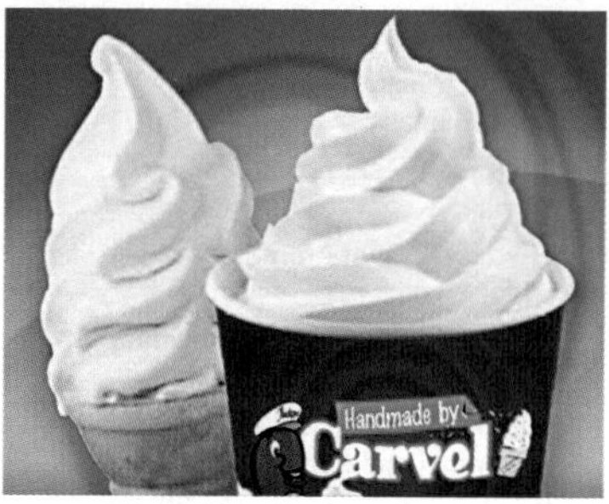


▲ Power Foods — *PointsPlus*™ value

|  | *PointsPlus*™ value |
|---|---|
| **No Fat Classic Sundae (Strawberry),** 1 regular | 8 |
| **Strawberry,** 1 regular | 16 |
| **Strawberry,** 1 large | 21 |

## DASHERS

|  | *PointsPlus*™ value |
|---|---|
| **Banana Barge®,** 1 | 27 |
| **Bananas Foster,** 1 | 18 |
| **Fudge Brownie,** 1 | 23 |
| **Mint Chocolate Chip,** 1 | 22 |
| **Peanut Butter Cup,** 1 | 27 |
| **Strawberry Shortcake,** 1 | 17 |

## FOUNTAIN DRINKS

|  | *PointsPlus*™ value |
|---|---|
| **Caramel Macchiato Freeze,** 1 small | 18 |
| **Caramel Macchiato Freeze - Light,** 1 small | 12 |
| **Carvelanche®, Butterfinger,** 1 small | 21 |
| **Carvelanche®, Cake Mix,** 1 small | 21 |
| **Carvelanche®, Cookies & Cream,** 1 small | 17 |
| **Carvelanche®, M&M,** 1 small | 21 |
| **Carvelanche®, Reese's,** 1 small | 21 |
| **Coffee Freeze,** 1 small | 19 |
| **Coffee Freeze - Light,** 1 small | 10 |
| **Cookie Dough Arctic Blender,** 1 small | 25 |

Fountain Drinks (cont'd)

| ▲ Power Foods | PointsPlus™ value |
|---|---|
| **Cookie Dough Arctic Blender - Light,** 1 small | 18 |
| **Fried Ice Cream Arctic Blender,** 1 small | 23 |
| **Fried Ice Cream Arctic Blender - Light,** 1 small | 16 |
| **Ice Cream Soda Float - Chocolate Ice Cream and Coke,** 1 small | 10 |
| **Ice Cream Soda Float - Chocolate Ice Cream and Soda Water,** 1 small | 12 |
| **Ice Cream Soda Float - Vanilla Ice Cream and Coke,** 1 small | 10 |
| **Ice Cream Soda Float - Vanilla Ice Cream and Soda Water,** 1 small | 12 |
| **Mocha Freeze,** 1 small | 17 |
| **Mocha Freeze - Light,** 1 small | 10 |
| **No Fat Carvelanche® (Strawberry),** 1 small | 11 |
| **No Fat Chocolate Shake,** 1 small | 12 |
| **No Fat Mocha Shake,** 1 small | 11 |
| **No Fat Vanilla Shake,** 1 small | 8 |
| **Peanut Butter Arctic Blender,** 1 small | 19 |
| **Peanut Butter Arctic Blender - Light,** 1 small | 13 |
| **Thick Chocolate Shake,** 1 small | 18 |
| **Thick Shake Float - Chocolate,** 1 small | 22 |
| **Thick Shake Float - Strawberry,** 1 small | 20 |
| **Thick Shake Float - Vanilla,** 1 small | 22 |
| **Thick Strawberry Shake,** 1 small | 16 |
| **Thick Vanilla Shake,** 1 small | 18 |

## NOVELTIES

| ▲ Power Foods | PointsPlus™ value |
|---|---|
| **98% Fat Free Flying Saucer®, Chocolate,** 1 | 5 |
| **98% Fat Free Flying Saucer®, Vanilla,** 1 | 5 |
| **Brown Bonnet®,** 1 | 11 |
| **Chipsters®,** 1 | 9 |
| **Deluxe Flying Saucer® (Sprinkles),** 1 | 10 |
| **Flying Saucer®, Chocolate,** 1 | 6 |
| **Flying Saucer®, Vanilla,** 1 | 7 |
| **Mini Sundae (Chocolate Syrup),** 1 | 6 |
| **No Fat Miniature Sundae,** 1 | 5 |
| **No Fat Olde Fashion Sundae,** 1 serving | 8 |
| **No Fat Parfait,** 1 serving | 5 |
| **No Sugar Added Miniature Sundae,** 1 | 6 |
| **No Sugar Added Olde Fashion Sundae,** 1 serving | 10 |
| **No Sugar Added Parfait,** 1 serving | 6 |
| **Olde Fashion Sundae,** 1 | 9 |
| **Sinful Love Bar™,** 1 | 13 |
| **Sprinkle Cup,** 1 | 7 |

## ITALIAN ICES

| ▲ Power Foods | PointsPlus™ value |
|---|---|
| **Bubble Gum,** 1 small | 3 |
| **Cherry,** 1 small | 4 |
| **Cherry Swirl,** 1 small | 13 |
| **Guava,** 1 small | 4 |
| **Lemon,** 1 small | 4 |
| **Mango,** 1 small | 4 |
| **Mango Swirl,** 1 small | 13 |
| **Passion Fruit,** 1 small | 4 |
| **Passion Fruit Swirl,** 1 small | 13 |
| **Sour Blue Raspberry,** 1 small | 4 |
| **Strawberry,** 1 small | 3 |

## SMOOTHIE

| ▲ Power Foods | PointsPlus™ value |
|---|---|
| **Berry Times Square,** 1 small | 9 |
| **Broadway Banana,** 1 small | 8 |
| **Rockefeller Raspberry,** 1 small | 8 |

▲ Power Foods | *PointsPlus*™ value

## GRANDE SALADS

|  | *PointsPlus*™ value |
|---|---|
| ▲ **Beans a la Charra (no cheese or pico de gallo),** 1 serving | 4 |
| **Santa Fe Chop,** 1 serving | 17 |
| **Santa Fe Chop (no cheese or bacon),** 1 serving | 9 |
| **Santa Fe Chop (no cheese),** 1 serving | 12 |
| **Santa Fe Chop (no cheese, bacon or avocado),** 1 serving | 7 |
| **Tostada Salad with Chicken,** 1 serving | 41 |
| **Tostada Salad with Chicken (no tortilla strips or cheese),** 1 serving | 25 |
| **Tostada Salad with Chicken (no tortilla strips),** 1 serving | 37 |
| **Tostada Salad with Chicken (no tortilla strips, cheese or sour cream),** 1 serving | 24 |
| **Tostada Salad with Chicken (no tortilla strips, cheese, sour cream or guacamole),** 1 serving | 23 |

## SIZZLING FAJITAS

|  | *PointsPlus*™ value |
|---|---|
| **Famous Chicken Fajitas (no tortillas, tamalito, rice, sour cream or guacamole),** 1 serving | 13 |
| **Juicy Shrimp Fajitas (no tortillas or tamalito),** 1 serving | 28 |
| **Juicy Shrimp Fajitas (no tortillas),** 1 serving | 30 |
| **Juicy Shrimp Fajitas (no tortillas, tamalito or rice),** 1 serving | 24 |
| **Juicy Shrimp Fajitas (no tortillas, tamalito, rice or sour cream),** 1 serving | 22 |
| **Juicy Shrimp Fajitas (no tortillas, tamalito, rice, sour cream or guacamole),** 1 serving | 21 |

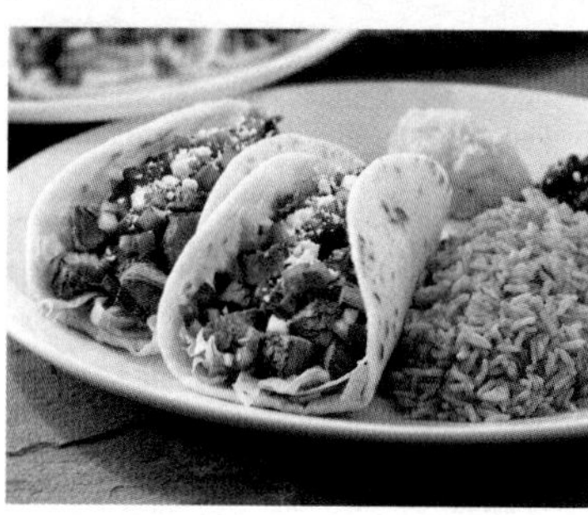

▲ Power Foods | *PointsPlus*™ value

|  | *PointsPlus*™ value |
|---|---|
| **Mix and Match Fajitas - Chicken and Steak (no tortillas or tamalito),** 1 serving | 22 |
| **Mix and Match Fajitas - Chicken and Steak (no tortillas),** 1 serving | 24 |
| **Mix and Match Fajitas - Chicken and Steak (no tortillas, tamalito or rice),** 1 serving | 18 |
| **Mix and Match Fajitas - Chicken and Steak (no tortillas, tamalito, rice or sour cream),** 1 serving | 16 |
| **Mix and Match Fajitas - Chicken and Steak (no tortillas, tamalito, rice, sour cream or guacamole),** 1 serving | 15 |
| **Original Famous Chicken Fajitas (no tortillas or tamalito or rice or sour cream),** 1 serving | 14 |
| **Original Famous Chicken Fajitas (no tortillas or tamalito or rice),** 1 serving | 16 |
| **Original Famous Chicken Fajitas (no tortillas or tamalito),** 1 serving | 20 |
| **Original Famous Chicken Fajitas (no tortillas),** 1 serving | 23 |
| **Portabella Mushroom and Asparagus Fajita (no tortillas),** 1 serving | 24 |
| **Portabella Mushroom and Asparagus Fajitas (no tortillas or tamalito),** 1 serving | 21 |

*Sizzling Fajitas (cont'd)*

| ▲ Power Foods | *PointsPlus*™ value |
|---|---|
| **Portabella Mushroom and Asparagus Fajitas (no tortillas, tamalito or rice),** 1 serving | 17 |
| **Portabella Mushroom and Asparagus Fajitas (no tortillas, tamalito, rice or sour cream),** 1 serving | 15 |
| **Portabella Mushroom and Asparagus Fajitas (no tortillas, tamalito, rice, sour cream or guacamole),** 1 serving | 14 |
| **Sizzling Steak Fajitas (no tortillas or tamalito),** 1 serving | 23 |
| **Sizzling Steak Fajitas (no tortillas or tamalito, rice, sour cream or guacamole),** 1 serving | 16 |
| **Sizzling Steak Fajitas (no tortillas),** 1 serving | 26 |
| **Sizzling Steak Fajitas (no tortillas, tamalito or rice),** 1 serving | 19 |
| **Sizzling Steak Fajitas (no tortillas, tamalito, rice or sour cream),** 1 serving | 17 |

## GRILLED TACOS

| ▲ Power Foods | *PointsPlus*™ value |
|---|---|
| **Chicken Tacos,** 1 serving | 26 |
| **Chicken Tacos (no tamalito or rice),** 1 serving | 19 |
| **Chicken Tacos (no tamalito),** 1 serving | 23 |
| **Chicken Tacos (no tamalito, rice or cheese),** 1 serving | 18 |
| **Fish Tacos - Salmon,** 1 serving | 26 |
| **Fish Tacos - Salmon (no tamalito or rice),** 1 serving | 20 |
| **Fish Tacos - Salmon (no tamalito),** 1 serving | 24 |
| **Fish Tacos - Salmon (no tamalito, rice or cheese),** 1 serving | 19 |
| **Fish Tacos - Sea Bass,** 1 serving | 25 |
| **Fish Tacos - Sea Bass (no tamalito or rice),** 1 serving | 18 |
| **Fish Tacos - Sea Bass (no tamalito),** 1 serving | 22 |
| **Fish Tacos - Sea Bass (no tamalito, rice or cheese),** 1 serving | 17 |
| **Fish Tacos - Sea Bass (no tamalito, rice, cheese or chipotle aioli),** 1 serving | 15 |
| **Fresh Fish Tacos - Salmon (no tamalito, rice, cheese or guacamole),** 1 serving | 17 |
| **Steak Tacos,** 1 serving | 27 |
| **Steak Tacos (no tamalito or rice),** 1 serving | 21 |
| **Steak Tacos (no tamalito),** 1 serving | 25 |
| **Steak Tacos (no tamalito, rice or cheese),** 1 serving | 20 |

## HOMEMADE BEANS

| ▲ Power Foods | *PointsPlus*™ value |
|---|---|
| **Beans a la Charra,** 1 serving | 5 |
| **Beans a la Charra (no cheese),** 1 serving | 5 |
| ▲ **Black Bean,** 1 serving | 4 |
| ▲ **Black Bean (no cheese),** 1 serving | 4 |
| ▲ **Black Beans (no cheese or pico de gallo),** 1 serving | 4 |
| **Refried Beans,** 1 serving | 7 |
| **Refried Beans (no cheese or pico de gallo),** 1 serving | 7 |
| **Refried Beans (no cheese),** 1 serving | 7 |

| ▲ Power Foods | *PointsPlus™* value |
|---|---|
| **CLASSICS** | |
| **Chick-fil-A® Chick-n-Strips®,** 3 strips | 9 |
| **Chick-fil-A® Chargrilled Chicken Sandwich,** 1 sandwich | 6 |
| **Chick-fil-A® Chargrilled Chicken Club Sandwich,** 1 sandwich | 10 |
| **Chick-fil-A® Chicken Sandwich,** 1 sandwich | 11 |
| **Chick-fil-A® Chicken Salad Sandwich,** 1 sandwich | 13 |
| **Chick-fil-A® Nuggets,** 8 nuggets | 7 |
| **COOL WRAP®** | |
| **Chargrilled Chicken Cool Wrap®,** 1 wrap | 11 |
| **Chicken Caesar Cool Wrap®,** 1 wrap | 12 |
| **Spicy Chicken Cool Wrap®,** 1 wrap | 11 |
| **SALADS** | |
| **Chick-fil-A® Chargrilled Chicken & Fruit Salad,** 1 salad | 6 |
| **Chick-fil-A® Chargrilled Chicken Garden Salad,** 1 salad | 4 |
| **Chick-fil-A® Chick-n-Strips® Salad,** 1 salad | 12 |
| **Chick-fil-A® Southwest Chargrilled Chicken Salad,** 1 salad | 6 |
| **Garlic Butter Croutons,** 1 packet | 2 |
| **Harvest Nut Granola,** 1 packet | 2 |
| **Honey Roasted Sunflower Kernels,** 1 packet | 2 |
| **Tortilla Strips,** 1 packet | 2 |

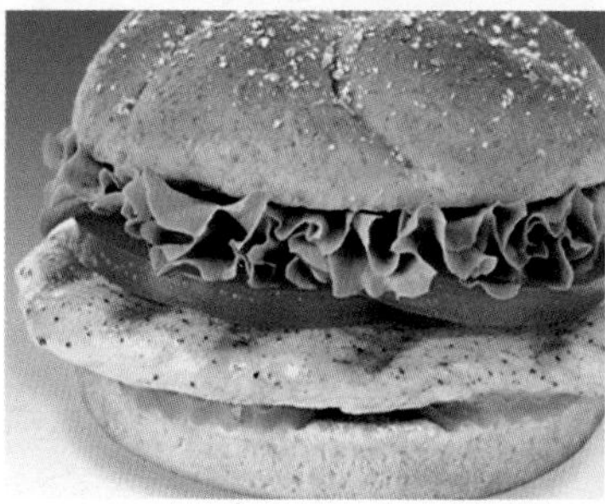

| ▲ Power Foods | *PointsPlus™* value |
|---|---|
| **DRESSINGS & SAUCES** | |
| **Blue Cheese Dressing,** 2 Tbsp | 4 |
| **Buttermilk Ranch Dressing,** 2 Tbsp | 4 |
| **Caesar Dressing,** 2 Tbsp | 5 |
| **Fat Free Honey Mustard Dressing,** 2 Tbsp | 2 |
| **Light Italian Dressing,** 2 Tbsp | 0 |
| **Reduced Fat Berry Balsamic Vinaigrette,** 2 Tbsp | 2 |
| **Spicy Dressing,** 2 Tbsp | 4 |
| **Thousand Island Dressing,** 2 Tbsp | 4 |
| **Barbecue Sauce,** 1 packet | 1 |
| **Buttermilk Ranch Sauce,** 1 serving | 3 |
| **Chick-fil-A® Sauce,** 1 packet | 4 |
| **Honey Mustard Sauce,** 1 packet | 1 |
| **Honey Roasted BBQ Sauce,** 1 packet | 2 |
| **Polynesian Sauce,** 1 packet | 3 |
| **SIDE ITEMS** | |
| **Carrot & Raisin Salad,** 1 salad portion | 7 |
| **Chick-fil-A® Waffle Potato Fries®,** 1 small serving | 8 |
| **Cole Slaw,** 1 small serving | 10 |
| ▲ **Fruit Cup,** 1 cup | 2 |
| **Hearty Breast of Chicken Soup,** 1 small serving | 4 |
| **Side Salad,** 1 salad | 2 |

# CHICK-FIL-A®

| ▲ Power Foods | *PointsPlus*™ value |
|---|---|
| **BREAKFAST** | |
| **Bacon, Egg & Cheese Biscuit,** 1 | 13 |
| **Chicken Breakfast Burrito,** 6 1/2 oz | 11 |
| **Chicken, Egg & Cheese on Sunflower Multigrain Bagel,** 7 1/2 oz | 13 |
| **Chick-fil-A® Chicken Biscuit,** 1 | 12 |
| **Chick-fil-A® Chick-n-Minis™ 3-count,** 1 serving | 7 |
| **Chick-fil-A® Chick-n-Minis™ 4-count,** 1 serving | 9 |
| **Cinnamon Cluster,** 1 | 11 |
| **Hash Browns,** 1 | 8 |
| **Hot Buttered Biscuit,** 1 | 8 |
| **Sausage Biscuit,** 5 1/4 oz | 16 |
| **Sausage Breakfast Burrito,** 6 1/2 oz | 13 |
| **Sunflower Multigrain Bagel,** 1 | 6 |
| **DESSERTS** | |
| **Cheesecake,** 1 slice | 9 |
| **Fudge Nut Brownie,** 1 brownie | 10 |
| **Icedream® Cone,** 1 cone | 5 |
| **Icedream® Cup,** 1 cup | 8 |
| **Lemon Pie,** 1 slice | 10 |
| **Chocolate Milkshake,** 1 small | 18 |
| **Chocolate Milkshake,** 1 large | 21 |
| **Strawberry Milkshake,** 1 small | 17 |
| **Strawberry Milkshake,** 1 large | 21 |
| **Vanilla Milkshake,** 1 small | 15 |
| **Vanilla Milkshake,** 1 large | 18 |
| **BEVERAGES** | |
| **Chick-fil-A® Diet Lemonade,** 1 small | 1 |
| **Chick-fil-A® Lemonade,** 1 small | 5 |
| **Coca-Cola® Classic,** 1 small container | 4 |
| **Sweet Tea,** 1 small cup | 3 |

▲ Power Foods — *PointsPlus*™ value

## GUILTLESS GRILL® (WITH SIDES)

|  | *PointsPlus*™ value |
|---|---|
| **Guiltless Grilled Chicken Sandwich (grilled chicken breast topped with low-fat ranch, shredded lettuce, tomato, and sauteed onions; served on whole wheat bun),** 1 | 9 |
| **Guiltless Grilled Chicken Sandwich, with no-fat honey mustard, with steamed seasonal veggies topped with parmesan cheese,** 1 serving | 15 |
| **Guiltless Grilled Salmon, with garlic and herbs, with rice, with steamed seasonal veggies topped with parmesan cheese,** 1 serving | 14 |

## GRILLED ENTRÉE

|  | *PointsPlus*™ value |
|---|---|
| **Margarita Grilled Chicken (grilled margarita-marinated chicken breast, rice & kettle black beans),** 1 serving | 13 |

## HOT OFF THE GRILL

|  | *PointsPlus*™ value |
|---|---|
| **Chili's Classic Sirloin (with toast, no sides),** 1 serving | 12 |

## FAJITAS (WITHOUT CONDIMENTS OR TORTILLAS)

|  | *PointsPlus*™ value |
|---|---|
| **Cadillac Style (rice & black beans only),** 1 serving | 7 |
| **Classic Chicken Fajitas (with sizzling onions and bell peppers),** 1 skillet | 9 |

## TORTILLAS & CONDIMENTS FOR FAJITAS

|  | *PointsPlus*™ value |
|---|---|
| **Fajita Condiments,** 1 serving | 6 |
| **Flour Tortilla for Fajitas,** 1 serving (3 each) | 10 |

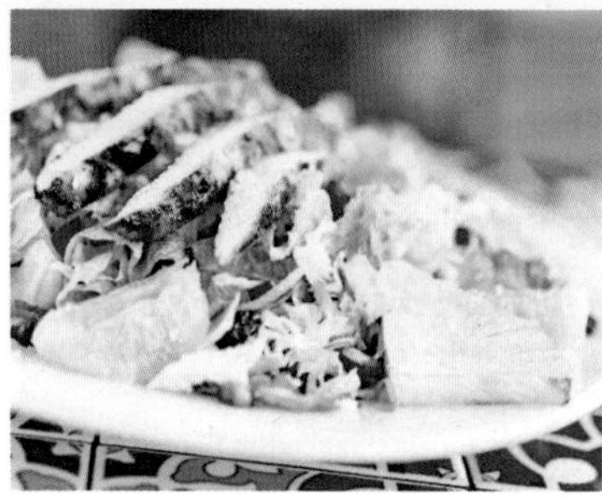

▲ Power Foods — *PointsPlus*™ value

## KID'S ENTRÉES (SIDES NOT INCLUDED)

|  | *PointsPlus*™ value |
|---|---|
| **Cheese Pizza,** 1 pizza | 15 |
| **Grilled Chicken Platter,** 1 serving | 4 |
| **Grilled Chicken Sandwich,** 1 serving | 6 |
| **Little Mouth Burger,** 1 serving | 9 |
| **Macaroni & Cheese,** 1 serving | 14 |

## SALADS

|  | *PointsPlus*™ value |
|---|---|
| **Dinner House Salad, without dressing,** 1 serving | 3 |
| **Guiltless Grill Asian Salad,** 1 serving | 10 |
| **Guiltless Grill Caribbean Salad,** 1 serving | 13 |
| **Mesquite Chicken Salad (without dressing),** 1 serving | 19 |
| **Quesadilla Explosion Salad, with Ranch dressing,** 1 serving | 27 |
| **Quesadilla Explosion Salad, without dressing (with 4 cheese quesadillas),** 1 serving | 28 |
| **Quesadilla Explosion Salad, without dressing (without quesadillas),** 1 serving | 15 |
| **Side House Salad, without dressing,** 1 serving | 3 |

| ▲ Power Foods | *PointsPlus*™ value |
|---|---|
| **NOT "JUST" SIDES** | |
| **Cinnamon Apples,** 1 serving | 6 |
| **Honey Mustard Dressing, No Fat,** 1 serving | 6 |
| ▲ **Kettle Black Beans,** 1 serving | 2 |
| **Ranch Dressing, Low Fat,** 1 serving | 1 |
| **Rice,** 1 serving | 4 |
| **Salsa Picante Sauce/Hot Sauce,** 1 serving | 1 |
| **SIDES & EXTRAS - GUILTLESS GRILL®** | |
| **Guiltless Steamed Veggies with Parmesan,** 1 serving | 1 |
| **SOUPS** (WITHOUT CRACKERS) | |
| **Chicken and Green Chile,** 1 cup | 3 |
| **Chicken and Green Chile,** 1 bowl | 5 |
| **TREAT YOURSELF** | |
| **Sweet Shot - Key Lime Pie,** 1 serving | 7 |
| **Sweet Shot - Red Velvet Cake,** 1 serving | 7 |

▲ Power Foods — *PointsPlus*™ value

## BUILD YOUR OWN BURRITO, FAJITA, TACO OR BOWL

|  | PointsPlus™ value |
|---|---|
| **Barbacoa,** 1 serving | 4 |
| ▲ **Black Beans,** 1 serving | 3 |
| **Carnitas,** 1 serving | 5 |
| **Cheese,** 1 serving | 3 |
| **Chicken,** 1 serving | 5 |
| ▲ **Fajita Vegetables,** 1 serving | 1 |
| ▲ **Pinto Beans,** 1 serving | 2 |
| ▲ **Romaine Lettuce (salad),** 1 serving | 0 |
| ▲ **Romaine Lettuce (tacos),** 1 serving | 0 |
| ▲ **Steak,** 1 serving | 5 |

## SALSAS

|  | PointsPlus™ value |
|---|---|
| ▲ **Corn Salsa,** 1 serving | 2 |
| ▲ **Green Tomatillo Salsa,** 1 serving | 0 |
| ▲ **Red Tomatillo Salsa,** 1 serving | 1 |
| ▲ **Tomato Salsa,** 1 serving | 0 |

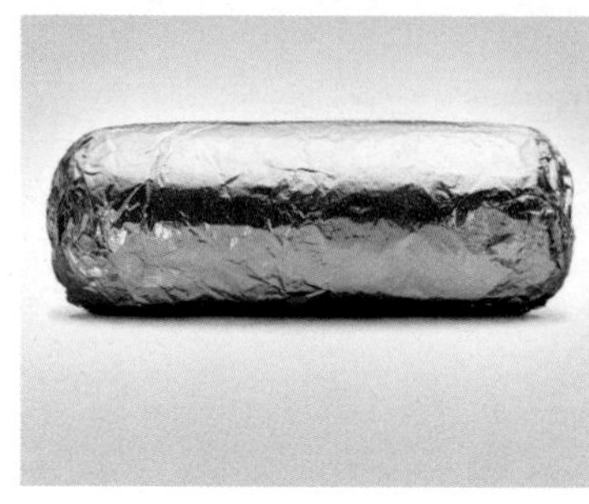

▲ Power Foods — *PointsPlus*™ value

## EXTRAS

|  | PointsPlus™ value |
|---|---|
| **Chips,** 1 serving | 15 |
| **Cilantro-Lime Rice,** 1 serving | 3 |
| **Guacamole,** 1 serving | 4 |
| **Sour Cream,** 1 serving | 3 |
| **Vinaigrette,** 1 serving | 8 |

## TORTILLAS & SHELLS

|  | PointsPlus™ value |
|---|---|
| **Crispy Taco Shell,** 1 | 1 |
| **Flour Tortilla (burrito),** 1 | 8 |
| **Flour Tortilla (taco),** 1 | 2 |

# CHURCH'S CHICKEN®

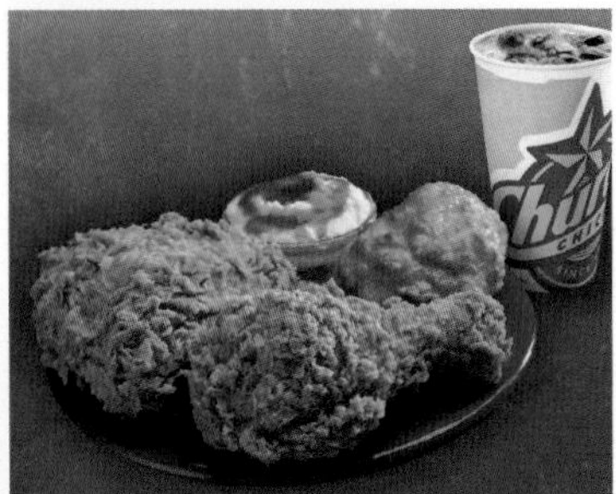

| ▲ Power Foods | *PointsPlus™* value |
|---|---|
| **MAIN COURSE** | |
| **Bigger Better Chicken Sandwich,** 1 | 13 |
| **Crunchy Tender Strip,** 1 strip | 3 |
| **Original Breast,** 1 (as served with skin) | 5 |
| **Original Leg,** 1 (as served with skin) | 3 |
| **Original Thigh,** 1 (as served with skin) | 9 |
| **Original Wing,** 1 (as served with skin) | 8 |
| **Spicy Breast,** 1 (as served with skin) | 8 |
| **Spicy Crunchy Tenders,** 1 | 3 |
| **Spicy Leg,** 1 (as served with skin) | 5 |
| **Spicy Thigh,** 1 (as served with skin) | 13 |
| **Spicy Wing,** 1 (as served with skin) | 11 |
| **SIDES** | |
| **Cajun Rice,** 1 regular | 4 |
| **Cole Slaw,** 1 regular | 4 |
| ▲ **Collard Greens,** 1 regular | 0 |
| ▲ **Corn on the Cob,** 1 serving | 3 |
| **French Fries,** 1 regular | 8 |
| **Honey Butter Biscuit,** 1 (plain) | 6 |
| **Jalapeño Cheese Bombers®,** 4 | 6 |
| **Macaroni & Cheese,** 1 regular | 6 |
| **Mashed Potatoes & Gravy,** 1 regular | 2 |
| **Okra,** 1 regular | 9 |
| **Sweet Corn Nuggets,** 1 regular | 16 |
| ▲ **Whole Jalapeno Peppers,** 2 | 0 |

| ▲ Power Foods | *PointsPlus™* value |
|---|---|
| **CONDIMENTS** | |
| **BBQ Sauce,** 1 package | 1 |
| **Creamy Jalapeno Sauce,** 1 package | 3 |
| **Honey Mustard Sauce,** 1 package | 3 |
| **Purple Pepper Sauce™,** 1 package | 1 |
| **Ranch Sauce,** 1 package | 3 |
| **DESSERT** | |
| **Apple Pie,** 1 serving | 7 |

# CICI'S PIZZA BUFFET

| ▲ Power Foods | *PointsPlus*™ value |
|---|---|
| **PIZZA** | |
| **Alfredo Pizza,** 1 slice | 3 |
| **Bacon Cheddar Pizza,** 1 slice | 4 |
| **BBQ Pizza,** 1 slice | 4 |
| **Beef Pizza,** 1 slice | 4 |
| **Buffalo Chicken,** 1 slice | 4 |
| **Cheese Pizza,** 1 slice | 4 |
| **Chicken Pizza,** 1 slice | 4 |
| **Ham and Pineapple Pizza,** 1 slice | 4 |
| **Ham Pizza,** 1 slice | 3 |
| **Mac & Cheese Pizza,** 1 slice | 4 |
| **Ole Pizza,** 1 slice | 3 |
| **Pepperoni & Jalapeno Pizza,** 1 slice | 4 |
| **DESSERT** | |
| **Brownies,** 1 piece | 4 |

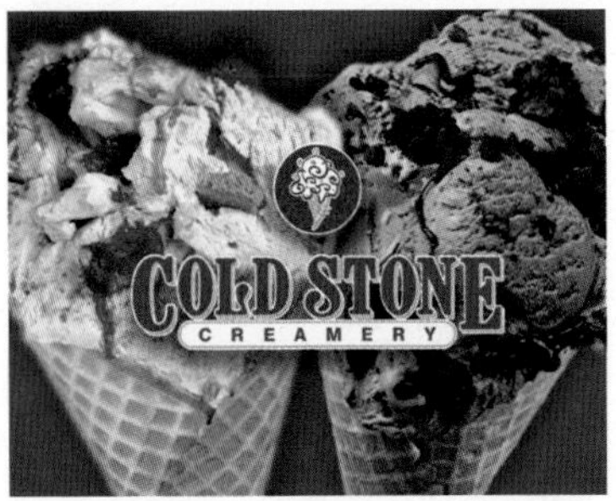


| ▲ Power Foods | *PointsPlus™* value |
|---|---|
| **ICE CREAM** | |
| **Amaretto Ice Cream,** 1 Gotta Have It | 22 |
| **Banana Ice Cream,** 1 Gotta Have It | 21 |
| **Black Cherry Ice Cream,** 1 Gotta Have It | 22 |
| **Blueberry Muffin Ice Cream,** 1 Gotta Have It | 23 |
| **Butter Pecan Ice Cream,** 1 Gotta Have It | 22 |
| **Cake Batter Ice Cream™,** 1 Gotta Have It | 23 |
| **Cheesecake Ice Cream,** 1 Gotta Have It | 22 |
| **Chocolate Cake Batter Ice Cream™,** 1 Gotta Have It | 23 |
| **Chocolate Ice Cream,** 1 Gotta Have It | 22 |
| **Chocolate Raspberry Truffle Ice Cream,** 1 Like It | 9 |
| **Cinnamon Bun Ice Cream,** 1 Gotta Have It | 25 |
| **Cinnamon Ice Cream,** 1 Gotta Have It | 22 |
| **Coconut Ice Cream,** 1 Gotta Have It | 22 |
| **Coffee Ice Cream,** 1 Gotta Have It | 22 |
| **Cookie Batter Ice Cream,** 1 Gotta Have It | 25 |

| ▲ Power Foods | *PointsPlus™* value |
|---|---|
| **Cotton Candy Ice Cream,** 1 Gotta Have It | 22 |
| **Dark Chocolate Ice Cream,** 1 Gotta Have It | 21 |
| **Dark Chocolate Peppermint Ice Cream,** 1 Gotta Have It | 22 |
| **Egg Nog Ice Cream,** 1 Gotta Have It | 17 |
| **French Toast Ice Cream,** 1 Gotta Have It | 22 |
| **French Vanilla Ice Cream,** 1 Gotta Have It | 23 |
| **Ghiradelli Chocolate Ice Cream,** 1 Gotta Have It | 25 |
| **Gingerbread Ice Cream,** 1 Like It | 9 |
| **Irish Cream Ice Cream,** 1 Gotta Have It | 22 |
| **JELL-O® Chocolate Pudding Ice Cream,** 1 Gotta Have It | 24 |
| **Macadamia Nut Ice Cream,** 1 Gotta Have It | 22 |
| **Mango Ice Cream,** 1 Gotta Have It | 21 |
| **Marshmallow Ice Cream,** 1 Gotta Have It | 22 |
| **Mint Ice Cream,** 1 Gotta Have It | 22 |
| **Mocha Ice Cream,** 1 Gotta Have It | 22 |
| **Nutter Butter Ice Cream,** 1 Like It | 11 |
| **Oatmeal Cookie Batter Ice Cream,** 1 Gotta Have It | 22 |
| **Orange Dreamsicle Ice Cream,** 1 Gotta Have It | 22 |
| **Peach Ice Cream,** 1 Like It | 9 |
| **Peanut Butter Ice Cream,** 1 Gotta Have It | 25 |
| **Pecan Praline Ice Cream,** 1 Gotta Have It | 22 |
| **Pistachio Ice Cream,** 1 Gotta Have It | 22 |
| **Pumpkin Ice Cream,** 1 Gotta Have It | 19 |
| **Raspberry Ice Cream,** 1 Gotta Have It | 22 |
| **Sinless Cake Batter Ice Cream,** 1 Gotta Have It | 13 |

| ▲ Power Foods | *PointsPlus*™ value |
|---|---|
| **Sinless Sans Fat™ Sweet Cream,** 1 Gotta Have It | 10 |
| **Strawberry Ice Cream,** 1 Gotta Have It | 21 |
| **Sweet Cream Ice Cream,** 1 Gotta Have It | 22 |
| **Vanilla Bean Ice Cream,** 1 Gotta Have It | 21 |
| **White Chocolate Ice Cream,** 1 Gotta Have It | 22 |

## GRAB & GO ICE CREAM

| ▲ Power Foods | *PointsPlus*™ value |
|---|---|
| **Cake Batter Batter, Batter™**, 1/2 cup | 6 |
| **Chocolate Devotion™**, 1/2 cup | 6 |
| **Coffee Lovers Only®**, 1/2 cup | 6 |
| **Crème De La Berry™**, 1/2 cup | 5 |
| **Founder's Favorite®**, 1/2 cup | 6 |
| **Peanut Butter Cup Perfection™**, 1/2 cup | 6 |
| **Rocky Off Road™**, 1/2 cup | 7 |
| **Shock-A-Cone™**, 1/2 cup | 6 |
| **Zenilla™**, 1/2 cup | 5 |

## SORBET & YOGURT

| ▲ Power Foods | *PointsPlus*™ value |
|---|---|
| **Countrytime Pink Lemonade Sorbet,** 1 Gotta Have It | 15 |
| **Fudge Brownie Batter Ice Cream,** 1 Gotta Have It | 24 |
| **Lemon Sorbet,** 1 Gotta Have It | 10 |
| **Nrgize Berry Yogurt,** 1 Like It | 4 |
| **Nrgize Yogurt,** 1 Like It | 4 |
| **Raspberry Sorbet,** 1 Gotta Have It | 11 |
| **Tangy and Tart Berry Yogurt,** 1 Gotta Have It | 10 |
| **Tart and Tangy Yogurt,** 1 Gotta Have It | 9 |
| **Watermelon Sorbet,** 1 Gotta Have It | 11 |

## CAKES & PIES

| ▲ Power Foods | *PointsPlus*™ value |
|---|---|
| **A Cheesecake Named Desire™**, 1 slice (1/14 of an 8" round) | 11 |
| **A Cheesecake Named Desire™**, 1 slice (1/8 of 6" round) | 12 |
| **Cake Batter Confetti™**, 1 slice (1/14 of an 8" round) | 11 |
| **Cake Batter Confetti™**, 1 slice (1/8 of 6" round) | 12 |
| **Chocolate Chipper™**, 1 slice (1/8 of 6" round) | 13 |
| **Chocolate Chipper™**, 1 slice (1/14 of an 8" round) | 12 |
| **Coffeehouse Crunch™**, 1 slice (1/14 of an 8" round) | 13 |
| **Coffeehouse Crunch™**, 1 slice (1/8 of 6" round) | 15 |
| **Cookie Dough Delirium™**, 1 slice (1/14 of an 8" round) | 12 |
| **Cookie Dough Delirium™**, 1 slice (1/8 of 6" round) | 14 |
| **Cookies & Creamery™**, 1 slice (1/14 of an 8" round) | 10 |
| **Cookies & Creamery™**, 1 slice (1/8 of 6" round) | 11 |
| **Midnight Delight™**, 1 slice (1/14 of an 8" round) | 13 |
| **Midnight Delight™**, 1 slice (1/8 of 6" round) | 14 |
| **MMMMMM Chip™**, 1 slice (1/8 of 6" round) | 11 |
| **MMMMMM Chip™**, 1 slice (1/14 of an 8" round) | 10 |
| **Peanut Butter Playground™**, 1 slice (1/14 of an 8" round) | 14 |
| **Peanut Butter Playground™**, 1 slice (1/8 of 6" round) | 16 |
| **Strawberry Passion™**, 1 slice (1/14 of an 8" round) | 12 |
| **Strawberry Passion™**, 1 slice (1/8 of 6" round) | 12 |

# COLD STONE CREAMERY

| ▲ Power Foods | PointsPlus™ value |
|---|---|
| **SINLESS SMOOTHIES** | |
| **2 to Mango™**, 1 Gotta Have It | 7 |
| **Berry Lemony™**, 1 Gotta Have It | 6 |
| **Berry Trinity™**, 1 Gotta Have It | 6 |
| **Citrus Sunsation™**, 1 Gotta Have It | 7 |
| **Man-Go Bananas™**, 1 Gotta Have It | 8 |
| **On The YoGo™**, 1 Gotta Have It | 7 |
| **Strawberry Bananza™**, 1 Gotta Have It | 7 |
| **LIFESTYLE SMOOTHIES** | |
| **Banana Banana,** 1 Gotta Have It | 14 |
| **Banana Strawberry,** 1 Gotta Have It | 13 |
| **Blueberry Banana,** 1 Gotta Have It | 11 |
| **Blueberry Pineapple,** 1 Gotta Have It | 10 |
| **Mango Pineapple,** 1 Gotta Have It | 14 |
| **Mango Strawberry,** 1 Gotta Have It | 17 |
| **Pineapple Coconut Orange,** 1 Gotta Have It | 16 |
| **Raspberry Banana,** 1 Gotta Have It | 12 |
| **Strawberry Raspberry,** 1 Gotta Have It | 12 |
| **LOWER CALORIE SIGNATURE SMOOTHIES** | |
| **Man-Go Bananas™**, 1 Like It | 8 |
| **SHAKES** | |
| **Cake'n Shake™**, 1 Gotta Have It | 47 |
| **Cherry Cheeseshake™**, 1 Gotta Have It | 44 |
| **Cream de Menthe™**, 1 Gotta Have It | 47 |
| **Lotta Caramel Latte™**, 1 Like It | 50 |
| **Milk and Cookies™**, 1 Gotta Have It | 47 |
| **Oh Fudge!™**, 1 Gotta Have It | 54 |
| **PB&C™**, 1 Gotta Have It | 56 |
| **Savory Strawberry™**, 1 Gotta Have It | 41 |

| ▲ Power Foods | PointsPlus™ value |
|---|---|
| **CANDY** | |
| **Almond Joy®**, 1 piece | 5 |
| **Butterfinger®**, 1/2 bar | 4 |
| **Chocolate Chips,** 1 oz | 4 |
| **Chocolate Shavings,** 1 serving | 2 |
| **Ghirardelli Caramel Square,** 1 | 2 |
| **Gumballs,** 1 oz | 2 |
| **Gummi Bears,** 1 oz | 3 |
| **Heath Bar®**, 1 bar | 3 |
| **Kit Kat®**, 1/2 bar | 3 |
| **M & M's®**, 1 oz | 5 |
| **Nestle Crunch® Bar,** 1/2 bar | 4 |
| **Peanut M & M's®**, 1 oz | 4 |
| **Reese's Pieces®**, 1 oz | 5 |
| **Reese's™ Peanut Butter Cup®**, 1 piece | 5 |
| **Snickers®**, 1/2 bar | 5 |
| **Twix®**, 1 piece | 4 |
| **White Chocolate Chips,** 1 oz | 4 |
| **Whoppers® Candy,** 1 serving | 3 |
| **York Peppermint Patties®**, 2 pieces | 3 |
| **FRUIT** | |
| **Apple Pie Filling,** 3/4 oz | 2 |
| ▲ **Bananas,** 3/4 oz | 0 |
| **Black Cherries,** 3/4 oz | 2 |
| ▲ **Blackberries,** 3/4 oz | 0 |
| ▲ **Blueberries,** 3/4 oz | 0 |
| **Cherry Pie Filling,** 3/4 oz | 1 |
| **Maraschino Cherries,** 1 | 0 |
| **Peach Pie Filling,** 1 oz | 2 |
| ▲ **Pineapple Chunks,** 3/4 oz | 0 |
| **Raisins,** 1 oz | 2 |
| ▲ **Raspberries,** 3/4 oz | 0 |
| ▲ **Strawberries,** 3/4 oz | 0 |

| ▲ Power Foods | PointsPlus™ value |
|---|---|
| **MIX-INS** | |
| **Brownies,** 1 piece | 4 |
| **Coconut,** 1/2 oz | 2 |
| **Cookie Dough,** 1 piece | 5 |
| **Graham Cracker Pie Crust,** 1 oz | 3 |
| **Granola,** 1 oz | 3 |
| **Marshmallows,** 1 oz | 3 |
| **Nilla Wafers,** 3 | 2 |
| **OREO® Cookies,** 2 | 3 |
| **OREO® Pie Crust,** 1 oz | 4 |
| **Peanut Butter,** 3/4 oz | 4 |
| **Toasted Coconut,** 1/2 oz | 3 |
| **Yellow Cake,** 1 piece | 2 |
| **NUTS** | |
| **Cashews,** 1 oz | 5 |
| **Macadamia Nuts,** 1 oz | 5 |
| **Peanuts,** 1 oz | 6 |
| **Pecan Pralines,** 1 oz | 6 |
| **Pecans,** 1 oz | 4 |
| **Pistachio Nuts,** 1 oz | 6 |
| **Roasted Almonds,** 1 oz | 4 |
| **Sliced Almonds,** 1 oz | 6 |
| **Walnuts,** 1 oz | 4 |
| **SUPPLEMENTS** | |
| **Nrgize Antioxidant/Immune Supplement,** 1 packet | 0 |
| **Nrgize Anti-Stress,** 1 packet | 0 |
| **Nrgize Energy Supplement,** 1 packet | 0 |
| **Nrgize Whey Protein Supplement,** 1 packet | 1 |

| ▲ Power Foods | PointsPlus™ value |
|---|---|
| **TOPPINGS** | |
| **Butterscotch Fat Free,** 1 oz | 2 |
| **Caramel,** 1 oz | 3 |
| **Caramel Fat Free,** 1 oz | 2 |
| **Chocolate Sprinkles,** 1 oz | 1 |
| **Cinnamon,** 1/8 tsp | 0 |
| **Fudge,** 1 oz | 3 |
| **Fudge Fat Free,** 1 oz | 2 |
| **Honey,** 1 oz | 3 |
| **Marshmallow Créme,** 1 oz | 3 |
| **Rainbow Sprinkles,** 1 oz | 1 |
| **Reddi Wip® Original,** 1 dollop | 1 |
| **WAFFLE PRODUCTS** | |
| **Dipped Waffle,** 1 | 9 |
| **Sugar Cone,** 1 | 1 |
| **Waffle Cone or Bowl,** 1 | 4 |

# CORNER BAKERY CAFE®

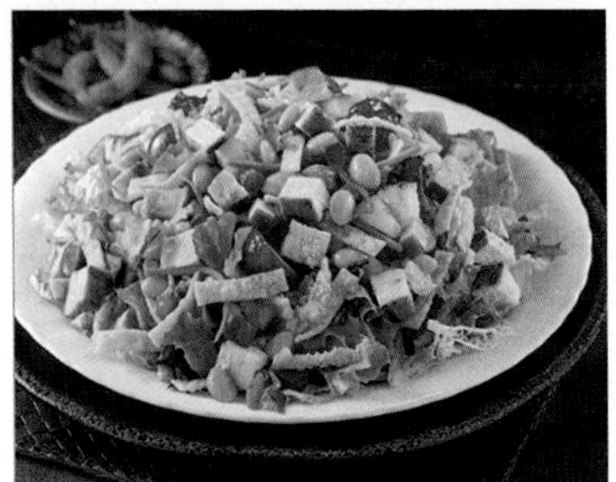

| ▲ Power Foods | *PointsPlus™* value |
|---|---|
| **BREAKFAST FOODS** | |
| **Anaheim Scrambler with Egg Whites, Fresh Fruit Salad Medley (substitute for potatoes) and Harvest Toast,** 1 serving | 13 |
| **Farmer's Scrambler with Egg Whites, Fresh Fruit Salad Medley (substitute for potatoes) and Harvest Toast,** 1 serving | 11 |
| **Fresh Berry Parfait,** 1 serving | 9 |
| **Loaded Oatmeal (hearty old-fashioned oatmeal made with skim milk and topped with brown sugar, dried Zante currants, dried cranberries, toasted almonds and walnuts; without sweet crisp),** 1 serving | 8 |
| ▲ **Oatmeal (hearty old-fashioned oatmeal made with skim milk),** 1 serving | 4 |
| **Seasonal Fresh Fruit Salad Medley (cantaloupe, honeydew, pineapple, and seedless red grapes),** 1 serving | 2 |
| **Swiss Oatmeal (chilled cereal with rolled oats, green apples, bananas, currants, dried cranberries, low-fat yogurt, and skim milk),** 1 serving | 10 |

| ▲ Power Foods | *PointsPlus™* value |
|---|---|
| **CAFE SALADS** | |
| **Chopped Cafe Salad with Chicken (no dressing),** 1 | 6 |
| **Chopped Cafe Salad with Chicken (with house dressing),** 1 | 10 |
| **Santa Fe Ranch Cafe Salad with Chicken (with light ranch dressing),** 1 | 12 |
| **Santa Fe Ranch Cafe Salad with Chicken (without dressing),** 1 | 10 |
| **ENTRÉE SALADS** | |
| **Chopped Salad with Chicken (with house dressing),** 1 | 21 |
| **Chopped Salad with Chicken (without dressing),** 1 | 13 |
| **Sante Fe Ranch Salad with Chicken (with light ranch dressing),** 1 | 21 |
| **Sante Fe Ranch Salad with Chicken (without light ranch dressing),** 1 | 18 |
| **TRIO SALAD** | |
| **Tuna Salad, Seasonal Fresh Fruit Salad Medley and Mixed Green Salad with House Dressing (without café roll),** 1 serving | 13 |
| **PASTA** | |
| **Penne with Marinara (penne pasta and all-vegetable marinara sauce),** 1 serving | 15 |
| **SANDWICHES** | |
| **Bavarian Ham on Pretzel Bread,** 1/2 sandwich | 9 |
| **Bavarian Turkey on Pretzel Bread,** 1/2 sandwich | 9 |
| **Tomato Mozzarella on Ciabatta Ficelle Bread,** 1/2 sandwich | 8 |

| ▲ Power Foods | PointsPlus™ value |
|---|---|
| **Tuna Salad on Harvest Bread,** 1 | 12 |
| **Turkey Frisco on Asiago Cheese Bread,** 1/2 sandwich | 11 |
| **Uptown Turkey on Harvest Bread,** 1/2 sandwich | 8 |

## SIDE SALADS

| | |
|---|---|
| **DC Chicken Salad,** 1 serving | 10 |
| **Large Mixed Green Salad (with house dressing),** 1 | 12 |
| **Large Mixed Green Salad (without dressing),** 1 | 4 |
| **Seasonal Fresh Fruit Salad Medley (cantaloupe, honeydew, pineapple, and seedless red grapes),** 1 | 2 |
| **Side Mixed Green Salad (with house dressing),** 1 | 6 |
| **Side Mixed Green Salad (without dressing),** 1 serving | 2 |
| **Tuna Salad,** 1 serving | 7 |

## SOUPS

| | |
|---|---|
| **Chicken Tortilla (without tortilla strips),** 1 small serving | 5 |
| **Chicken Tortilla (without tortilla strips),** 1 large serving | 8 |
| **Mom's Chicken Noodle,** 1 small serving | 4 |
| **Roasted Tomato Basil (without croutons),** 1 small serving | 4 |

## BREAD

| | |
|---|---|
| **Cafe Roll,** 1 | 3 |
| **Garlic Bread (served with pasta entrées),** 1 serving | 3 |
| **Harvest Crisp,** 1 | 1 |
| **Sweet Crisp,** 1 | 4 |

| ▲ Power Foods | PointsPlus™ value |
|---|---|

## DESSERTS

| | |
|---|---|
| **Fudge Brownie Bite,** 1 serving | 2 |
| **Mini Chocolate Chip Cookie,** 1 | 2 |

# COUNTRY KITCHEN® RESTAURANT

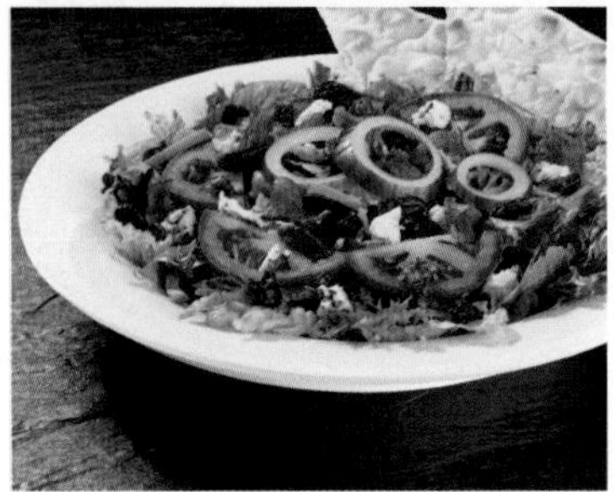

| ▲ Power Foods | *PointsPlus*™ value |
|---|---|
| **BREAKFAST** | |
| **Bacon,** 4 slices | 7 |
| ▲ **Ham Steak,** 1 steak | 3 |
| **Sausage Links,** 4 links | 9 |
| **Sausage Patties,** 2 patties | 6 |
| **Bagel (plain),** 1 | 7 |
| **Cream Cheese,** 1 packet | 3 |
| **Jams, Jelly, Preserves,** 1 packet | 1 |
| **Pancake Syrup,** 1/4 cup | 5 |
| **LIGHTER APPETITES** | |
| **Chicken Breast (without sides and roll),** 1 serving | 3 |
| **SALADS & SALAD DRESSINGS** | |
| **Garden Salad, Side (without dressing),** 1 serving | 1 |
| **Blue Cheese Dressing,** 2 Tbsp | 4 |
| **Honey Mustard Dressing,** 2 Tbsp | 3 |
| **Thousand Island Dressing,** 2 Tbsp | 4 |

| ▲ Power Foods | *PointsPlus*™ value |
|---|---|
| **SIDES** | |
| **Baked Potato,** 1 | 5 |
| **Carrots,** 1/2 cup | 1 |
| **Corn,** 1/2 cup | 2 |
| **Dinner Roll,** 1 roll | 2 |
| **Garlic Bread,** 2 slices | 9 |
| **Green Beans,** 1/2 cup | 0 |
| **Mixed Vegetables,** 1/2 cup | 1 |
| **Old Fashioned Calico Bean Soup®,** 1 cup | 3 |

| ▲ Power Foods | *PointsPlus*™ value |
|---|---|
| **BETTER BUNCH™ (WITHOUT MAYO, CHEESE, OR ADDED SALT)** | |
| **Chicken Breast,** 7 1/2" sub | 9 |
| **Club,** 7 1/2" sub | 10 |
| **Garden Veggie,** 7 1/2" sub | 7 |
| **Ham,** 7 1/2" sub | 8 |
| **Hot Veggie,** 7 1/2" sub | 7 |
| **Mini Club,** 5" sub | 5 |
| **Mini Garden Veggie,** 5" sub | 4 |
| **Mini Ham,** 5" sub | 4 |
| **Mini Hot Veggie,** 5" sub | 4 |
| **Mini Turkey Breast,** 5" sub | 5 |
| **Roast Beef,** 7 1/2" sub | 10 |
| **Turkey Breast,** 7 1/2" sub | 8 |
| **BETTER BUNCH™ SALADS (WITHOUT CROUTONS, CHEESE, OR DRESSING)** | |
| **Chef Salad,** 1 | 3 |
| **Garden Salad,** 1 | 1 |
| **Garden Salad with Chicken Breast,** 1 | 3 |
| ▲ **Side Salad,** 1 | 0 |
| **MINI SUBS** | |
| **Mini BLT,** 5" sub | 8 |
| **Mini Chicken Cheddar Deluxe,** 5" sub | 9 |
| **Mini Chicken Salad,** 5" sub | 7 |
| **Mini Club,** 5" sub | 9 |
| **Mini Garden Veggie,** 5" sub | 6 |
| **Mini Ham & Provolone,** 5" sub | 9 |
| **Mini Hot Veggie,** 5" sub | 7 |
| **Mini Italian Special,** 5" sub | 11 |
| **Mini Meatball & Provolone,** 5" sub | 10 |
| **Mini Pepperoni Melt,** 5" sub | 10 |
| **Mini Pizza Sub,** 5" sub | 9 |
| **Mini Seafood with Crab,** 5" sub | 9 |
| **Mini Three Cheese,** 5" sub | 10 |
| **Mini Tuna,** 5" sub | 9 |
| **Mini Turkey Breast,** 5" sub | 8 |

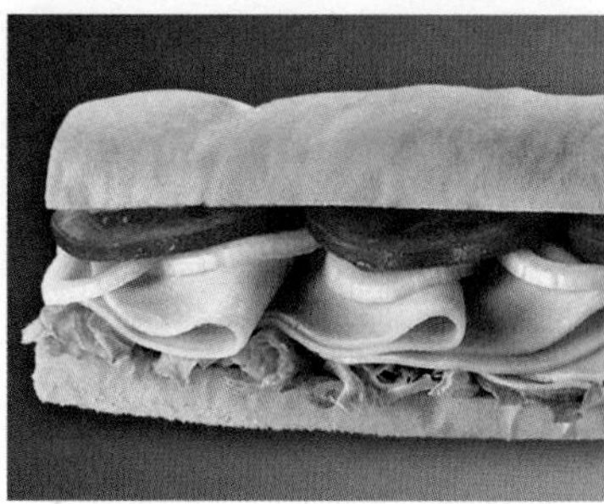

| ▲ Power Foods | *PointsPlus*™ value |
|---|---|
| **SUB SANDWICHES** | |
| **BLT,** 7 1/2" sub | 17 |
| **Cheese Steak,** 7 1/2" sub | 13 |
| **Chicken Breast,** 7 1/2" sub | 15 |
| **Chicken Cheddar Deluxe,** 7 1/2" sub | 19 |
| **Chicken Salad,** 7 1/2" sub | 15 |
| **Club,** 7 1/2" sub | 18 |
| **Double Cheese Steak,** 7 1/2" sub | 19 |
| **Garden Veggie,** 7 1/2" sub | 10 |
| **Gyro,** 7 1/2" sub | 20 |
| **Ham & Provolone,** 7 1/2" sub | 17 |
| **Hot Veggie,** 7 1/2" sub | 12 |
| **Italian Special,** 7 1/2" sub | 22 |
| **Meatball & Provolone,** 7 1/2" sub | 19 |
| **Pepperoni Melt,** 7 1/2" sub | 20 |
| **Philly Cheese Steak,** 7 1/2" sub | 14 |
| **Pizza Sub,** 7 1/2" sub | 19 |
| **Roast Beef,** 7 1/2" sub | 16 |
| **Seafood with Crab,** 7 1/2" sub | 18 |
| **Spicy Chicken Sedona,** 7 1/2" sub | 14 |
| **Three Cheese,** 7 1/2" sub | 19 |
| **Tuna,** 7 1/2" sub | 18 |
| **Turkey Breast,** 7 1/2" sub | 15 |

| ▲ Power Foods | *PointsPlus*™ value |
|---|---|
| **SALADS** (WITHOUT DRESSING) | |
| **Chef Salad,** 1 serving | 9 |
| **Chicken Sedona Salad,** 1 serving | 5 |
| **Garden Salad,** 1 serving | 6 |
| **Garden Salad with Chicken Breast,** 1 serving | 9 |
| **Italian Salad,** 1 serving | 11 |
| **Seafood Salad,** 1 serving | 8 |
| **Side Salad,** 1 serving | 4 |
| **Tuna Salad,** 1 serving | 18 |
| **FRENCH FRIES** | |
| **French Fries,** 1 large serving | 13 |
| **SOUPS** | |
| **Beef Steak & Noodle Soup,** 1 large | 4 |
| **Cheddar Cauliflower Soup,** 1 large | 4 |
| **Cheddar Cheese Soup,** 1 large | 9 |
| **Chicken & Dumplings,** 1 large | 6 |
| **Chicken Noodle Soup,** 1 large | 5 |
| **Chicken with Wild Rice Soup,** 1 large | 7 |
| **Chili,** 1 large | 8 |
| **Cream of Broccoli with Cheese Soup,** 1 large | 6 |
| **Cream of Mushroom Soup,** 1 large | 7 |
| **Cream of Potato Soup,** 1 large | 7 |
| **Eight Bean Soup with Ham,** 1 large | 4 |
| **Fiesta Tortilla Soup with Chicken,** 1 large | 5 |
| **New England Clam Chowder,** 1 large | 6 |
| **Tomato Basil Soup with Raviolini,** 1 large | 4 |
| **Vegetable Beef Soup,** 1 large | 3 |

| ▲ Power Foods | *PointsPlus*™ value |
|---|---|
| **BREADS** | |
| **Flour Tortilla Wrap,** 1 | 6 |
| **Garlic Herb Bread,** 7 1/2" | 6 |
| **Italian Bread,** 7 1/2" | 6 |
| **Mini Garlic Herb Bread,** 5" | 3 |
| **Mini Italian Bread,** 5" | 3 |
| **Mini Parmesan-Asiago Bread,** 5" | 3 |
| **Mini Wheat Bread,** 5" | 3 |
| **Parmesan-Asiago Bread,** 7 1/2" | 6 |
| **Wheat Bread,** 7 1/2" | 6 |
| **COOKIES** | |
| **Chocolate Chip Cookie,** 1 | 6 |
| **Chocolate Chip Cookie with M&M's,** 1 | 5 |
| **Coconut Toffee Chip Cookie,** 1 | 5 |
| **Double Chocolate Chip Cookie,** 1 | 5 |
| **Oatmeal Cranberry Walnut Cookie,** 1 | 5 |
| **Oatmeal Raisin Cookie,** 1 | 5 |
| **Peanut Butter with Reese's Pieces Cookie,** 1 | 6 |
| **Snickerdoodle Cookie,** 1 | 5 |
| **Sugar Cookie,** 1 | 5 |
| **White Chunk Macadamia Nut Cookie,** 1 | 6 |

# CRACKER BARREL OLD COUNTRY STORE®

▲ Power Foods — *PointsPlus™* value

## COUNTRY DINNER PLATES

| Item | *PointsPlus™* value |
|---|---|
| **BBQ, Pulled Pork,** 1 serving | 9 |
| **Catfish (fried),** 1 fillet | 5 |
| **Catfish, Spicy Grilled,** 1 fillet | 3 |
| **Chicken n' Dumplins,** 1 serving | 7 |
| **Chicken Tenderloin (fried),** 4 pieces | 10 |
| **Chicken Tenderloin, Grilled,** 4 pieces | 4 |
| **City Ham, Grilled,** 1 slice | 4 |
| **Country Ham, Grilled,** 1 slice | 7 |
| **Pork Chop, Grilled,** 1 | 6 |

## FANCY FIXINS

| Item | *PointsPlus™* value |
|---|---|
| **Catfish (spicy grilled),** 2 fillets | 6 |
| **Chicken n' Dumplins,** 1 serving | 10 |
| **Chicken Tenderloin (grilled),** 6 pieces | 6 |
| **Country Fried Steak (with gravy),** 1 serving | 16 |
| **Country Fried Steak (without gravy),** 1 serving | 14 |
| **Roast Beef & Gravy,** 1 serving | 13 |
| **Sirloin Steak,** 1 serving | 8 |

## SANDWICH

| Item | *PointsPlus™* value |
|---|---|
| **Homemade Chicken Salad Sandwich (sourdough white bread),** 1 | 13 |

## SALADS/DRESSINGS

| Item | *PointsPlus™* value |
|---|---|
| **House Salad,** 1 serving | 8 |
| ▲ **Tossed Salad,** 1 serving | 0 |
| **Fat Free Honey Mustard Dressing,** 2 packets | 3 |
| **Fat Free Italian Dressing,** 2 packets | 1 |
| **Fat Free Ranch Dressing,** 2 packets | 2 |
| **Fat Free Thousand Island Dressing,** 2 packets | 3 |

▲ Power Foods — *PointsPlus™* value

## SOUPS

| Item | *PointsPlus™* value |
|---|---|
| **Beef Stew,** 1 cup | 3 |
| **Chicken & Rice Soup,** 1 cup | 4 |
| **Chicken Noodle Soup,** 1 cup | 2 |
| **Potato Soup,** 1 cup | 2 |
| **Turkey Noodle Soup,** 1 cup | 3 |
| **Vegetable Soup,** 1 bowl | 3 |

## VEGETABLES N' SIDES

| Item | *PointsPlus™* value |
|---|---|
| **Applesauce,** 1 serving | 3 |
| **Boiled Cabbage,** 1 serving | 2 |
| **Broccoli casserole,** 1 serving | 5 |
| **Brown Rice,** 1 serving | 3 |
| ▲ **Carrots,** 1 serving | 0 |
| **Cole Slaw,** 1 serving | 7 |
| **Corn,** 1 serving | 5 |
| **Cornbread Dressing,** 1 serving | 8 |
| **Dumplings,** 1 serving | 5 |
| **Fried Apples,** 1 serving | 4 |
| **Green Beans,** 1 serving | 1 |
| **Hashbrown Casserole,** 1 serving | 5 |
| **Lima Beans,** 1 serving | 7 |
| **Macaroni n' Cheese,** 1 serving | 7 |
| **Mashed Potatoes,** 1 serving | 5 |
| **Okra, Fried,** 1 serving | 6 |
| ▲ **Pinto Beans,** 1 bowl (12 oz) | 10 |
| ▲ **Pinto Beans,** 1 serving | 3 |
| **Red Skin Potatoes, Boiled,** 1 serving | 4 |
| **Sweet Potato Casserole,** 1 serving | 5 |
| **Turnip Greens,** 1 serving | 2 |
| **Yellow Rice,** 1 serving | 7 |

# CRACKER BARREL OLD COUNTRY STORE®

| ▲ Power Foods | *PointsPlus™* value |
|---|---|
| **BREAD** | |
| **Biscuit,** 1 | 4 |
| **Cornbread Muffin,** 1 | 5 |
| **Promise® Spread Butter Cup,** 1 packet | 1 |
| **Regular Wheat Bread,** 1 slice | 2 |
| **Regular White Bread,** 1 slice | 2 |
| **Toast - Sourdough Wheat,** 1 slice | 3 |
| **Toast - Sourdough White,** 1 slice | 4 |
| **Whipped Butter Cup,** 1 packet | 1 |
| **BREAKFAST MENU** | |
| **Bacon,** 3 slices | 5 |
| ▲ **Egg Beaters, Scrambled,** 1 serving | 1 |
| **Eggs, Fried,** 2 eggs | 5 |
| ▲ **Eggs, Poached,** 2 eggs | 3 |
| **Eggs, Scrambled,** 2 eggs | 4 |
| **Eggs, Scrambled with Cheese (2 eggs),** 1 serving | 6 |
| **Grits (plain),** 1 serving | 2 |
| **Natural Syrup,** 1 bottle | 3 |
| **Natural Syrup, Sugar Free,** 1 bottle | 1 |
| ▲ **Oatmeal, Plain,** 1 serving | 3 |
| **Pancakes (no butter),** 2 | 11 |
| **Sawmill Gravy,** 1 serving | 4 |
| **Smoked Sausage Patties,** 2 | 6 |
| **Smoked Sausage Patties (half order),** 1 patty | 3 |
| **Turkey Sausage,** 2 patties | 3 |

| ▲ Power Foods | *PointsPlus™* value |
|---|---|

## BUTTERBURGERS®

| | |
|---|---|
| **BBQ Bacon Cheddar ButterBurger, Double,** 1 | 22 |
| **ButterBurger, Cheese, Single,** 1 | 11 |
| **ButterBurger, Cheese, Double,** 1 | 16 |
| **ButterBurger, Cheese, Triple,** 1 | 21 |
| **ButterBurger, Low Carb,** 1 | 12 |
| **ButterBurger, the Original, Single,** 1 | 9 |
| **ButterBurger, The Original, Double,** 1 | 13 |
| **ButterBurger, the Original, Triple,** 1 | 16 |
| **Cheddar ButterBurger, Single,** 1 | 11 |
| **Cheddar ButterBurger, Double,** 1 | 17 |
| **Cheddar ButterBurger with Bacon, Double,** 1 | 20 |
| **Cheddar ButterBurger, Triple,** 1 | 22 |
| **Mushroom & Swiss, Single,** 1 | 11 |
| **Mushroom & Swiss Double,** 1 | 17 |
| **Mushroom & Swiss, Triple,** 1 | 22 |
| **Sourdough Melt, Single,** 1 | 11 |
| **Sourdough Melt, Double,** 1 | 17 |
| **Sourdough Melt, Triple,** 1 | 22 |
| **The Culver's Bacon Deluxe, Single,** 1 | 16 |
| **The Culver's Bacon Deluxe, Double,** 1 | 20 |
| **The Culver's Bacon Deluxe, Triple,** 1 | 25 |
| **The Culver's Deluxe, Single,** 1 | 14 |
| **The Culver's Deluxe, Double,** 1 | 18 |
| **The Culver's Deluxe, Triple,** 1 | 23 |
| **Wisconsin Swiss Melt, Single,** 1 | 11 |
| **Wisconsin Swiss Melt, Double,** 1 | 16 |
| **Wisconsin Swiss Melt, Triple,** 1 | 22 |

## DAILY FEATURES

| | |
|---|---|
| **BBQ Chicken,** 1 | 9 |
| **BBQ Pork,** 1 | 11 |

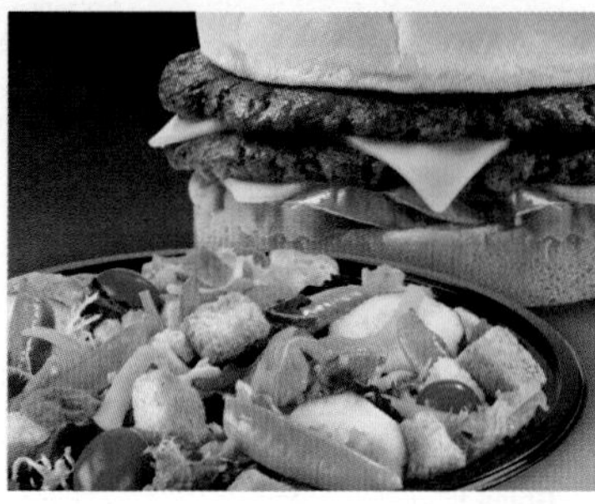

| ▲ Power Foods | *PointsPlus™* value |
|---|---|
| **BLT,** 1 | 13 |
| **Chicken Salad on Grilled Sourdough,** 1 | 14 |
| **Chili Cheese Hot Dog,** 1 | 14 |
| **Fish n' Chips,** 6 pieces | 36 |
| **Pork Tenderloin, Grilled,** 1 | 12 |
| **Tuna Salad on Grilled Sourdough,** 1 | 13 |
| **Ultimate Grilled Cheese,** 1 | 18 |

## FAVORITES

| | |
|---|---|
| **Angus Philly Steak Sandwich,** 1 | 13 |
| **Beef Pot Roast Sandwich,** 1 | 10 |
| **Cheese Hot Dog,** 1 | 13 |
| **Chicken Tenders, Breaded,** 4 pieces | 12 |
| **Chili Dog,** 1 | 11 |
| **Flame Roasted Chicken Breast,** 1 | 10 |
| **Flame Roasted Chicken Filet Sandwich,** 1 | 17 |
| **Grilled Ham 'n Swiss on Rye,** 1 | 13 |
| **Grilled Rueben Melt,** 1 | 16 |
| **Hot Dog,** 1 | 11 |
| **North Atlantic Cod Filet Sandwich,** 1 | 20 |
| **Pork Tenderloin Sandwich,** 1 | 16 |
| **Turkey BLT,** 1 | 15 |
| **Turkey, Stacked, Sandwich,** 1 | 12 |

# CULVER'S®

| ▲ Power Foods | *PointsPlus*™ value |
|---|---|
| **SIDES** | |
| **Chili Cheddar Fries,** 1 serving | 18 |
| **Coleslaw,** 1 serving | 9 |
| **Crinkle Cut Fries, Small,** 1 serving | 7 |
| **Crinkle Cut Fries, Regular,** 1 serving | 10 |
| **Crinkle Cut Fries, Large,** 1 serving | 13 |
| **Dairyland Cheese Curds,** 1 serving | 18 |
| **Dinner Roll,** 1 | 4 |
| **Green Beans,** 1 serving | 6 |
| **Mashed Potatoes,** 1 serving | 3 |
| **Mashed Potatoes & Gravy,** 1 serving | 3 |
| **Onion Rings, Breaded,** 1 serving | 17 |
| **DINNER PLATES** | |
| **Beef Pot Roast Dinner,** 1 serving | 22 |
| **Butterfly Crispy Shrimp,** 6 pieces | 34 |
| **Chicken Basket,** 2 pieces | 34 |
| **Chopped Steak Dinner,** 1 serving | 23 |
| **Fresh Fried Chicken,** 4 pieces | 58 |
| **Fresh Fried Chicken,** 2 pieces | 47 |
| **North Atlantic Cod Filet,** 2 pieces | 49 |
| **North Atlantic Cod Filet,** 3 pieces | 57 |
| **Walleye Filet,** 2 pieces | 48 |
| **Walleye Filet,** 3 pieces | 55 |
| **GARDEN FRESH SALADS** | |
| **Avocado Pecan Bleu with Blackened Chicken,** 1 serving | 15 |
| **Chicken Cashew with Flame Roasted Chicken,** 1 serving | 12 |
| **Classic Caesar with Flame Roasted Chicken,** 1 serving | 9 |
| **Crispy Chicken Salad,** 1 serving | 17 |
| **Garden Fresco,** 1 serving | 6 |
| **Side Caesar,** 1 serving | 2 |
| **Side Salad,** 1 serving | 2 |

| ▲ Power Foods | *PointsPlus*™ value |
|---|---|
| **SALAD DRESSING** | |
| **Bleu Cheese Fancy Chunky,** 1 serving | 9 |
| **Caesar Dressing,** 1 serving | 6 |
| **French,** 1 serving | 5 |
| **French, Reduced Calorie,** 1 serving | 4 |
| **Ranch, Buttermilk, Gourmet,** 1 serving | 7 |
| **Ranch, Reduced Calorie,** 1 serving | 4 |
| **Raspberry Vinaigrette,** 1 serving | 1 |
| **Reduced Calorie Raspberry Vinaigrette Dressing,** 1 serving | 1 |
| **Sesame Ginger Dressing,** 1 serving | 2 |
| **Thousand Island, Gourmet,** 1 serving | 6 |
| **SOUPS** | |
| **Baja Chicken Enchilada,** 1 serving | 9 |
| **Bean with Ham,** 1 serving | 4 |
| **Boston Clam Chowder,** 1 serving | 7 |
| **Broccoli Cheese with Florets,** 1 serving | 6 |
| **Cauliflower Cheese,** 1 serving | 7 |
| **Cheesy Chicken Tortilla,** 1 serving | 5 |
| **Chicken & Dumpling,** 1 serving | 8 |
| **Chicken Gumbo,** 1 serving | 3 |
| **Chicken Noodle,** 1 serving | 3 |
| **Corn Chowder,** 1 serving | 7 |
| **Cream of Broccoli,** 1 serving | 5 |
| **French Onion,** 1 serving | 4 |
| **George's Chili,** 1 serving | 9 |
| **George's Chili Supreme,** 1 serving | 12 |
| **Italian Style Wedding,** 1 serving | 7 |
| **Lumberjack Mixed Vegetable,** 1 serving | 4 |
| **Minestrone,** 1 serving | 2 |
| **Mushroom Medley,** 1 serving | 7 |
| **Oven Roasted Turkey Noodle,** 1 serving | 4 |
| **Potato Au Gratin,** 1 serving | 10 |

| Power Foods | PointsPlus™ value |
|---|---|
| **Potato with Bacon,** 1 serving | 6 |
| **Split Pea with Ham,** 1 serving | 6 |
| **Stuffed Green Pepper with Beef,** 1 serving | 4 |
| **Tomato Basil Ravioletti,** 1 serving | 3 |
| **Tomato Florentine,** 1 serving | 3 |
| **Vegetable Beef & Barley,** 1 serving | 3 |
| **Wild & Brown Rice with Chicken,** 1 serving | 12 |
| **Wisconsin Cheese,** 1 serving | 10 |

## KID'S MEALS

| | |
|---|---|
| **ButterBurger,** 1 | 9 |
| **ButterBurger, Cheese,** 1 | 11 |
| **Chicken Tenders, Breaded,** 2 pieces | 6 |
| **Corn Dog,** 1 | 7 |
| **Crinkle Cut Fries,** 1 serving | 7 |
| **Grilled Cheese on Sourdough,** 1 | 8 |
| **Hot Dog with Bun,** 1 | 10 |

## CONDIMENTS & SAUCES

| | |
|---|---|
| **BBQ Sauce,** 1 serving | 1 |
| **Honey Mustard,** 1 serving | 4 |
| **Horseradish Sauce,** 1 serving | 4 |
| **Picante Sauce, Mild and Medium,** 1 serving | 0 |
| **Shrimp Cocktail Sauce,** 1 serving | 1 |
| **Steak Sauce,** 1 serving | 0 |
| **Sweet & Sour Dipping Sauce,** 1 serving | 2 |
| **Tartar Sauce,** 1 serving | 5 |

## CLASSIC SUNDAES

| | |
|---|---|
| **Banana Split,** 2 scoops | 30 |
| **Banana Split,** 3 scoops | 37 |
| **Bananas Foster Sundae,** 1 scoop | 11 |
| **Bananas Foster Sundae,** 2 scoops | 21 |

| Power Foods | PointsPlus™ value |
|---|---|
| **Bananas Foster Sundae,** 3 scoops | 28 |
| **Caramel Cashew,** 1 scoop | 16 |
| **Caramel Cashew,** 2 scoops | 26 |
| **Caramel Cashew,** 3 scoops | 31 |
| **Fudge Pecan Sundae,** 1 scoop | 17 |
| **Fudge Pecan Sundae,** 2 scoops | 27 |
| **Fudge Pecan Sundae,** 3 scoops | 32 |
| **Turtle Sundae,** 1 scoop | 17 |
| **Turtle Sundae,** 2 scoops | 27 |
| **Turtle Sundae,** 3 scoops | 32 |

## CONES & FROZEN CUSTARD

| | |
|---|---|
| **Chocolate Cake Cone,** 1 scoop | 8 |
| **Chocolate Cake Cone,** 2 scoops | 16 |
| **Chocolate Cake Cone,** 3 scoops | 20 |
| **Chocolate Dipped Waffle Cone,** 1 | 7 |
| **Chocolate Dipped Waffle Cone,** 1 scoop | 15 |
| **Chocolate, Dish,** 1 small scoop | 8 |
| **Chocolate, Waffle Cone,** 1 scoop | 10 |
| **Chocolate, Waffle Cone,** 2 scoops | 18 |
| **Chocolate, Waffle Cone,** 3 scoops | 22 |
| **Mini Scoop Chocolate Cake Cone,** 1 | 5 |
| **Mini Scoop Vanilla Cake Cone,** 1 | 5 |
| **No Sugar Added Caramel Fudge Swirl,** 1 | 6 |
| **Oreo Frozen Custard Sandwich, Chocolate,** 1 | 8 |
| **Oreo Frozen Custard Sandwich, Mint,** 1 | 8 |
| **Oreo Frozen Custard Sandwich, Vanilla,** 1 | 8 |
| **Plain Cake Cone,** 1 | 1 |
| **Plain Waffle Cone,** 1 | 3 |
| **Vanilla, Cake Cone,** 1 scoop | 9 |
| **Vanilla, Cake Cone,** 2 scoops | 17 |
| **Vanilla, Cake Cone,** 3 scoops | 21 |
| **Vanilla, Chocolate Dipped Waffle Cone,** 1 scoop | 15 |

*Cones & Frozen Custard (cont'd)*

| ▲ Power Foods | *PointsPlus*™ value |
|---|---|
| **Vanilla, Dish,** 1 scoop | 8 |
| **Vanilla, Waffle Cone,** 1 scoop | 11 |
| **Vanilla, Waffle Cone,** 2 scoops | 19 |
| **Vanilla, Waffle Cone,** 3 scoops | 23 |

## CONCRETE MIXERS

| ▲ Power Foods | *PointsPlus*™ value |
|---|---|
| **Chocolate Concrete Mixer,** 1 short | 22 |
| **Turtle Concrete,** 1 short | 25 |
| **Vanilla Concrete Mixer,** 1 short | 19 |
| **Vanilla Concrete Mixer,** 1 medium | 23 |
| **Vanilla Concrete Mixer,** 1 tall | 27 |

## MALTS, SHAKES, FLOATS

| ▲ Power Foods | *PointsPlus*™ value |
|---|---|
| **Chocolate Malt,** 1 short | 20 |
| **Chocolate Shake,** 1 short | 21 |
| **Culver's Root Beer Float,** 1 | 13 |
| **Old Fashioned Cherry Soda,** 1 | 14 |
| **Vanilla Malt,** 1 short | 18 |
| **Vanilla Shake,** 1 short | 17 |

## SPECIAL TREATS

| ▲ Power Foods | *PointsPlus*™ value |
|---|---|
| **Cookie Dough Craving Concrete Cake,** 1 serving | 8 |
| **Cookies & Cream Concrete Cake,** 1 serving | 7 |
| **Lemon Ice,** 1 | 4 |
| **Lemon Ice Cooler,** 1 | 8 |
| **Lemon Ice Smoothie,** 1 | 11 |
| **Turtle Concrete Cake,** 1 serving | 8 |

## TOPPINGS

| ▲ Power Foods | *PointsPlus*™ value |
|---|---|
| **Almond,** 1 serving | 2 |
| **Andes Crème De Menthe Thins,** 1 serving | 4 |
| **Blackberry,** 1 serving | 0 |
| **Blueberry,** 1 serving | 0 |
| **Brownie Pieces,** 1 serving | 10 |
| **Butterfinger®,** 1 serving | 3 |
| **Butterscotch,** 1 serving | 1 |
| **Cashew,** 1 serving | 2 |
| **Cherry, Red,** 1 serving | 1 |
| **Chocolate Chip Cookie Dough,** 1 serving | 3 |
| **Chocolate Syrup,** 1 serving | 2 |
| **Crème De Menthe,** 1 serving | 1 |
| **Heath® Toffee Chunks,** 1 serving | 4 |
| **Hershey's Take Five,** 1 serving | 4 |
| **Hot Caramel,** 1 serving | 1 |
| **Hot Fudge,** 1 serving | 1 |
| **M&M Minis,** 1 serving | 4 |
| **Marshmallow Crème,** 1 serving | 1 |
| **Milk Chocolate Flakes,** 1 serving | 4 |
| **Nestle Crunch,** 1 serving | 4 |
| **Novelty Coating,** 1 serving | 2 |
| **Oreo® Cookie Crumbs,** 1 serving | 2 |
| **Peach,** 1 serving | 0 |
| **Peanut Butter,** 1 serving | 5 |
| **Pecan Halves,** 1 serving | 3 |
| **Pineapple,** 1 serving | 1 |
| **Raspberry,** 1 serving | 0 |
| **Reese's Pieces® Minis,** 1 serving | 4 |
| **Reese's® Peanut Butter Cups,** 1 serving | 4 |
| **Snickers® Candy Bar Pieces,** 1 serving | 2 |
| **Spanish Peanuts,** 1 serving | 5 |
| **Sprinkles, Blue and White,** 1 serving | 4 |
| **Strawberry, Sliced,** 1 serving | 0 |

## DRINKS

| ▲ Power Foods | *PointsPlus*™ value |
|---|---|
| **Culver's® Root Beer,** 1 | 9 |
| **Mocha N'iced Coffee, Short,** 1 | 5 |
| **Mocha N'iced Coffee, Medium,** 1 | 8 |
| **Mocha N'iced Coffee, Tall,** 1 | 14 |
| **Vanilla N'iced Coffee, Short,** 1 | 5 |
| **Vanilla N'iced Coffee, Medium,** 1 | 8 |
| **Vanilla N'iced Coffee, Tall,** 1 | 13 |

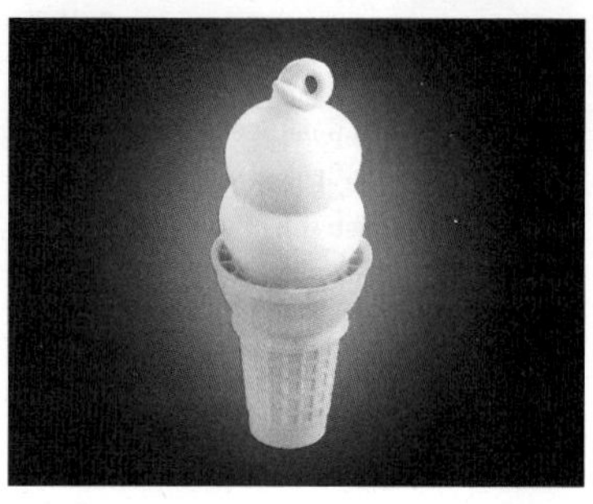

▲ Power Foods — *PointsPlus*™ value

## BLIZZARD® TREATS

|  | *PointsPlus*™ value |
|---|---|
| **Banana Cream Pie Blizzard,** 1 large | 30 |
| **Banana Split Blizzard,** 1 small | 12 |
| **Banana Split Blizzard,** 1 medium | 15 |
| **Banana Split Blizzard,** 1 large | 21 |
| **Butterfinger® Blizzard,** 1 large | 27 |
| **Cappuccino Heath® Blizzard,** 1 large | 34 |
| **Cherry CheeseQuake Blizzard,** 1 large | 26 |
| **Choco Cherry Love Blizzard,** 1 large | 25 |
| **Chocolate Chip Blizzard,** 1 large | 35 |
| **Chocolate Dipped Strawberry Blizzard,** 1 large | 30 |
| **Chocolate Xtreme Blizzard,** 1 large | 40 |
| **Cookie Dough Blizzard,** 1 small | 20 |
| **Cookie Dough Blizzard,** 1 medium | 28 |
| **Cookie Dough Blizzard,** 1 large | 36 |
| **French Silk Pie Blizzard,** 1 large | 37 |
| **Georgia Mud Fudge Blizzard,** 1 large | 41 |
| **Hawaiian Blizzard,** 1 large | 22 |
| **Heath® Blizzard,** 1 large | 35 |
| **M&M's Chocolate Candy Blizzard,** 1 large | 31 |
| **Midnight Truffle Blizzard,** 1 large | 37 |
| **Mint Oreo Blizzard,** 1 large | 29 |
| **Mocha Chip Blizzard,** 1 large | 30 |
| **Oreo Cheesequake Blizzard,** 1 large | 31 |
| **Oreo® Cookies Blizzard,** 1 small | 15 |
| **Oreo® Cookies Blizzard,** 1 medium | 18 |
| **Oreo® Cookies Blizzard,** 1 large | 27 |
| **Peanut Butter Butterfinger Blizzard,** 1 large | 41 |
| **Raspberry Truffle Blizzard,** 1 large | 30 |
| **Reese's® Peanut Butter Cups Blizzard,** 1 small | 15 |
| **Snickers® Blizzard,** 1 large | 31 |
| **Strawberry Cheesequake Blizzard,** 1 small | 14 |
| **Tropical Blizzard,** 1 small | 14 |
| **Turtle Pecan Cluster Blizzard,** 1 large | 41 |

## MOOLATTE®

|  | *PointsPlus*™ value |
|---|---|
| **Cappuccino MooLatte,** 16 oz | 13 |
| **Caramel MooLatte,** 16 oz | 17 |
| **French Vanilla MooLatte,** 16 oz | 15 |
| **Mocha MooLatte,** 16 oz | 16 |

## ROYAL TREATS®

|  | *PointsPlus*™ value |
|---|---|
| **Banana Split,** 1 serving | 14 |
| **Brownie Earthquake,** 1 serving | 21 |
| **Peanut Buster Parfait,** 1 serving | 19 |
| **Peanut Butter Blast,** 1 serving | 18 |
| **Strawberry Shortcake,** 1 serving | 13 |

## NOVELTIES

|  | *PointsPlus*™ value |
|---|---|
| **Buster Bar,** 1 serving | 14 |
| **Butterscotch Dilly Bar,** 1 serving | 6 |
| **Cherry Dilly Bar,** 1 serving | 6 |
| **Cherry Starkiss,** 1 serving | 2 |
| **Chocolate Dilly Bar,** 1 serving | 7 |
| **Chocolate Mint Dilly Bar,** 1 serving | 7 |
| **DQ Home-Pak,** 1 serving | 31 |

*Novelties (cont'd)*

| ▲ Power Foods | PointsPlus™ value |
|---|---|
| **DQ Sandwich,** 1 serving | 5 |
| **Fudge Bar,** 1 serving | 1 |
| **Heath Dilly Bar,** 1 serving | 6 |
| **No Sugar Added Dilly Bar,** 1 serving | 6 |
| **Stars and Stripes Starkiss Bar,** 1 serving | 2 |
| **Vanilla Orange Bar,** 1 serving | 2 |

## MALTS, SHAKES & ARCTIC RUSH®

| ▲ Power Foods | PointsPlus™ value |
|---|---|
| **Arctic Rush, All Flavors,** 1 small | 5 |
| **Arctic Rush, All Flavors,** 1 medium | 7 |
| **Arctic Rush, All Flavors,** 1 large | 10 |
| **Blue Raspberry Arctic Rush,** 1 large | 10 |
| **Blue Raspberry Arctic Rush Float,** 1 large | 18 |
| **Blue Raspberry Arctic Rush Freeze,** 1 large | 23 |
| **Butterscotch Malt,** 1 large | 37 |
| **Butterscotch Shake,** 1 large | 32 |
| **Caramel Shake,** 1 large | 33 |
| **Cherry Arctic Rush,** 1 large | 10 |
| **Cherry Arctic Rush Float,** 1 large | 18 |
| **Cherry Arctic Rush Freeze,** 1 large | 23 |
| **Grape Arctic Rush,** 1 large | 11 |
| **Grape Arctic Rush Float,** 1 large | 18 |
| **Grape Arctic Rush Freeze,** 1 large | 23 |
| **Kiwi Strawberry Arctic Rush,** 1 large | 11 |
| **Kiwi Strawberry Arctic Rush Float,** 1 large | 18 |
| **Kiwi Strawberry Arctic Rush Freeze,** 1 large | 23 |
| **Lemon-Lime Arctic Rush,** 1 large | 10 |
| **Lemon-Lime Arctic Rush Float,** 1 large | 18 |
| **Lemon-Lime Arctic Rush Freeze,** 1 large | 23 |
| **Malt, Banana,** 1 small | 15 |
| **Malt, Caramel,** 1 large | 37 |
| **Malt, Cherry,** 1 small | 16 |
| **Malt, Cherry,** 1 medium | 22 |
| **Malt, Cherry,** 1 large | 32 |
| **Malt, Chocolate,** 1 small | 17 |
| **Malt, Chocolate,** 1 medium | 24 |
| **Malt, Chocolate,** 1 large | 35 |
| **Malt, Hot Fudge,** 1 large | 37 |
| **Malt, Pineapple,** 1 small | 15 |
| **Malt, Pineapple,** 1 medium | 21 |
| **Malt, Pineapple,** 1 large | 30 |
| **Malt, Strawberry,** 1 small | 15 |
| **Peanut Butter Malt,** 1 small | 24 |
| **Peanut Butter Malt,** 1 medium | 33 |
| **Peanut Butter Malt,** 1 large | 47 |
| **Peanut Butter Shake,** 1 small | 21 |
| **Peanut Butter Shake,** 1 medium | 30 |
| **Peanut Butter Shake,** 1 large | 43 |
| **Shake Hot Fudge,** 1 large | 33 |
| **Shake, Banana,** 1 small | 13 |
| **Shake, Caramel,** 1 small | 16 |
| **Shake, Cherry,** 1 large | 27 |
| **Shake, Chocolate,** 1 small | 15 |
| **Shake, Chocolate,** 1 medium | 21 |
| **Shake, Chocolate,** 1 large | 30 |
| **Shake, Pineapple,** 1 small | 13 |
| **Shake, Pineapple,** 1 medium | 18 |
| **Shake, Pineapple,** 1 large | 26 |
| **Shake, Strawberry,** 1 large | 26 |
| **Shake, Vanilla,** 1 large | 31 |

## SUNDAES

| ▲ Power Foods | PointsPlus™ value |
|---|---|
| **Butterscotch Sundae,** 1 large | 16 |
| **Peanut Butter Sundae,** 1 large | 21 |

## WAFFLE TREATS

| ▲ Power Foods | PointsPlus™ value |
|---|---|
| **Chocolate Coated Waffle Cone with Soft Serve,** 1 serving | 15 |

| ▲ Power Foods | PointsPlus™ value |
|---|---|
| **Chocolate Covered Strawberry Waffle Bowl Sundae,** 1 serving | 21 |
| **Fab Fudge Waffle Bowl Sundae,** 1 serving | 20 |
| **Fudge Brownie Temptation Waffle Bowl Sundae,** 1 serving | 26 |
| **Nut N' Fudge Waffle Bowl,** 1 serving | 24 |
| **Plain Waffle Cone with Soft Serve,** 1 serving | 12 |
| **Turtle Waffle Bowl Sundae,** 1 serving | 22 |

## DQ® CAKES

| ▲ Power Foods | PointsPlus™ value |
|---|---|
| **Cake,** 10", 1/10 of the cake | 14 |
| **Cake,** 8", 1/8 of the cake | 11 |
| **Choco Cherry Love 10" Blizzard Cake,** 1/10 of the cake | 18 |
| **Choco Cherry Love 8" Blizzard Cake,** 1/8 of the cake | 15 |
| **Chocolate Chip Cookie Dough Blizzard Cake,** 10", 1/10 of the cake | 20 |
| **Chocolate Chip Cookie Dough Blizzard Cake,** 8", 1/8 of the cake | 17 |
| **Chocolate Dipped Strawberry 10" Blizzard Cake,** 1/10 of the cake | 19 |
| **Chocolate Dipped Strawberry 8" Blizzard Cake,** 1/8 of the cake | 16 |
| **Chocolate Xtreme Blizzard Cake,** 10", 1/10 of the cake | 21 |
| **Chocolate Xtreme Blizzard Cake,** 8", 1/8 of the cake | 18 |
| **Cotton Candy 10" Blizzard Cake,** 1/10 of the cake | 17 |
| **Cotton Candy 8" Blizzard Cake,** 1/8 of the cake | 16 |
| **Girl Scouts Thin Mint Cookie 10" Blizzard Cake,** 1/10 of the cake | 17 |
| **Girl Scouts Thin Mint Cookie 8" Blizzard Cake,** 1/8 of the cake | 13 |
| **Heart Cake,** 1/10 of the cake | 8 |
| **Log Cake,** 1/8 of the cake | 8 |
| **Oreo Blizzard Cake,** 10", 1/10 of the cake | 21 |
| **Oreo Blizzard Cake,** 8", 1/8 of the cake | 17 |
| **Pumpkin Pie 10" Blizzard Cake,** 1/10 of the cake | 17 |
| **Pumpkin Pie 8" Blizzard Cake,** 1/8 of the cake | 15 |
| **Reeses Peanut Butter Cup 10" Blizzard Cake,** 1/10 of the cake | 20 |
| **Reeses Peanut Butter Cup 8" Blizzard Cake,** 1/8 of the cake | 16 |
| **Sheet Cake,** 1/24 of the cake | 9 |
| **Strawberry CheeseQuake Blizzard Cake,** 10", 1/10 of the cake | 17 |
| **Strawberry CheeseQuake Blizzard Cake,** 8", 1/8 of the cake | 14 |

## DQ® CONES

| ▲ Power Foods | PointsPlus™ value |
|---|---|
| **Chocolate Cone,** 1 small | 6 |
| **Chocolate Cone,** 1 medium | 9 |
| **Chocolate Cone,** 1 child's | 4 |
| **Dipped Cone, Butterscotch,** 1 child's | 5 |
| **Dipped Cone, Cherry,** 1 child's | 5 |
| **Dipped Cone, Chocolate,** 1 small | 9 |
| **Dipped Cone, Chocolate,** 1 medium | 13 |
| **Dipped Cone, Chocolate,** 1 large | 18 |
| **Vanilla Cone,** 1 small | 6 |
| **Vanilla Cone,** 1 medium | 9 |
| **Vanilla Cone,** 1 large | 13 |
| **Vanilla Cone,** 1 child's | 4 |

## DQ® SUNDAES

| ▲ Power Foods | PointsPlus™ value |
|---|---|
| **Banana,** 1 small | 6 |
| **Caramel,** 1 large | 16 |
| **Cherry,** 1 large | 14 |
| **Chocolate,** 1 small | 7 |
| **Chocolate,** 1 medium | 11 |
| **Chocolate,** 1 large | 15 |

DQ® Sundaes (cont'd)

| ▲ Power Foods | PointsPlus™ value |
|---|---|
| **Hot Fudge,** 1 large | 16 |
| **Marshmallow,** 1 large | 16 |
| **Pineapple,** 1 large | 13 |
| **Strawberry,** 1 small | 7 |
| **Strawberry,** 1 medium | 9 |
| **Strawberry,** 1 large | 13 |

## XTRA STUFF

| ▲ Power Foods | PointsPlus™ value |
|---|---|
| **Almond Pieces,** 1 serving | 2 |
| ▲ **Banana Slices,** 1 serving | 0 |
| **Blackberry Topping,** 1 serving | 2 |
| **Blueberry Topping,** 1 serving | 2 |
| **Butterfinger Pieces,** 1 serving | 3 |
| **Butterscotch Cone Coating,** 1 serving | 6 |
| **Butterscotch Topping,** 1 serving | 2 |
| **Caramel Topping,** 1 serving | 2 |
| **Cheesecake Pieces,** 1 serving | 3 |
| **Cherry Cone Coating,** 1 serving | 6 |
| **Cherry Topping,** 1 serving | 1 |
| **Chewy Baked Brownie Pieces,** 1 serving | 3 |
| **Choco Chunks,** 1 serving | 4 |
| **Chocolate Chip Cookie Dough Pieces,** 1 serving | 4 |
| **Chocolate Topping,** 1 serving | 2 |
| **Cocoa Fudge,** 1 serving | 4 |
| **Coconut Flakes,** 1 serving | 2 |
| **Heath Pieces,** 1 serving | 4 |
| **Hot Fudge Topping,** 1 serving | 2 |
| **M&M Chocolate Candies,** 1 serving | 4 |
| **Maple Walnut Topping,** 1 serving | 4 |
| **Marshmallow Topping,** 1 serving | 2 |
| **Oreo Pieces,** 1 serving | 4 |
| **Peanut Butter Topping,** 1 serving | 5 |
| **Peanuts,** 1 serving | 2 |
| **Pecan Pieces,** 1 serving | 3 |
| **Pineapple Topping,** 1 serving | 1 |
| **Rainbow Sprinkles,** 1 serving | 2 |
| **Red Raspberry Topping,** 1 serving | 1 |
| **Reese's Peanut Butter Cup Pieces,** 1 serving | 4 |
| **Snickers Pieces,** 1 serving | 4 |
| **Strawberry Topping,** 1 serving | 1 |
| **Whipped Topping,** 1 serving | 3 |

## GRILLBURGER®

| ▲ Power Foods | PointsPlus™ value |
|---|---|
| **1/4 Lb Classic GrillBurger,** 1 serving | 13 |
| **1/4 Lb Classic GrillBurger with Cheese,** 1 serving | 14 |
| **1/4 Lb FlameThrower GrillBurger,** 1 serving | 20 |
| **1/2 Lb GrillBurger,** 1 serving | 22 |
| **1/2 Lb GrillBurger with Cheese,** 1 serving | 24 |
| **1/2 Lb Classic Grillburger with Cheese,** 1 serving | 22 |
| **1/2 Lb FlameThrower GrillBurger,** 1 serving | 28 |
| **Bacon Cheddar GrillBurger,** 1 serving | 20 |
| **Bacon Double Cheeseburger,** 1 serving | 18 |
| **Cheeseburger,** 1 serving | 10 |
| **Double Cheeseburger,** 1 serving | 15 |
| **Double Hamburger,** 1 serving | 13 |
| **Hamburger,** 1 serving | 9 |

## SANDWICHES/BASKETS

| ▲ Power Foods | PointsPlus™ value |
|---|---|
| **Chicken Strip Basket™ (4 breaded chicken strips, country gravy and Texas toast),** 1 | 30 |
| **Chicken Strip Basket™ (6 breaded strips, country gravy and Texas toast),** 1 | 36 |

▲ Power Foods — PointsPlus™ value

## HOT DOGS

|  | PointsPlus™ value |
|---|---|
| **All Beef Cheese Dog,** 1 serving | 9 |
| **All Beef Chili & Cheese Dog,** 1 serving | 10 |
| **All Beef Chili & Cheese Foot Long Dog,** 1 serving | 18 |
| **All Beef Chili Dog,** 1 serving | 9 |
| **All Beef Foot Long Hot Dog,** 1 serving | 15 |
| **All Beef Hot Dog,** 1 serving | 8 |

## SIDES

|  | PointsPlus™ value |
|---|---|
| **French Fries,** 1 regular | 8 |
| **French Fries,** 1 large | 13 |
| **French Fries,** 1 child's | 5 |
| **Onion Rings,** 1 serving | 10 |
| ▲ **Side Salad,** 1 serving | 0 |

## REGIONAL FAVORITE TREATS

|  | PointsPlus™ value |
|---|---|
| **Barbecue Beef Sandwich,** 1 serving | 7 |
| **Barbecue Pork Sandwich,** 1 serving | 9 |
| **Breaded Mushrooms,** 1 serving | 7 |
| **California GrillBurger,** 1 serving | 15 |
| **Chili Cheese Fries,** 1 serving | 27 |
| **Deluxe Cheeseburger,** 1 serving | 10 |
| **Deluxe Double Cheeseburger,** 1 serving | 16 |
| **Deluxe Double Hamburger,** 1 serving | 13 |
| **Deluxe Hamburger,** 1 serving | 9 |
| **DQ Ultimate® Burger,** 1 serving | 20 |
| **Fish Filet Sandwich,** 1 serving | 11 |
| **Fish Filet Sandwich with Cheese,** 1 serving | 13 |
| **Mushroom Swiss GrillBurger,** 1 serving | 16 |
| **Pecan Mudslide,** 1 serving | 18 |
| **White Cheese Kurds,** 1 serving | 15 |

## IRON GRILLED SANDWICHES, BASKETS & MORE FOOD

|  | PointsPlus™ value |
|---|---|
| **Chicken Strip Basket - 4 Piece with Country Gravy,** 1 serving | 29 |
| **Chicken Strip Basket - 6 Piece with Country Gravy,** 1 serving | 32 |
| **Crispy Chicken Salad,** 1 serving | 9 |
| **Crispy Chicken Sandwich,** 1 serving | 14 |
| **Crispy Chicken Sandwich with Cheese,** 1 serving | 15 |
| **Crispy FlameThrower Chicken Sandwich,** 1 serving | 22 |
| **FlameThrower Crispy Chicken Wrap,** 1 serving | 7 |
| **Grilled Chicken Salad,** 1 serving | 6 |
| **Grilled Chicken Sandwich,** 1 serving | 10 |
| **Grilled Chicken Wrap,** 1 serving | 5 |
| **Grilled FlameThrower Chicken Sandwich,** 1 serving | 16 |
| **Iron Grilled Cheese Sandwich,** 1 serving | 8 |
| **Iron Grilled Chicken Quesadilla Basket,** 1 serving | 31 |
| **Iron Grilled Classic Club Sandwich,** 1 serving | 15 |
| **Iron Grilled Supreme BLT Sandwich,** 1 serving | 15 |
| **Iron Grilled Turkey Sandwich,** 1 serving | 13 |
| **Iron Grilled Veggie Quesadilla Basket,** 1 serving | 27 |
| **Shrimp Basket,** 1 serving | 26 |

▲ Power Foods — *PointsPlus™* value

## SALAD DRESSINGS & CONDIMENTS

|  | PointsPlus™ value |
|---|---|
| **Fat Free Italian Dressing,** 1 serving | 0 |
| **Fat Free Ranch Dressing,** 1 serving | 1 |
| **Fat Free Red French Dressing,** 1 serving | 1 |
| **Fat Free Thousand Island Dressing,** 1 serving | 2 |
| **BBQ Sauce Dipping Cup,** 1 serving | 0 |
| **Bleu Cheese Dipping Sauce,** 1 serving | 6 |
| **Honey Mustard Dipping Sauce,** 1 serving | 7 |
| **Ketchup Packet,** 1 serving | 0 |
| **Mayonnaise,** 1 serving | 3 |
| **Mustard Packet,** 1 serving | 0 |
| **Peppered Gravy,** 1 serving | 7 |
| **Ranch Dipping Sauce,** 1 serving | 9 |
| **Sweet and Sour Dipping Sauce,** 1 serving | 3 |
| **Wild Buffalo Sauce,** 1 serving | 3 |

## KID'S MEALS

|  | PointsPlus™ value |
|---|---|
| **All Beef Hot Dog Kid's Meal,** 1 serving | 12 |
| **All Beef Hot Dog Kid's Meal with Applesauce,** 1 serving | 10 |
| **Cheeseburger Kid's Meal,** 1 serving | 15 |
| **Cheeseburger Kid's Meal with Applesauce,** 1 serving | 12 |
| **Chicken Strip Kid's Meal,** 1 serving | 11 |
| **Chicken Strip Kid's Meal with Applesauce,** 1 serving | 8 |
| **Hamburger Kid's Meal,** 1 serving | 15 |
| **Hamburger Kid's Meal with Apple Sauce,** 1 serving | 11 |

▲ Power Foods — *PointsPlus™* value

## SOFT DRINKS

|  | PointsPlus™ value |
|---|---|
| **Barq's Root Beer,** 1 small | 5 |
| **Bottled Water,** 1 serving | 0 |
| **Cherry Coca-Cola,** 1 small | 5 |
| **Coca Cola,** 1 small | 5 |
| **Coffee,** 8 oz | 0 |
| **Diet Coca Cola,** 1 small | 0 |
| **Diet Pepsi,** 1 small | 0 |
| **Dr. Pepper,** 1 small | 5 |
| **Milk, whole,** 8 oz | 4 |
| **Mountain Dew,** 1 small | 6 |
| **Mug Root Beer,** 1 small | 5 |
| **Pepsi,** 1 small | 5 |
| **Sierra Mist,** 1 small | 5 |
| **Sprite,** 1 small | 5 |

| ▲ Power Foods | *PointsPlus*™ value |
|---|---|

## SUBS

| | |
|---|---|
| **BLT & Cheese,** 1 small | 13 |
| **Capicola & Cheese,** 1 small | 11 |
| **Cheese,** 1 small | 16 |
| **Cheeseburger,** 1 small | 14 |
| **Chicken Club,** 1 small | 16 |
| **Chicken Honey Dijon,** 1 small | 13 |
| **Chicken Salad,** 1 small | 18 |
| **Chicken Stir Fry,** 1 small | 12 |
| **Classic Veggie,** 1 small | 12 |
| **Grilled Chicken,** 1 small | 9 |
| **Ham,** 1 small | 8 |
| **Ham & Cheese,** 1 small | 10 |
| **Ham & Salami,** 1 small | 12 |
| **Hamburger,** 1 small | 12 |
| **Italian,** 1 small | 14 |
| **Lobster,** 1 small | 14 |
| **Lobster Roll,** 1 small | 10 |
| **Lobster, Baked Stuffed,** 1 small | 17 |
| **Meatball,** 1 small | 18 |
| **Meatball & Cheese,** 1 small | 21 |
| **Mortadella & Cheese,** 1 small | 16 |
| **Number 9,** 1 small | 12 |
| **Pastrami,** 1 small | 17 |
| **Pastrami & Cheese,** 1 small | 17 |
| **Pepperoni,** 1 small | 16 |
| **Roast Beef,** 1 small | 8 |
| **Roast Beef,** 1 small | 8 |
| **Salad,** 1 small | 7 |
| **Salami & Cheese,** 1 small | 16 |
| **Seafood Salad,** 1 small | 13 |
| **Steak,** 1 small | 13 |
| **Steak & Cheese,** 1 small | 15 |
| **Steak Bomb,** 1 small | 18 |
| **Steak Tip,** 1 small | 14 |
| **Surf n' Turf,** 1 small | 21 |
| **Toasted Pastrami,** 1 small | 20 |
| **Toasted Pastrami Ruben,** 1 small | 20 |
| **Toasted RB & Ched,** 1 small | 16 |
| **Toasted Roast Beef & Cheddar,** 1 small | 15 |
| **Toasted Spicy MB,** 1 small | 23 |
| **Toasted Spicy Meatball,** 1 small | 27 |
| **Toasted Tuna & Swiss,** 1 small | 22 |
| **Toasted Turkey & Ham,** 1 small | 15 |
| **Toasted Turkey Thanksgiving,** 1 small | 16 |
| **Tuna,** 1 small | 19 |
| **Turkey,** 1 small | 8 |
| **Turkey Club,** 1 small | 11 |

## ONE POUNDER

| | |
|---|---|
| **Number 9,** 1 | 38 |
| **Steak,** 1 | 30 |
| **Steak and Cheese,** 1 | 34 |
| **Steak Bomb,** 1 | 42 |

## WRAPS

| | |
|---|---|
| **BLT & Cheese,** 1 | 15 |
| **Buffalo Chicken Salad,** 1 | 21 |
| **Caesar Salad,** 1 | 20 |
| **Capicola & Cheese,** 1 | 13 |
| **Cheese,** 1 | 18 |
| **Cheeseburger,** 1 | 16 |
| **Chicken Ceasar Salad,** 1 | 23 |
| **Chicken Club,** 1 | 19 |
| **Chicken Cobb,** 1 | 24 |
| **Chicken Filet & Bacon,** 1 | 19 |
| **Chicken Honey Dijon,** 1 | 16 |
| **Chicken Salad,** 1 | 20 |
| **Chicken Stir Fry,** 1 | 14 |
| **Classic Veggie,** 1 | 14 |

# D'ANGELO GRILLED SANDWICHES

*Wraps (cont'd)*

| ▲ Power Foods | *PointsPlus*™ value |
|---|---|
| **Greek,** 1 | 25 |
| **Grilled Chicken,** 1 | 11 |
| **Ham & Cheese,** 1 | 12 |
| **Ham & Salami,** 1 | 15 |
| **Hamburger,** 1 | 16 |
| **Italian,** 1 | 16 |
| **Lobster,** 1 | 17 |
| **Meatball,** 1 | 20 |
| **Mortadella & Cheese,** 1 | 18 |
| **Number 9,** 1 | 18 |
| **Pastrami,** 1 | 19 |
| **Pepperoni,** 1 | 15 |
| **Roast Beef,** 1 | 11 |
| **Salad,** 1 | 9 |
| **Salami & Cheese,** 1 | 17 |
| **Seafood Salad,** 1 | 14 |
| **Steak,** 1 | 17 |
| **Steak & Cheese,** 1 | 17 |
| **Steak Bomb,** 1 | 19 |
| **Steak Tip,** 1 | 11 |
| **Tuna,** 1 | 20 |
| **Turkey,** 1 | 10 |
| **Turkey Club,** 1 | 13 |

## POKKETS

| ▲ Power Foods | *PointsPlus*™ value |
|---|---|
| **BLT & Cheese,** 1 | 12 |
| **Caesar Salad,** 1 | 16 |
| **Capicola & Cheese,** 1 | 9 |
| **Cheese,** 1 | 14 |
| **Cheeseburger,** 1 | 12 |
| **Chicken Ceasar Salad,** 1 | 19 |
| **Chicken Club,** 1 | 14 |
| **Chicken Honey Dijon,** 1 | 12 |
| **Chicken Salad,** 1 | 16 |
| **Chicken Stir Fry,** 1 | 10 |
| **Classic Vegetable,** 1 | 10 |
| **Classic Veggie (no cheese),** 1 | 5 |
| **Greek,** 1 | 21 |
| **Grilled Chicken,** 1 | 7 |
| **Ham,** 1 | 6 |
| **Ham & Cheese,** 1 | 8 |
| **Ham & Salami,** 1 | 10 |
| **Hamburger,** 1 | 10 |
| **Italian,** 1 | 12 |
| **Lobster,** 1 | 13 |
| **Meatball,** 1 | 16 |
| **Mortadella & Cheese,** 1 | 14 |
| **Number 9,** 1 | 13 |
| **Pastrami,** 1 | 12 |
| **Pastrami & Cheese,** 1 | 15 |
| **Pepperoni,** 1 | 11 |
| **Roast Beef,** 1 | 7 |
| **Salad,** 1 | 5 |
| **Salami & Cheese,** 1 | 14 |
| **Seafood Salad,** 1 | 12 |
| **Steak,** 1 | 13 |
| **Steak & Cheese,** 1 | 13 |
| **Steak Bomb,** 1 | 16 |
| **Steak Tip,** 1 | 11 |
| **Tuna,** 1 | 17 |
| **Turkey,** 1 | 6 |
| **Turkey Club,** 1 | 9 |

## QUESADILLAS

| ▲ Power Foods | *PointsPlus*™ value |
|---|---|
| **Chicken Stir Fry,** 1 | 9 |
| **Number 9,** 1 | 10 |
| **Veggie,** 1 | 8 |
| **Salsa,** 1 | 0 |
| **Sour Cream,** 1 | 3 |

| ▲ Power Foods | *PointsPlus*™ value |
|---|---|
| **KIDZ MENU** | |
| **Cheeseburger Sub,** 1 | 8 |
| **Ham & Cheese Sub,** 1 | 6 |
| **Kidz Tuna Sub,** 1 | 10 |
| **Meatball Sub,** 1 | 9 |
| **Chocolate Chip Cookie,** 1 | 5 |
| **BREADS** | |
| **Honey Wheat Roll,** 1 small | 6 |
| **Honey Wheat Roll,** 1 medium | 9 |
| **Honey Wheat Roll,** 1 large | 13 |
| **Honey Whole Wheat Wrap,** 1 | 9 |
| **Plain Wrap,** 1 | 8 |
| **Pokket, Plain,** 1 | 5 |
| **Traditional Roll,** 1 small | 6 |
| **Traditional Roll,** 1 medium | 10 |
| **Traditional Roll,** 1 large | 12 |
| **White Roll,** 1 small | 6 |
| **White Pokket Bread,** 1 | 4 |
| **Wraps, Honey Wheat,** 1 | 9 |
| **Wraps, Plain,** 1 | 8 |
| **TOPPINGS** | |
| **Bacon,** 1 serving | 2 |
| **Buffalo Sauce,** 1 serving | 0 |
| ▲ **Cucumber,** 3 slices | 0 |
| **Fat Free Mayonnaise,** 1 packet | 0 |
| ▲ **Hot Peppers,** 3/4 oz | 0 |
| ▲ **Lettuce,** 1 oz | 0 |
| **Mayonnaise,** 2 Tbsp | 7 |
| ▲ **Mushrooms,** 1 oz | 0 |
| **Mustard - Yellow,** 2 Tbsp | 0 |
| **Mustard (Honey Dijon),** 1 serving | 2 |
| **Mustard Yellow,** 1 serving | 0 |
| **Olive Oil Blends,** 2 Tbsp | 7 |

| ▲ Power Foods | *PointsPlus*™ value |
|---|---|
| ▲ **Onions,** 1/2 oz | 0 |
| **Pickles,** 8 slice | 0 |
| **Processed American Cheese,** 1 oz | 3 |
| **Provolone Cheese,** 1 oz | 3 |
| ▲ **Sweet Peppers,** 1 oz | 0 |
| **Swiss Cheese,** 1 oz | 3 |
| ▲ **Tomato Slices,** 3 slices | 0 |
| **Turkey Gravy,** 1 serving | 13 |
| **Vinegar,** 1 serving | 0 |
| **White Cheddar Cheese,** 1 oz | 3 |
| **SALAD ENTRÉE** | |
| **Caesar,** 1 serving | 18 |
| **Chicken Caesar,** 1 serving | 19 |
| **Chicken Stir Fry,** 1 serving | 4 |
| **Greek,** 1 serving | 21 |
| **Greek (no dressing),** 1 serving | 9 |
| **SALADS** | |
| **Antipasto,** 1 serving | 7 |
| **Chicken Stir Fry Salad,** 1 serving | 4 |
| **Cobb,** 1 serving | 8 |
| **Lobster,** 1 serving | 10 |
| **Roast Beef,** 1 serving | 4 |
| **Steak Tip Caesar,** 1 serving | 18 |
| **Tossed,** 1 serving | 1 |
| **Turkey,** 1 serving | 4 |
| **SALAD DRESSINGS** | |
| **Balsamic,** 1 serving | 6 |
| **Bleu Cheese,** 1 serving | 4 |
| **Caesar,** 1 serving | 12 |
| **Creamy Italian,** 1 serving | 10 |
| **Fat Free Caesar,** 1 serving | 1 |
| **Greek,** 1 serving | 7 |

*Salad Dressings (cont'd)*

| ▲ Power Foods | *PointsPlus*™ value |
|---|---|
| **Greek with Feta Cheese,** 1 serving | 7 |
| **Honey Mustard,** 1 serving | 4 |
| **Lite Ranch,** 1 serving | 6 |
| **Olive Oil Vinaigrette,** 1 serving | 5 |

## SOUP

| | |
|---|---|
| **Beef Stew,** 1 small | 5 |
| **Broccoli & Cheddar,** 1 small serving | 7 |
| **Broccoli & Cheddar,** 1 large serving | 10 |
| **Chicken Noodle,** 1 small | 3 |
| **Extra Broccoli & Cheddar Cheese,** 1 small | 7 |
| **Hearty Vegetable,** 1 small | 1 |
| **Italian Wedding,** 1 small | 3 |
| **Lobster Bisque,** 1 small | 10 |
| **New England Clam Chowder,** 1 small | 9 |
| **Portuguese Kale,** 1 small | 4 |
| **NE Clam Chowder,** 1 small | 9 |
| **NE Clam Chowder,** 1 large | 13 |

| ▲ Power Foods | PointsPlus™ value |
|---|---|
| **TACOS** | |
| **Big Fat Chicken Taco™**, 1 | 9 |
| **Big Fat Steak Taco™**, 1 | 10 |
| **Carne Asada Taco**, 1 | 5 |
| **Chicken Soft Taco**, 1 | 6 |
| **Chicken Taco Del Carbon™**, 1 | 4 |
| **Crispy Fish Taco™**, 1 | 8 |
| **Macho Taco®**, 1 | 8 |
| **Shredded Beef Taco Del Carbon™**, 1 | 5 |
| **Soft Taco**, 1 | 5 |
| **Steak Taco Del Carbon™**, 1 | 5 |
| **Taco**, 1 | 3 |
| **TOSTADA** | |
| **Tostada**, 1 | 7 |
| **BURRITOS** | |
| **Chicken Works Burrito**, 1 | 14 |
| **Del Beef Burrito™**, 1 | 12 |
| **Del Combo Burrito**, 1 | 12 |
| **Deluxe Combo Burrito™**, 1 | 15 |
| **Deluxe Del Beef Burrito™**, 1 | 13 |
| **Macho Beef Burrito™**, 1 | 25 |
| **Macho Chicken Burrito™**, 1 | 23 |
| **Macho Combo Burrito™**, 1 | 25 |
| **Shredded Beef Combo Burrito**, 1 | 17 |
| **Steak Works Burrito**, 1 | 16 |
| **Veggie Works Burrito**, 1 | 16 |
| **NACHOS** | |
| **Macho Nachos®**, 1 | 26 |

| ▲ Power Foods | PointsPlus™ value |
|---|---|
| **QUESADILLAS** | |
| **Cheddar Quesadilla**, 1 | 12 |
| **Spicy Jack Quesadilla**, 1 | 12 |
| **BURGERS** | |
| **Bacon Double Del® Cheeseburger**, 1 | 20 |
| **Bun Taco**, 1 | 11 |
| **Cheeseburger**, 1 | 11 |
| **Double Del® Cheeseburger**, 1 | 15 |
| **Hamburger**, 1 | 9 |
| **FRENCH FRIES** | |
| **French Fries**, 1 small serving | 8 |
| **French Fries**, 1 medium serving | 10 |
| **French Fries**, 1 macho serving | 19 |
| **Kids Fries**, 1 kids serving | 4 |
| **Chili Cheddar Fries**, 1 serving | 13 |
| **Deluxe Chili Cheese Fries™**, 1 serving | 16 |
| **SALADS** | |
| **Deluxe Chicken Salad**, 1 | 19 |
| **Deluxe Taco Salad™**, 1 | 21 |
| **Mexican Caesar Salad (large) + Chicken with Dressing**, 1 | 13 |
| **Mexican Caesar Salad (large) with Dressing**, 1 | 12 |
| **Mexican Caesar Salad (large) without Dressing**, 1 | 5 |
| **Mexican Caesar Salad (large) without Dressing + Chicken**, 1 | 10 |
| **Mexican Caesar Salad (large) without Dressing + Steak**, 1 | 7 |
| **Mexican Caesar Salad (side)**, 1 | 10 |
| **Mexican Caesar Salad (side) without Dressing**, 1 | 2 |

# DEL TACO®

| ▲ Power Foods | *PointsPlus*™ value |
|---|---|
| **Mexican Caesar Salad + Steak (large),with Dressing,** 1 | 16 |
| **Taco Salad,** 1 | 10 |

## BREAKFAST FOODS

| | |
|---|---|
| **5-Piece Hash Brown Sticks,** 1 serving | 6 |
| **8-Piece Hash Brown Sticks,** 1 serving | 9 |
| **Bacon & Egg Quesadilla,** 1 | 11 |
| **Big Fat Breakfast Taco,** 1 | 10 |
| **Breakfast Burrito,** 1 | 7 |
| **Egg & Cheese Burrito,** 1 | 10 |
| **Macho Bacon & Egg Burrito™,** 1 | 24 |
| **Shredded Beef Breakfast Burrito,** 1 | 18 |
| **Side of Bacon (2 slices),** 1 serving | 1 |
| **Steak & Egg Burrito,** 1 | 13 |

## SIDES

| | |
|---|---|
| **Beans 'n Cheese Cup,** 1 serving | 6 |
| **Medium Chips and Salsa,** 1 serving | 4 |
| **Large Chips and Salsa,** 1 serving | 11 |
| **Rice Cup,** 1 serving | 4 |

## SHAKES

| | |
|---|---|
| **Chocolate Shake,** 1 | 18 |
| **Strawberry Shake,** 1 | 16 |
| **Vanilla Shake,** 1 | 16 |

| ▲ Power Foods | *PointsPlus*™ value |
|---|---|

## APPETIZERS
(WITHOUT DIPPING SAUCES OR DRESSINGS)

| Item | *PointsPlus*™ value |
|---|---|
| **Buffalo Chicken Strips, celery sticks,** 5 strips | 19 |
| **Buffalo Wings,** 9 wings | 8 |
| **Chicken Strips, plain with celery,** 5 strips | 19 |
| **Mozzarella Sticks,** 8 sticks | 33 |
| **Nachos,** 1 platter | 31 |
| **Sampler™,** 1 platter | 38 |
| **Strips and sticks,** 1 serving | 34 |
| **Sweet & Tangy BBQ Chicken Strips,** 1 serving | 21 |
| **Sweet & Tangy BBQ Chicken Wings,** 1 serving | 9 |
| **Sweet & Tangy BBQ Shrimp,** 1 serving | 9 |

## DENNY'S® FAMOUS SLAMS

| Item | *PointsPlus*™ value |
|---|---|
| **All-American Slam®, without choice of hashed browns, grits, or bread,** 1 serving | 22 |
| **French Toast Slam®, without syrup or margarine,** 1 serving | 25 |
| **Lumberjack Slam®,** 1 serving | 22 |

## BURGERS & SANDWICHES

| Item | *PointsPlus*™ value |
|---|---|
| **Bacon-Cheddar Burger,** 1 | 30 |
| **Bacon, Lettuce & Tomato Sandwich,** 1 | 15 |
| **Boca Burger®,** 1 | 13 |
| **Breaded Chicken Sandwich with Honey Mustard Dressing,** 1 | 30 |
| **Chicken Ranch Melt,** 1 | 24 |
| **Classic Burger with Cheese,** 1 | 25 |
| **Club Sandwich,** 1 | 17 |
| **Crispy Chicken Sandwich,** 1 serving | 25 |
| **Double Cheeseburger,** 1 | 41 |
| **Fabulous French Toast Platter,** 3 pieces | 27 |
| **Fit Fare Boca Burger,** 1 | 9 |
| **Fit-Fare Chicken Sandwich with Fruit,** 1 serving | 12 |
| **Grilled Chicken Sandwich with Honey Mustard Dressing,** 1 serving | 26 |
| **Mushroom-Swiss Burger,** 1 | 24 |
| **Spicy Buffalo Chicken Melt,** 1 | 25 |
| **The Super Bird® Sandwich,** 1 | 15 |
| **Western Burger,** 1 | 35 |

## DINNERS
(WITHOUT SIDE DISHES OR CHOICE OF BREAD)

| Item | *PointsPlus*™ value |
|---|---|
| **Chicken Strips,** 1 serving | 15 |
| **Country Fried Steak,** 1 serving | 27 |
| **Fit Fare Grilled Chicken Dinner with Green Beans & Tomato Slices,** 1 serving | 9 |
| **Fit Fare Grilled Tilapia with Rice Pilaf, Corn & Tomato Slices,** 1 serving | 15 |
| ▲ **Grilled Chicken Dinner,** 1 serving | 6 |
| **Grilled Shrimp Skewers with Rice Pilaf,** 1 serving | 10 |
| **Grilled Tilapia Dinner with Rice Pilaf,** 1 serving | 14 |
| **Homestyle Meatloaf with gravy,** 1 serving | 14 |
| **Lemon Pepper Tilapia with Rice Pilaf,** 1 serving | 16 |
| **Mushroom Swiss Chop'd Steak with Gravy,** 1 serving | 25 |
| **T-bone Steak & Breaded Shrimp Dinner,** 1 serving | 25 |
| **T-bone Steak & Shrimp Skewer Dinner,** 1 serving | 22 |
| **T-bone Steak Dinner,** 1 serving | 20 |
| **Top Sirloin Steak & Breaded Shrimp,** 1 serving | 11 |
| **Top Sirloin Steak & Shrimp Skewers,** 1 serving | 7 |
| **Top Sirloin Steak Dinner,** 1 serving | 5 |

▲ Power Foods — *PointsPlus*™ value

## SIDES

| Item | PointsPlus™ value |
|---|---|
| **Breaded Shrimp,** 6 pieces | 5 |
| **Cinnamon Apples,** 1 serving | 3 |
| **Corn,** 1 serving | 4 |
| **Cottage Cheese,** 1 serving | 2 |
| **Dinner Rolls,** 1 serving | 7 |
| **French Fries, salted,** 1 serving | 12 |
| **Garlic Dinner Bread,** 1 serving | 5 |
| **Grilled Shrimp Skewer,** 1 | 2 |
| **Hashed Browns,** 1 serving | 5 |
| **Mashed Potatoes, plain,** 1 serving | 10 |
| **Mixed Vegetables,** 1 serving | 1 |
| **Onion Rings,** 1 serving | 15 |
| **Seasoned Fries,** 1 serving | 14 |
| **Smothered Cheese Fries,** 1 serving | 23 |
| ▲ **Tomato Slices,** 3 slices | 0 |
| **Vegetable Rice Pilaf,** 1 serving | 5 |

## SALADS (WITHOUT BREAD)

| Item | PointsPlus™ value |
|---|---|
| **Chicken Strip Salad Deluxe,** 1 | 16 |
| **Coleslaw,** 1 serving | 7 |
| **Fit-Fare Grilled Chicken Breast Salad with Lemon or Lime Wedges,** 1 | 7 |
| **Garden Side Salad, without dressing,** 1 | 3 |
| **Grilled Chicken Deluxe Salad,** 1 | 7 |
| **Croutons (for salad),** 1 serving | 3 |

## SALAD DRESSINGS

| Item | PointsPlus™ value |
|---|---|
| **Blue Cheese Dressing,** 1 serving | 5 |
| **Caesar Dressing,** 1 serving | 3 |
| **Fat Free Italian,** 1 serving | 0 |
| **Fat Free Ranch Dressing,** 1 serving | 0 |
| **French Dressing,** 1 serving | 2 |
| **Honey Mustard Dressing,** 1 serving | 4 |
| **Ranch Dressing,** 1 serving | 4 |
| **Thousand Island Dressing,** 1 serving | 3 |

## SOUPS

| Item | PointsPlus™ value |
|---|---|
| **Chicken Noodle Soup,** 1 bowl | 5 |
| **Clam Chowder,** 1 bowl | 4 |
| **Vegetable Beef Soup,** 1 bowl | 4 |

## CONDIMENTS, SAUCES & GRAVIES

| Item | PointsPlus™ value |
|---|---|
| **BBQ Sauce,** 1 serving | 2 |
| ▲ **Pico de Gallo,** 1 serving | 0 |
| **Sour Cream,** 1 serving | 3 |

## OMELETTES (WITHOUT HASH BROWNS, GRITS OR BREAD)

| Item | PointsPlus™ value |
|---|---|
| **Ham & Cheddar Omelette,** 1 serving | 15 |
| **Ultimate Omelette®,** 1 serving | 18 |
| **Veggie-Cheese Omelette,** 1 serving | 13 |
| **Veggie-Cheese Omelette with Egg Whites,** 1 serving | 10 |

## BREAKFAST SIDES

| Item | PointsPlus™ value |
|---|---|
| **Applesauce Musselman's®,** 1 serving | 2 |
| **Bacon,** 4 strip | 5 |
| **Bagel, with 1 oz cream cheese,** 1 | 9 |
| ▲ **Banana,** 1 serving | 0 |
| **Biscuit,** 1 | 5 |
| **Biscuit & Sausage Gravy,** 1 serving | 15 |
| **Country Fried Potatoes,** 1 serving | 10 |
| **Egg,** 1 | 3 |
| ▲ **Egg Whites Egg Substitute,** 1 serving | 1 |
| **English Muffin, with margarine,** 1 | 4 |
| ▲ **Grapes,** 1 serving | 0 |
| **Grits, with margarine,** 1 serving | 7 |
| **Ham, Grilled, Honey Smoked,** 1 slice | 3 |
| **Hashed Browns with Cheddar Cheese,** 1 serving | 8 |
| **Hashed Browns with Onions, Cheese, Gravy,** 1 serving | 13 |
| **Quaker® Oatmeal with 8 oz Milk,** 1 serving | 7 |

| ▲ Power Foods | *PointsPlus*™ value |
|---|---|
| **Sausage,** 4 links | 10 |
| **Toast, dry,** 1 slice | 2 |

## OTHER BREAKFAST PLATTERS

| | |
|---|---|
| **Belgian Waffle Platter,** 1 serving | 18 |
| **Country Fried Steak & Eggs, without choice of bread,** 1 serving | 17 |
| **Heartland Scramble,** 1 serving | 31 |
| **Meat Lover's Scramble,** 1 serving | 30 |
| **Moons Over My Hammy®, without choice of potatoes or grits,** 1 serving | 20 |
| **Pancakes,** 3 | 11 |

## OTHER BREAKFAST PLATTERS

| | |
|---|---|
| **Southwestern Sizzlin Skillet,** 1 serving | 26 |
| **T-bone Steak & Eggs, without choice of hashed browns, grits, or bread,** 1 serving | 20 |
| **Top Sirloin Steak & Eggs, without choice of hashed browns, grits, or bread,** 1 serving | 10 |
| **Two Egg Breakfast,** 1 serving | 5 |

## SENIOR DINNER (WITHOUT VEGETABLE, SOUP, SALAD, FRUIT OR BREAD)

| | |
|---|---|
| **Senior Country Fried Steak with Gravy,** 1 serving | 14 |
| ▲ **Senior Grilled Chicken Breast,** 1 serving | 3 |
| **Senior Grilled Tilapia,** 1 serving | 6 |
| **Senior Home Style Meatloaf,** 1 serving | 7 |
| **Senior Meatloaf with Gravy,** 1 serving | 15 |
| **Senior Shrimp Skewer with Rice,** 1 serving | 7 |

## SENIOR LUNCH (WITHOUT FRENCH FRIES OR HASHED BROWNS)

| ▲ Power Foods | *PointsPlus*™ value |
|---|---|
| **Grilled Cheese Deluxe Sandwich,** 1 | 15 |
| **Senior Bacon Cheddar Burger,** 1 | 17 |
| **Senior Club,** 1 | 15 |

## SENIOR BREAKFAST

| | |
|---|---|
| **Senior Belgian Waffle Slam®, with egg,** 1 serving | 12 |
| **Senior French Toast Slam with 1 Egg,** 1 serving | 8 |
| **Senior Omelette, without choice of hashed browns, grits, or bread,** 1 serving | 13 |
| **Senior Scrambled Egg & Cheddar with Pancakes,** 1 serving | 21 |
| **Senior Starter™,** 1 serving | 6 |

## KID'S D-ZONE (WITHOUT SIDES)

| | |
|---|---|
| ▲ **Anti-Gravity Grapes,** 1 serving | 0 |
| **Astronaut Applesauce,** 1 serving | 3 |
| **Big Dipper French Toastix™ & Whipped Topping (no meat),** 1 serving | 8 |
| **Big Dipper French Toastix™ with Meat & Whipped Topping,** 1 serving | 12 |
| **Cosmic Cheese Burger,** 1 serving | 10 |
| **Flying Saucer Pizza,** 1 serving | 9 |
| **Galactic Grilled Cheese,** 1 serving | 9 |
| **Goldfish® Galaxy,** 1 serving | 4 |
| **Junior Grand Slam®,** 1 serving | 10 |
| **Little Dipper Sampler (no dressing or marinara sauce),** 1 serving | 16 |
| **Macaroni & Cheese,** 1 serving | 9 |
| **Mini Hot Dog in a Bun,** 1 | 9 |
| **Moon Crater Mashed Potatoes with Brown Gravy,** 1 serving | 7 |

*Kid's D-Zone (cont'd)*

| ▲ Power Foods | PointsPlus™ value |
|---|---|
| **Moons & Stars Chicken Nuggets & BBQ Sauce,** 1 serving | 8 |
| **Smiley Alien Hotcakes with Meat,** 1 serving | 11 |
| **Smiley Alien Hotcakes without Meat,** 1 serving | 9 |
| **Space Saucers,** 1 serving | 12 |

## KID'S SIDES & DESSERTS

| | |
|---|---|
| **Cosmos Milkshake - all flavors,** 1 serving | 13 |
| **Deep Space French Fries,** 1 serving | 12 |
| **Delicious Dip Sundae,** 1 serving | 8 |
| **Far Out Fruit Medley,** 1 serving | 2 |
| **Neutron Brownie (kids),** 1 serving | 11 |
| **Orbits of Oreo Sundae,** 1 serving | 11 |
| **Oreo Blender Blaster,** 1 kids serving | 19 |
| **Solar S'Cream - all flavors,** 1 serving | 3 |

## ICE CREAM

| | |
|---|---|
| **Double Scoop Sundae,** 1 | 11 |
| **Single Scoop/Sundae (delicious dip),** 1 | 8 |

## SUNDAES, SHAKES & FLOATS

| | |
|---|---|
| **Banana Split,** 1 serving | 22 |
| **Floats (root beer or cola),** 1 | 12 |
| **Milkshake (vanilla/chocolate),** 1 | 16 |
| **Oreo Blender Blaster,** 1 | 25 |

## SYRUPS & TOPPINGS

| ▲ Power Foods | PointsPlus™ value |
|---|---|
| **Cherry Topping,** 3 oz | 2 |
| **Maple-Flavored Syrup,** 3 Tbsp | 4 |
| **Strawberry Topping,** 2 oz | 2 |
| **Sugar-Free Maple-Flavored Syrup,** 3 Tbsp | 1 |
| **Whipped Cream,** 2 Tbsp | 1 |
| **Whipped Margarine,** 1 serving | 1 |

## DESSERTS

| | |
|---|---|
| **Apple Crisp a la Mode,** 1 slice | 20 |
| **Apple Pie,** 1 slice | 14 |
| **Carrot Cake,** 1 slice | 23 |
| **Cheesecake,** 1 slice | 18 |
| **Cheesecake (no sugar added),** 1 slice | 9 |
| **Coconut Cream Pie,** 1 slice | 18 |
| **French Silk Pie,** 1 slice | 21 |
| **Hershey's Chocolate Cake,** 1 slice | 16 |
| **Hot Fudge Brownie a la Mode,** 1 serving | 27 |
| **Oreo Sundae,** 1 serving | 21 |

## DESSERT TOPPINGS

| | |
|---|---|
| **Chocolate Topping,** 1 serving | 4 |
| **Fudge Topping,** 1 serving | 6 |

## BEVERAGES

| | |
|---|---|
| **Cappuccino French Vanilla,** 1 | 4 |
| **Cherry Limeade,** 1 | 5 |
| **Hot Chocolate,** 1 | 4 |
| **Island Fizz,** 1 | 5 |
| **Lemonade with Ice,** 1 | 4 |
| **OJ Mango,** 1 | 7 |
| **Pineapple Dream,** 1 | 5 |
| **Raspberry Iced Tea,** 1 | 2 |
| **Razzdango,** 1 | 5 |
| **Strawberry Mango Pucker,** 1 | 6 |
| **Very Double Berry,** 1 | 7 |

# DIPPIN' DOTS

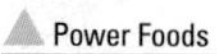 Power Foods — *PointsPlus*™ value

## ICE CREAM

|  | *PointsPlus*™ value |
|---|---|
| **Banana Split,** 1/2 cup | 5 |
| **Bubble Gum,** 1/2 cup | 4 |
| **Candy Bar Crunch,** 1/2 cup | 7 |
| **Caramel Brownie Sundae,** 1/2 cup | 5 |
| **Chocolate,** 1/2 cup | 4 |
| **Chocolate Chip Cookie Dough,** 1/2 cup | 6 |
| **Cookies 'n Cream with Oreo,** 1/2 cup | 5 |
| **Cotton Candy,** 1/2 cup | 5 |
| **Horchata,** 1/2 cup | 5 |
| **Java Delight,** 1/2 cup | 5 |
| **Mint Chocolate,** 1/2 cup | 4 |
| **Moose Tracks,** 1/2 cup | 6 |
| **No Sugar Added Fudge Ice Cream (fat free),** 1/2 cup | 2 |
| **No Sugar Added Vanilla Ice Cream (reduced fat),** 1/2 cup | 3 |
| **Peanut Butter Chip,** 1/2 cup | 4 |
| **Root Beer Float,** 1/2 cup | 3 |
| **Strawberry,** 1/2 cup | 5 |
| **Tropical Tie Dye,** 1/2 cup | 5 |
| **Vanilla,** 1/2 cup | 5 |
| **Yogurt (Strawberry Cheese),** 1/2 cup | 3 |

## SHERBET

|  | *PointsPlus*™ value |
|---|---|
| **Lemon Lime Sherbet,** 1/2 cup | 3 |
| **Orange Sherbet,** 1/2 cup | 3 |
| **Raspberry Sherbet,** 1/2 cup | 3 |

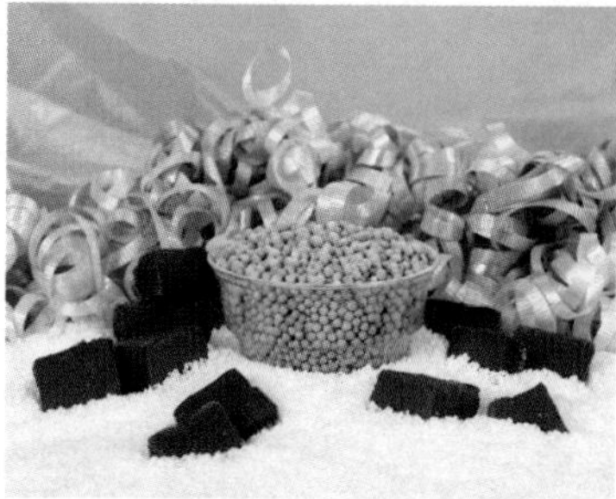

Power Foods — *PointsPlus*™ value

## DOTS 'N CREAM

|  | *PointsPlus*™ value |
|---|---|
| **Banana Split,** 1/2 cup | 6 |
| **Caramel Cappuccino**™, 1/2 cup | 5 |
| **Mint Chocolate,** 1/2 cup | 7 |
| **Orange Crème de la Crème**™, 1/2 cup | 5 |
| **Vanilla Over the Rainbow**™, 1/2 cup | 6 |
| **Wild About Chocolate**™, 1/2 cup | 7 |

## FLAVORED ICE

|  | *PointsPlus*™ value |
|---|---|
| **Cherry Berry Ice,** 1/2 cup | 2 |
| **Liberty Ice,** 1/2 cup | 2 |
| **Pink Lemonade Ice,** 1/2 cup | 2 |
| **Rainbow Ice,** 1/2 cup | 2 |
| **Watermelon Ice,** 1/2 cup | 2 |

# DOMINO'S PIZZA®

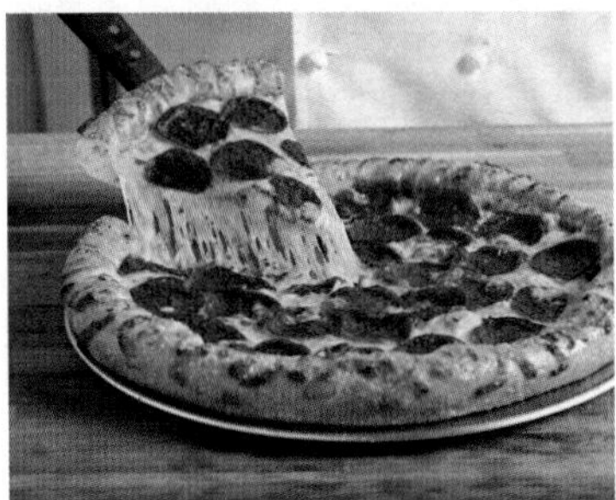

▲ Power Foods

| MEDIUM PIZZA (INCLUDES CRUST, SAUCE & CHEESE) | *PointsPlus™* value |
|---|---|
| **Deep Dish,** 1/8 of the 12" medium pizza | 6 |
| **Hand-Tossed,** 1/8 of the 12" medium pizza | 5 |
| **Thin Crust,** 1/8 of the 12" medium pizza | 4 |

| PIZZA TOPPINGS (FOR MEDIUM PIZZA) | *PointsPlus™* value |
|---|---|
| **American Cheese,** topping for 1/8 of the 12" pizza | 1 |
| **Anchovies,** toppings for 1/8 of the 12" medium pizza | 0 |
| **Bacon,** topping for 1/8 of the 12" medium pizza | 1 |
| ▲ **Banana Peppers,** topping for 1/8 of the 12" pizza | 0 |
| **Beef,** topping for 1/8 of the 12" medium pizza | 1 |
| **Black Olives,** topping for 1/8 of the 12" medium pizza | 0 |
| **Cheddar Cheese,** topping for 1/8 of the 12" pizza | 1 |
| **Chicken,** topping for 1/8 of the 12" pizza | 0 |
| **Extra Cheese,** topping for 1/8 of the 12" medium pizza | 1 |
| **Garlic,** topping for 1/8 of the 12" medium pizza | 0 |
| ▲ **Green Chile Peppers,** topping for 1/8 of the 12" pizza | 0 |
| **Green Olives,** topping for 1/8 of the 12" pizza | 0 |
| ▲ **Green Pepper,** topping for 1/8 of the 12" medium pizza | 0 |
| **Ham,** topping for 1/8 of the 12" medium pizza | 0 |
| ▲ **Jalapeno,** topping for 1/8 of the 12" pizza | 0 |
| ▲ **Mushrooms,** topping for 1/8 of the 12" medium pizza | 0 |
| ▲ **Onions,** topping for 1/8 of the 12" medium pizza | 0 |
| **Pepperoni,** topping for 1/8 of the 12" medium pizza | 1 |
| ▲ **Philly Meat,** topping for 1/8 of the 12" pizza | 0 |
| ▲ **Pineapple,** topping for 1/8 of the 12" medium pizza | 0 |
| **Provolone Cheese,** topping for 1/8 of the 12" pizza | 1 |
| **Sausage,** topping for 1/8 of the 12" medium pizza | 1 |
| ▲ **Tomatoes,** topping for 1/8 of the 12" medium pizza | 0 |

| LARGE PIZZA (INCLUDES CRUST, SAUCE & CHEESE) | *PointsPlus™* value |
|---|---|
| **Deep Dish,** 1/8 of the 14" large pizza | 9 |
| **Hand-Tossed,** 1/8 of the 14" large pizza | 7 |
| **Thin Crust,** 1/8 of the 14" large pizza | 5 |

| PIZZA TOPPINGS (FOR LARGE PIZZA) | *PointsPlus™* value |
|---|---|
| **American Cheese,** topping for 1/8 of the 14" pizza | 1 |
| **Anchovies,** topping for 1/8 of the 14" large pizza | 0 |

# DOMINO'S PIZZA®

| ▲ Power Foods | *PointsPlus*™ value |
|---|---|
| **Bacon,** topping for 1/8 of the 14" large pizza | 1 |
| ▲ **Banana Peppers,** toppings for 1/8 of the 14" pizza | 0 |
| **Beef,** topping for 1/8 of the 14" large pizza | 1 |
| **Black Olives,** topping for 1/8 of the 14" large pizza | 0 |
| **Cheddar Cheese,** topping for 1/8 of the 14" pizza | 1 |
| **Chicken,** topping for 1/8 of the 14" pizza | 1 |
| **Extra Cheese,** topping for 1/8 of the 14" large pizza | 1 |
| **Garlic,** topping for 1/8 of the 14" pizza | 0 |
| ▲ **Green Chile Peppers,** toppings for 1/8 of the 14" pizza | 0 |
| **Green Olives,** topping for 1/8 of the 14" pizza | 1 |
| ▲ **Green Pepper,** topping for 1/8 of the 14" large pizza | 0 |
| **Ham,** topping for 1/8 of the 14" large pizza | 0 |
| ▲ **Jalapeno,** topping for 1/8 of the 14" pizza | 0 |
| ▲ **Mushrooms,** topping for 1/8 of the 14" large pizza | 0 |
| ▲ **Onions,** topping for 1/8 of the 14" large pizza | 0 |
| **Pepperoni,** topping for 1/8 of the 14" large pizza | 1 |
| ▲ **Philly Meat,** topping for 1/8 of the 14" pizza | 0 |
| ▲ **Pineapple,** topping for 1/8 of the 14" large pizza | 0 |
| **Provolone Cheese,** topping for 1/8 of the 14" pizza | 2 |
| **Sausage,** topping for 1/8 of the 14" large pizza | 2 |
| ▲ **Tomatoes,** topping for 1/8 of the 14" large pizza | 0 |

| ▲ Power Foods | *PointsPlus*™ value |
|---|---|
| **PIZZA TOPPINGS (FOR MEDIUM FEAST PIZZA)** | |
| **America's Favorite Feast®,** topping for 1/8 of the 12" medium pizza | 3 |
| **Bacon Cheeseburger Feast®,** topping for 1/8 of the 12" medium pizza | 4 |
| **Barbecue Feast,** topping for 1/8 of the 12" medium pizza | 4 |
| **Deluxe Feast®,** topping for 1/8 of the 12" medium pizza | 3 |
| **ExtravaganZZa Feast®,** topping for 1/8 of the 12" medium pizza | 4 |
| **Hawaiian Feast®,** topping for 1/8 of the 12" medium pizza | 3 |
| **MeatZZa Feast®,** topping for 1/8 of the 12" medium pizza | 4 |
| **Pepperoni Feast®,** topping for 1/8 of the 12" medium pizza | 4 |
| **Philly Cheese Steak Feast,** topping for 1/8 of the 12" medium pizza | 3 |
| **Vegi Feast®,** topping for 1/8 of the 12" medium pizza | 2 |
| **CRUST OPTIONS (FOR MEDIUM FEAST PIZZA)** | |
| **Deep Dish (shell only),** 1/8 of the pizza | 4 |
| **Hand Tossed (dough only),** 1/8 of the pizza | 3 |
| **Thin Crust (shell only),** 1/8 of the pizza | 2 |

# DOMINO'S PIZZA®

| ▲ Power Foods | PointsPlus™ value |
|---|---|
| **PIZZA TOPPINGS** (FOR LARGE FEAST PIZZA) | |
| **America's Favorite Feast®,** topping for 1/8 of the 14" large pizza | 5 |
| **Bacon Cheeseburger Feast®,** topping for 1/8 of the 14" large pizza | 5 |
| **Barbecue Feast,** topping for 1/8 of the 14" large pizza | 5 |
| **Deluxe Feast®,** topping for 1/8 of the 14" large pizza | 4 |
| **ExtravaganZZa Feast®,** topping for 1/8 of the 14" large pizza | 6 |
| **Hawaiian Feast®,** topping for 1/8 of the 14" large pizza | 3 |
| **MeatZZa Feast®,** topping for 1/8 of the 14" large pizza | 5 |
| **Pepperoni Feast®,** topping for 1/8 of the 14" large pizza | 5 |
| **Philly Cheese Steak Feast,** toppings for 1/8 of the 14" large pizza | 3 |
| **Vegi Feast®,** topping for 1/8 of the 14" large pizza | 3 |
| **CRUST OPTIONS** (FOR LARGE FEAST PIZZA) | |
| **Deep Dish (shell only),** 1/8 of the pizza | 6 |
| **Thin Crust (shell only),** 1/8 of the pizza | 3 |
| **AMERICAN LEGENDS PIZZA** (SMALL) | |
| **Buffalo Chicken Hand Tossed Crust,** 1/6 of a 10" small pizza | 7 |
| **Buffalo Chicken Thin Crust,** 1/4 of a 10" small pizza | 6 |
| **Cali Chicken Bacon Ranch Hand Tossed,** 1/6 of a 10" small pizza | 8 |
| **Cali Chicken Bacon Ranch Thin Crust,** 1/4 of a 10" small pizza | 8 |
| **Honolulu Hawaiian Hand Tossed,** 1/6 of a 10" small pizza | 7 |
| **Honolulu Hawaiian Thin Crust,** 1/4 of a 10" small pizza | 6 |
| **Memphis BBQ Chicken Hand Tossed,** 1/6 of a 10" small pizza | 7 |
| **Memphis BBQ Chicken Thin Crust,** 1/4 of a 10" small pizza | 6 |
| **Pacific Veggie Hand Tossed,** 1/6 of a 10" small pizza | 6 |
| **Pacific Veggie Thin Crust,** 1/4 of a 10" small pizza | 5 |
| **Philly Cheese Steak Hand Tossed,** 1/6 of a 10" small pizza | 7 |
| **Philly Cheese Steak Thin Crust,** 1/4 of a 10" small pizza | 6 |
| **AMERICAN LEGENDS PIZZA** (MEDIUM) | |
| **Buffalo Chicken Deep Dish,** 1/8 of a 12" medium pizza | 8 |
| **Buffalo Chicken Hand Tossed,** 1/8 of a 12" medium pizza | 7 |
| **Buffalo Chicken Thin Crust,** 1/8 of a 12" medium pizza | 10 |
| **Cali Chicken Bacon Ranch Deep Dish,** 1/8 of a 12" medium pizza | 9 |
| **Cali Chicken Bacon Ranch Hand Tossed,** 1/8 of a 12" medium pizza | 8 |
| **Cali Chicken Bacon Ranch Thin Crust,** 1/8 of a 12" medium pizza | 13 |
| **Honolulu Hawaiian Deep Dish,** 1/8 of a 12" medium pizza | 7 |
| **Honolulu Hawaiian Hand Tossed,** 1/8 of a 12" medium pizza | 7 |
| **Honolulu Hawaiian Thin Crust,** 1/8 of a 12" medium pizza | 10 |
| **Memphis BBQ Chicken Deep Dish,** 1/8 of a 12" medium pizza | 8 |

| ▲ Power Foods | PointsPlus™ value |
|---|---|
| **Memphis BBQ Chicken Hand Tossed,** 1/8 of a 12" medium pizza | 7 |
| **Memphis BBQ Chicken Thin Crust,** 1/4 of a 12" medium pizza | 10 |
| **Pacific Veggie Deep Dish,** 1/8 of a 12" medium pizza | 7 |
| **Pacific Veggie Hand Tossed,** 1/8 of a 12" medium pizza | 6 |
| **Pacific Veggie Thin Crust,** 1/4 of a 12" medium pizza | 9 |
| **Philly Cheese Steak Deep Dish,** 1/8 of a 12" medium pizza | 8 |
| **Philly Cheese Steak Hand Tossed,** 1/8 of a 12" medium pizza | 7 |
| **Philly Cheese Steak Thin Crust,** 1/4 of a 12" medium pizza | 10 |

## AMERICAN LEGENDS PIZZA (LARGE)

| | |
|---|---|
| **Buffalo Chicken Deep Dish,** 1/8 of a 14" large pizza | 11 |
| **Buffalo Chicken Hand Tossed,** 1/8 of a 14" large pizza | 9 |
| **Buffalo Chicken Thin Crust,** 1/8 of a 14" large pizza | 7 |
| **Cali Chicken Bacon Ranch Deep Dish,** 1/8 of a 14" large pizza | 13 |
| **Cali Chicken Bacon Ranch Hand Tossed,** 1/8 of a 14" large pizza | 12 |
| **Cali Chicken Bacon Ranch Thin Crust,** 1/8 of a 14" large pizza | 9 |
| **Honolulu Hawaiian Deep Dish,** 1/8 of a 14" large pizza | 11 |
| **Honolulu Hawaiian Hand Tossed,** 1/8 of a 14" large pizza | 9 |
| **Honolulu Hawaiian Thin Crust,** 1/8 of a 14" large pizza | 7 |
| **Memphis BBQ Chicken Deep Dish,** 1/8 of a 14" large pizza | 12 |
| **Memphis BBQ Chicken Hand Tossed,** 1/8 of a 14" large pizza | 10 |

| ▲ Power Foods | PointsPlus™ value |
|---|---|
| **Memphis BBQ Chicken Thin Crust,** 1/8 of a 14" large pizza | 7 |
| **Pacific Veggie Deep Dish,** 1/8 of a 14" large pizza | 10 |
| **Pacific Veggie Hand Tossed,** 1/8 of a 14" large pizza | 8 |
| **Pacific Veggie Thin Crust,** 1/8 of a 14" large pizza | 6 |
| **Philly Cheese Steak Deep Dish,** 1/8 of a 14" large pizza | 11 |
| **Philly Cheese Steak Hand Tossed,** 1/8 of a 14" large pizza | 9 |
| **Philly Cheese Steak Thin Crust,** 1/8 of a 14" large pizza | 6 |

## BROOKLYN STYLE PIZZAS

| | |
|---|---|
| **Cheese Only Pizza,** 1/6 of the 14" large pizza | 6 |
| **Cheese Only Pizza,** 1/6 of the 16" extra large pizza | 10 |
| **Add Pepperoni,** topping for 1/6 of the 14" large pizza | 1 |
| **Add Pepperoni,** topping for 1/6 of 16" extra-large pizza | 2 |

## OVEN BAKED SANDWICHES

| | |
|---|---|
| **Chicken Bacon Ranch,** 1 | 24 |
| **Chicken Parmesan,** 1 | 20 |
| **Italian,** 1 | 23 |
| **Philly Cheese Steak,** 1 | 18 |
| **Extra Cheese,** 1 serving | 2 |
| **Extra Chicken,** 1 serving | 2 |
| **Extra Italian Meat,** 1 serving | 3 |
| ▲ **Extra Philly Meat,** 1 serving | 1 |
| ▲ **Extra Veggies, Italian,** 1 serving | 0 |
| ▲ **Extra Veggies, Philly,** 1 serving | 0 |

# DOMINO'S PIZZA®

| ▲ Power Foods | *PointsPlus*™ value |
|---|---|
| **CHICKEN SIDES** | |
| **Barbecue Buffalo Wings,** 2 pieces | 6 |
| **Buffalo Chicken Kickers®,** 2 pieces | 3 |
| **Hot Buffalo Wings,** 2 pieces | 5 |
| **Blue Cheese Dipping Sauce,** 1 container | 6 |
| **Hot Dipping Sauce,** 1 container | 1 |
| **Ranch Dipping Sauce,** 1 container | 6 |
| **BREAD SIDES** | |
| **Breadstick,** 1 piece | 3 |
| **Cheesy Bread,** 1 piece | 3 |
| **Cinna Stix®,** 1 piece | 3 |
| **Garlic Dipping Sauce,** 1 container | 7 |
| **Italian Dipping Sauce,** 1 serving | 1 |
| **Marinara Dipping Sauce,** 1 container | 1 |
| **Parmesan Peppercorn Dipping Sauce,** 1 serving | 6 |
| **Sweet Icing,** 1 container | 7 |
| **SALADS & DRESSINGS** | |
| **Garden Fresh Salad,** 1/2 container | 2 |
| **Grilled Chicken Caesar,** 1/2 container | 3 |
| **Blue Cheese Dressing,** 1 package | 7 |
| **Buttermilk Ranch Dressing,** 1 package | 6 |
| **Creamy Caesar Dressing,** 1 package | 6 |
| **Golden Italian Dressing,** 1 package | 6 |
| **Italian Light Dressing,** 1 package | 0 |
| **Croutons,** 1 package | 1 |

| ▲ Power Foods | *PointsPlus*™ value |
|---|---|
| **APPETIZERS** | |
| **Garlic Wings,** 5 | 19 |
| **Plain Wings,** 5 | 15 |
| **Spicy Garlic Wings,** 5 | 20 |
| **Wedge Fries,** 1 side portion | 7 |
| **SIGNATURE PIZZA** | |
| **Chicken Spinach Mozzarella, Bakery Crust,** 2 slices | 10 |
| **Chicken Spinach Mozzarella, No Dough,** 1/4 pizza or 1 individual size pizza | 16 |
| **Chicken Spinach Mozzarella, Thicker Crust,** 1/4 pizza or 1 individual size pizza | 11 |
| **Chicken Spinach Mozzarella, Thin Crust,** 1/4 pizza or 1 individual size pizza | 17 |
| **Margherita, Bakery Crust,** 2 slices | 10 |
| **Margherita, No Dough,** 1 pizza | 17 |
| **Margherita, Thicker Crust,** 1/4 pizza or 1 individual size pizza | 21 |
| **Margherita, Thin Crust,** 1/4 pizza or 1 individual size pizza | 17 |
| **NO DOUGH PIZZAS** | |
| **BBQ Chicken,** 1 whole pizza | 13 |
| **Fresh Mozzarella Meatball,** 1 whole pizza | 13 |
| **Pepperoni Zinger,** 1 whole pizza | 16 |
| **LARGE THICKER CRUST PIZZA** | |
| **BBQ Chicken,** 1/8 of the large pizza | 11 |
| **Fresh Mozzarella Meatball,** 1/4 pizza or 1 individual size pizza | 24 |
| **Pepperoni Zinger,** 1/8 of the large pizza | 11 |

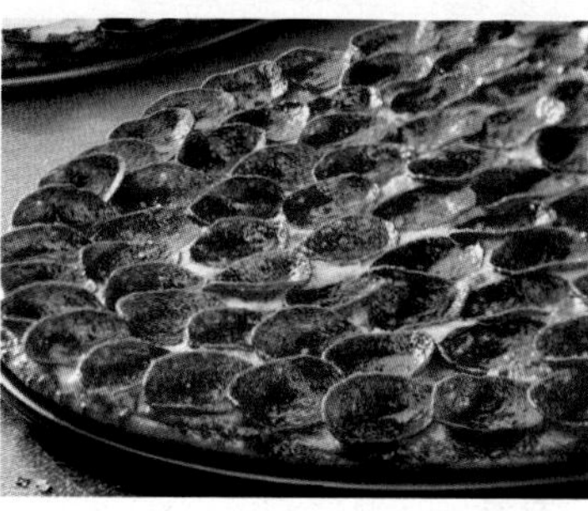

| ▲ Power Foods | *PointsPlus*™ value |
|---|---|
| **LARGE THIN CRUST PIZZA** | |
| **BBQ Chicken,** 1/8 of the large pizza | 8 |
| **Fresh Mozzarella Meatball,** 1/4 pizza or 1 individual size pizza | 19 |
| **Pepperoni Zinger, Thin Crust,** 1/8 of the large pizza | 9 |
| **OVEN-BAKED SUBS** | |
| **Big Don Italian - Wheat Roll,** 1 sub | 19 |
| **Big Don Italian - White Roll,** 1 sub | 19 |
| **Big Don Sausage Italian - Wheat Roll,** 1 sub | 26 |
| **Big Don Sausage Italian - White Roll,** 1 sub | 26 |
| **Big Don Sausage with Pizza Sauce - Wheat Roll,** 1 sub | 24 |
| **Big Don Sausage with Pizza Sauce - White Roll,** 1 sub | 25 |
| **Big Don with Pizza Sauce - Wheat Roll,** 1 sub | 17 |
| **Big Don with Pizza Sauce - White Roll,** 1 sub | 17 |
| **Big Ham and Cheese - Wheat Roll,** 1 sub | 16 |
| **Big Ham and Cheese Sub - White Roll,** 1 sub | 16 |

*Oven-Baked Subs (cont'd)*

| ▲ Power Foods | ***PointsPlus***™ value |
|---|---|
| **Big Steak Hoagie with Mushroom Gravy - Wheat Roll (select markets only),** 1 sub | 21 |
| **Big Steak Hoagie with Mushroom Gravy - White Roll,** 1 sub | 21 |
| **Big Steak Hoagie with Pizza Sauce - Wheat Roll (select markets only),** 1 sub | 21 |
| **Big Steak Hoagie with Pizza Sauce - White Roll,** 1 sub | 21 |
| **Chicken Bacon Cheddar - Wheat Roll,** 1 sub | 21 |
| **Chicken Bacon Cheddar - White Roll,** 1 sub | 21 |
| **Fresh Vegy - Wheat Roll,** 1 sub | 14 |
| **Fresh Vegy - White Roll,** 1 sub | 14 |
| **Meatball - Wheat Roll,** 1 sub | 30 |
| **Meatball on White Roll,** 1 sub | 30 |
| **Roast Beef & Provolone - Wheat Roll,** 1 sub | 21 |
| **Roast Beef & Provolone - White Roll,** 1 sub | 21 |
| **Turkey Club - Wheat Roll,** 1 sub | 19 |
| **Turkey Club - White Roll,** 1 sub | 19 |

## SALADS (WITHOUT DRESSING)

| | |
|---|---|
| **Chicken Harvest Salad (entrée),** 1 | 11 |
| **Harvest Salad (side),** 1 | 2 |
| **Italian Chef Salad (entrée),** 1 | 7 |
| **Italian Salad (side),** 1 | 3 |

## STROMBOLI

| | |
|---|---|
| **3 Meat,** 1/2 | 9 |
| **Deluxe,** 1/2 | 8 |
| **Pepperoni,** 1/2 | 9 |
| **Vegy,** 1/2 | 8 |

| ▲ Power Foods | *PointsPlus*™ value |
|---|---|
| **DONUTS** | |
| **Boston Kreme Donut,** 1 | 7 |
| **Chocolate Frosted Donut,** 1 | 6 |
| **Chocolate Glazed Cake Donut,** 1 | 8 |
| **French Cruller,** 1 | 7 |
| **Glazed Donut,** 1 | 6 |
| **Jelly Filled Donut,** 1 | 7 |
| **Old Fashioned Cake Donut,** 1 | 8 |
| **MUNCHKINS** | |
| **Glazed Cake Munchkin,** 1 | 2 |
| **Glazed Chocolate Cake Munchkin,** 1 | 2 |
| **Jelly Filled Munchkin,** 1 | 2 |
| **MUFFINS** | |
| **Blueberry Muffin,** 1 | 14 |
| **Coffee Cake Muffin,** 1 | 17 |
| **English Muffin,** 1 | 4 |
| **Reduced Fat Blueberry Muffin,** 1 | 12 |
| **FANCIES** | |
| **Coffee Roll,** 1 | 11 |
| **OVEN TOASTED BREAKFAST SANDWICHES** | |
| **Egg & Cheese on English Muffin,** 1 | 8 |
| **Egg & Cheese Wake Up Wrap,** 1 wrap | 5 |
| **Egg White & Cheese Wake Up Wrap,** 1 wrap | 4 |
| **Ham, Egg & Cheese on English Muffin,** 1 | 9 |
| **Sausage, Egg & Cheese on English Muffin,** 1 | 13 |

| ▲ Power Foods | *PointsPlus*™ value |
|---|---|
| **OVEN TOASTED FLATBREAD SANDWICHES** | |
| **Egg White Turkey Sausage Flatbread Sandwich,** 1 | 7 |
| **Egg White Veggie Flatbread Sandwich,** 1 | 7 |
| **Grilled Cheese Flatbread,** 1 | 12 |
| **Turkey Cheddar & Bacon Flatbread,** 1 | 11 |
| **OTHER OVEN TOASTED ITEMS** | |
| **Hash Browns,** 9 pieces | 5 |
| **BAGELS** | |
| **Cinnamon Raisin Bagel,** 1 | 9 |
| **Multigrain Bagel,** 1 | 10 |
| **Plain Bagel,** 1 | 10 |
| **CREAM CHEESES** | |
| **Plain Cream Cheese,** 1 serving | 4 |
| **Reduced Fat Blueberry Cream Cheese,** 1 serving | 4 |
| **Reduced Fat Cream Cheese,** 1 serving | 3 |
| **Reduced Fat Strawberry Cream Cheese,** 1 serving | 4 |

*Cream Cheeses (cont'd)*

| ▲ Power Foods | *PointsPlus™* value |
|---|---|
| **Reduced Fat Veggie Cream Cheese,** 1 serving | 3 |

## COFFEE

| | |
|---|---|
| **Coffee,** 1 small | 0 |
| **Coffee with Milk,** 1 small | 1 |
| ▲ **Coffee with Skim Milk,** 1 small | 1 |
| **Iced Coffee,** 1 small | 0 |
| **Iced Coffee with Cream,** 1 small | 2 |
| **Iced Coffee with Milk,** 1 small | 1 |
| ▲ **Iced Coffee with Skim Milk,** 1 small | 1 |

## COOLATTA®

| | |
|---|---|
| **Coffee Coolatta® with Cream,** 1 small | 9 |
| **Coffee Coolatta® with Milk,** 1 small | 5 |
| **Coffee Coolatta® with Skim Milk,** 1 small | 4 |
| **Strawberry Fruit Coolatta®,** 1 small | 8 |
| **Tropicana Orange Coolatta®,** 1 small | 6 |

## FLAVORED COFFEE

| | |
|---|---|
| **Blueberry Coffee,** 1 small | 0 |
| **Caramel Coffee,** 1 small | 0 |
| **Cinnamon Coffee,** 1 small | 0 |
| **Coconut Coffee,** 1 small | 0 |
| **French Vanilla Coffee,** 1 small | 0 |
| **Hazelnut Coffee,** 1 small | 0 |
| **Raspberry Coffee,** 1 small | 0 |
| **Toasted Almond Coffee,** 1 small | 0 |

## HOT ESPRESSO DRINKS

| ▲ Power Foods | *PointsPlus™* value |
|---|---|
| **Cappuccino Small,** 10 fl oz | 2 |
| **Caramel Swirl Latte,** 1 small | 6 |
| **Caramel Swirl Latte with Skim Milk,** 1 small | 5 |
| **Espresso,** 2 oz | 0 |
| **Latte,** 1 small | 3 |
| ▲ **Latte Lite,** 1 small | 2 |
| **Mocha Swirl Latte,** 1 small | 6 |
| **Mocha Swirl Latte with Skim Milk,** 1 small serving | 5 |
| **Turbo Hot™,** 1 small | 4 |

## ICED ESPRESSO DRINKS

| | |
|---|---|
| **Iced Caramel Swirl Latte,** 1 small | 6 |
| **Iced Caramel Swirl Latte with Skim Milk,** 1 small | 5 |
| **Iced Latte,** 1 small | 3 |
| ▲ **Iced Latte Lite,** 1 small | 2 |
| ▲ **Iced Latte with Skim Milk,** 1 small | 2 |
| **Iced Mocha Swirl Latte,** 1 small | 6 |
| **Iced Mocha Swirl Latte with Skim Milk,** 1 small | 5 |
| **Turbo Ice™,** 1 small | 4 |

## TEA

| | |
|---|---|
| **Decaffeinated Tea,** 10 fl oz | 0 |
| **Freshly Brewed Plain Iced Tea,** 16 fl oz | 0 |
| **Freshly Brewed Sweetened Iced Tea,** 16 fl oz | 2 |
| **Freshly Brewed Unsweetened Tea,** 10 fl oz | 0 |
| **Green Tea,** 10 fl oz | 0 |
| **Peach Flavored Iced Tea,** 16 fl oz | 0 |
| **Peach Flavored Sweetened Iced Tea,** 16 fl oz | 2 |
| **Raspberry Flavored Iced Tea,** 16 fl oz | 0 |
| **Raspberry Flavored Sweetened Iced Tea,** 16 fl oz | 2 |

## OTHER BEVERAGES

| | |
|---|---|
| **Dunkaccino®,** 1 small | 7 |
| **Hot Chocolate,** 1 small | 6 |
| **White Hot Chocolate,** 1 small | 7 |

| ▲ Power Foods | PointsPlus™ value |
|---|---|
| **GET IT STARTED** | |
| **Baby Calamari,** 1 serving | 13 |
| **Caprese Flatbread,** 1 serving | 8 |
| **Chili Chicken,** 1 serving | 16 |
| **Crispy Chicken Tenders (without fries),** 1 serving | 9 |
| **Dynamite Shrimp Rolls,** 1 serving | 8 |
| **Edamame Beans,** 1 serving | 1 |
| **Flatbread Duo,** 1 serving | 16 |
| **Hummus Flatbread,** 1 serving | 8 |
| **Leroy's Crispy Dry Ribs,** 1 serving | 18 |
| **Los Cabos Chicken Tacos,** 1 serving | 7 |
| **One Pound Wings & Dip,** 1 serving | 23 |
| **One Pound Wings (without dip),** 1 serving | 17 |
| **Smoked Salmon and Tuna Roll,** 1 serving | 22 |
| **BURGERS & SANDWICHES** | |
| **Cajun Chicken Cheddar Sandwich (without fries or salad),** 1 serving | 21 |
| **Earls Bigger Better 1/2 Pound Burger (without fries or salad),** 1 serving | 20 |
| **Earls Bigger Better 1/2 Pound Burger with Cheddar & Bacon (without fries or salad),** 1 serving | 26 |
| **Earls Bigger Better 1/2 Pound Burger with Cheddar (without fries or salad),** 1 serving | 23 |
| **Earls Bigger Better 1/2 Pound Burger with Mushrooms (without fries or salad),** 1 serving | 24 |
| **Grilled Chicken and Baked Brie on Ciabatta (without fries or salad),** 1 serving | 20 |
| **Los Cabos Chicken Tacos,** 1 serving | 11 |
| **Roasted Chicken Quesadilla (without fries or salad),** 1 serving | 18 |
| **Short Rib Beef Dip,** 1 serving | 26 |
| **Tuna/Cheddar Melt,** 1 serving | 28 |

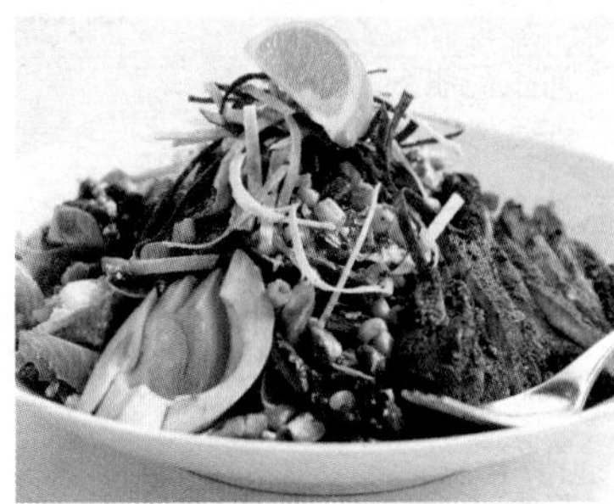

| ▲ Power Foods | PointsPlus™ value |
|---|---|
| **CHICKEN & RIBS** | |
| **Braised Hickory Back Ribs,** 1 serving | 32 |
| **Cajun Blackened Chicken,** 1 serving | 14 |
| **Ribs & Chicken Combo - Full,** 1 serving | 46 |
| **Ribs & Chicken Combo - Half,** 1 serving | 23 |
| **Roast Chicken with Dijon,** 1 serving | 12 |
| **FROM THE WATER** | |
| **Brown Sugar Mustard Salmon,** 1 serving | 12 |
| **Cajun Salmon,** 1 serving | 12 |
| **Cajun Salmon with Honeydew Pear Salsa,** 1 serving | 18 |
| **Soy Ginger Salmon,** 1 serving | 18 |
| **PASTAS** | |
| **Mediterranean Linguini with Chicken,** 1 serving | 29 |
| **Penne Alfredo (without chicken or shrimp),** 1 serving | 42 |
| **Penne Alfredo with Chicken,** 1 serving | 48 |
| **Penne Alfredo with Shrimp,** 1 serving | 47 |

Pastas (cont'd)

| ▲ Power Foods | PointsPlus™ value |
| --- | --- |
| **Prawn and Scallop Linguini,** 1 serving | 31 |

## PIZZAS

| | |
| --- | --- |
| **Margherita Pizza,** 1 serving | 20 |
| **The Californian,** 1 serving | 28 |
| **The Sicilian,** 1 serving | 29 |

## STEAKS

| | |
| --- | --- |
| **10 oz California Cut New York Striploin,** 1 serving | 11 |
| **10 oz Peppercorn California Cut New York Striploin,** 1 serving | 16 |
| **7 oz Top Sirloin,** 1 serving | 7 |

## BIG BOWLS

| | |
| --- | --- |
| **Hunan Kung Pao (without chicken or shrimp),** 1 serving | 27 |
| **Hunan Kung Pao with Chicken,** 1 serving | 31 |
| **Hunan Kung Pao with Shrimp,** 1 serving | 34 |
| **Jeera Chicken Curry (with rice and naan bread),** 1 serving | 36 |
| **Pad Thai,** 1 serving | 30 |
| **Spicy Thai Green Curry with Shrimp,** 1 serving | 30 |
| **Thai Green Curry with Chicken,** 1 serving | 41 |

## SALADS

| | |
| --- | --- |
| **Caesar Salad,** 1 serving | 16 |
| **Champagne Berry Salad,** 1 serving | 16 |
| **Market Salad,** 1 serving | 51 |
| **Organic Greens,** 1 serving | 6 |

| ▲ Power Foods | PointsPlus™ value |
| --- | --- |
| **Santa Fe Chicken Salad,** 1 serving | 24 |
| **Starter Caesar Salad (side Caesar portion),** 1 serving | 6 |
| **Warm Beet and Spinach Salad,** 1 serving | 14 |
| **West Coast Prawn Salad,** 1 serving | 24 |

## SOUPS & BREADS

| | |
| --- | --- |
| **Clam Chowder,** 1 serving | 39 |
| **Grilled Garlic Bread,** 1 serving | 16 |
| **Rosemary-Oregano Pan Bread,** 1 serving | 19 |

## ACCOMPANIMENTS

| | |
| --- | --- |
| **Coleslaw,** 1 serving | 8 |
| **Earl's 8 oz. Fries - Yukon Gold,** 1 serving | 21 |
| **Garlic Mashed Potatoes,** 1 serving | 13 |
| **Mediterranean Vegetables,** 1 serving | 3 |
| **Roast Potatoes,** 1 serving | 11 |
| **Side Ceasar Salad,** 1 serving | 6 |
| **Warm Potato Salad,** 1 serving | 12 |

## DESSERTS

| | |
| --- | --- |
| **Campfire Smores,** 1 serving | 19 |
| **Chocolate Sticky Toffee Pudding,** 1 serving | 19 |
| **Sundae - Caramel,** 1 serving | 25 |
| **Sundae - Mocha Kahlua,** 1 serving | 46 |
| **Sundae - Strawberry,** 1 serving | 20 |

▲ Power Foods — *PointsPlus™* value

## APPETIZERS

| Item | PointsPlus value |
|---|---|
| **Breaded Zucchini,** 1 serving | 11 |
| **Cheese Sticks,** 1 serving | 11 |
| **Chicken Quesadilla,** 1 serving | 24 |
| **Onion Rings,** 1 serving | 6 |

## SALADS/DRESSINGS

| Item | PointsPlus value |
|---|---|
| **Buffalo Chicken Salad,** 1 serving | 18 |
| **Chicken & Strawberry Salad,** 1 serving | 5 |
| **Chicken and Spinach Salad,** 1 serving | 9 |
| **Chicken Portabella Salad,** 1 serving | 8 |
| **Fruit Salad with Sherbet,** 1 serving | 8 |
| **Garden Salad,** 1 serving | 3 |
| **Grilled Chicken Salad,** 1 serving | 11 |
| **Bleu Cheese Dressing,** 2 Tbsp | 3 |
| **Caesar Dressing,** 2 Tbsp | 7 |
| **French Fat Free Dressing,** 2 Tbsp | 2 |
| **Fruit Salad Dressing,** 2 Tbsp | 4 |
| **House Salad Dressing,** 2 Tbsp | 3 |
| **Italian Dressing,** 2 Tbsp | 4 |
| **Italian Fat Free Dressing,** 2 Tbsp | 0 |
| **Poppyseed Dressing,** 2 Tbsp | 7 |
| **Thousand Island Dressing,** 2 Tbsp | 3 |

## BURGERS

| Item | PointsPlus value |
|---|---|
| **Black Angus American Grill Burger,** 1 | 16 |
| **Black Angus Bacon Cheddar Burger,** 1 | 24 |
| **Black Angus Bacon Cheeseburger,** 1 | 15 |
| **Black Angus Cheeseburger,** 1 | 13 |
| **Black Angus Hamburger,** 1 | 12 |
| **Black Angus Mushroom & Onion Burger,** 1 | 19 |

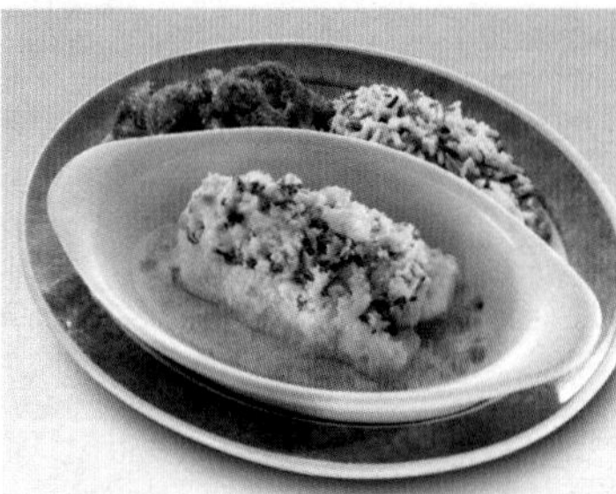

▲ Power Foods — *PointsPlus™* value

| Item | PointsPlus value |
|---|---|
| **Black Angus Superburger,** 1 | 29 |
| **Classic Gardenburger,** 1 | 9 |
| **Original Superburger®,** 1 | 19 |

## BREAKFAST

| Item | PointsPlus value |
|---|---|
| **Bacon,** 1 slice | 1 |
| **Banana's Foster French Toast,** 1 serving | 16 |
| **Cereal (with milk),** 1 serving | 10 |
| **Egg (fried),** 1 | 3 |
| ▲ **Egg (poached),** 1 | 2 |
| ▲ **Egg Beaters®,** 1 serving | 2 |
| **French Toast,** 1 slice | 3 |
| **Fruit Cup,** 1 | 2 |
| **Ham,** 1 serving | 3 |
| **Hash Browns,** 1 serving | 6 |
| **Homefries,** 1 serving | 6 |
| ▲ **Oatmeal (plain),** 1 serving | 4 |
| **Oatmeal (with milk),** 1 serving | 6 |
| **Omelette (bacon & cheese),** 1 serving | 13 |
| **Omelette (cheese),** 1 serving | 10 |
| **Omelette (ham & cheese),** 1 serving | 12 |
| **Omelette (meat lovers),** 1 serving | 19 |
| **Omelette (supreme),** 1 serving | 11 |
| **Omelette (western),** 1 serving | 9 |

*Breakfast (cont'd)*

| ▲ Power Foods | *PointsPlus™* value |
|---|---|
| **Pancake,** 1 | 6 |
| **Pancake (blueberry),** 1 | 7 |
| **Sausage,** 1 | 4 |
| **Toast (buttered),** 1 serving | 7 |
| **Waffles (Belgian),** 1 serving | 17 |

## BREADS

| ▲ Power Foods | *PointsPlus™* value |
|---|---|
| **Bagel (plain),** 1 | 8 |
| **Bun (hoagie),** 1 | 5 |
| **Bun (hot dog),** 1 | 3 |
| **Bun (superburger),** 1 | 5 |
| **Bun (three cheese hoagie),** 1 | 13 |
| **English Muffin,** 1 | 3 |
| **Italian Bread,** 1 slice | 1 |
| **Roll (kaiser),** 1 | 5 |
| **Rye,** 1 serving | 2 |
| **SnoTop,** 1 | 3 |
| **Sourdough,** 1 serving | 2 |
| **Sticky Loaf,** 2 | 8 |
| **Toast (dry),** 1 serving | 3 |
| **Toast (raisin, buttered),** 1 serving | 7 |
| **Toast (rye, buttered),** 1 serving | 7 |
| **Toast (sourdough, buttered),** 1 serving | 6 |
| **Toast (whole wheat, buttered),** 1 serving | 7 |
| **White Bread,** 1 serving | 2 |
| **Whole Wheat Bread,** 1 serving | 2 |
| **Yellow Bread,** 1 serving | 3 |

## DINNERS

| ▲ Power Foods | *PointsPlus™* value |
|---|---|
| **Baked Lemon Sole,** 1 serving | 7 |
| **Chargrilled Chicken,** 2 breasts | 4 |
| **Chicken Fillets,** 5 | 14 |
| **Chicken Parmesan Marinara,** 1 serving | 22 |
| **Chicken Stir-Fry,** 1 serving | 13 |
| **Fish (breaded),** 2 fillets | 24 |
| **Ground Sirloin,** 1 serving | 11 |
| ▲ **Liver,** 1 serving | 7 |
| ▲ **Nantucket Cod,** 1 serving | 8 |
| **Pork Chops (sesame),** 2 chops | 8 |
| **Rosemary Chicken,** 2 breasts | 9 |
| ▲ **Salmon (Alaskan sockeye),** 1 serving | 7 |
| **Scrod (baked),** 2 fillets | 11 |
| ▲ **Scrod (Floridian),** 1 regular serving | 3 |
| **Spaghetti (marinara),** 1 serving | 16 |
| **T-Bone,** 1 serving | 15 |

## SMALLER PORTIONS

| ▲ Power Foods | *PointsPlus™* value |
|---|---|
| **Baked Scrod (Floridian),** 1 fillet | 3 |
| **Banana's Foster French Toast,** 1 serving | 13 |
| **Chargrilled Chicken,** 1 breast | 4 |
| **Chicken Fillet,** 4 pieces | 11 |
| **Fish (breaded),** 1 fillet | 12 |
| **French Toast,** 2 pieces | 12 |
| **Hot Turkey Sandwich,** 1 serving | 4 |
| **Pork Chop (sesame),** 1 chop | 4 |
| **Pot Roast Sandwich,** 1 serving | 7 |
| **Rosemary Chicken,** 1 breast | 5 |
| **Scrod (baked),** 1 fillet | 9 |
| **Spaghetti (marinara),** 1 serving | 8 |
| **Spaghetti (meat sauce),** 1 serving | 11 |

## SANDWICHES

| ▲ Power Foods | *PointsPlus™* value |
|---|---|
| **BLT,** 1 | 8 |
| **Buffalo Chicken Sandwich,** 1 | 21 |
| **Chicken (chargrilled),** 1 | 9 |
| **Chicken Portabella Hoaggie,** 1 | 23 |
| **Grilled Cheese,** 1 | 14 |
| **Hot Turkey,** 1 | 6 |
| **Reuben,** 1 | 19 |

| ▲ Power Foods | *PointsPlus*™ value |
|---|---|
| **Santa Fe Turkey and Bacon,** 1 | 23 |
| **Shredded Pot Roast,** 1 | 14 |
| **Steak'n Cheese,** 1 | 27 |
| **Turkey Club,** 1 | 20 |
| **Whale of a Cod Sandwich,** 1 | 23 |

## SIDES

| ▲ Power Foods | *PointsPlus*™ value |
|---|---|
| **Applesauce,** 1 serving | 3 |
| ▲ **Banana,** 1 large | 0 |
| ▲ **Banana,** 1 medium | 0 |
| **Broccoli Soup,** 1 cup | 6 |
| **Broccoli Soup,** 1 bowl | 11 |
| **Buttered Noodles,** 1 serving | 7 |
| **Chicken Noodle Soup,** 1 cup | 3 |
| **Chicken Noodle Soup,** 1 bowl | 7 |
| **Chili,** 1 cup | 3 |
| **Chili,** 1 bowl | 5 |
| **Clam Chowder,** 1 cup | 4 |
| **Clam Chowder,** 1 bowl | 9 |
| **Coleslaw,** 1 serving | 6 |
| ▲ **Cottage Cheese,** 1 serving | 3 |
| **French Fries,** 1 serving | 9 |
| **Gravy (beef),** 1 serving | 1 |
| **Gravy (turkey),** 1 serving | 1 |
| **Macaroni & Cheese,** 1 serving | 7 |
| **Onion Rings,** 10 | 3 |
| ▲ **Potato (baked),** 1 | 5 |
| **Potato (scalloped),** 1 serving | 6 |
| **Potato (whipped),** 1 serving | 8 |
| **Potato Soup,** 1 cup | 6 |
| **Potato Soup,** 1 bowl | 9 |
| **Rice (Mexican),** 1 serving | 3 |
| **Rice (white),** 1 serving | 4 |
| **Rice Pilaf,** 1 serving | 4 |
| **Rice Pudding,** 1 serving | 4 |
| ▲ **Strawberries (fresh cup),** 1 cup | 0 |
| ▲ **Sugar Snap Peas,** 1 serving | 0 |
| **Wedding Soup,** 1 cup | 3 |
| **Wedding Soup,** 1 bowl | 5 |

## BAKERY

| ▲ Power Foods | *PointsPlus*™ value |
|---|---|
| **Bear Claw,** 1 | 14 |
| **Biscuit,** 1 | 6 |
| **Biscuit (cheese),** 1 | 3 |
| **Cookie (Christmas),** 1 | 7 |
| **Cookie (Easter),** 1 | 7 |
| **Cookie (Halloween),** 1 | 7 |
| **Cookie (shamrock),** 1 | 7 |
| **Cookie (smiley),** 1 | 7 |
| **Cookie (steeler/penguin/pirate),** 1 | 7 |
| **Cookie (valentine),** 1 | 7 |
| **Cornbread,** 1 serving | 3 |
| **Crumby Buns,** 1 | 5 |
| **Garlic Toast,** 1 serving | 12 |
| **Honey Bun,** 1 | 5 |
| **Muffin (apple raisin),** 1 | 7 |
| **Muffin (banana nut),** 1 | 8 |
| **Muffin (blueberry),** 1 | 7 |
| **Muffin (chocolate nut),** 1 | 9 |
| **Muffin (corn),** 1 | 6 |
| **Muffin (cranberry),** 1 | 7 |
| **Muffin (oatbran apple raisin),** 1 | 8 |
| **Muffin (oatbran),** 1 | 9 |
| **Muffin (strawberry creme),** 1 | 7 |
| **Muffin (strawberry filled),** 1 | 8 |
| **Pastry Bite,** 1 | 3 |
| **Raisin Bread,** 1 serving | 2 |

## DESSERTS

| ▲ Power Foods | *PointsPlus*™ value |
|---|---|
| **Cheesecake,** 1 slice | 14 |
| **Cheesecake (with strawberries),** 1 slice | 21 |
| **Grilled Stickies a La Mode (loaf),** 1 serving | 13 |
| **Ice Cream,** 2 scoops | 8 |
| **Pie (apple cranberry),** 1 slice | 18 |

Desserts (cont'd)

| ▲ Power Foods | *PointsPlus™* value |
|---|---|
| **Pie (apple),** 1 slice | 13 |
| **Pie (banana crème),** 1 slice | 12 |
| **Pie (blackberry),** 1 slice | 14 |
| **Pie (blueberry),** 1 slice | 12 |
| **Pie (cherry),** 1 slice | 13 |
| **Pie (coconut crème),** 1 slice | 13 |
| **Pie (lemon meringue),** 1 slice | 7 |
| **Pie (oreo cream),** 1 slice | 14 |
| **Pie (peachberry),** 1 slice | 11 |
| **Pie (pumpkin),** 1 slice | 11 |
| **Pie (strawberry),** 1 slice | 10 |
| **Sherbet (plain),** 1 serving | 3 |
| **Sundae (chocolate),** 1 serving | 15 |
| **Sundae (chocolate),** 1 junior | 8 |
| **Sundae (hot fudge),** 1 serving | 18 |
| **Sundae (hot fudge),** 1 junior | 10 |
| **Sundae (strawberry),** 1 serving | 17 |

## CHILDREN'S

| ▲ Power Foods | *PointsPlus™* value |
|---|---|
| **Cheeseburger,** 1 | 10 |
| **Fish Plank,** 1 serving | 8 |
| **French Toast (bacon),** 1 serving | 9 |
| **French Toast (sausage),** 1 serving | 15 |
| **Giggle (bacon),** 1 serving | 10 |
| **Giggle (sausage),** 1 serving | 16 |
| **Grilled Cheese,** 1 | 14 |
| **Hot Dog,** 1 | 10 |
| **Macaroni & Cheese,** 1 serving | 4 |
| **Pizza,** 1 slice | 11 |
| **Spaghetti,** 1 serving | 9 |

## CONDIMENTS

| ▲ Power Foods | *PointsPlus™* value |
|---|---|
| **BBQ Sauce,** 1 serving | 2 |
| **Cheese Sauce,** 1 serving | 4 |
| **Chipotle BBQ Sauce,** 1 serving | 5 |
| **Cocktail Sauce,** 1 serving | 2 |
| **Lite Soy Sauce,** 1 serving | 0 |
| **Reduced Maple Syrup,** 1 serving | 1 |
| **Sour Cream,** 1 serving | 1 |
| **Sugar-Free Syrup,** 1 serving | 1 |
| **Supreme Sauce,** 1 serving | 4 |
| **Sweet'n Sour Sauce,** 1 serving | 2 |
| **Teriyaki Sauce,** 2 Tbsp | 0 |

## BEVERAGES

| ▲ Power Foods | *PointsPlus™* value |
|---|---|
| **Cappuccino,** 1 small | 3 |
| **Cappuccino,** 1 medium | 5 |
| **Cappuccino,** 1 grande | 6 |
| **Chai,** 1 small | 3 |
| **Chai,** 1 grande | 5 |
| **Chai, Iced,** 1 serving | 2 |
| **Latte,** 1 small | 5 |
| **Latte,** 1 medium | 6 |
| **Latte,** 1 grande | 8 |
| **Latte, Iced,** 1 serving | 5 |
| **Milkshake (Chai Tea),** 1 | 16 |
| **Milkshake (Mocha Java),** 1 | 18 |
| **Milkshake (Vanilla Latte),** 1 | 18 |

# EL POLLO LOCO

| ▲ Power Foods | *PointsPlus*™ value |
|---|---|
| **HEALTHLY DINING** | |
| **BRC Burrito,** 1 | 11 |
| **Caesar Pollo Salad without Dressing,** 1 | 5 |
| ▲ **Chicken Breast, Skinless,** 1 serving | 4 |
| **Chicken Tortilla Soup,** 1 serving | 6 |
| **Chicken Tortilla Soup (no tortilla strips),** 1 serving | 4 |
| **Chicken Tostada without Shell,** 1 | 10 |
| ▲ **Fresh Vegetables (without margarine),** 1 serving | 1 |
| **Garden Salad (without tortilla strips),** 1 | 2 |
| **Original Pollo Bowl®,** 1 | 13 |
| ▲ **Pinto Beans,** 1 serving | 3 |
| ▲ **Skinless Breast Meal (no tortilla strips on salad),** 1 serving | 7 |
| ▲ **Skinless Breast Meal Special Request,** 1 serving | 7 |
| **Spanish Rice,** 1 serving | 4 |
| **Taco al Carbon,** 1 | 4 |
| **FLAME-GRILLED CHICKEN** | |
| ▲ **Chicken Breast, Skinless,** 1 serving | 4 |
| ▲ **Chopped Breast Meat,** 1 serving | 2 |
| **Leg,** 1 serving | 2 |
| **Thigh,** 1 serving | 6 |
| **Wing,** 1 serving | 2 |
| **BOWLS & SALADS** | |
| **Caesar Bowl,** 1 | 14 |
| **Caesar Pollo Salad,** 1 | 14 |
| **Caesar Pollo Salad without Dressing,** 1 | 5 |
| **Chicken Ceasar Bowl,** 1 serving | 13 |

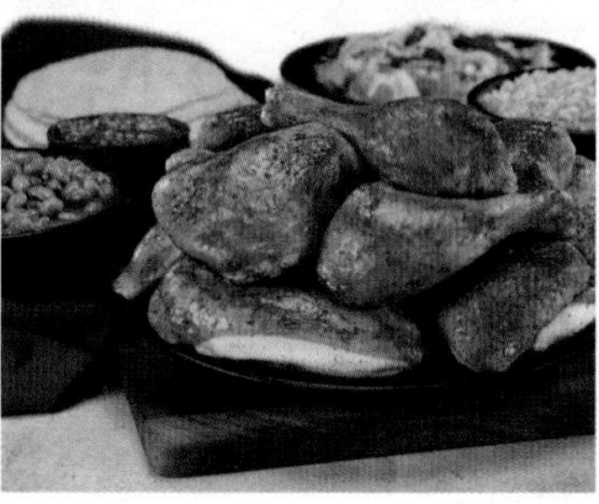

| ▲ Power Foods | *PointsPlus*™ value |
|---|---|
| **Chicken Ceasar Salad (no dressing),** 1 serving | 6 |
| **Chicken Tostada Salad (no dressing),** 1 serving | 22 |
| **Chicken Tostada Salad (no dressing, no shell),** 1 serving | 10 |
| **Garden Salad,** 1 | 3 |
| **Loco Salad with Creamy Cilantro Dressing,** 1 | 5 |
| **Original Pollo Bowl®,** 1 | 13 |
| **Small Garden Salad (no dressing),** 1 serving | 2 |
| **Small Garden Salad (no dressing, no tortilla strips),** 1 serving | 1 |
| **Ultimate Pollo Bowl,** 1 | 22 |
| **DRESSINGS** | |
| **Creamy Cilantro,** 1 serving | 6 |
| **Light Italian,** 1 serving | 0 |
| **Lite Creamy Cilantro Dressing,** 1 serving | 2 |
| **Ranch,** 1 serving | 6 |
| **Thousand Island,** 1 serving | 6 |

# EL POLLO LOCO

| ▲ Power Foods | *PointsPlus™* value |
| --- | --- |
| **BURRITOS** | |
| **BRC Burrito,** 1 | 11 |
| **Classic Chicken Burrito®,** 1 | 14 |
| **Pollo Asada Burrito,** 1 | 16 |
| **Twice Grilled Burrito®,** 1 | 22 |
| **Ultimate Grilled Burrito®,** 1 | 17 |
| **MEXICAN FAVORITES** | |
| **Chicken Soft Taco,** 1 | 6 |
| **Chicken Tortilla Soup,** 1 serving | 6 |
| **Chicken Verde Quesadilla,** 1 | 16 |
| **Crunchy Chicken Taco,** 1 | 5 |
| **Grilled Chicken Nachos,** 1 serving | 21 |
| **Grilled Chicken Tortilla Rolls,** 1 | 10 |
| **TACO COMBOS (INCLUDES CHIPS & BEANS)** | |
| **6.5" Flour Tortilla,** 2 | 5 |
| **6" Corn Tortilla,** 2 | 3 |
| **Tortilla Chips,** 1 serving | 6 |
| **LOCAL FAVORITES VALUE MEALS** | |
| **BRC Burrito,** 1 | 10 |
| **Cheese Quesadilla,** 1 | 11 |
| **Chicken Taquito,** 1 | 5 |
| **Loco Nachos,** 1 serving | 8 |
| **Loco Salad with Creamy Cilantro Dressing,** 1 | 5 |
| **Taco al Carbon,** 1 | 4 |
| **Two Churros,** 1 serving | 8 |
| **SIDES (SMALL)** | |
| **BBQ Black Beans,** 1 | 5 |
| **Cole Slaw,** 1 serving | 3 |
| ▲ **Corn Cobbette,** 1 | 2 |
| **French Fries,** 1 kids serving | 6 |
| **Fresh Vegetables (with margarine),** 1 serving | 2 |
| ▲ **Fresh Vegetables (without margarine),** 1 serving | 1 |
| **Garden Salad,** 1 | 3 |
| **Macaroni and Cheese,** 1 serving | 8 |
| **Mashed Potatoes,** 1 serving | 3 |
| ▲ **Pinto Beans,** 1 serving | 5 |
| **Refried Beans (with cheese),** 1 | 6 |
| **Spanish Rice,** 1 serving | 6 |
| **SALSAS & MORE** | |
| **Avocado Salsa (hot),** 1 serving | 1 |
| ▲ **Chipotle Salsa (hot),** 1 serving | 0 |
| **Fried Serrano Pepper,** 1 serving | 1 |
| **Guacamole,** 1 serving | 1 |
| ▲ **House Salsa (mild),** 1 serving | 0 |
| **Jack & Poblano Queso,** 1 serving | 3 |
| **Jalapeño Hot Sauce,** 1 packet | 0 |
| **Ketchup,** 1 packet | 0 |
| ▲ **Pico de Gallo Salsa (medium),** 1 serving | 0 |
| **Sour Cream,** 1 serving | 1 |
| **KIDS MEAL** | |
| **Cheese Quesadilla,** 1 | 11 |
| **French Fries,** 1 kids serving | 6 |
| **Leg,** 1 serving | 2 |
| **Popcorn Chicken,** 1 serving | 5 |
| **BBQ Sauce,** 1 serving | 1 |
| **DESSERTS** | |
| **Caramel Flan,** 1 serving | 7 |
| **Vanilla Kid Cone,** 1 cone | 5 |
| **Vanilla Large Cone,** 1 cone | 13 |
| **Vanilla Regular Cone,** 1 cone | 9 |
| **Vanilla Soft Serve,** 1 cup | 8 |

| ▲ Power Foods | *PointsPlus*™ value |
|---|---|
| **HELP ME LOSE WEIGHT** | |
| **Low Carb,** 1 | 8 |
| **Power Fuel,** 1 | 11 |
| **Slim N Fit,** 1 | 9 |
| **Zone Zinger,** 1 | 11 |
| **LOW SUGAR** | |
| **Fruity Supreme,** 1 | 7 |
| **Island Breeze,** 1 | 6 |
| **Pacific Splash,** 1 | 6 |
| **Zip Zip,** 1 | 6 |
| **NO FAT** | |
| **Apple Andie,** 1 | 6 |
| **Blueberry Blast,** 1 | 9 |
| **Mango Mania,** 1 | 10 |
| **Orange Twister,** 1 | 3 |
| **Peach Pleasure,** 1 | 7 |
| **Pineapple Bliss,** 1 | 5 |
| **BOOST MY IMMUNE SYSTEM** | |
| **Cranberry Delight,** 1 | 15 |
| **Grape Escape,** 1 | 13 |
| **Immunity Nectar,** 1 | 10 |
| **Quick Start,** 1 | 6 |
| **Rejuvenator,** 1 | 8 |
| **Sambazon,** 1 | 12 |
| **BULK ME UP** | |
| **Mega Mass,** 1 | 16 |
| **Nutty Banana,** 1 | 19 |
| **The Builder,** 1 | 33 |
| **LAYERED SMOOTHIES** | |
| **Blueberry Layered Smoothie,** 1 | 11 |

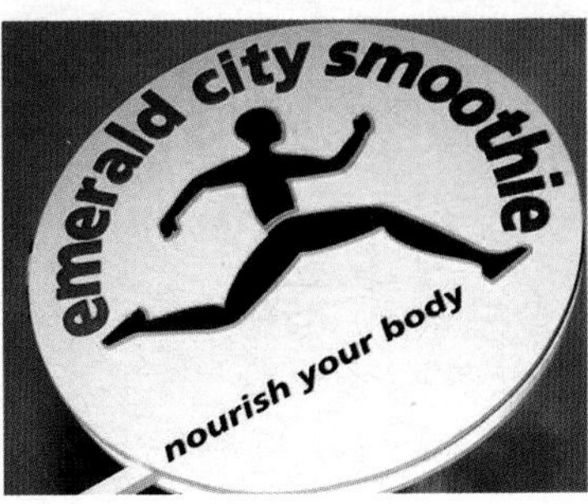


| ▲ Power Foods | *PointsPlus*™ value |
|---|---|
| **Peach Layered Smoothie,** 1 | 8 |
| **Pineapple Banana Layered Smoothie,** 1 | 9 |
| **Sambazon Layered Smoothie,** 1 | 12 |
| **Strawberry Orange Layered Smoothie,** 1 | 11 |
| **MRP** | |
| **Lean Body,** 1 | 8 |
| **Lean-Out,** 1 | 15 |
| **Mini Mass,** 1 | 13 |
| **TREAT MY BODY** | |
| **Berry Berry,** 1 | 8 |
| **Coconut Passion,** 1 | 16 |
| **Energizer,** 1 | 8 |
| **Guava Sunrise,** 1 | 11 |
| **Kiwi Kic,** 1 | 11 |
| **Marionberry Fuel,** 1 | 9 |
| **Mocha Bliss,** 1 | 14 |
| **PB&J,** 1 | 16 |
| **Peanut Passion,** 1 | 14 |
| **Raspberry Dream,** 1 | 10 |
| **Topical Paradise,** 1 | 12 |
| **Zesty Lemon,** 1 | 11 |

# FAMOUS DAVE'S

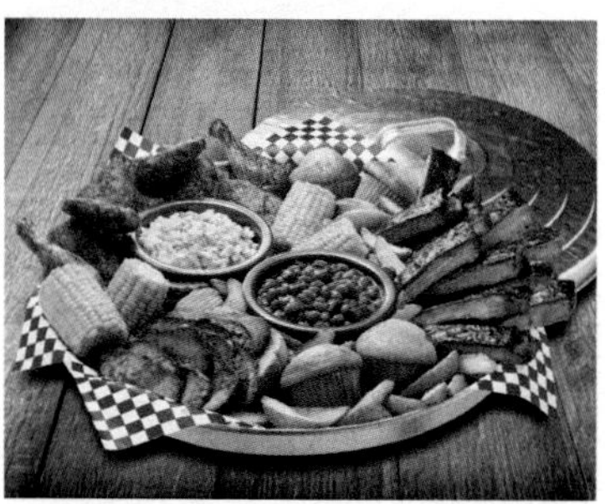

| ▲ Power Foods | *PointsPlus™* value |
|---|---|
| **APPETIZERS** | |
| **BBQ Chicken Wings,** 12 pieces | 29 |
| **BBQ Chicken Wings,** 24 pieces | 58 |
| **Buffalo Chicken Wings,** 12 pieces | 29 |
| **Buffalo Chicken Wings,** 24 pieces | 59 |
| **Chicken Tenders with Sweet Soul Jalapeno Sauce,** 1 order | 21 |
| **Onion Strings Served with Remoulade Sauce,** 1 order | 48 |
| **Rib Tips Served on a Bed of Famous Fries,** 1 order | 54 |
| **Sampler Platter,** 1 order | 69 |
| **Smoked Salmon Spread Served with Fire-Grilled Flatbread,** 1 order | 31 |
| **Sweetwater Catfish Fingers with Remoulade & Sweet Soul Jalapeno Sauces,** 1 order | 22 |
| **AWARD WINNING ST. LOUIS RIBS** (NOT INCLUDING CORNBREAD, MUFFIN, CORN-ON-THE-COB OR SIDE DISHES) | |
| **Half-Slab,** 1 order (6 ribs) | 18 |
| **Regular Ribs,** 4 ribs | 12 |
| **St. Louis Style - The Big Slab,** 1 order (12 ribs) | 37 |

| ▲ Power Foods | *PointsPlus™* value |
|---|---|
| **BARBEQUE CLASSICS** (NOT INCLUDING CORNBREAD, MUFFIN, CORN-ON-THE-COB OR SIDE DISHES) | |
| **Barbeque Chicken,** 1 order | 23 |
| **BBQ Chicken Wings,** 1 order | 29 |
| **Buffalo Chicken Wings with Blue Cheese Dipping Sauce,** 1 order | 29 |
| **Chicken Tenders with Sweet Soul Jalapeno Sauce,** 1 order | 26 |
| **Country Roasted Chicken,** 1 order | 22 |
| **Georgia Chopped Pork,** 1 order | 17 |
| **Hot Link Sausage,** 1 order | 38 |
| **Rib Tips,** 1 order | 48 |
| **Texas Beef Brisket,** 1 order | 22 |
| **BBQ COMBOS** (NOT INCLUDING CORNBREAD, MUFFIN, CORN-ON-THE-COB OR SIDE DISHES) | |
| **St. Louis Rib n' Meat BBQ Combo with BBQ Chicken,** 1 order | 29 |
| **St. Louis Rib n' Meat BBQ Combo with BBQ Chicken Wings,** 1 order | 33 |
| **St. Louis Rib n' Meat BBQ Combo with Beef Brisket,** 1 order | 25 |
| **St. Louis Rib n' Meat BBQ Combo with Buffalo Chicken Wings,** 1 order | 33 |
| **St. Louis Rib n' Meat BBQ Combo with Chicken Tenders,** 1 order | 30 |
| **St. Louis Rib n' Meat BBQ Combo with Chopped Pork,** 1 order | 22 |
| **St. Louis Rib n' Meat BBQ Combo with Hot Link Sausage,** 1 order | 31 |
| **St. Louis Rib n' Meat BBQ Combo with Rib Tips,** 1 order | 60 |
| **St. Louis Rib n' Meat BBQ Combo with Roasted Chicken,** 1 order | 27 |
| **St. Louis Rib n' Meat BBQ Combo with Sweetwater Catfish,** 1 order | 31 |

| ▲ Power Foods | PointsPlus™ value |
|---|---|
| **Two-Meat BBQ Combo with BBQ Chicken,** 1 order | 13 |
| **Two-Meat BBQ Combo with BBQ Chicken Wings,** 1 order | 21 |
| **Two-Meat BBQ Combo with Beef Brisket,** 1 order | 13 |
| **Two-Meat BBQ Combo with Buffalo Chicken Wings,** 1 order | 21 |
| **Two-Meat BBQ Combo with Chicken Tenders,** 1 order | 18 |
| **Two-Meat BBQ Combo with Chopped Pork,** 1 order | 10 |
| **Two-Meat BBQ Combo with Hot Link Sausage,** 1 order | 19 |
| **Two-Meat BBQ Combo with Rib Tips,** 1 order | 48 |
| **Two-Meat BBQ Combo with Roasted Chicken,** 1 order | 11 |
| **Two-Meat BBQ Combo with Sweetwater Catfish,** 1 order | 19 |

## CHAR-GRILLED BURGERS

| | |
|---|---|
| **Char Grilled Cheeseburger,** 1 | 24 |
| **Dave's Favorite,** 1 | 28 |
| **Devil's Spit Burger,** 1 | 28 |
| **Ultimate BBQ Burger,** 1 | 32 |

## DAVE'S FAMOUS FISH
(NOT INCLUDING CORNBREAD, MUFFIN, CORN-ON-THE-COB OR SIDE DISHES)

| | |
|---|---|
| **Sweet & Sassy Grilled Salmon Served on a Bed of Fried Onion Strings,** 1 order | 25 |
| **Sweetwater Catfish Served with Remoulade & Sweet Soul Jalapeno Sauce,** 1 order | 26 |

| ▲ Power Foods | PointsPlus™ value |
|---|---|

## ENTRÉE SALADS

| | |
|---|---|
| **Classic Caesar Salad,** 1 | 18 |
| **Crispy Chicken Salad,** 1 | 27 |
| **Dave's Sassy BBQ Salad with BBQ Chicken,** 1 | 20 |
| **Dave's Sassy BBQ Salad with BBQ Pork,** 1 | 21 |
| **Dave's Sassy BBQ Salad with Beef,** 1 | 24 |
| **Grilled Caesar Salad Chicken,** 1 | 23 |
| **Smoked Salmon Caesar Salad,** 1 | 24 |

## LUNCH - EARLY BIRD SPECIALS
(NOT INCLUDING SIDE DISHES)

| | |
|---|---|
| **BBQ Stuffed Potato with BBQ Chicken,** 1 order | 21 |
| **BBQ Stuffed Potato with Georgia Chopped Pork,** 1 order | 22 |
| **BBQ Stuffed Potato with Texas Beef Brisket,** 1 order | 24 |
| **Combo Special - BBQ Chicken,** 1 order | 13 |
| **Combo Special - BBQ Chicken Wings,** 1 order | 22 |
| **Combo Special - Buffalo Chicken Wings,** 1 order | 22 |
| **Combo Special - Chicken Tenders,** 1 order | 14 |
| **Combo Special - Country Roasted Chicken,** 1 order | 11 |
| **Combo Special - Georgia Chopped Pork,** 1 order | 8 |
| **Combo Special - Hot Link Sausage,** 1 order | 19 |
| **Combo Special - Rib Tips,** 1 order | 26 |

*Lunch - Early Bird Specials (cont'd)*

| ▲ Power Foods | *PointsPlus™* value |
|---|---|
| **Combo Special - Sweetwater Catfish,** 1 order | 17 |
| **Combo Special - Texas Beef Brisket,** 1 order | 11 |
| **Crispy Chicken Salad,** 1 | 16 |
| **Dave's Sassy BBQ Salad with BBQ Chicken,** 1 | 12 |
| **Dave's Sassy BBQ Salad with BBQ Pork,** 1 | 12 |
| **Dave's Sassy BBQ Salad with Texas Beef Brisket,** 1 | 14 |
| **Fresh Garden Salad, without dressing,** 1 | 8 |
| **Georgia Chopped Pork,** 1 order | 10 |
| **Grilled Caesar Salad Chicken,** 1 | 13 |
| **Loaded Baked Potato,** 1 order | 18 |
| **Platter Special - Barbeque Chicken,** 1 order | 13 |
| **Platter Special - BBQ Chicken Wings,** 1 order | 22 |
| **Platter Special - Buffalo Chicken Wings,** 1 order | 22 |
| **Platter Special - Chicken Tenders,** 1 order | 18 |
| **Platter Special - Country Roasted Chicken,** 1 order | 11 |
| **Platter Special - Hot Link Sausage,** 1 order | 19 |
| **Platter Special - Rib Tips,** 1 order | 26 |
| **Platter Special - St. Louis Style Spareribs,** 1 order | 9 |
| **Platter Special - Sweetwater Catfish,** 1 order | 19 |
| **Platter Special - Texas Beef Brisket,** 1 order | 13 |
| **Real Que Sandwich - Georgia Chopped Pork,** 1 order | 13 |
| **Real Que Sandwich Special - Pulled BBQ Chicken with Jack Cheese,** 1 | 15 |
| **Side Caesar Salad,** 1 salad | 9 |
| **Smoked Salmon Caesar Salad,** 1 | 15 |

| ▲ Power Foods | *PointsPlus™* value |
|---|---|
| **REAL QUE SANDWICHES** | |
| **Barbeque Chicken Sandwich,** 1 order | 20 |
| **BBQ Buddies,** 1 order | 26 |
| **Georgia Chopped Pork Sandwich,** 1 order | 17 |
| **Texas Beef Brisket Sandwich,** 1 order | 22 |
| **Texas Manhandler,** 1 order | 23 |
| **TONGUE TICKLIN' CHICKEN SANDWICHES** | |
| **Cajun Chicken Sandwich,** 1 order | 33 |
| **Char Grilled Chicken Sandwich,** 1 order | 13 |
| **Hickory Chicken Sandwich,** 1 order | 20 |
| **TASTE TEMPTING SIDE DISHES** | |
| **Carrot & Celery Sticks with Ranch Dressing - Lil' Wilbur,** 1 side | 12 |
| **Corn Bread Muffin,** 1 muffin | 11 |
| **Corn on the Cob,** 1 | 6 |
| **Creamy Coleslaw,** 1 side | 8 |
| **Dave's Cheesy Mac & Cheese,** 1 side order | 10 |
| **Drunkin' Apples,** 1 side | 4 |
| **Famous Fries,** 1 regular | 11 |
| **Garlic Red Skin Mashed Potatoes,** 1 side | 4 |
| **Potato Salad,** 1 side | 6 |
| **Southern-Style Green Beans,** 1 side order | 8 |
| **Wilbur Beans,** 1 side | 4 |

| ▲ Power Foods | *PointsPlus*™ value |
| --- | --- |
| **SOUPS, CHILI & SALADS** | |
| **Chicken Wild Rice Soup,** 1 cup | 6 |
| **Dave's Famous Chili,** 1 cup | 10 |
| **Fresh Garden Salad (without dressing),** 1 order | 8 |
| **Side Caesar Salad,** 1 order | 9 |
| **Cup of Chili with Caesar Salad,** 1 order | 19 |
| **Cup of Chili with Garden Salad, no dressing,** 1 order | 18 |
| **Cup of Wild Rice Soup with Caesar Salad,** 1 order | 12 |
| **Cup of Wild Rice Soup with Garden Salad, no dressing,** 1 order | 14 |
| **LIL' WILBUR MEALS (DOES NOT INCLUDE SIDES)** | |
| **BBQ Chicken,** 1 order | 13 |
| **Chicken Tenders,** 1 order | 12 |
| **Country-Roasted Chicken,** 1 order | 11 |
| **Georgia Chopped Pork Sandwich,** 1 order | 11 |
| **Kid's Burger,** 1 order | 12 |
| **Kid's Cheeseburger,** 1 order | 14 |
| **Macaroni & Cheese,** 1 order | 9 |
| **Mini Corn Dogs,** 1 order | 11 |
| **Real Que Sandwich Specials - Texas Beef Brisket,** 1 order | 16 |
| **Rib Dinner,** 1 order | 6 |
| **Root Beer Float,** 1 | 6 |
| **Ice Cream Sundae,** 1 | 7 |
| **Oreo Cookies,** 1 packet | 3 |

| ▲ Power Foods | *PointsPlus*™ value |
| --- | --- |
| **SAUCES** | |
| **Devil's Spit Sauce,** 1 serving | 2 |
| **Georgia Mustard Sauce,** 1 serving | 1 |
| **Rich & Sassy Dave's Original Recipe Sauce,** 1 serving | 3 |
| **Sweet & Zesty Sauce,** 1 serving | 3 |
| **Texas Pit Sauce,** 1 serving | 2 |
| **HOMESTYLE DESSERTS** | |
| **Better Than Mom's Pecan Pie,** 1 order | 34 |
| **Dave's Famous Bread Pudding,** 1 order | 40 |
| **Famous Sundae,** 1 order | 35 |
| **Hot Fudge Kahula Brownie,** 1 order | 47 |

# FAZOLI'S® RESTAURANTS

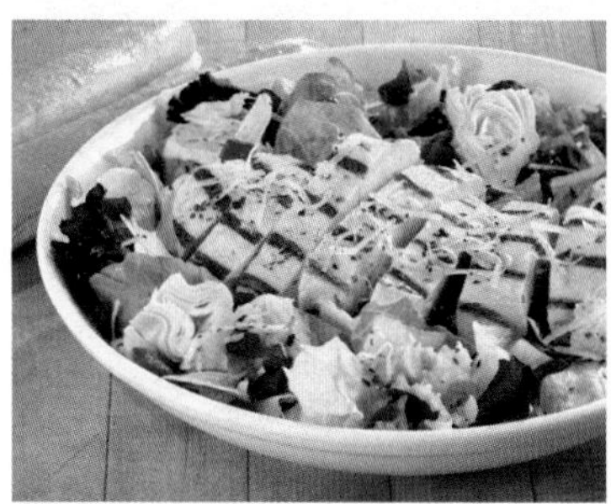

| ▲ Power Foods | PointsPlus™ value |
|---|---|

## SUBMARINOS®

| | |
|---|---|
| **Club Italiano,** 1 | 20 |
| **Fazoli's® Original,** 1 | 23 |
| **Ham and Swiss Supremo,** 1 | 18 |
| **Italian Beef Gorgonzola,** 1 | 20 |
| **Italian Four Cheese & Tomato,** 1 | 19 |
| **Roasted Red Pepper Chicken,** 1 | 20 |
| **Smoked Turkey Basil,** 1 | 20 |

## CLASSIC PASTAS

| ▲ Power Foods | PointsPlus™ value |
|---|---|
| **Classic Sampler Platter,** 1 serving | 23 |
| **Fettuccine with Alfredo - Small,** 1 serving | 16 |
| **Fettuccine with Alfredo - Regular,** 1 serving | 23 |
| **Fettuccine with Marinara - Small,** 1 serving | 11 |
| **Fettuccine with Marinara - Regular,** 1 serving | 16 |
| **Fettuccine with Meat Sauce - Small,** 1 serving | 13 |
| **Fettuccine with Meat Sauce - Regular,** 1 serving | 19 |
| **Penne with Alfredo - Small,** 1 serving | 16 |
| **Penne with Alfredo - Regular,** 1 serving | 23 |
| **Penne with Marinara - Small,** 1 serving | 11 |
| **Penne with Marinara - Regular,** 1 serving | 16 |
| **Penne with Meat Sauce - Small,** 1 serving | 13 |
| **Penne with Meat Sauce - Regular,** 1 serving | 19 |
| **Ravioli with Marinara Sauce,** 1 serving | 13 |
| **Ravioli with Meat Sauce,** 1 serving | 15 |
| **Spaghetti with Alfredo - Small,** 1 serving | 16 |
| **Spaghetti with Alfredo - Regular,** 1 serving | 23 |
| **Spaghetti with Marinara - Small,** 1 serving | 11 |
| **Spaghetti with Marinara - Regular,** 1 serving | 16 |
| **Spaghetti with Meat Sauce - Small,** 1 serving | 13 |
| **Spaghetti with Meat Sauce - Regular,** 1 serving | 19 |
| **Ultimate Sampler Platter,** 1 serving | 29 |

## OVEN BAKED PASTAS

| | |
|---|---|
| **Baked Spaghetti,** 1 serving | 16 |
| **Baked Spaghetti with Italian Sausage,** 1 serving | 25 |
| **Baked Spaghetti with Meatballs,** 1 serving | 23 |
| **Chicken Broccoli Penne Bake,** 1 serving | 23 |
| **Chicken Parmigano,** 1 serving | 26 |
| **Creamy Chicken Florentine,** 1 serving | 23 |
| **Fazoli's® Deep Dish Pasta,** 1 serving | 22 |
| **Penne with Creamy Basil Chicken,** 1 serving | 25 |
| **Rigatoni Romano,** 1 serving | 23 |
| **Tortellini Robusto,** 1 serving | 27 |
| **Twice Baked Lasagna,** 1 serving | 18 |

# FAZOLI'S® RESTAURANTS

| ▲ Power Foods | *PointsPlus*™ value |
|---|---|

## SPECIALTY PASTA

| | |
|---|---|
| **Chicken Carbonara,** 1 serving | 20 |
| **Chicken Piccata,** 1 serving | 23 |
| **Creamy Chicken Basil,** 1 serving | 23 |
| **Penne Rosa with Savory Chicken,** 1 serving | 17 |
| **Tortellini & Sun-Dried Tomato Rustico,** 1 serving | 23 |

## PASTA TOPPINGS

| | |
|---|---|
| ▲ **Broccoli,** 1 serving | 0 |
| ▲ **Broccoli and Fire-Roasted Tomatoes,** 1 serving | 0 |
| **Meatballs,** 1 serving | 6 |
| ▲ **Sliced Grilled Chicken,** 1 serving | 3 |
| **Sliced Italian Sausage,** 1 serving | 5 |

## PIZZA

| | |
|---|---|
| **Cheese Slice,** 1 slice | 7 |
| **Pepperoni Slice,** 1 slice | 8 |

## SALADS (WITHOUT DRESSING)

| | |
|---|---|
| **Antipasto Salad,** 1 serving | 7 |
| **Chicken & Pasta Caesar,** 1 serving | 11 |
| **Chicken Caprese,** 1 serving | 9 |
| **Cranberry & Walnut Chicken,** 1 serving | 9 |
| **Crispy Chicken BLT,** 1 serving | 13 |
| **Grilled Chicken Artichoke,** 1 serving | 5 |
| **Side Caesar Salad,** 1 serving | 1 |
| ▲ **Side Garden Salad,** 1 serving | 1 |
| **Side Italian Salad,** 1 serving | 2 |
| **Side Pasta Salad,** 1 side serving | 8 |

## SALAD DRESSINGS

| ▲ Power Foods | *PointsPlus*™ value |
|---|---|
| **Balsamic Dressing,** 1 serving | 5 |
| **Caesar,** 1 serving | 7 |
| **Creamy Parmesan Peppercorn Ranch,** 1 serving | 6 |
| **Croutons (Pack),** 1 package | 2 |
| **Honey French,** 1 serving | 6 |
| **Italian,** 1 serving | 4 |
| **Lemon Basil,** 1 serving | 3 |
| **Lite Ranch,** 1 serving | 3 |
| **Red Wine Vinaigrette,** 1 serving | 3 |

## BREAKSTICKS

| | |
|---|---|
| **Breadstick, Dry,** 1 serving | 3 |
| **Garlic Breadstick,** 1 serving | 4 |

## KID'S MEALS

| | |
|---|---|
| **Cheese Pizza,** 1 | 7 |
| **Fettuccini Alfredo,** 1 serving | 7 |
| **Meat Lasagna,** 1 serving | 7 |
| **Pepperoni Pizza,** 1 | 8 |
| **Ravioli with Marinara Sauce,** 1 serving | 6 |
| **Ravioli with Meat Sauce,** 1 serving | 7 |
| **Spaghetti with Marinara Sauce,** 1 serving | 5 |
| **Spaghetti with Meat Sauce,** 1 serving | 6 |
| **Spaghetti with Meatballs,** 1 serving | 8 |

## DESSERTS

| | |
|---|---|
| **Choco-Lato Mousse,** 1 serving | 17 |
| **Chocolate Chip Cannolis,** 1 serving | 5 |
| **Chocolate Chunk Cookie,** 1 | 14 |
| **Chocolate Layer Cake,** 1 serving | 20 |
| **NY Style Cheesecake with Strawberry Topping,** 1 serving | 18 |

## DRINKS

| | |
|---|---|
| **Italian Lemon Ice,** 1 regular serving | 5 |
| **Italian Lemon Ice with Strawberry,** 1 | 8 |

# FIREHOUSE SUBS

| ▲ Power Foods | *PointsPlus™* value |
|---|---|
| **MEDIUM SUBS (WITHOUT MAYONNAISE AND CHEESE)** | |
| **Chicken Salad,** 1 sandwich | 21 |
| **Club On A Sub,** 1 sandwich | 12 |
| **Corned Beef,** 1 sandwich | 12 |
| **Engine Company,** 1 sandwich | 10 |
| **Engineer,** 1 sandwich | 9 |
| **Ham,** 1 sandwich | 10 |
| **Hero,** 1 sandwich | 11 |
| **Hook & Ladder,** 1 sandwich | 11 |
| **Italian,** 1 sandwich | 14 |
| **Meatball,** 1 sandwich | 20 |
| **NY Steamer,** 1 sandwich | 10 |
| **Pastrami,** 1 sandwich | 11 |
| **Roast Beef,** 1 sandwich | 9 |
| **Sliced Deli Chicken,** 1 sandwich | 9 |
| **Smokehouse Beef & Cheddar,** 1 sandwich | 20 |
| **Steak,** 1 sandwich | 13 |
| **Tuna Salad,** 1 sandwich | 17 |
| **Turkey,** 1 sandwich | 9 |
| **Veggie,** 1 sandwich | 8 |
| **Veggie (no meat),** 1 medium | 8 |
| **LARGE SUBS (WITHOUT MAYONNAISE AND CHEESE)** | |
| **Chicken Salad,** 1 sandwich | 38 |
| **Club On A Sub,** 1 sandwich | 22 |
| **Corned Beef,** 1 sandwich | 20 |
| **Engine Company,** 1 sandwich | 18 |
| **Engineer,** 1 sandwich | 18 |
| **Ham,** 1 sandwich | 16 |
| **Hero,** 1 sandwich | 18 |
| **Hook & Ladder,** 1 sandwich | 18 |
| **Italian,** 1 sandwich | 27 |
| **Meatball,** 1 sandwich | 33 |
| **NY Steamer,** 1 sandwich | 21 |
| **Pastrami,** 1 sandwich | 17 |
| **Roast Beef,** 1 sandwich | 22 |
| **Sliced Deli Chicken,** 1 sandwich | 14 |
| **Smokehouse Beef & Cheddar,** 1 sandwich | 28 |
| **Steak,** 1 sandwich | 21 |
| **Tuna Salad,** 1 sandwich | 29 |
| **Turkey,** 1 sandwich | 15 |
| **Veggie,** 1 sandwich | 13 |
| **Veggie (no meat),** 1 large | 13 |
| **CHILI & SALADS** | |
| **Chief's Salad with Chicken Salad,** 1 | 19 |
| **Chief's Salad with Ham, without dressing,** 1 salad | 9 |
| **Chief's Salad with Sliced Deli Chicken,** 1 salad | 7 |
| **Chief's Salad with Tuna Salad,** 1 salad | 15 |
| **Chief's Salad with Turkey, without dressing,** 1 salad | 8 |
| **Chili,** 1 bowl | 10 |
| **SALAD DRESSINGS** | |
| **Balsamic Vinaigrette,** 1 packet | 5 |
| **Fat Free Ranch,** 1 packet | 1 |
| **Fat Free Raspberry Vinaigrette,** 1 packet | 1 |
| **Italian,** 1 packet | 6 |
| **Ranch,** 1 packet | 8 |
| **Thousand Island,** 1 packet | 5 |
| **BREAD** | |
| **Wheat,** 8" | 6 |
| **White,** 12" | 10 |

| ▲ Power Foods | *PointsPlus*™ value |
| --- | --- |
| **DESSERTS** | |
| **Brownies,** 1 piece | 12 |
| **Chocolate Chip Cookie,** 1 | 8 |
| **Oatmeal Raisin Cookie,** 1 | 8 |
| **Peanut Butter Cookie,** 1 | 10 |

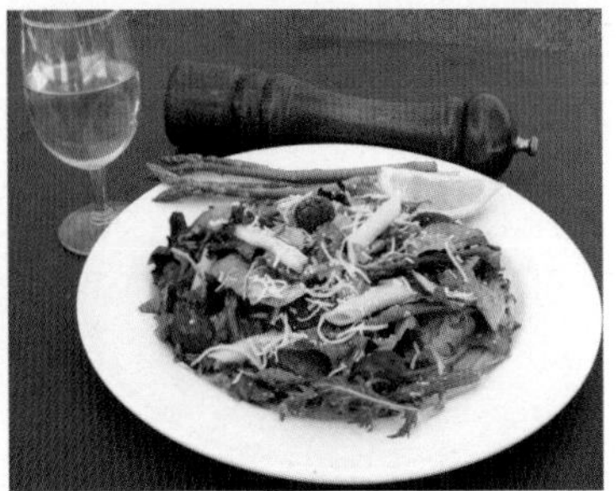

▲ Power Foods — *PointsPlus™* value

## BAKERY - MUFFINS, BISCUITS & BREADS

|  | PointsPlus™ value |
|---|---|
| **Apple Raisin Honey Bran,** 1 | 4 |
| **Blueberry,** 1 | 5 |
| **Corn,** 1 | 5 |
| **Country Herbed Biscuit,** 1 | 7 |
| **Louisiana Sweet Potato Biscuit,** 1 | 8 |
| **Pumpkin Cranberry,** 1 | 6 |
| **Pumpkin Cranberry Crunch Muffin,** 1 | 8 |
| **Pumpkin Raisin Muffin,** 1 | 6 |
| **Pumpkin Spice,** 1 | 5 |
| **Raspberry Orange,** 1 | 5 |
| **Raspberry Orange Muffin (low fat),** 1 | 4 |
| **Raspberry Peach,** 1 | 5 |
| **Zucchini, Carrot & Raisin,** 1 | 6 |

## BUILD YOUR OWN SALAD BAR

|  | PointsPlus™ value |
|---|---|
| ▲ **Beets, Julienne,** 2 Tbsp | 0 |
| **Blue Cheese,** 2 Tbsp | 2 |
| ▲ **Broccoli,** 2 Tbsp | 0 |
| ▲ **Cabbage,** 2 Tbsp | 0 |
| ▲ **Carrots,** 2 Tbsp | 0 |
| ▲ **Cauliflower,** 2 Tbsp | 0 |
| ▲ **Celery,** 2 Tbsp | 0 |
| ▲ **Corn Kernels,** 2 Tbsp | 1 |
| **Cottage Cheese, 2%,** 2 Tbsp | 1 |
| ▲ **Cucumber,** 4 slices | 0 |
| ▲ **Edamame,** 2 Tbsp | 1 |
| ▲ **Garbanzo Beans,** 2 Tbsp | 1 |
| ▲ **Green Beans - Fresh,** 2 Tbsp | 0 |
| ▲ **Green Bell Pepper,** 2 Tbsp | 0 |
| ▲ **Green Onions,** 2 Tbsp | 0 |
| ▲ **Greens: Iceberg lettuce,** 1/2 cup | 0 |
| ▲ **Greens: Romaine Lettuce,** 1/2 cup | 0 |
| ▲ **Greens: Spinach,** 1/2 cup | 0 |
| ▲ **Greens: Spring Mix,** 1/2 cup | 0 |
| ▲ **Hard Boiled Egg,** 2 Tbsp | 1 |
| ▲ **Hominy,** 2 Tbsp | 0 |
| ▲ **Jalapeno Peppers,** 2 Tbsp | 0 |
| ▲ **Jicama,** 2 Tbsp | 0 |
| ▲ **Kidney Beans,** 2 Tbsp | 1 |
| ▲ **Mushrooms,** 2 Tbsp | 0 |
| **Olives,** 2 Tbsp | 1 |
| ▲ **Peas,** 2 Tbsp | 0 |
| ▲ **Pepperoncini,** 2 Tbsp | 0 |
| ▲ **Radishes,** 2 Tbsp | 0 |
| **Rainbow Rotini,** 2 Tbsp | 0 |
| **Raisins,** 2 Tbsp | 2 |
| ▲ **Red Bell Pepper,** 2 Tbsp | 0 |
| ▲ **Red Onions,** 2 Tbsp | 0 |
| ▲ **Snap Peas - Fresh,** 2 Tbsp | 0 |
| **Sunflower Seeds,** 2 Tbsp | 3 |
| ▲ **Sweet Corn,** 2 Tbsp | 1 |
| ▲ **Tofu,** 2 Tbsp | 1 |
| ▲ **Tomatoes,** 2 Tbsp | 0 |
| ▲ **Zucchini,** 2 Tbsp | 0 |
| **Protein Toppers: Honey Lime Chipotle Chicken,** 2 oz | 4 |
| ▲ **Protein Toppers: Icelandic Shrimp,** 1 serving | 2 |
| ▲ **Protein Toppers: Mesquite Grilled Chicken,** 2 oz | 2 |

| ▲ Power Foods | PointsPlus™ value |
|---|---|
| **Protein Toppers: Sesame Ginger Chicken,** 2 oz | 4 |
| **Protein Toppers: Spicy Cajun Chicken,** 2 oz | 2 |
| **Protein Toppers: Szechuan Beef,** 2 oz | 3 |
| ▲ **Protein Toppers: Tuna,** 2 oz | 1 |

## PREPARED SALADS

| ▲ Power Foods | PointsPlus™ value |
|---|---|
| **Almond Chicken Pasta,** 1/2 cup | 6 |
| **Antipasto Salad,** 1/2 cup | 4 |
| **Artichoke and Bowtie Pasta,** 1/2 cup | 3 |
| **Asian Broccoli Slaw,** 1/2 cup | 2 |
| **Asian Edamame and Pasta,** 1/2 cup | 4 |
| **Asian Slaw,** 1/2 cup | 1 |
| **Basil Aioli with Wild Rice,** 1/2 cup | 5 |
| **Black Bean Fresca,** 1/2 cup | 2 |
| **Broccoli Almondine,** 1/2 cup | 4 |
| **Caesar Pasta,** 1/2 cup | 3 |
| **Caribbean Cole Slaw,** 1/2 cup | 3 |
| **Carrot Coriander Salad,** 1/2 cup | 1 |
| **Cavatappi Pesto Salad,** 1/2 cup | 3 |
| **Chayote Pineapple Picante Slaw,** 1/2 cup | 1 |
| **Chicken Basil Aioli,** 1/2 cup | 5 |
| **Chicken Pesto Penne,** 1/2 cup | 3 |
| **Chili Lime Fiesta Medley,** 1/2 cup | 0 |
| **Classic Carrot Raisin,** 1/2 cup | 4 |
| **Classic Picnic Slaw,** 1/2 cup | 2 |
| **Country Picnic Potato,** 1/2 cup | 6 |
| **Creamy Citrus Slaw,** 1/2 cup | 2 |
| **Creamy Dijon Potato,** 2/3 cup | 3 |
| **Creamy Dill Potato,** 1/2 cup | 3 |
| **Creamy Italian Ranch Pasta,** 1/2 cup | 3 |
| **Creamy Peanut Slaw,** 1/2 cup | 4 |
| **Creole Corn & Black-Eyed Pea Relish,** 1/2 cup | 5 |
| **Crisp Apple Pineapple,** 1/2 cup | 2 |
| **Curried Cous Cous,** 1/2 cup | 3 |
| **Eggplant Dip,** 2 Tbsp | 0 |
| **Fat-Free Marinated Cucumber Salad,** 1/2 cup | 0 |
| ▲ **Fresh Vegetable Medley,** 1/2 cup | 0 |
| **Ginger Soy Long Noodle,** 1/2 cup | 4 |
| **Greek Goddess Medley,** 1/2 cup | 3 |
| **Honey Citrus Slaw,** 1/2 cup | 1 |
| **Honey Lime Chipotle Slaw,** 1/2 cup | 2 |
| ▲ **Italian Tomato and Cucumber,** 1/2 cup | 0 |
| ▲ **Italian Vegetable Medley,** 1/2 cup | 0 |
| **Jicama Citrus,** 1/2 cup | 1 |
| **Lemon Garlic Pasta,** 1/2 cup | 2 |
| **Low Carb Broccoli Obsession,** 1/2 cup | 0 |
| **Madras Curried Rice,** 1/2 cup | 4 |
| ▲ **Marinated Cucumber,** 1/2 cup | 1 |
| **Marinated Sesame Cucumber,** 1/2 cup | 1 |
| **Mexicali Pasta,** 1/2 cup | 2 |
| **Mom's Mac,** 1/2 cup | 6 |
| **Montego Bay,** 1/2 cup | 3 |
| **New Delhi Turkey,** 1/2 cup | 6 |
| **No Fry Stir Fry Rice,** 1/2 cup | 5 |
| **Orecchiette with Bacon Ranch,** 1/2 cup | 5 |
| **Palermo Pasta,** 1/2 cup | 3 |
| **Pasta Classica,** 1/2 cup | 5 |
| **Pasta Pomodoro,** 1/2 cup | 4 |
| **Pina Colada Slaw,** 1/2 cup | 3 |
| **Radiatore Pasta,** 1/2 cup | 4 |
| **Rice with Artichoke,** 1/2 cup | 2 |
| **Roasted Red Potato,** 1/2 cup | 3 |
| **Roasted Vegetable,** 1/2 cup | 4 |
| **Santa Fe Corn Relish,** 1/2 cup | 4 |
| **Seafood Pasta,** 1/2 cup | 6 |

*Prepared Salads (cont'd)*

| ▲ Power Foods | *PointsPlus*™ value |
|---|---|
| **Smashed Potato,** 1/2 cup | 6 |
| **Summer Garden Pasta,** 1/2 cup | 1 |
| **Sundried Tomato Cous Cous,** 1/2 cup | 3 |
| **Sweet and Sour Broccoli,** 1/2 cup | 4 |
| **Tabouli,** 1/2 cup | 3 |
| **Thai Shredded Slaw,** 1/2 cup | 1 |
| **Thai Shrimp and Snow Peas,** 1/2 cup | 3 |
| **Tuna Taragon,** 1/2 cup | 7 |
| **Waldorf Lite,** 1/2 cup | 2 |
| ▲ **Wild Rice,** 1/2 cup | 2 |
| **Wild Rice & Cranberry Salad,** 1/2 cup | 3 |
| **Wild Rice Chicken,** 1/2 cup | 4 |

## SPECIALTY SALADS

| ▲ Power Foods | *PointsPlus*™ value |
|---|---|
| **Antipasto Salad,** 1 cup | 5 |
| **Autumn Mixed Greens with Roasted Beet,** 1 cup | 5 |
| **Azteca Ensalada,** 1 cup | 5 |
| **California Fresh Toss Salad,** 1 cup | 5 |
| **Caribbean Chicken Salad,** 1 cup | 6 |
| **Chinese Chicken Salad,** 1 cup | 6 |
| ▲ **Classic Caesar,** 1 cup | 0 |
| **Cool Raspberry Crunch,** 1 cup | 4 |
| **Fall Mixed Greens with Balsamic Vinaigrette,** 1 cup | 3 |
| **Fuji Apple & Papaya Wasabi Toss,** 1 cup | 3 |
| **Mediterranean Roasted Veggie Salad,** 1 cup | 3 |
| **Raspberry and Walnut,** 1 cup | 4 |
| **Raspberry Walnut Chicken Salad,** 1 cup | 4 |
| **Shanghai Chicken Salad,** 1 cup | 5 |
| **Spinach Dijon,** 1 cup | 2 |
| **Summer Citrus Splash Salad,** 1 cup | 5 |

## DRESSINGS

| ▲ Power Foods | *PointsPlus*™ value |
|---|---|
| **1000 Island,** 2 Tbsp | 4 |
| **Bleu Cheese,** 2 Tbsp | 4 |
| **Chinese Chicken Salad Dressing,** 2 Tbsp | 4 |
| **Fat Free French,** 2 Tbsp | 1 |
| **Fat Free Honey Dijon,** 2 Tbsp | 1 |
| **Fat Free Italian,** 2 Tbsp | 0 |
| **Fat Free Ranch,** 2 Tbsp | 1 |
| **Parmesan Peppercorn,** 2 Tbsp | 4 |
| **Ranch,** 2 Tbsp | 4 |

## PASTAS & SAUCES

| ▲ Power Foods | *PointsPlus*™ value |
|---|---|
| **Alfredo,** 2 oz | 5 |
| **Bowtie Pesto Primavera (oven baked pasta),** 1/2 cup | 6 |
| **Carbonara Oven Baked Pasta,** 1/2 cup | 6 |
| **Chicken Piccata Oven Baked Pasta,** 1/2 cup | 6 |
| **Chile Con Queso Oven Baked Pasta,** 1/2 cup | 4 |
| **Classic Vermicelli with Italian Meat Sauce,** 1/2 cup | 4 |
| **Creamy Garlic Alfredo,** 1/4 cup | 5 |
| **Penne Pomodoro (oven baked pasta),** 1/2 cup | 3 |
| **Spicy Szechuan Noodle,** 1/2 cup | 5 |
| **Tomato Bacon Oven Bake Pasta,** 1/2 cup | 5 |
| **Vegetarian Jambalaya,** 1/2 cup | 4 |
| **Yankee Doodle Cheddar & Macaroni,** 1/2 cup | 5 |
| **Sauce - Italian Meat Sauce,** 2 fl oz | 1 |
| **Sauce - Macaroni and Cheese Sauce,** 2 fl oz | 3 |
| **Sauce - Pomodoro,** 1/4 cup | 0 |

| ▲ Power Foods | *PointsPlus™* value |
|---|---|

## PIZZA

| | |
|---|---|
| **California Fresh Veggie Pizza,** 1 slice | 4 |
| **Cheese Pizza,** 1 slice | 3 |
| **Fresh Roma Tomato & Basil Pizza,** 1 slice | 3 |
| **Pepperoni Pizza,** 1 slice | 4 |
| **Pesto Ranch with Smoked Bacon,** 1 slice | 4 |

## RICE

| | |
|---|---|
| **Herb Rice,** 1/2 cup | 3 |
| **Peking Rice,** 1/2 cup | 4 |
| **White Rice,** 1/2 cup | 3 |

## SOUPS

| | |
|---|---|
| **Baked Potato,** 1 cup | 8 |
| **Bayou Black Eyed Pea and Ham,** 1 cup | 5 |
| **Broccoli Cheese,** 1 cup | 4 |
| **Cajun Black Bean Chili,** 1 cup | 5 |
| **Carrot Ginger,** 1 cup | 2 |
| **Chile Verde,** 1 cup | 5 |
| **Confetti Bean Chili,** 1 cup | 4 |
| **Corn Beef and Cabbage,** 1 cup | 5 |
| **Cream of Asparagus,** 1 cup | 8 |
| **Cream of Broccoli,** 1 cup | 5 |
| **Cream of Mushroom,** 1 cup | 6 |
| **Creamy Potato Leek with Bacon,** 1 cup | 9 |
| **Creamy Thai Vegetable Soup,** 1 cup | 7 |
| **Creamy Tomato and Shrimp Bisque,** 1 cup | 7 |
| **Creamy Tomato Bisque,** 1 cup | 7 |
| **Fall Harvest Butternut Squash,** 1 cup | 7 |
| **Fettuccine Chicken Noodle,** 1 cup | 3 |
| **Firehouse Chili,** 1 cup | 7 |
| **French Onion,** 1 cup | 3 |
| **Grandma's Chicken & Dumplings,** 1 cup | 5 |
| **Greek Artichoke and Lemon Rice,** 1 cup | 3 |
| **Green Chili and Corn Chowder,** 1 cup | 3 |
| **Harvest Vegetable,** 1 cup | 2 |
| **Hearty Garden Vegetable Barley,** 1 cup | 2 |
| ▲ **Hearty Vegetable,** 1 cup | 0 |
| **Italian Split Pea,** 1 cup | 3 |
| **Mushroom Bean and Barley,** 1 cup | 3 |
| **Navy Bean and Ham,** 1 cup | 4 |
| **New England Clam Chowder,** 1 cup | 8 |
| **New Orleans Gumbo,** 1 cup | 5 |
| **Pho Noodle Bowl,** 1 cup | 3 |
| **Pho Noodle Bowl (vegetarian),** 1 cup | 3 |
| **Potato Cheddar,** 1 cup | 10 |
| **Ratatouille Stew,** 1 cup | 2 |
| **Red Bean Chili,** 1 cup | 5 |
| **Roasted Sirloin Chili,** 1 cup | 5 |
| **San Jose Chicken Chili,** 1 cup | 4 |
| **Savory Bean,** 1 cup | 5 |
| **Smoke House Potato Cheddar,** 1 cup | 14 |
| **Sopa Albondigas,** 1 cup | 6 |
| **Southern Lentil,** 1 cup | 4 |
| **Southwest Corn Chowder,** 1 cup | 8 |
| **Southwestern Black Bean with Andouille,** 1 cup | 4 |
| **Spicy Texas Chili Con Carne,** 1 cup | 5 |
| **Spicy Vegetable Gumbo,** 1 cup | 2 |
| **Split Pea with Ham,** 1 cup | 4 |
| ▲ **Summer Squash,** 1 cup | 0 |
| **Texas Chicken Tortilla,** 1 cup | 4 |
| **Thai Coconut Ginger,** 1 cup | 6 |
| **Tomato Basil Florentine,** 1 cup | 2 |
| **Turkey and Wild Rice Soup,** 1 cup | 3 |
| **Turkey Chili,** 1 cup | 5 |

*Soups (cont'd)*

| ▲ Power Foods | *PointsPlus*™ value |
|---|---|
| **Turkey Gumbo,** 1 cup | 2 |
| **Tuscan Tortellini Minestrone,** 1 cup | 4 |
| **Tuscan White Bean and Vegetable,** 1 cup | 3 |
| **Vegetable Minestrone,** 1 cup | 2 |
| **Vegetarian Vegetable,** 1 cup | 2 |
| **Wild Rice Chicken,** 1 cup | 4 |

## DESSERTS

| | |
|---|---|
| **Apple Spice Cake,** 1 piece | 4 |
| **Apple Streusel Cake,** 1 piece | 12 |
| **Apricot Streusel Cake,** 1 piece | 11 |
| **Aunt Janet's Pumpkin Spice Cake,** 1 piece | 4 |
| **Blueberry Streusal Cake,** 1 piece | 12 |
| **Caramel Crème Custard Ole,** 1/2 cup | 6 |
| **Chocolate Pudding,** 1/2 cup | 4 |
| **Chocolate Soft Serve,** 1 serving | 3 |
| **Coconut Cream Pie Pudding,** 1/2 cup | 7 |
| ▲ **Fruit Salad/Grapes,** 1/2 cup | 0 |
| ▲ **Fruit Salad/Watermelon,** 1/2 cup | 0 |
| **Key Lime Pie Pudding,** 1/2 cup | 7 |
| **Lemon Pudding Cake,** 1 | 4 |
| **Miss Barbara's Famous Carrot Cake,** 1 piece | 6 |
| **Old Fashioned Bread Pudding,** 1 piece | 4 |
| **Orangesicle Cake,** 1 | 4 |
| **Peach Streusal Cake,** 1 piece | 11 |
| **Pumpkin Cream Pie Pudding,** 1/2 cup | 6 |
| **Smore Cake,** 1 | 4 |
| ▲ **Sugar Free Gelatin,** 1/2 cup | 0 |
| **Tapioca Pudding,** 1/2 cup | 4 |
| **Triple Berry Lemon Shortcake,** 1 piece | 8 |
| **Triple Decadence Brownie,** 1 | 4 |
| **Vanilla Soft Serve,** 1 serving | 3 |
| **Warm Gingerbread,** 1 piece | 3 |
| **Whipped Topping,** 2 Tbsp | 0 |

| ▲ Power Foods | *PointsPlus*™ value |
|---|---|
| **ENERGY SMOOTHIES** | |
| **Acai Energy,** 1 serving | 8 |
| **All That Razz,** 1 serving | 9 |
| **Berry Breeze,** 1 serving | 8 |
| **Caribbean Craze,** 1 serving | 8 |
| **High Test Energizer,** 1 serving | 8 |
| **Jamaican Jammer,** 1 serving | 9 |
| **Mango Beach,** 1 serving | 5 |
| **Maui Mango,** 1 serving | 8 |
| **Mystic Mango,** 1 serving | 10 |
| **OJ Sunrise,** 1 serving | 10 |
| **Orange Passion,** 1 serving | 5 |
| **Peach Sunset,** 1 serving | 7 |
| **Peachy Pineapple,** 1 serving | 9 |
| **Peanut Butter Energizer,** 1 serving | 13 |
| **Pineapple Paradise,** 1 serving | 9 |
| **Strawberry Oasis,** 1 serving | 5 |
| **Strawberry Shooter,** 1 serving | 7 |
| **Strawberry Squeeze,** 1 serving | 8 |
| **Strawberry Sunrise,** 1 serving | 5 |

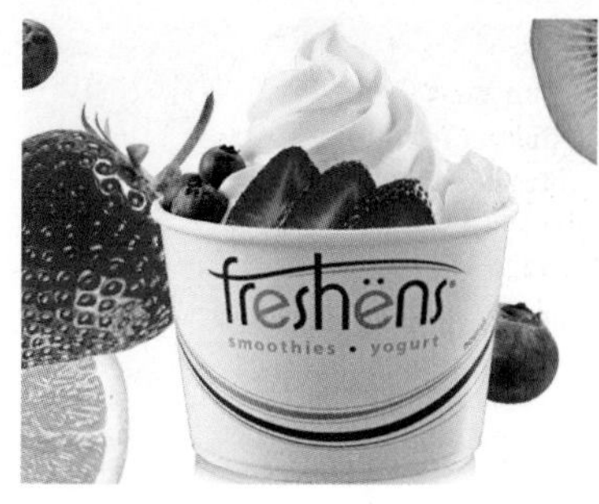


| ▲ Power Foods | *PointsPlus*™ value |
|---|---|
| **FROZEN TREATS** | |
| **JavaBoost - Caramel,** 1 | 13 |
| **JavaBoost - Caramel Light,** 1 | 9 |
| **JavaBoost - Double Chocolate,** 1 | 22 |
| **JavaBoost - Java Chip,** 1 | 20 |
| **JavaBoost - Mocha,** 1 | 12 |
| **JavaBoost - Mocha Light,** 1 | 8 |
| **JavaBoost - Strawberry Crème,** 1 | 13 |
| **JavaBoost - Strawberry Crème Light,** 1 | 8 |
| **JavaBoost - Vanilla Crème,** 1 | 12 |
| **JavaBoost - Vanilla Crème Light,** 1 | 7 |
| **Acai Energy Bowl,** 1 serving | 11 |

# GODFATHER'S PIZZA®

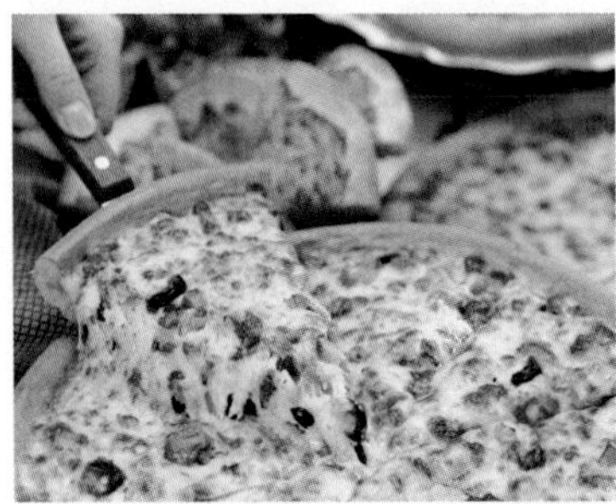

| ▲ Power Foods | *PointsPlus™* value |
|---|---|
| **ORIGINAL CRUST PIZZA** | |
| **All Meat Combo,** 1/10 of the jumbo pizza | 13 |
| **All Meat Combo,** 1/4 of the mini pizza | 6 |
| **All Meat Combo,** 1/10 of the large pizza | 10 |
| **All Meat Combo,** 1/8 of the medium pizza | 9 |
| **Bacon Cheeseburger,** 1/10 of the jumbo pizza | 12 |
| **Bacon Cheeseburger,** 1/4 of the mini pizza | 6 |
| **Bacon Cheeseburger,** 1/10 of the large pizza | 10 |
| **Bacon Cheeseburger,** 1/8 of the medium pizza | 8 |
| **Cheese Pizza,** 1/10 of the jumbo pizza | 9 |
| **Cheese Pizza,** 1/10 of the large pizza | 7 |
| **Cheese Pizza,** 1/8 of the medium pizza | 6 |
| **Cheese Pizza,** 1/4 of the mini pizza | 4 |
| **Combo Pizza,** 1/4 of the mini pizza | 5 |
| **Combo Pizza,** 1/10 of the jumbo pizza | 12 |
| **Combo Pizza,** 1/8 of the medium pizza | 9 |
| **Combo Pizza,** 1/10 of the large pizza | 10 |
| **Hawaiian,** 1/10 of the jumbo pizza | 9 |
| **Hawaiian,** 1/4 of the mini pizza | 4 |

| ▲ Power Foods | *PointsPlus™* value |
|---|---|
| **Hawaiian,** 1/10 of the large pizza | 8 |
| **Hawaiian,** 1/8 of the medium pizza | 7 |
| **Hot Stuff,** 1/10 of the jumbo pizza | 13 |
| **Hot Stuff,** 1/4 of the mini pizza | 5 |
| **Hot Stuff,** 1/10 of the large pizza | 10 |
| **Hot Stuff,** 1/8 of the medium pizza | 9 |
| **Humble Pie,** 1/10 of the jumbo pizza | 13 |
| **Humble Pie,** 1/10 of the large pizza | 10 |
| **Humble Pie,** 1/8 of the medium pizza | 9 |
| **Humble Pie,** 1/4 of the mini pizza | 6 |
| **Pepperoni,** 1/10 of the jumbo pizza | 10 |
| **Pepperoni,** 1/8 of the medium pizza | 7 |
| **Pepperoni,** 1/4 of the mini pizza | 4 |
| **Pepperoni,** 1/10 of the large pizza | 8 |
| **Super Combo,** 1/10 of the jumbo pizza | 13 |
| **Super Combo,** 1/10 of the large pizza | 11 |
| **Super Combo,** 1/4 of the mini pizza | 6 |
| **Super Combo,** 1/8 of the medium pizza | 9 |
| **Super Hawaiian,** 1/10 of the large pizza | 8 |
| **Super Hawaiian,** 1/10 of the jumbo pizza | 10 |
| **Super Hawaiian,** 1/8 of the medium pizza | 7 |
| **Super Hawaiian,** 1/4 of the mini pizza | 4 |
| **Super Taco,** 1/10 of the jumbo pizza | 14 |
| **Super Taco,** 1/10 of the large pizza | 12 |
| **Super Taco,** 1/8 of the medium pizza | 10 |
| **Super Taco,** 1/4 of the mini pizza | 6 |
| **Taco,** 1/10 of the jumbo pizza | 13 |
| **Taco,** 1/10 of the large pizza | 11 |
| **Taco,** 1/8 of the medium pizza | 10 |
| **Taco,** 1/4 of the mini pizza | 6 |
| **Veggie,** 1/10 of the jumbo pizza | 9 |
| **Veggie,** 1/10 of the large pizza | 8 |
| **Veggie,** 1/8 of the medium pizza | 7 |
| **Veggie,** 1/4 of the mini pizza | 4 |

| ▲ Power Foods | *PointsPlus*™ value |
|---|---|

## THIN CRUST PIZZA

| | |
|---|---|
| **All Meat Combo,** 1/8 of the medium pizza | 7 |
| **All Meat Combo,** 1/10 of the large pizza | 8 |
| **Bacon Cheeseburger,** 1/8 of the medium pizza | 7 |
| **Bacon Cheeseburger,** 1/10 of the large pizza | 7 |
| **Cheese,** 1/8 of the medium pizza | 4 |
| **Cheese,** 1/10 of the large pizza | 5 |
| **Combo,** 1/8 of the medium pizza | 6 |
| **Combo,** 1/10 of the large pizza | 7 |
| **Hawaiian,** 1/8 of the medium pizza | 5 |
| **Hawaiian,** 1/10 of the large pizza | 6 |
| **Hot Stuff,** 1/8 of the medium pizza | 7 |
| **Hot Stuff,** 1/10 of the large pizza | 8 |
| **Humble Pie,** 1/8 of the medium pizza | 7 |
| **Humble Pie,** 1/10 of the large pizza | 8 |
| **Pepperoni,** 1/8 of the medium pizza | 5 |
| **Pepperoni,** 1/10 of the large pizza | 6 |
| **Super Combo,** 1/10 of the large pizza | 8 |
| **Super Combo,** 1/8 of the medium pizza | 7 |
| **Super Hawaiian,** 1/8 of the medium pizza | 6 |
| **Super Hawaiian,** 1/10 of the large pizza | 6 |
| **Super Taco,** 1/10 of the large pizza | 9 |
| **Super Taco,** 1/8 of the medium pizza | 8 |
| **Taco,** 1/10 of the large pizza | 7 |
| **Taco,** 1/8 of the medium pizza | 7 |
| **Veggie,** 1/10 of the large pizza | 5 |
| **Veggie,** 1/8 of the medium pizza | 4 |

## GOLDEN CRUST PIZZA

| | |
|---|---|
| **All Meat Combo,** 1/8 of the medium pizza | 8 |
| **All Meat Combo,** 1/10 of the large pizza | 9 |
| **Bacon Cheeseburger,** 1/8 of the medium pizza | 7 |
| **Bacon Cheeseburger,** 1/10 of the large pizza | 6 |
| **Cheese Pizza,** 1/10 of the large pizza | 6 |
| **Cheese Pizza,** 1/8 of the medium pizza | 6 |
| **Combo Pizza,** 1/10 of the large pizza | 8 |
| **Combo Pizza,** 1/8 of the medium pizza | 7 |
| **Hawaiian,** 1/8 of the medium pizza | 6 |
| **Hawaiian,** 1/10 of the large pizza | 7 |
| **Hot Stuff,** 1/8 of the medium pizza | 8 |
| **Hot Stuff,** 1/10 of the large pizza | 8 |
| **Humble Pie,** 1/8 of the medium pizza | 8 |
| **Humble Pie,** 1/10 of the large pizza | 9 |
| **Pepperoni,** 1/8 of the medium pizza | 7 |
| **Pepperoni,** 1/10 of the large pizza | 7 |
| **Super Combo,** 1/8 of the medium pizza | 8 |
| **Super Combo,** 1/10 of the large pizza | 9 |
| **Super Hawaiian,** 1/10 of the large pizza | 7 |
| **Super Hawaiian,** 1/8 of the medium pizza | 6 |
| **Super Taco,** 1/8 of the medium pizza | 9 |
| **Super Taco,** 1/10 of the large pizza | 10 |
| **Taco,** 1/10 of the large pizza | 9 |
| **Taco,** 1/8 of the medium pizza | 8 |
| **Veggie Pizza,** 1/8 of the medium pizza | 6 |
| **Veggie Pizza,** 1/10 of the large pizza | 7 |

## SIDE ORDERS

| | |
|---|---|
| **Cheesesticks,** 1/6 of the pan | 3 |
| **Monkey Bread,** 1/6 of the pan | 3 |
| **Potato Wedges,** 1 serving | 5 |

## DESSERT

| | |
|---|---|
| **Cinnamon Streusel,** 1/6 of the aluminum pan | 4 |

# GOLDEN CORRAL® BUFFET & GRILL

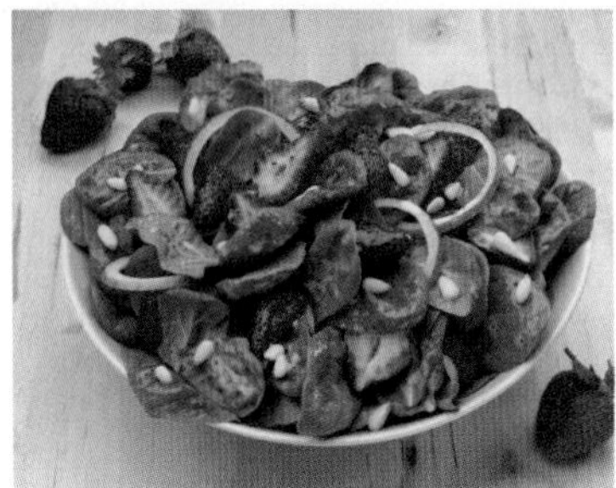

| ▲ Power Foods | *PointsPlus™* value |
|---|---|
| **MEATS/FISH** | |
| **Awesome Pot Roast,** 1 serving | 5 |
| **Barbeque Pork,** 1 serving | 4 |
| **Barbeque Pork Spareribs,** 1 | 6 |
| **Battered Pollock Fish Fillet,** 1 serving | 5 |
| **Bourbon Street Chicken,** 1 serving | 5 |
| **Breaded Butterflied Shrimp,** 6 | 6 |
| **Breaded Shrimp,** 16 | 5 |
| **Chicken Breast Fillet, Marinated,** 1 serving | 3 |
| **Chicken Tenders,** 1 serving | 5 |
| **Country Fried Steak,** 1 serving | 4 |
| **Fresh Fried Chicken (Leg/Thigh),** 1 piece | 7 |
| **Hot Steamed Shrimp,** 1 cup | 0 |
| **Meatloaf,** 1 serving | 5 |
| **Pork Roast,** 1 serving | 6 |
| **Pork Steaks,** 1 serving | 6 |
| **Rotisserie Chicken (Breast/Wing),** 1 piece | 8 |
| **Salmon Steaks, with Lemon Herb Butter Sauce,** 1 serving | 5 |

| ▲ Power Foods | *PointsPlus™* value |
|---|---|
| **HOT CHOICE** | |
| **Brown Gravy,** 1 serving | 3 |
| **Chicken & Pastry Noodles,** 1 serving | 2 |
| **Macaroni & Beef,** 1 cup | 7 |
| **Macaroni & Cheese,** 1 cup | 11 |
| **Mashed Potatoes (made-from-scratch),** 1 serving | 3 |
| **Poultry Gravy,** 1 serving | 3 |
| **Spaghetti Pasta,** 1 serving | 5 |
| **Spaghetti Sauce,** 1/2 cup | 3 |
| **Tamales, Beef,** 2 | 6 |
| **COLD CHOICE** | |
| **Cocktail Sauce,** 1/4 cup | 2 |
| **Creamy Caesar Dressing,** 2 Tbsp | 3 |
| **Dijon Honey Mustard Salad Dressing,** 2 Tbsp | 4 |
| **Fat Free Ranch Dressing,** 2 Tbsp | 0 |
| **Fat Free Red French Dressing,** 2 Tbsp | 1 |
| **Fat Free Thousand Island Dressing,** 2 Tbsp | 1 |
| **French Salad Dressing,** 2 Tbsp | 3 |
| **Honey Butter,** 1 individual cup | 2 |
| **Hot Bacon Dressing,** 2 Tbsp | 4 |
| **Lite Olive Oil Vinaigrette,** 2 Tbsp | 2 |
| **Poppyseed Dressing,** 2 Tbsp | 3 |
| **Red French Salad Dressing,** 2 Tbsp | 3 |
| **Sesame Oriental Dressing,** 2 Tbsp | 5 |
| **Sliced Yellow Peaches,** 1/2 cup | 0 |
| **Tartar Sauce,** 2 Tbsp | 4 |
| **Turkey - Dark, Julienne,** 1 serving | 2 |
| **Turkey - White, Julienne,** 1 serving | 2 |

| ▲ Power Foods | *PointsPlus*™ value |
|---|---|
| **VEGETABLES** | |
| **Asian Beans,** 1 cup | 0 |
| **Brussels Sprouts,** 6 | 0 |
| **Collard Greens,** 1 serving | 1 |
| **Creamed Corn,** 1 serving | 2 |
| **Creamed Spinach,** 1/2 cup | 5 |
| **Escalloped Apples,** 2/3 cup | 5 |
| ▲ **Spinach,** 1/3 cup | 0 |
| ▲ **Turnip Greens,** 2/3 cup | 0 |
| **Yams & Apples,** 1/2 cup | 4 |
| **PIZZA** | |
| **Pizza,** 1 slice | 6 |
| **SOUP** | |
| **Broccoli Cheese with Florets,** 1/2 cup | 3 |
| **Chicken Gumbo,** 1/2 cup | 2 |
| **Chicken Noodle,** 1/2 cup | 2 |
| **Clam Chowder,** 1/2 cup | 4 |
| **Potato with Bacon,** 1/2 cup | 3 |
| **Timberline Chili,** 1 cup | 7 |
| **Vegetable Beef,** 1/2 cup | 3 |
| **SUNRISE BREAKFAST BUFFET®** | |
| **Apple Juice,** 1 serving | 1 |
| **Bacon,** 1 piece | 2 |
| **Corned Beef Hash,** 1 cup | 11 |
| **Creamed Chipped Beef,** 1/2 cup | 5 |
| **Eggs, Scrambled,** 1 serving | 4 |
| **Orange Juice,** 1 serving | 1 |
| **Orange-Guava-Passion Fruit Juice,** 1 serving | 1 |
| **Sausage Gravy,** 1 serving | 1 |
| **Sausage Patties,** 1 | 7 |
| **Split Smoked Sausage,** 1 | 7 |

| ▲ Power Foods | *PointsPlus*™ value |
|---|---|
| **BRASS BELL BAKERY®** | |
| **Caramel Topping,** 1 serving | 9 |
| **Carrot Cake,** 1 serving | 11 |
| **Chocolate Chip Cookie,** 1 | 3 |
| **Chocolate Soft Serve,** 1/2 cup | 3 |
| **Chocolate Syrup,** 1 serving | 7 |
| **Chocolate White Chip Cookie,** 1 | 3 |
| **Coconut Cookie,** 1 | 3 |
| **Cornbread (Skillet),** 1 | 3 |
| **Hot Fudge Topping,** 1 serving | 9 |
| **Oatmeal Bar,** 1 square | 2 |
| **Oatmeal Raisin Cookie,** 1 | 2 |
| **Peanut Butter with Nuts Cookie,** 1 | 3 |
| **Sherbet,** 1/2 cup | 3 |
| **Strawberry Topping,** 1 serving | 5 |
| **Sugar Free Chocolate Chocolate Chip Cookie,** 1 | 2 |
| **Turtle Coating,** 1 serving | 18 |
| **Vanilla Cake,** 1 slice | 4 |
| **Vanilla Soft Serve,** 1/2 cup | 3 |
| **Yeast Rolls (without butter),** 1 | 5 |

# GOLDEN SPOON® FROZEN YOGURT

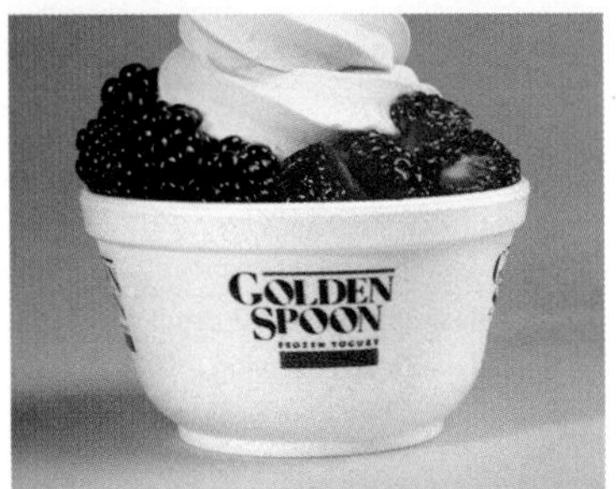


| ▲ Power Foods | *PointsPlus*™ value |
|---|---|

## FROZEN YOGURT

| | |
|---|---|
| **Heath Bar® Low-Fat Frozen Yogurt,** 1 mini cup | 3 |
| **Low-Fat Frozen Yogurt (all flavors except Heath Bar®),** 1 mini cup | 3 |
| **Non-Fat Frozen Yogurt (all flavors except Heath Bar®),** 1 mini cup | 3 |

| ▲ Power Foods | *PointsPlus*™ value |
|---|---|

## CONES

| | |
|---|---|
| **Cake Cone,** 1 cone | 0 |
| **Cake Cone with Heath Bar® Low-Fat Frozen Yogurt,** 1 small | 4 |
| **Cake Cone with Heath Bar® Low-Fat Frozen Yogurt,** 1 regular | 6 |
| **Cake Cone with Non-Fat Frozen Yogurt (all flavors except Heath Bar®),** 1 small | 3 |
| **Cake Cone with Non-Fat Frozen Yogurt (all flavors except Heath Bar®),** 1 regular | 4 |
| **Waffle Cone with Heath Bar®,** 1 serving | 8 |
| **Waffle Cone with Non-Fat Frozen Yogurt (all flavors except Heath Bar®),** 1 serving | 6 |

| ▲ Power Foods | *PointsPlus™* value |
|---|---|
| **DAILY SOUPS** | |
| **Chicken Vegetable,** 1 serving | 2 |
| **Gazpacho,** 1 serving | 1 |
| **Green and Yellow Split Pea,** 1 serving | 6 |
| **Ten Vegetable,** 1 serving | 2 |
| **Three Lentil Chili,** 1 serving | 4 |
| **Tuscan White Bean,** 1 serving | 4 |
| **DAILY SPECIALS** | |
| **7 Herb Bistro Chicken,** 1 serving | 4 |
| **Asparagus Potato Leek,** 1 serving | 2 |
| **Asparagus White Mushroom,** 1 serving | 3 |
| **Autumn Minestrone,** 1 serving | 4 |
| **Baja Shrimp,** 1 serving | 4 |
| **BBQ Beef and Cheddar,** 1 serving | 10 |
| **Beef Barley,** 1 serving | 5 |
| **Beef Stroganoff,** 1 serving | 6 |
| **Black Lentil with Double Bacon,** 1 serving | 5 |
| **Black Lentil with Meatballs,** 1 serving | 3 |
| **Black Lentil with Smoked Turkey,** 1 serving | 3 |
| **Boston Shrimp Chowder,** 1 serving | 6 |
| **Broccoli Cheddar,** 1 serving | 8 |
| **Broccoli Cheddar Mashed,** 1 serving | 8 |
| **Campfire Vegetarian Chili,** 1 serving | 5 |
| **Carrot Ginger Bisque,** 1 serving | 4 |
| **Cauliflower Cheddar,** 1 serving | 8 |
| **Chicken and Mushroom Egg Barley,** 1 serving | 3 |
| **Chicken and Sausage Jambalaya,** 1 serving | 4 |
| **Chicken and Wild Mushroom Stew,** 1 serving | 6 |

| ▲ Power Foods | *PointsPlus™* value |
|---|---|
| **Chicken Asparagus Bisque,** 1 serving | 5 |
| **Chicken Barley,** 1 serving | 3 |
| **Chicken Black Bean Chili,** 1 serving | 5 |
| **Chicken Cacciatore,** 1 serving | 3 |
| **Chicken Chili,** 1 serving | 7 |
| **Chicken Corn Bisque,** 1 serving | 7 |
| **Chicken Fagioli,** 1 serving | 5 |
| **Chicken Marsala,** 1 serving | 3 |
| **Chicken Mole Poblano,** 1 serving | 6 |
| **Chicken Mushroom Wild Rice,** 1 serving | 3 |
| **Chicken Pot Pie,** 1 serving | 5 |
| **Chicken Sausage and Seafood Paella,** 1 serving | 6 |
| **Chicken Tomato Florentine,** 1 serving | 5 |
| **Chicken Tortilla,** 1 serving | 4 |
| **Chicken Wild Mushroom Bisque,** 1 serving | 6 |
| **Chicken with Sweet Italian Sausage,** 1 serving | 5 |
| **Chili Macaroni and Cheese,** 1 serving | 12 |
| **Chilled Asparagus Potato Leek,** 1 serving | 2 |
| **Chilled Carrot Dill,** 1 serving | 2 |
| **Chilled Carrot Ginger,** 1 serving | 2 |
| **Chilled Cucumber Yogurt Dill,** 1 serving | 2 |
| **Chilled Curried Corn,** 1 serving | 5 |
| **Chilled Potato Leek,** 1 serving | 5 |
| **Chilled Roasted Pepper Vichyssoise,** 1 serving | 5 |
| **Chilled Spring Pea with Mint,** 1 serving | 5 |
| **Chilled Summer Tomato,** 1 serving | 4 |
| **Chilled Tomato Orange,** 1 serving | 4 |
| **Chunky Chicken Chowder,** 1 serving | 6 |
| **Chunky Potato Leek,** 1 serving | 6 |

Daily Specials (cont'd)

| ▲ Power Foods | PointsPlus™ value |
|---|---|
| **Classic Beef Stew,** 1 serving | 5 |
| **Classic Black Bean,** 1 serving | 4 |
| **Classic Lentil,** 1 serving | 4 |
| **Classic Minestrone,** 1 serving | 3 |
| **Coconut Chicken,** 1 serving | 5 |
| **Coconut Shrimp,** 1 serving | 8 |
| **Crab and Spring Pea,** 1 serving | 6 |
| **Crab and Tomato,** 1 serving | 2 |
| **Crab Asparagus Bisque,** 1 serving | 4 |
| **Crab Bisque,** 1 serving | 5 |
| **Cream of Asparagus,** 1 serving | 4 |
| **Cream of Broccoli,** 1 serving | 7 |
| **Cream of Carrot,** 1 serving | 5 |
| **Cream of Chicken with Rice,** 1 serving | 4 |
| **Cream of Spring Vegetable,** 1 serving | 7 |
| **Cream of Tomato,** 1 serving | 7 |
| **Cream of Tomato Chicken Orzo,** 1 serving | 6 |
| **Cream of Tomato with Pasta and Meatballs,** 1 serving | 9 |
| **Cream of Wild Mushroom,** 1 serving | 5 |
| **Creamy Chicken Broccoli,** 1 serving | 5 |
| **Creamy Chicken with Wild Rice and Marsala,** 1 serving | 6 |
| **Creole Gumbo,** 1 serving | 6 |
| **Cuban Black Bean,** 1 serving | 7 |
| **Curried Cauliflower and Chickpea,** 1 serving | 3 |
| **Curried Shrimp and Corn Bisque,** 1 serving | 9 |
| **Curried Vegetables,** 1 serving | 4 |
| **Curry Chicken Chowder,** 1 serving | 6 |
| **Curry Chicken Tomato,** 1 serving | 5 |
| **Fall Apple Cheddar,** 1 serving | 6 |
| **Fall Harvest Vegetable,** 1 serving | 3 |
| **French Onion Cheddar,** 1 serving | 7 |

| ▲ Power Foods | PointsPlus™ value |
|---|---|
| **Ginger Butternut Squash,** 1 serving | 6 |
| **Ginger Carrot Artichoke,** 1 serving | 2 |
| **Ginger Crab and Corn,** 1 serving | 4 |
| **Golden Summer Tomato,** 1 serving | 1 |
| **Hearty Lamb Barley,** 1 serving | 5 |
| **Hearty Tomato Vegetable,** 1 serving | 2 |
| **Hungarian Beef Goulash,** 1 serving | 5 |
| **Hungarian Wild Mushroom,** 1 serving | 3 |
| **Italian County Chicken with Truffle,** 1 serving | 3 |
| **Italian Lentil with Pastini,** 1 serving | 2 |
| **Italian Tomato and White Bean,** 1 serving | 3 |
| **Italian Vegetable with Rice,** 1 serving | 2 |
| **Italian Wedding Soup,** 1 serving | 4 |
| **Italian White Bean with Escarole,** 1 serving | 5 |
| **Loaded Baked Potato,** 1 serving | 9 |
| **Lobster Bisque,** 1 serving | 5 |
| **Macaroni and Cheese with Beef,** 1 serving | 11 |
| **Manhattan Clam Chowder,** 1 serving | 4 |
| **Maryland Crab,** 1 serving | 3 |
| **Mediterranean Vegetable with Pesto,** 1 serving | 4 |
| **Mexican Chicken Pozole,** 1 serving | 3 |
| **Moroccan Chicken,** 1 serving | 5 |
| **Moroccan Lamb,** 1 serving | 4 |
| **Moroccan Red Lentil,** 1 serving | 4 |
| **Mulligatawny,** 1 serving | 9 |
| **Mushroom Artichoke,** 1 serving | 2 |
| **New England Clam Chowder,** 1 serving | 7 |
| **Old Fashioned Chicken and Dumpling,** 1 serving | 4 |
| **Pasta Bolognese,** 1 serving | 7 |
| **Pasta e Fagioli,** 1 serving | 4 |

| ▲ Power Foods | *PointsPlus*™ value |
|---|---|
| **Pasta Primavera,** 1 serving | 4 |
| **Potato Italian Sausage,** 1 serving | 5 |
| **Potato Wild Mushroom,** 1 serving | 6 |
| **Red Lentil with Cumin and Lemon,** 1 serving | 4 |
| **Rhode Island Clam Chowder,** 1 serving | 6 |
| **Roadhouse Chili,** 1 serving | 6 |
| **Roasted Butternut Squash,** 1 serving | 6 |
| **Roasted Pumpkin Bisque,** 1 serving | 5 |
| **Roasted Vegetable Chowder,** 1 serving | 2 |
| **Roman Tomato Sausage and Pepper,** 1 serving | 4 |
| **Roman Tomato with Pastini,** 1 serving | 3 |
| **Seafood Chowder,** 1 serving | 7 |
| **Seafood Jambalaya,** 1 serving | 4 |
| **Seafood Pot Pie,** 1 serving | 5 |
| **Senegalese Chicken,** 1 serving | 8 |
| **Shrimp and Asparagus Bisque,** 1 serving | 5 |
| **Shrimp and Black Bean Chili,** 1 serving | 6 |
| **Shrimp Bisque,** 1 serving | 7 |
| **Shrimp Creole,** 1 serving | 3 |
| **Sloppy Joe,** 1 serving | 7 |
| **Smoked Turkey Corn Chowder,** 1 serving | 5 |
| **Southwest Chicken Cheddar,** 1 serving | 7 |
| **Southwest Shrimp Corn Chowder,** 1 serving | 6 |
| **Spanish Lentil with Chorizo,** 1 serving | 6 |
| **Spiced Coconut Pumpkin Bisque,** 1 serving | 5 |
| **Spiced Lentil with Spinach,** 1 serving | 4 |

| ▲ Power Foods | *PointsPlus*™ value |
|---|---|
| **Spiced Shrimp and Sweet Potato,** 1 serving | 8 |
| **Spicy Crab and Corn,** 1 serving | 4 |
| **Spicy Shrimp and Vegetables,** 1 serving | 3 |
| **Spinach Artichoke Cheddar,** 1 serving | 9 |
| **Spinach Bisque,** 1 serving | 5 |
| **Spinach Mushroom and Leek,** 1 serving | 2 |
| **Split Pea with Rosemary,** 1 serving | 5 |
| **Split Pea with Smoked Turkey,** 1 serving | 5 |
| **Steak and Potato,** 1 serving | 5 |
| **Summer Beef Vegetable,** 1 serving | 4 |
| **Summer Vegetable,** 1 serving | 2 |
| **Sweet Corn and Tomato Chowder,** 1 serving | 7 |
| **Sweet Corn Chowder,** 1 serving | 9 |
| **Sweet Crab Chowder,** 1 serving | 4 |
| **Sweet Potato Bisque,** 1 serving | 6 |
| **Sweet Potato Chicken Chowder,** 1 serving | 6 |
| **Tailgate Chili,** 1 serving | 8 |
| **Tarragon Chicken,** 1 serving | 5 |
| **Texas Beef Chili,** 1 serving | 7 |
| **Three Bean Chili,** 1 serving | 3 |
| **Tomato Basil with Rice,** 1 serving | 3 |
| **Tomato Bisque,** 1 serving | 5 |
| **Tomato Cheddar,** 1 serving | 10 |
| **Tomato Clam Pennette,** 1 serving | 5 |
| **Tomato Eggplant,** 1 serving | 2 |
| **Tomato Florentine,** 1 serving | 3 |
| **Tomato Lentil,** 1 serving | 3 |
| **Tomato Seafood Bisque,** 1 serving | 6 |
| **Tomato Wild Rice,** 1 serving | 6 |

*Daily Specials (cont'd)*

▲ Power Foods

| | ***PointsPlus***™ value |
|---|---|
| **Tomato Zucchini,** 1 serving | 1 |
| **Tortellini en Brodo with Chicken,** 1 serving | 2 |
| **Tortellini with Wild Mushroom,** 1 serving | 7 |
| **Turkey Chili,** 1 serving | 6 |
| **Turkey Dinner,** 1 serving | 5 |
| **Turkey Pot Pie,** 1 serving | 5 |
| **Turkey Provencal,** 1 serving | 4 |
| **Tuscan Chicken,** 1 serving | 3 |
| **Two Cheddar Chowder w/ Double Smoked Bacon,** 1 serving | 10 |
| **Vegetable Barley,** 1 serving | 3 |
| **Vegetable Jambalaya,** 1 serving | 3 |
| **Vegetarian Black Lentil,** 1 serving | 2 |
| **Vegetarian Split Pea,** 1 serving | 4 |
| **Vegetarian Sweet Corn Chowder,** 1 serving | 7 |
| **Vegetarian Tomato Cheddar,** 1 serving | 10 |
| **White Bean Broccoli SDT,** 1 serving | 4 |
| **Wild Mushroom Barley,** 1 serving | 2 |
| **Wild Mushroom Fagioli,** 1 serving | 4 |
| **Wild Mushroom Lentil,** 1 serving | 3 |
| **Winter Chicken,** 1 serving | 4 |
| **Winter Russian Beef,** 1 serving | 6 |
| **Winter Vegetable,** 1 serving | 3 |
| **Yellow Lentil with Curried Chicken,** 1 serving | 4 |
| **Yucatan Chicken Lime and Orzo,** 1 serving | 4 |
| **Yukon Potato with 4 Cheeses,** 1 serving | 10 |
| **Zucchini Eggplant Chickpea,** 1 serving | 3 |

UARANTEED
LOWEST
RATE!

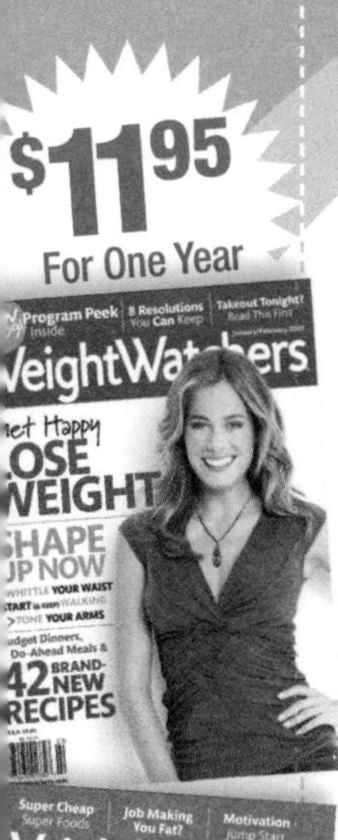


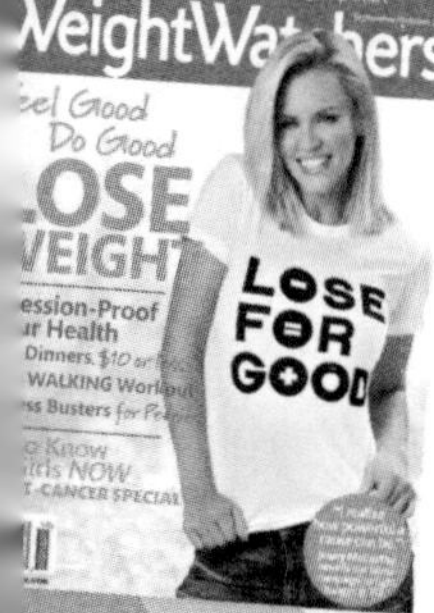


To subscribe call
800-978-2400,visit
WeightWatchers.com/magazine,
r mail attached card today!

eightWatchers

Special Members' Only Rate

# Subscribe & SAVE!

☐ *Yes*, please send me one year (6 issues) of ***Weight Watchers*** Magazine for only $11.95 – that's an incredible 32% savings off the cover price.

☐ **Payment enclosed - $11.95**    ☐ **Please bill me**

NAME (Please print)

ADDRESS APT.#

CITY

STATE ZIP

☐ Please check this box if you wish to receive information or promotional material by e-mail from Weight Watchers International Inc, its subsidiaries or affiliates.

EMAIL U11MEMDG

Please allow 6 to 8 weeks for delivery of first issue. Offer valid in U.S. only. In Canada: a 1-year subscription (6 issues) is $24.95 USD.

WeightWatchers

WHAT HAVE YOU GOT TO LOSE?



**To subscribe call 800-978-2400,
visit www.WeightWatchers.com/magazine,
or mail attached card today!**

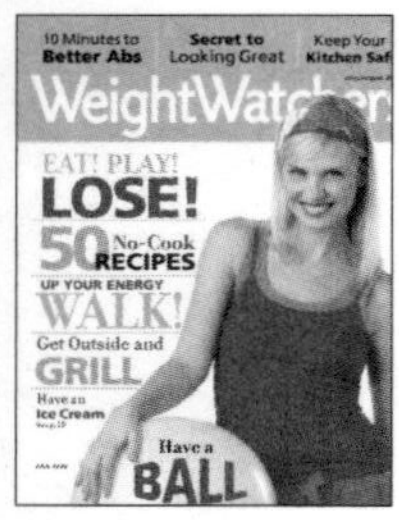

**BUSINESS REPLY MAIL**

FIRST-CLASS MAIL PERMIT NO. 449 RED OAK, IA

POSTAGE WILL BE PAID BY ADDRESSEE

**WeightWatchers**

PO BOX 8569
RED OAK, IA 51591-3569

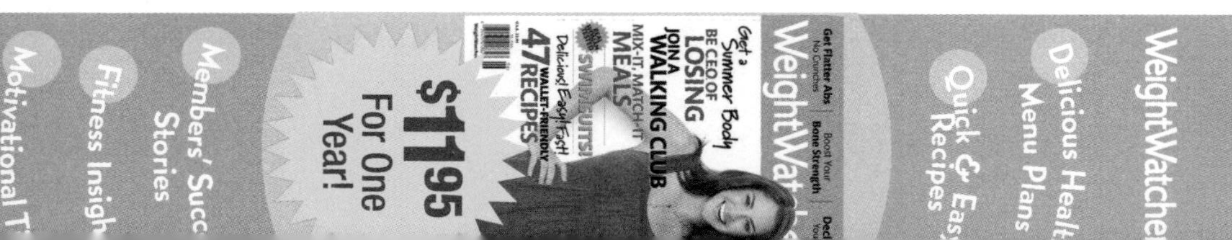

▲ Power Foods — *PointsPlus™* value

## THICKBURGERS & SANDWICHES

|  | PointsPlus™ value |
|---|---|
| **1/3 Lb. Bacon Cheese Thickburger™,** 1 | 25 |
| **1/3 Lb. Cheeseburger,** 1 | 18 |
| **1/3 Lb. Low Carb Thickburger™,** 1 | 11 |
| **1/3 Lb. Mushroom & Swiss™ Thickburger™,** 1 | 19 |
| **1/3 Lb. Original Thickburger™,** 1 | 25 |
| **1/2 Lb. Grilled Sourdough Thickburger™,** 1 | 28 |
| **1/2 Lb. Six Dollar Burger,** 1 | 28 |
| **2/3 Lb. Double Bacon Cheese Thickburger™,** 1 | 35 |
| **2/3 Lb. Double Thickburger™,** 1 | 33 |
| **2/3 Lb. Monster Thickburger™,** 1 | 38 |
| **BBQ Chicken Sandwich,** 1 | 9 |
| **Big Chicken Fillet Sandwich™,** 1 | 21 |
| **Big Hot Ham 'N' Cheese™,** 1 | 14 |
| **Big Roast Beef™ Sandwich,** 1 | 13 |
| **Charbroiled Chicken Club Sandwich,** 1 | 14 |
| **Cheeseburger,** 1 small | 9 |
| **Hamburger,** 1 small | 8 |
| **Hot Dog,** 1 | 11 |
| **Hot Ham 'N' Cheese™ Sandwich,** 1 | 11 |
| **Kid's Meal - Cheeseburger,** 1 | 16 |
| **Kid's Meal - Chicken Strips (no sauce),** 1 | 13 |
| **Kid's Meal - Hamburger,** 1 | 15 |
| **Low Carb Charbroiled Chicken Club Sandwich,** 1 | 10 |
| **Regular Roast Beef Sandwich,** 1 | 9 |
| **Spicy Chicken Sandwich,** 1 | 11 |

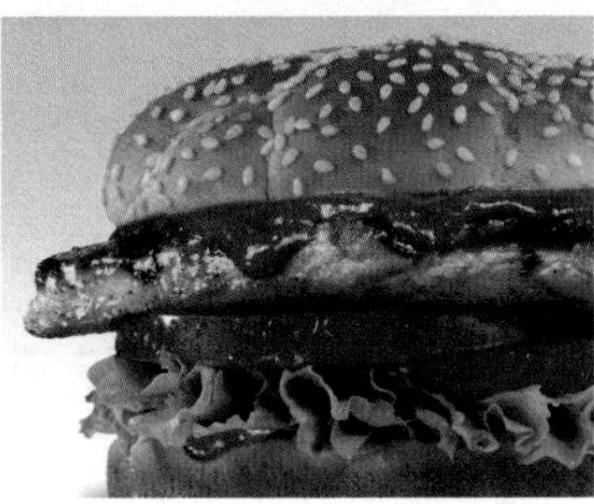

▲ Power Foods — *PointsPlus™* value

## CHICKEN

|  | PointsPlus™ value |
|---|---|
| **Chicken Strips,** 3 pieces | 10 |
| **Chicken Strips,** 5 pieces | 17 |
| **Fried Chicken Breast,** 1 (as served with skin) | 10 |
| **Fried Chicken Leg,** 1 (as served with skin) | 5 |
| **Fried Chicken Thigh,** 1 (as served with skin) | 9 |
| **Fried Chicken Wing,** 1 (as served with skin) | 5 |

## SIDES

|  | PointsPlus™ value |
|---|---|
| **Coleslaw,** 1 small serving | 5 |
| **Crispy Curls™,** 1 small | 9 |
| **Crispy Curls™,** 1 medium | 11 |
| **Crispy Curls™,** 1 large | 13 |
| **Mashed Potatoes, without gravy,** 1 small serving | 2 |
| **Natural Cut French Fries,** 1 small | 9 |
| **Natural Cut French Fries,** 1 medium | 12 |
| **Natural Cut French Fries,** 1 large | 13 |
| **Natural Cut French Fries,** 1 kids serving | 5 |
| **Side Salad (no dressing),** 1 | 3 |

# HARDEE'S®

| ▲ Power Foods | *PointsPlus*™ value |
| --- | --- |
| **BREAKFAST** | |
| **Bacon, Egg & Cheese Biscuit,** 1 | 15 |
| **Big Country® Breakfast Platter - Bacon,** 1 | 26 |
| **Biscuit 'N' Gravy™,** 1 serving | 15 |
| **Biscuit 'N' Gravy™ Breakfast Bowl,** 1 | 21 |
| **Chicken Fillet Biscuit,** 1 | 16 |
| **Cinnamon 'N' Raisin™ Biscuit,** 1 | 8 |
| **Country Ham Biscuit,** 1 | 12 |
| **Country Steak Biscuit,** 1 | 17 |
| **Frisco Breakfast Sandwich®,** 1 | 11 |
| **Ham, Egg and Cheese Biscuit,** 1 | 15 |
| **Jelly Biscuit,** 1 | 12 |
| **Loaded Breakfast Burrito,** 1 | 21 |
| **Loaded Omelet Biscuit,** 1 | 17 |
| **Low Carb Breakfast Bowl®,** 1 | 17 |
| **Made From Scratch™ Biscuit,** 1 | 10 |
| **Monster Biscuit™,** 1 | 19 |
| **Pancakes without Syrup,** 3 | 8 |
| **Pork Chop Biscuit,** 1 | 19 |
| **Sausage & Egg Biscuit,** 1 | 17 |
| **Sausage Biscuit,** 1 | 15 |
| **Sunrise Croissant™ with Ham,** 1 | 12 |
| **BREAKFAST SIDES** | |
| **Grits,** 1 serving | 3 |
| **Hash Rounds™ Potatoes,** 1 small serving | 7 |
| **DESSERTS** | |
| **Apple Turnover,** 1 | 8 |
| **Chocolate Chip Cookie,** 1 | 8 |
| **Hand Scooped Malt,** 1 | 21 |
| **Hand Scooped Shake,** 1 | 19 |
| **Peach Cobbler,** 1 small serving | 8 |
| **Single Scoop Ice Cream Bowl,** 1 | 7 |
| **Single Scoop Ice Cream Cone,** 1 | 8 |

| ▲ Power Foods | *PointsPlus™* value |
|---|---|
| **HIGH TECH BURRITOS** | |
| **Baja Shrimp,** 1 serving | 22 |
| **Breakfast Burrito,** 1 serving | 21 |
| **Breakfast Burrito - Chicken,** 1 serving | 26 |
| **Breakfast Burrito - Pork,** 1 serving | 27 |
| **Breakfast Burrito - Steak,** 1 serving | 26 |
| **Cabo Supreme - Chicken,** 1 serving | 19 |
| **Cabo Supreme - Pork,** 1 serving | 20 |
| **Cabo Supreme - Steak,** 1 serving | 19 |
| **Curry Chicken,** 1 serving | 15 |
| **Godzilla,** 1 serving | 27 |
| **Grilled Fajita - Chicken Breast,** 1 serving | 23 |
| **Grilled Fajita - Steak,** 1 serving | 24 |
| **Hawaiian Teriyaki - Chicken,** 1 serving | 15 |
| **Hawaiian Teriyaki - Steak,** 1 serving | 16 |
| **Low Fat Chicken,** 1 serving | 15 |
| **Spicy Cajun - Chicken Breast,** 1 serving | 24 |
| **Spicy Cajun - Shrimp,** 1 serving | 23 |
| **Surf & Turf,** 1 serving | 24 |
| **Thai Chicken,** 1 serving | 27 |
| **Tuscan Pesto™, Chicken,** 1 serving | 25 |
| **Tuscan Pesto™, Prawn,** 1 serving | 24 |
| **Ya-hoo Bbq - Chicken,** 1 serving | 23 |
| **Ya-hoo Bbq - Pork,** 1 serving | 25 |
| **Ya-hoo Bbq - Steak,** 1 serving | 24 |
| **CLASSIC BURRITOS** | |
| **Carnitas Pork,** 1 serving | 21 |
| **Chicken,** 1 small serving | 14 |
| **Chicken,** 1 regular serving | 23 |
| **Grilled Steak,** 1 serving | 19 |
| **HTB™, Steak & Chicken,** 1 serving | 24 |
| **Large Bean & Cheese,** 1 serving | 23 |

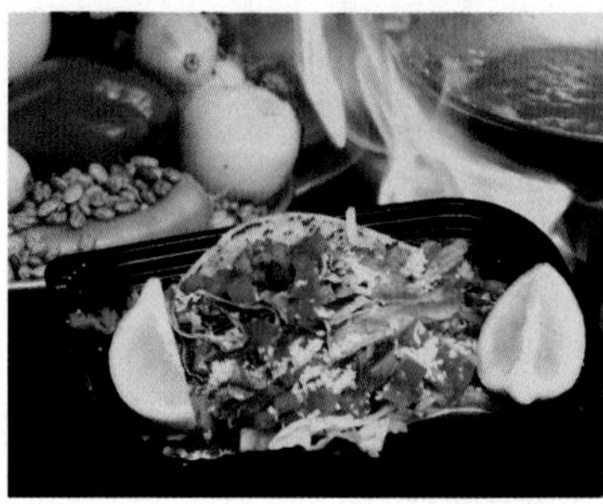

| ▲ Power Foods | *PointsPlus™* value |
|---|---|
| **Pork,** 1 small serving | 14 |
| **Steak,** 1 small serving | 14 |
| **HEALTHLY GRILL** | |
| **Asian Pan Seared Shrimp,** 1 serving | 9 |
| **Braised Tofu,** 1 serving | 13 |
| **California,** 1 serving | 13 |
| **Curry Shrimp,** 1 serving | 11 |
| **Fresh Veggie,** 1 serving | 13 |
| **Grilled Chicken Breast,** 1 serving | 8 |
| **Low Fat Chicken Burrito,** 1 | 14 |
| **Steak Fiesta,** 1 serving | 8 |
| **OTHER STUFF** | |
| **High Tech® Quesadilla,** 1 serving | 22 |
| **TACOS & QUESADILLAS** | |
| **Fish Tacos,** 1 serving | 14 |
| **Street Tacos - Chicken,** 1 serving | 7 |
| **Street Tacos - Pork,** 1 serving | 8 |
| **Street Tacos - Steak,** 1 serving | 7 |
| **Quesadilla - Chicken,** 1 serving | 25 |
| **Quesadilla - No Meat,** 1 serving | 20 |
| **Quesadilla - Pork,** 1 serving | 26 |
| **Quesadilla - Steak,** 1 serving | 25 |

# HIGH TECH BURRITOS

| ▲ Power Foods | *PointsPlus*™ value |
|---|---|
| **KIDS STUFF** | |
| **Burrito Dog,** 1 serving | 16 |
| **Itty Bitty Beanie,** 1 serving | 11 |
| **Itty Bitty Chicken,** 1 serving | 11 |
| **Quesarito,** 1 serving | 11 |
| **SIDES** | |
| **Guacamole, Fresh,** 1 serving | 2 |
| **Mild Salsa,** 1 serving | 0 |

▲ Power Foods — *PointsPlus*™ value

## APPETIZERS

|  | PointsPlus™ value |
|---|---|
| **Blackened Chicken Quesadilla,** 1 serving | 30 |
| **Bruschetta,** 1 serving | 17 |
| **Bruschetta and Shrimp,** 1 serving | 36 |
| **Calamari,** 1 serving | 11 |
| **Chicken Finger - Buffalo Style,** 1 serving | 19 |
| **Chicken Finger - Traditional,** 1 serving | 14 |
| **Chicken Wings - Buffalo Style,** 1 serving | 25 |
| **Chicken Wings - Thai Chile Style,** 1 serving | 30 |
| **Chipotle Chicken Nachos,** 1 serving | 60 |
| **Grilled Vegetable Pizza,** 1 serving | 20 |
| **Jumbo Stuffed Shrooms,** 1 serving | 32 |
| **Lettuce Wraps,** 1 serving | 14 |
| **Miniature Burger Threesome,** 1 serving | 31 |
| **Seared Rare Tuna Wontons,** 1 serving | 9 |
| **Shrimp Cocktail with Cocktail Sauce,** 1 serving | 13 |
| **Spinach Dip with Lavosh Crackers,** 1 serving | 37 |
| **Steamed Mussels with Andouille,** 1 serving | 16 |
| **Add Asian Dipping Sauce,** 1 serving | 1 |
| **Add Bleu Cheese Dressing,** 1 serving | 10 |
| **Add Cocktail Sauce,** 1 serving | 2 |
| **Add Honey Mustard Sauce,** 1 serving | 7 |
| **Add Horseradish Sauce,** 1 serving | 10 |

▲ Power Foods — *PointsPlus*™ value

## OMELETTES, FRITTATAS, PANCAKES & FRENCH TOAST

|  | PointsPlus™ value |
|---|---|
| **Cobb Omelette,** 1 serving | 26 |
| **French Toast,** 1 serving | 33 |
| **Ham and Cheese Omelette,** 1 serving | 25 |
| **Pot Roast Frittata,** 1 serving | 29 |
| **Southwest Frittata,** 1 serving | 31 |
| **Sweet Potato Pancakes,** 1 serving | 23 |
| **Wild Mushroom and Brie Omelette,** 1 serving | 31 |

## BRUNCH

|  | PointsPlus™ value |
|---|---|
| **BBLT,** 1 sandwich | 20 |
| **Smoked Salmon and Pretzel Bread,** 1 serving | 23 |
| **Smoked Salmon Starter,** 1 serving | 5 |

## BRUNCH – SIDE CHOICES

|  | PointsPlus™ value |
|---|---|
| **Bacon,** 1 serving | 3 |
| **Chicken Sausage,** 1 serving | 2 |

## LUNCH ENTRÉES

|  | PointsPlus™ value |
|---|---|
| **Honey Mustard Sauce,** 1 serving | 7 |
| **Lunch Chicken Enchiladas,** 1 serving | 28 |
| **Lunch Chicken Finger Entrée,** 1 serving | 14 |
| **Lunch Crisp Fried Shrimp,** 1 serving | 8 |
| **Lunch Pot Roast,** 1 serving | 12 |
| **Peanut Ginger Slaw,** 1 serving | 6 |

# HOULIHAN'S

▲ Power Foods — *PointsPlus™* value

## LUNCH COMBOS

|  | PointsPlus™ value |
|---|---|
| **Asia Tuna Salad,** 1 small | 17 |
| **BBQ Salmon Salad,** 1 small | 17 |
| **Buffalo Bleu Salad,** 1 small | 26 |
| **Chicken Salad Sandwich Combo,** 1 serving | 11 |
| **Down Home Pot Roast Combo,** 1 serving | 12 |
| **Fish Tacos Combo,** 1 serving | 11 |
| **French Dip Sandwich Combo,** 1 serving | 11 |
| **Fried Shrimp Combo with Fries and Slaw,** 1 serving | 17 |
| **Grilled Chicken Caesar Salad,** 1 small | 20 |
| **Grilled Shrimp Combo (with asparagus and pa),** 1 serving | 11 |
| **Grilled Vegetable Pizza,** 1 serving | 20 |
| **Heartland Chicken Salad - Fried,** 1 small | 24 |
| **Heartland Chicken Salad - Grilled,** 1 small | 18 |
| **Mini Burgers,** 2 burgers | 20 |
| **Southwest Grilled Chicken Wrap Combo,** 1 serving | 12 |
| **Tandoori Chicken Wrap Combo,** 1 serving | 6 |
| **Tillamook Roast Beef Combo,** 1 serving | 9 |
| **Veggie Club Combo,** 1 serving | 7 |
| **Whole Grain Club Sandwich Combo,** 1 sandwich | 10 |

## LUNCH COMBOS – SIDE CHOICES

|  | PointsPlus™ value |
|---|---|
| **Chicken Fingers Combo (with fries and slaw),** 1 serving | 25 |
| **Chipotle Smoked Chicken Enchiladas Combo,** 1 serving | 20 |
| **French Fries,** 1 serving | 7 |
| **Tortilla Chips with Salsa,** 1 serving | 4 |

▲ Power Foods — *PointsPlus™* value

## LUNCH HALF SANDWICH WITH SOUP OR SALAD

|  | PointsPlus™ value |
|---|---|
| **Club Sandwich,** 1 serving | 10 |
| **Fish Tacos,** 1 serving | 12 |
| **French Dip Sandwich,** 1 serving | 13 |
| **Honey Dijon Chicken Salad Sandwich,** 1 serving | 11 |
| **Side Caesar Salad,** 1 serving | 14 |
| **Side House Salad Blue Cheese,** 1 serving | 5 |
| **Side House Salad Cheddar Cheese,** 1 serving | 5 |
| **Southwest Grilled Chicken Wrap,** 1 serving | 12 |
| **Tillamook Beef Sandwich,** 1 serving | 9 |
| **Veggie Club Sandwich,** 1 serving | 7 |

## LUNCH SOUP/SALAD COMBOS

|  | PointsPlus™ value |
|---|---|
| **Entrée Caesar Salad,** 1 serving | 28 |
| **Focaccia Bread,** 1 serving | 4 |
| **French Onion Soup,** 1 serving | 7 |
| **Large House Salad Blue Cheese,** 1 serving | 10 |
| **Large House Salad Cheddar Cheese,** 1 serving | 10 |
| **Large House Salad Cheddar Cheese (with balsamic dressing),** 1 serving | 8 |
| **Large House Salad Cheddar Cheese (with ranch dressing),** 1 serving | 10 |
| **Potato Soup,** 1 serving | 10 |
| **Small Asian Tuna Salad,** 1 serving | 17 |
| **Small BBQ Salmon Salad,** 1 serving | 13 |
| **Small Buffalo Blue Chicken Salad,** 1 serving | 24 |
| **Small Fried Heartland Chicken Salad,** 1 serving | 20 |
| **Small Grilled Chicken Caesar Salad,** 1 serving | 20 |
| **Small Grilled Heartland Chicken Salad,** 1 serving | 15 |
| **Tortilla Soup,** 1 serving | 4 |

| ▲ Power Foods | *PointsPlus*™ value |
|---|---|

## HOMEMADE SOUPS & SIDE SALADS

| | |
|---|---|
| **Caesar Salad,** 1 salad | 14 |
| **House Chop Salad (with bleu cheese),** 1 salad | 5 |
| **House Chop Salad (with cheddar cheese),** 1 salad | 5 |
| **Signature Tuscan Salad,** 1 salad | 9 |
| **Chicken Tortilla Soup,** 1 serving | 4 |
| **French Onion Soup (with provolone & croutons),** 1 serving | 7 |
| **Original Baked Potato Soup,** 1 serving | 10 |
| **Add Balsamic Vinaigrette Dressing,** 1 serving | 4 |
| **Add Ranch Dressing,** 1 serving | 5 |

## SANDWICHES

| | |
|---|---|
| **BBQ Veggie Melt,** 1 sandwich | 18 |
| **Brentwood Chicken Sandwich,** 1 sandwich | 20 |
| **Buffalo Chicken Sandwich,** 1 sandwich | 20 |
| **Build Your Own Burger,** 1 burger | 25 |
| **French Dip,** 1 serving | 25 |
| **Gorgonzola Chicken Sandwich,** 1 sandwich | 20 |
| **Honey Dijon Chicken Salad Sandwich,** 1 sandwich | 21 |
| **Low Carb Burger (with cauli mash & veg),** 1 burger | 22 |
| **Rueben,** 1 sandwich | 28 |
| **Southern California Fish Tacos,** 1 serving | 23 |
| **Southwest Grilled Chicken Wrap,** 1 wrap | 23 |
| **Tillamook Burger,** 1 burger | 32 |
| **Tillamook Roast Beef Sandwich,** 1 sandwich | 18 |
| **Veggie Club Sandwich,** 1 sandwich | 15 |
| **Whole Grain Club Club,** 1 sandwich | 15 |
| **Add Bacon Strips,** 1 serving | 3 |
| **Add Gorgonzola Cheese,** 1 serving | 2 |
| **Add Gouda Cheese,** 1 serving | 4 |
| **Add Provolone Cheese,** 1 serving | 4 |
| **Add Tillamook Cheese,** 1 serving | 5 |

## DINNER ENTRÉES

| | |
|---|---|
| **Almond Crusted Tilapia,** 1 serving | 24 |
| **Asian Noodle Bowl - Chicken,** 1 bowl | 19 |
| **Asian Noodle Bowl - Shrimp,** 1 bowl | 18 |
| **Atlantic Salmon - Mustard Encrusted,** 1 serving | 30 |
| **Atlantic Salmon - Simply Prepared,** 1 serving | 14 |
| **Atlantic Salmon - Wood Grilled,** 1 serving | 20 |
| **Chicken Fettucine Alfredo,** 1 serving | 36 |
| **Chicken Finger Platter,** 1 serving | 31 |
| **Chicken Parmesan,** 1 serving | 36 |
| **Chipotle Smoked Chicken Enchiladas,** 1 serving | 32 |
| **Down Home Pot Roast,** 1 serving | 24 |
| **Filet Mignon,** 1 serving | 34 |
| **Grilled Rosemary Chicken,** 1 serving | 18 |
| **Herb Grilled Chicken,** 1 serving | 12 |
| **Huge Panko Battered Shrimp,** 1 serving | 25 |
| **Jumbo Grilled Shrimp,** 1 serving | 14 |
| **Low Carb Shrimp wth Cauliflower Mashed,** 1 serving | 16 |
| **Meatloaf,** 1 serving | 30 |
| **New York Strip,** 1 serving | 38 |
| **Petite Sirloin,** 5-oz serving | 14 |
| **Prime Top Sirloin,** 5-oz serving | 27 |
| **Prime Top Sirloin,** 9-oz serving | 34 |
| **Prime Top Sirloin,** 10-oz serving | 36 |
| **Seared Scallops with Asparagus Risotto,** 1 serving | 15 |

*Dinner Entrées (cont'd)*

| ▲ Power Foods | *PointsPlus™* value |
|---|---|
| **Shrimp Scampi,** 1 serving | 32 |
| **Sizzling Fajitas - Chicken,** 1 serving | 34 |
| **Sizzling Fajitas - Combo,** 1 serving | 32 |
| **Sizzling Fajitas - Steak,** 1 serving | 37 |
| **Stir Fry - Chicken,** 1 serving | 27 |
| **Stir Fry - Shrimp,** 1 serving | 28 |
| **Stir Fry - Vegetable,** 1 serving | 26 |
| **Stuffed Chicken Breast,** 1 serving | 28 |
| **Tuscany Lemon Chicken Pasta,** 1 serving | 40 |
| **Wild Mushrooom Enchiladas,** 1 serving | 32 |

## ENTRÉE SALADS

| ▲ Power Foods | *PointsPlus™* value |
|---|---|
| **Buffalo Bleu Salad,** 1 salad | 38 |
| **Chicken Asian Chop Chop,** 1 salad | 26 |
| **Chicken Caesar,** 1 salad | 28 |
| **Fire Grilled Salmon Salad,** 1 salad | 31 |
| **Heartland Chicken Salad - Fried,** 1 salad | 36 |
| **Heartland Chicken Salad - Grilled,** 1 salad | 27 |
| **Large House Salad (with bleu cheese, no dressing),** 1 salad | 10 |
| **Large House Salad (with cheddar cheese, no dressing),** 1 salad | 10 |
| **Mandarin Chicken Salad,** 1 salad | 26 |
| **Prime Steak and Wedge Salad,** 1 salad | 37 |
| **Seared Ahi Tuna Salad,** 1 salad | 28 |

## SMALL PLATES (SELECT RESTAURANTS)

| ▲ Power Foods | *PointsPlus™* value |
|---|---|
| **BBQ Chicken Flatbread,** 1 serving | 9 |
| **Chilled Udon Noodles - Tandoori Chicken Skewer,** 1 serving | 10 |
| **Chilled Udon Noodles - Thai Shrimp,** 1 serving | 10 |
| **Chilled Udon Noodles - Vegetable,** 1 serving | 7 |
| **Chipotle Cheese Fries (Truck Stop Fries),** 1 serving | 13 |
| **Creamy Spinach Dip Mini with Tortilla Chips,** 1 serving | 17 |
| **Fried Shrimp Po Boy Sliders - Single,** 1 serving | 6 |
| **Goat Cheese Filled Artichoke Hearts,** 1 serving | 14 |
| **Grilled 4 oz Filet with Arugula Salad,** 1 serving | 12 |
| **Grilled 4 oz Salmon with Watercress Salad,** 1 serving | 8 |
| **Grilled Asparagus Salad,** 1 serving | 7 |
| **Grilled Side of Tandoori Chicken Skewers,** 2 | 3 |
| **Grilled Tandoori Chicken Skewers,** 3 | 6 |
| **Mini Cheese Burger - Single,** 1 serving | 11 |
| **Mini Crisp Fried Shrimp with Cocktail Sauce,** 3 | 6 |
| **Naked Pork Dumpling Skewers,** 5 | 14 |
| **Parmesan French Fries,** 1 serving | 8 |
| **Parmesan French Fries (with three dipping sauces),** 1 serving | 14 |
| **Pasta Bolognese,** 1 serving | 10 |
| **Pickle Fries,** 1 serving | 7 |
| **Pickle Fries (with two dipping sauces),** 1 serving | 15 |
| **Pot Roast Poutine (Disco Fries),** 1 serving | 15 |
| **Pot Roast Sliders - Single,** 1 serving | 7 |
| **Seared Sea Scallops with Watercress Salad,** 1 serving | 8 |
| **Shrimp & Gazpacho Shooters - Single,** 1 serving | 1 |
| **Shrimp Spring Rolls,** 1 serving | 5 |

| ▲ Power Foods | *PointsPlus*™ value |
|---|---|
| **Shrimp Spring Rolls (with three dipping sauces),** 1 serving | 8 |
| **Shroom's,** 3 | 13 |
| **Shroom's (with horseradish sauce),** 3 | 23 |
| **Slow Roasted Pork Flatbread,** 1 serving | 12 |
| **Smoked Pork Sliders - Single,** 1 serving | 8 |
| **Spicy Chicken & Avocado Eggrolls,** 1 serving | 9 |
| **Spicy Chicken & Avocado Eggrolls (with sour cream),** 1 serving | 11 |
| **Tomatillo Shrimp with Corn Tamale Cake,** 1 serving | 8 |
| **White Bean"Hummus",** 1 serving | 12 |
| **White Bean "Hummus" (with grilled pita bread),** 1 serving | 26 |
| **Wild Mushroom & Arugula Flatbread,** 1 serving | 10 |

## SIDES & CONDIMENTS

| ▲ Power Foods | *PointsPlus*™ value |
|---|---|
| **Chipotle Corn,** 1 serving | 8 |
| **Chipotle Ketchup,** 1 1/2 oz | 1 |
| **Cocktail Sauce,** 1 serving | 2 |
| **French Fries,** 1 small serving | 4 |
| **French Green Beans,** 1 serving | 3 |
| **Grey Poupon Mustard,** 1 Tbsp | 0 |
| **Grilled Asparagus,** 1 serving | 1 |
| **Grilled Asparagus with Roasted Tomatillo Vinaigrette,** 1 serving | 1 |
| **Grilled Garlic Zucchini,** 1 serving | 4 |
| **Loaded Baker,** 1 serving | 16 |
| **Mashed Potato,** 1 serving | 8 |
| **Mediterranean Orzo,** 1 serving | 4 |
| **Mediterranean Orzo Salad,** 1 serving | 4 |
| **Mustard,** 1 Tbsp | 0 |
| **Mustard Green Beans,** 1 serving | 3 |
| **Sugar Snap Peas,** 1 serving | 3 |
| **Tortilla Chips & Salsa,** 1 serving | 4 |
| **Tuscan Side Salad,** 1 serving | 9 |
| **Balsamic Dressing,** 1 serving | 4 |
| **Bleu Cheese Dressing,** 3 fl oz | 16 |
| **Creamy Garlic Ranch Dressing,** 2 fl oz | 10 |
| **Creamy Mango Dressing,** 2 fl oz | 7 |
| **Napa Dressing,** 1 1/2 fl oz | 7 |
| **Ranch Dressing,** 1 serving | 5 |
| **Rice Wine Vinaigrette,** 2 fl oz | 8 |

## DESSERTS

| ▲ Power Foods | *PointsPlus*™ value |
|---|---|
| **Bourbon Pecan Pie,** 1 piece | 26 |
| **Cappuccino Cake,** 1 serving | 17 |
| **Caramel Nut Crunch Pie,** 1 piece | 14 |
| **Crème Brulee,** 1 serving | 9 |
| **Italian Style Donuts,** 1 | 31 |
| **Smores,** 1 | 27 |
| **White Chocolate Banana Cream Pie,** 1 piece | 13 |

*Menu items vary by location.*

# HUHOT MONGOLIAN GRILL®

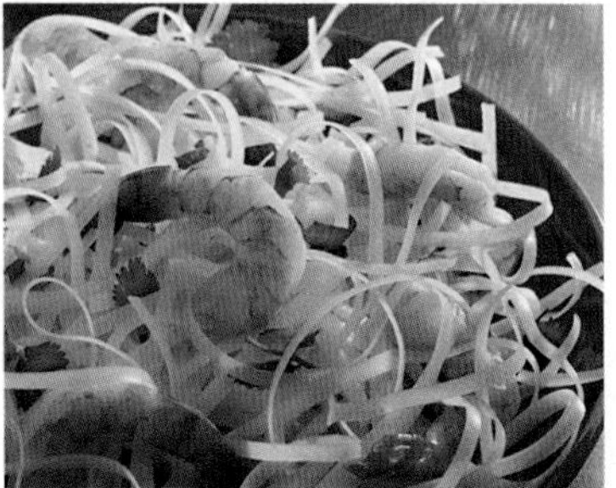

▲ Power Foods

| | *PointsPlus*™ value |
|---|---|
| **MEAT & POULTRY ENTRÉES** | |
| ▲ **Beef,** 1/4 cup | 1 |
| ▲ **Chicken,** 1/4 cup | 1 |
| **Mild Sausage,** 1/4 cup | 3 |
| ▲ **Pork,** 1/4 cup | 1 |
| **Spicy Sausage,** 1/4 cup | 3 |
| **SEAFOOD** | |
| ▲ **Calamari,** 1/4 cup | 1 |
| ▲ **Cod,** 1/4 cup | 1 |
| ▲ **Halibut,** 1/4 cup | 1 |
| ▲ **Krab,** 1/4 cup | 1 |
| ▲ **Mahi Mahi,** 1/4 cup | 1 |
| **Salmon,** 1/4 cup | 2 |
| ▲ **Scallops,** 1/4 cup | 1 |
| ▲ **Shrimp,** 1/4 cup | 1 |
| ▲ **Swordfish,** 1/4 cup | 1 |

▲ Power Foods

| | *PointsPlus*™ value |
|---|---|
| **VEGETABLES** | |
| ▲ **Baby Corn,** 1/4 cup | 0 |
| ▲ **Bamboo Shoots,** 1/4 cup | 0 |
| ▲ **Bean Sprouts,** 1/4 cup | 0 |
| ▲ **Black Beans,** 1/4 cup | 1 |
| ▲ **Broccoli,** 1/4 cup | 0 |
| ▲ **Cabbage,** 1/4 cup | 0 |
| ▲ **Carrots,** 1/4 cup | 0 |
| ▲ **Celery,** 1/4 cup | 0 |
| ▲ **Cilantro,** 1/4 cup | 0 |
| ▲ **Green Peppers,** 1/4 cup | 0 |
| ▲ **Mushrooms,** 1/4 cup | 0 |
| ▲ **Peas,** 1/4 cup | 0 |
| ▲ **Pineapple,** 1/4 cup | 0 |
| ▲ **Red Potatoes,** 1/4 cup | 1 |
| ▲ **Snow Peas,** 1/4 cup | 0 |
| ▲ **Spinach,** 1/4 cup | 0 |
| ▲ **Tofu,** 1/4 cup | 1 |
| ▲ **Tomatoes,** 1/4 cup | 0 |
| ▲ **Water Chestnuts,** 1/4 cup | 0 |
| ▲ **Yellow Onions,** 1/4 cup | 0 |
| ▲ **Yellow Squash,** 1/4 cup | 0 |
| ▲ **Zucchini,** 1/4 cup | 0 |
| **NOODLES & RICE** | |
| **Chinese Noodles,** 1/4 cup | 5 |
| **Pad Thai Noodles,** 1/4 cup | 5 |
| **Yakisoba Noodles,** 1/4 cup | 2 |

| ▲ Power Foods | *PointsPlus*™ value |
|---|---|
| **SALAD DRESSING** | |
| **Asian Vinaigrette,** 1 oz | 6 |
| **SAUCES** | |
| **Bekter's Ginger,** 1 oz | 0 |
| **Black Thai Peanut,** 1 oz | 3 |
| **Burn-Your-Village Barbeque,** 1 oz | 1 |
| **Feed the Hordes Hoisin,** 1 oz | 1 |
| **Five Village Fire Szechuan,** 1 oz | 0 |
| **Khan's Favorite,** 1 oz | 0 |
| **Kung Pao ... Yow!,** 1 oz | 0 |
| **Mean Bean Garlic Sauce,** 1 oz | 0 |
| **Mongol Mustard,** 1 oz | 1 |
| **Not-So-Sweet & Sour,** 1 oz | 1 |
| **Samurai Teriyaki,** 1 oz | 1 |
| **Yellow Belly Curry,** 1 oz | 2 |
| **SOUP** | |
| **Egg Drop Soup,** 8 oz | 1 |
| **Hot & Sour Soup,** 8 oz | 2 |

# IN-N-OUT BURGER®

| ▲ Power Foods | *PointsPlus*™ value |
|---|---|
| **HAMBURGERS** | |
| **Cheeseburger with Onion,** 1 | 13 |
| **Cheeseburger with Onion (with mustard & ketchup instead of spread),** 1 | 11 |
| **Cheeseburger with Onion Protein® Style (bun replaced with lettuce),** 1 | 9 |
| **Double-Double® Burger with Onion,** 1 | 18 |
| **Double-Double® Burger with Onion (with mustard & ketchup instead of spread),** 1 | 16 |
| **Double-Double® Burger with Onion Protein Style (bun replaced with lettuce),** 1 | 14 |
| **Hamburger with Onion,** 1 | 10 |
| **Hamburger with Onion (with mustard & ketchup instead of spread),** 1 | 8 |
| **Hamburger with Onion Protein® Style (bun replaced with lettuce),** 1 | 7 |
| **FRENCH FRIES** | |
| **French Fries,** 1 serving | 11 |
| **SHAKES** | |
| **Chocolate Shake,** 1 | 19 |
| **Strawberry Shake,** 1 | 19 |
| **Vanilla Shake,** 1 | 19 |

▲ Power Foods | *PointsPlus™* value

## START-UPS

| Item | PointsPlus value |
|---|---|
| **Bruschetta,** 1 serving | 17 |
| **Cheese Garlic Pan Bread,** 1 serving | 32 |
| **Goat Cheese Dip,** 1 serving | 25 |
| **Honey Garlic Wing Sauce,** 1 serving | 6 |
| **Jack's Ultimate Nachos, Vegetable,** 1 serving | 44 |
| **Lobster and Crab Dip,** 1 serving | 15 |
| **Mini Pork Souvlaki Pita,** 1 | 11 |
| **Add Fajita Beef Chili,** 1 serving | 2 |

## BETWEEN THE BUNS, BURGERS & SANDWICHES

| Item | PointsPlus value |
|---|---|
| **Chicken Focaccia,** 1 | 14 |
| **Classic Burger,** 1 | 22 |
| **Deluxe Bacon Cheeseburger,** 1 | 30 |
| **Le Montreal Special,** 1 | 8 |
| **Senor Jack's Jalapeno Burger,** 1 | 26 |
| **Smokey Jack's Burger,** 1 | 32 |
| **Topless Steak Sandwich,** 1 | 19 |
| **Shredded Cheddar Cheese,** 1 serving | 6 |
| **Shredded Monterey Jack,** 1 serving | 6 |
| **Shredded Smoked Mozzarella,** 1 serving | 4 |

## CHICKEN FINGER MEAL

| Item | PointsPlus value |
|---|---|
| **With Mild Finger Sauce,** 1 serving | 12 |
| **With Medium Finger Sauce,** 1 serving | 11 |
| **With Hot Finger Sauce,** 1 serving | 12 |
| **With Honey Chili Finger Sauce,** 1 serving | 9 |

▲ Power Foods | *PointsPlus™* value

## MEAT N' GREET

| Item | PointsPlus value |
|---|---|
| **Butter Brushed NY Steak (sides not included),** 1 | 16 |
| **Butter Brushed Sirloin Steak,** 1 | 8 |
| **Jack's Chicago Steak,** 1 | 20 |
| **Pepper Crusted NY Steak,** 1 | 20 |

## PIZZAS

| Item | PointsPlus value |
|---|---|
| **Chicken Club Pizza,** 1 serving | 31 |
| **Dueling Sausage Pizza,** 1 serving | 28 |
| **The Easy Sell Pizza,** 1 serving | 28 |
| **The Opa Pizza,** 1 serving | 28 |

## OLD & NEW FAITHFULS

| Item | PointsPlus value |
|---|---|
| **Beer Battered Fish & Chips,** 1 serving | 43 |
| **Chicken Fajitas (no sauce added),** 1 | 33 |
| **Chicken Fajitas, Lunch,** 1 | 23 |
| **Chicken Parmigana,** 1 serving | 32 |
| **Chicken Santorini,** 1 serving | 33 |
| **Grilled Chicken Rigatoni,** 1 serving | 27 |
| **Grilled Salmon Provencal,** 1 serving | 50 |
| **Parmesan Chicken Bowties,** 1 serving | 39 |
| **Steak Fajitas (no sauce added),** 1 | 35 |
| **Steak Fajitas, Lunch,** 1 | 24 |
| **Vegetable Fajitas (no sauce added),** 1 | 29 |
| **Vegetarian Fajitas, Lunch,** 1 serving | 21 |
| **BBQ Sauce,** 1 serving | 1 |
| **Cajun Spice,** 1 tsp | 0 |
| **Fajita Sauce,** 1 serving | 0 |
| **Red Eye Sauce,** 1 serving | 0 |
| **Teriyaki Sauce,** 1 serving | 1 |

| ▲ Power Foods | *PointsPlus™* value |
|---|---|
| **LUNCH COMBOS / 1/2 PIZZAS** | |
| **Chicken Club 1/2 Pizza,** 1 serving | 16 |
| **Chipotle Chicken Pita,** 1 | 15 |
| **Dueling Sausage 1/2 Pizza,** 1 serving | 14 |
| **Lunch Quesadilla,** 1 | 17 |
| **The Easy Sell 1/2 Pizza,** 1 serving | 14 |
| **The Opa 1/2 Pizza,** 1 serving | 13 |
| **LIGHTER FLARE** | |
| **NY Steak,** 1 | 15 |
| **Vegetable Fajita (no cheese),** 1 lunch portion | 18 |
| **WOK THE WOK** | |
| **Honey Sesame Chicken,** 1 serving | 26 |
| **Kung Pao Chicken,** 1 serving | 29 |
| **Kung Pao Vegetables,** 1 serving | 26 |
| **Kung Pao with Shrimp,** 1 serving | 28 |
| **Pad Thai,** 1 serving | 29 |
| **Pad Thai with Chicken,** 1 serving | 32 |
| **Sambal Oelek for Pad Thai,** 1 serving | 0 |
| **Soy Sauce for Pad Thai,** 1 serving | 0 |
| **Tamarind Chicken,** 1 serving | 42 |
| **Thai Chicken Coconut Curry,** 1 serving | 33 |
| **GET A LEAF** | |
| **Asian Grilled Salmon Salad,** 1 | 14 |
| **Beijing Beef Salad,** 1 | 16 |
| **Ceasar Salad,** 1 | 15 |
| **Chopstick Chicken Salad (no dressing),** 1 | 10 |

| ▲ Power Foods | *PointsPlus™* value |
|---|---|
| **SALAD DRESSINGS** | |
| **Blackberry Balsamic,** 1 serving | 1 |
| **Ginger Dressing,** 1 serving | 3 |
| **Sesame Dressing,** 1 serving | 3 |
| **SOUPS** | |
| **Carrot Soup Bowl,** 1 serving | 6 |
| **Carrot Soup Cup,** 1 serving | 3 |
| **Cheddar Cheese Soup Cup,** 1 serving | 4 |
| **Chicken Orzo Soup Bowl,** 1 serving | 4 |
| **Chicken Orzo Soup Cup,** 1 serving | 2 |
| **Crackers for Soup,** 1 packet | 1 |
| **Italian Wedding Soup Bowl,** 1 serving | 6 |
| **Moroccan Soup,** 1 cup | 1 |
| **Tomato Pepper Bisque,** 1 cup | 4 |
| **Wicked Chicken Soup,** 1 cup | 3 |
| **MISCELLANEOUS SIDES** | |
| **Baked Potato, Loaded,** 1 | 13 |
| **Chicken Focaccia,** 1 serving | 8 |
| **French Fries,** 1 serving | 19 |
| **Garlic Mashed Potatoes,** 1 serving | 9 |
| **Grilled Chicken Breasts (2 x 4 oz Plain),** 1 serving | 5 |
| **Jack's Vegetables,** 1 serving | 7 |
| **Jasmine Rice,** 1 serving | 10 |
| **Ketchup,** 1 serving | 1 |
| **Pork Souvlaki,** 1 | 11 |
| **Salmon Grilled (8 oz plain),** 1 serving | 13 |
| **Top Sirloin Steak (no butter),** 1 | 8 |

| ▲ Power Foods | *PointsPlus*™ value |
|---|---|

## BURGERS & MORE

| | |
|---|---|
| **Bacon Ultimate Cheeseburger,** 1 serving | 25 |
| **Big Cheeseburger,** 1 serving | 16 |
| **Double Bacon 'n' Cheese Ciabatta Burger,** 1 | 31 |
| **Hamburger,** 1 serving | 8 |
| **Hamburger Deluxe,** 1 serving | 10 |
| **Hamburger Deluxe with Cheese,** 1 serving | 12 |
| **Hamburger with Cheese,** 1 serving | 9 |
| **Jumbo Jack,** 1 serving | 15 |
| **Jumbo Jack w/ Cheese,** 1 serving | 17 |
| **Junior Bacon Cheeseburger,** 1 serving | 11 |
| **Mini Sirloin Burgers,** 1 serving | 20 |
| **Single Bacon 'n' Cheese Ciabatta Burger,** 1 | 24 |
| **Sirloin Cheeseburger,** 1 serving | 24 |
| **Sirloin Cheeseburger (with Bacon),** 1 serving | 26 |
| **Sirloin Swiss & Grilled Onions Burger,** 1 serving | 24 |
| **Sirloin Swiss & Grilled Onions Burger (with Bacon),** 1 serving | 26 |
| **Sourdough Jack,** 1 serving | 18 |
| **Sourdough Steak Melt,** 1 serving | 17 |
| **Sourdough Ultimate Cheeseburger,** 1 serving | 24 |
| **Ultimate Cheeseburger,** 1 serving | 24 |

## CHICKEN & FISH

| | |
|---|---|
| **Buffalo Ranch Chicken Mini,** 1 serving | 19 |
| **Chicken Fajita Pita Made with Whole Grain (no salsa),** 1 serving | 8 |
| **Chicken Fajita Pita Made with Whole Grain (with salsa),** 1 serving | 9 |
| **Chicken Sandwich,** 1 serving | 12 |

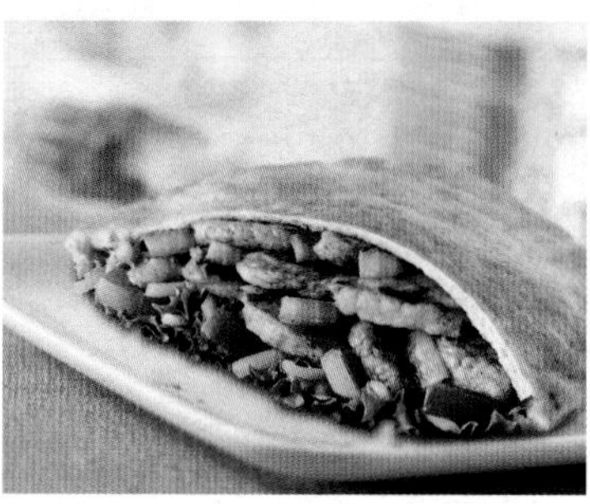

| ▲ Power Foods | *PointsPlus*™ value |
|---|---|
| **Chicken Sandwich with Bacon,** 1 serving | 13 |
| **Chipotle Chicken Ciabatta™ with Grilled Chicken,** 1 | 18 |
| **Chipotle Chicken Ciabatta™ with Spicy Crispy Chicken,** 1 | 20 |
| **Crispy Chicken Breast Strips,** 4 pieces | 15 |
| **Fish and Chips with Large Natural Cut Fries,** 1 serving | 27 |
| **Fish and Chips with Medium Natural Cut Fries,** 1 serving | 22 |
| **Fish and Chips with Small Natural Cut Fries,** 1 serving | 18 |
| **Fish Sandwich,** 1 serving | 12 |
| **Grilled Chicken Strips,** 4 pieces | 6 |
| **Homestyle Ranch Chicken Club,** 1 serving | 19 |
| **Jack's Spicy Chicken,** 1 serving | 15 |
| **Jack's Spicy Chicken (with cheese),** 1 serving | 17 |
| **Sourdough Grilled Chicken Club,** 1 serving | 15 |

## TERIYAKI BOWLS

| | |
|---|---|
| **Chicken Teriyaki Bowl,** 1 serving | 18 |
| **Steak Teriyaki Bowl,** 1 serving | 20 |

| ▲ Power Foods | *PointsPlus™* value |
|---|---|
| **VALUE MENU** | |
| **Two Tacos,** 1 serving | 10 |
| **SALADS** (WITHOUT DRESSING & CONDIMENTS) | |
| **Asian Chicken Salad with Crispy Chicken Strips,** 1 | 8 |
| ▲ **Asian Chicken Salad with Grilled Chicken Strips,** 1 | 4 |
| **Asian Chicken Salad with Spicy Bites,** 1 | 9 |
| **Chicken Club Salad with Crispy Chicken Strips,** 1 serving | 13 |
| **Chicken Club Salad with Grilled Chicken Strips,** 1 serving | 9 |
| **Chicken Club Salad with Spicy Bites,** 1 | 14 |
| **Side Salad,** 1 serving | 1 |
| **Southwest Chicken Salad with Crispy Chicken Strips,** 1 serving | 14 |
| **Southwest Chicken Salad with Grilled Chicken Strips,** 1 serving | 9 |
| **Gourmet Seasoned Croutons,** 1 serving | 4 |
| **Spicy Corn Sticks,** 1 serving | 4 |
| **SAUCES & DRESSINGS** | |
| **Asian Sesame Dressing,** 1 serving | 5 |
| **Bacon Ranch Dressing,** 1 serving | 7 |
| **Barbecue Dipping Sauce,** 1 serving | 1 |
| **Buttermilk House Dipping Sauce,** 2 Tbsp | 4 |
| **Chipotle Sauce,** 1 serving | 3 |
| **Creamy Ranch Sauce,** 1 serving | 2 |
| **Creamy Southwest Dressing,** 1 serving | 6 |
| **Fire Roasted Salsa,** 1 serving | 0 |
| **Frank's Red Hot Sauce,** 1 serving | 0 |
| **Frank's® Red Hot® Buffalo Dipping Sauce,** 1 serving | 0 |
| **Honey Mustard Dipping Sauce,** 1 serving | 2 |
| **Ketchup,** 1 serving | 0 |
| **Lite Ranch Dressing,** 1 serving | 4 |
| **Log Cabin® Syrup,** 1 serving | 5 |
| **Low Fat Balsamic Dressing,** 1 serving | 1 |
| **Mayo-onion,** 1 serving | 3 |
| **Peppercorn Mayo,** 1 serving | 5 |
| **Ranch Dressing,** 1 serving | 9 |
| **Smoky Cheddar Mayo,** 1 serving | 6 |
| **Sweet & Sour Dipping Sauce,** 1 serving | 1 |
| **Tartar Sauce,** 1 serving | 6 |
| **Teriyaki Dipping Sauce,** 1 serving | 2 |
| **Teriyaki Dipping Sauce,** 1 large serving | 3 |
| **Zesty Marinara Sauce,** 1 serving | 0 |
| **KID'S MEALS** | |
| **Applesauce (1 portion cup),** 1 | 3 |
| **Chicken Breast Strips,** 2 | 6 |
| **Crispy Chicken Strips,** 2 pieces | 7 |
| **French Toast Sticks,** 2 pieces | 8 |
| **Grilled Cheese,** 1 serving | 9 |
| **Grilled Chicken Strips,** 2 pieces | 3 |
| **Hamburger,** 1 serving | 8 |
| **Hamburger with Cheese,** 1 serving | 9 |
| **Natural Cut Fries - Kids,** 1 serving | 6 |
| **CONDIMENTS** | |
| **Country Crock® Spread,** 1 packet | 1 |
| **Roasted Slivered Almonds,** 1 serving | 3 |
| **Whipped Topping,** 1 serving | 3 |
| **Wonton Strips,** 1 serving | 3 |

| ▲ Power Foods | *PointsPlus*™ value |
| --- | --- |

## EXTRAS

| | |
| --- | --- |
| **Grape Jelly,** 1 serving | 1 |
| ▲ **Grilled Onions,** 1 serving | 0 |
| **Malt Vinegar,** 1 serving | 0 |
| **Mayonnaise,** 1 serving | 2 |
| **Mustard,** 1 serving | 0 |
| **Pride Margarine Spread,** 1 serving | 1 |
| **Red Onion,** 2 pieces | 0 |
| **Sour Cream,** 1 serving | 2 |
| **Strawberry Jelly,** 1 serving | 1 |
| **Stuffed Jalapeno,** 3 pieces | 6 |
| **Taco Sauce,** 1 serving | 0 |

## SNACKS & SIDES

| | |
| --- | --- |
| **Bacon Cheddar Potato Wedges,** 1 serving | 19 |
| **Beef Taco (regular),** 1 serving | 5 |
| **Egg Roll,** 3 pieces | 12 |
| **Egg Roll,** 1 piece | 4 |
| **Fruit Cup,** 1 serving | 2 |
| **Mozzarella Cheese Sticks,** 3 pieces | 7 |
| **Mozzarella Cheese Sticks,** 6 pieces | 15 |
| **Natural Cut Fries,** 1 small | 9 |
| **Onion Rings,** 8 pieces | 12 |
| **Pita Snack, Crispy Chicken,** 1 serving | 11 |
| **Pita Snack, Fish,** 1 serving | 10 |
| **Pita Snack, Grilled Chicken,** 1 serving | 8 |
| **Pita Snack, Steak,** 1 serving | 9 |
| **Sampler Trio,** 1 serving | 21 |
| **Seasoned Curly Fries,** 1 small | 7 |
| **Stuffed Jalapeños,** 3 pieces | 6 |
| **Stuffed Jalapeños,** 7 pieces | 14 |
| **Taco Nachos with Salsa,** 1 serving | 13 |
| **Taco Nachos without Salsa,** 1 serving | 13 |

| ▲ Power Foods | *PointsPlus*™ value |
| --- | --- |

## BREAKFAST

| | |
| --- | --- |
| **Bacon Breakfast Jack,** 1 serving | 8 |
| **Bacon, Egg & Cheese Biscuit,** 1 serving | 11 |
| **Breakfast Jack,** 1 serving | 7 |
| **Chorizo Sausage Burrito (no salsa),** 1 serving | 19 |
| **Chorizo Sausage Burrito (with salsa),** 1 serving | 19 |
| **Denver Breakfast Bowl,** 1 serving | 21 |
| **Extreme Sausage Sandwich,** 1 serving | 18 |
| **French Toast Sticks,** 4 pieces | 16 |
| **Hash Brown Sticks,** 5 pieces | 8 |
| **Hearty Breakfast Bowl,** 1 serving | 23 |
| **Homestyle Chicken Biscuit,** 1 serving | 15 |
| **Meaty Breakfast Burrito (no salsa),** 1 serving | 16 |
| **Meaty Breakfast Burrito (with salsa),** 1 serving | 17 |
| **Sausage Biscuit,** 1 serving | 13 |
| **Sausage Breakfast Jack,** 1 serving | 12 |
| **Sausage Croissant,** 1 serving | 15 |
| **Sausage, Egg & Cheese Biscuit,** 1 serving | 16 |
| **Sourdough Breakfast Sandwich,** 1 serving | 11 |
| **Spicy Chicken Biscuit,** 1 serving | 15 |
| **Steak & Egg Burrito (no salsa),** 1 serving | 22 |
| **Steak & Egg Burrito (with salsa),** 1 serving | 22 |
| **Supreme Croissant,** 1 serving | 12 |
| **Ultimate Breakfast Sandwich,** 1 serving | 13 |

## SHAKES & DESSERTS

| ▲ Power Foods | *PointsPlus*™ value |
|---|---|
| **Cheesecake,** 1 serving | 8 |
| **Chocolate Ice Cream Shake,** 1 large | 39 |
| **Chocolate Ice Cream Shake,** 1 regular | 21 |
| **Chocolate Overload Cake,** 1 serving | 8 |
| **Chocolate Shake with Whipped Topping,** 1 small | 22 |
| **Egg Nog Shake (seasonal only),** 24 oz | 39 |
| **Egg Nog Shake (seasonal only),** 16 oz | 20 |
| **Mini Churros,** 5 pieces | 9 |
| **Oreo Shake with Whipped Topping,** 1 small | 22 |
| **OREO® Cookie Ice Cream Shake,** 1 large | 39 |
| **OREO® Cookie Ice Cream Shake,** 1 regular | 21 |
| **Strawberry Ice Cream Shake,** 1 regular | 20 |
| **Strawberry Ice Cream Shake,** 1 large | 38 |
| **Strawberry Shake with Whipped Topping,** 1 small | 21 |
| **Vanilla Ice Cream Shake,** 1 large | 35 |
| **Vanilla Ice Cream Shake,** 1 regular | 18 |
| **Vanilla Shake with Whipped Topping,** 1 small | 19 |

## DRINKS

| ▲ Power Foods | *PointsPlus*™ value |
|---|---|
| **Barqs Root Beer,** 1 small | 7 |
| **Caramel Iced Coffee,** 1 small | 3 |
| **Dannon Spring Water,** 1 serving | 0 |
| **Diet Coke,** 1 small | 0 |
| **Dr Pepper,** 1 small | 7 |
| **Fanta Orange,** 1 small | 6 |
| **Fanta Strawberry,** 1 small | 6 |
| **Fresh Brewed Iced Tea,** 1 small | 0 |
| **Mango Flavored Iced Tea,** 24 oz | 2 |
| **Mango Smoothie,** 1 small | 8 |
| **Minute Maid Lemonade,** 1 small | 6 |
| **Minute Maid Orange Juice,** 10 fl oz | 4 |
| **Original Iced Coffee,** 1 small | 3 |
| **Peach Flavored Iced Tea,** 24 oz | 2 |
| **Raspberry Flavored Iced Tea,** 24 oz | 2 |
| **Regular Coke,** 1 small | 7 |
| **Smoothie, Orange Sunrise,** 16 fl oz | 8 |
| **Sprite,** 1 small | 6 |
| **Strawberry Banana Smoothie,** 1 small | 8 |
| **Tropical Smoothie,** 16 fl oz | 9 |
| **Tropical Smoothie,** 24 fl oz | 13 |
| **Vanilla Iced Coffee,** 1 small | 3 |

| ▲ Power Foods | *PointsPlus™* value |
|---|---|
| **BLENDED WITH A PURPOSE™** | |
| **Acai Super-Antioxidant™,** 16 fl oz | 7 |
| **Mango Metabolizer™,** 16 fl oz | 8 |
| **Pomegranate Heart Happy™,** 16 fl oz | 8 |
| **Protein Berry Workout™ with Soy,** 16 fl oz | 7 |
| **Protein Berry Workout™ with Whey,** 16 fl oz | 7 |
| **Strawberry Energizer™,** 16 fl oz | 7 |
| **Strawberry Nirvana®,** 16 fl oz | 4 |
| **The Coldbuster®,** 16 fl oz | 6 |
| **BREAKFAST BLENDS** | |
| **Mango Peach Topper,** 1 | 10 |
| **Orange Carrot Banana,** 1 | 4 |
| **Orange Mango Passion,** 1 | 4 |
| **CLASSICS** | |
| **Aloha Pineapple®,** 16 fl oz | 8 |
| **Banana Berry™,** 16 fl oz | 7 |
| **Caribbean Passion®,** 16 fl oz | 6 |
| **Mango-A-Go-Go®,** 16 fl oz | 7 |
| **Peach Pleasure®,** 16 fl oz | 7 |
| **Pomegranate Pick-Me-Up™,** 16 fl oz | 7 |
| **Razzmatazz®,** 16 fl oz | 7 |
| **Strawberries Wild®,** 16 fl oz | 7 |
| **Strawberry Surf Rider™,** 16 fl oz | 8 |

| ▲ Power Foods | *PointsPlus™* value |
|---|---|
| **FRESH SQUEEZED JUICES** | |
| **Carrot Juice,** 16 fl oz | 4 |
| **Orange Juice,** 16 fl oz | 6 |
| **HOT OATMEAL** | |
| **Apple Cinnamon Oatmeal,** 1 bowl | 8 |
| **Blueberry & Blackberry Oatmeal,** 1 bowl | 8 |
| **Brown Sugar Oatmeal,** 1 bowl | 6 |
| **Fresh Banana Oatmeal,** 1 bowl | 8 |
| **JAMBA ALL FRUIT™** | |
| **Mega Mango™,** 16 fl oz | 6 |
| **Peach Perfection™,** 16 fl oz | 6 |
| **Pomegranate Paradise™,** 16 fl oz | 6 |
| **Strawberry Whirl™,** 16 fl oz | 6 |
| **JAMBA LIGHT™** | |
| **Berry Fulfulling®,** 16 fl oz | 4 |
| **Mango Mantra®,** 16 fl oz | 4 |

# JERSEY MIKE'S® SUBS

| ▲ Power Foods | *PointsPlus™* value |
|---|---|
| **COLD SUBS** (DOES NOT INCLUDE VINEGAR, OIL OR MAYONNAISE) | |
| **#2 Jersey Shore Favorite in a Tub,** 1 | 7 |
| **#2 Jersey Shore Favorite on Wheat,** 1 mini | 8 |
| **#2 Jersey Shore Favorite on White,** 1 mini | 9 |
| **#3 American Classic in a Tub,** 1 | 7 |
| **#3 American Classic on Wheat,** 1 mini | 8 |
| **#3 American Classic on White,** 1 mini | 9 |
| **#5 Super Sub in a Tub,** 1 | 8 |
| **#5 Super Sub on Wheat,** 1 mini | 9 |
| **#5 Super Sub on White,** 1 mini | 9 |
| **#6 Roast Beef & Provolone in a Tub,** 1 | 11 |
| **#6 Roast Beef & Provolone on Wheat,** 1 mini | 11 |
| **#6 Roast Beef & Provolone on White,** 1 mini | 11 |
| **#7 Turkey Breast & Provolone in a Tub,** 1 | 6 |
| **#7 Turkey Breast & Provolone on Wheat,** 1 mini | 8 |
| **#7 Turkey Breast & Provolone on White,** 1 mini | 8 |
| **#8 Club Sub with Mayonnaise in a Tub,** 1 | 16 |
| **#8 Club Sub with Mayonnaise on Wheat,** 1 mini | 13 |
| **#8 Club Sub with Mayonnaise on White,** 1 mini | 14 |
| **#9 Club Supreme with Mayonnaise in a Tub,** 1 | 17 |
| **#9 Club Supreme with Mayonnaise on Wheat,** 1 mini | 14 |
| **#9 Club Supreme with Mayonnaise on White,** 1 mini | 15 |
| **#10 Albacore Tuna in a Tub,** 1 | 17 |
| **#10 Albacore Tuna on Wheat,** 1 mini | 14 |
| **#10 Albacore Tuna on White,** 1 mini | 15 |
| **#13 Original Italian in a Tub,** 1 | 10 |
| **#13 Original Italian on Wheat,** 1 mini | 11 |
| **#13 Original Italian on White,** 1 mini | 11 |
| **#14 Veggie in a Tub,** 1 | 12 |
| **#14 Veggie on Wheat,** 1 regular | 18 |
| **#14 Veggie on White,** 1 regular | 19 |
| **HOT SUBS** | |
| **#15 Meatball & Cheese on Wheat,** 1 regular | 23 |
| **#15 Meatball & Cheese on White,** 1 regular | 23 |
| **#17 Chicken Philly on Wheat,** 1 regular | 15 |
| **#17 Chicken Philly on White,** 1 regular | 16 |
| **#17 Steak Philly on Wheat,** 1 regular | 15 |
| **#17 Steak Philly on White,** 1 regular | 15 |
| **#18 Chicken Parmesan on Wheat,** 1 regular | 16 |
| **#18 Chicken Parmesan on White,** 1 regular | 16 |
| **#18 Grilled Chicken on Wheat,** 1 regular | 16 |
| **#18 Grilled Chicken on White,** 1 regular | 17 |
| **#19 BBQ Beef on Wheat,** 1 regular | 17 |
| **#19 BBQ Beef on White,** 1 regular | 18 |
| **#20 Pastrami & Swiss on Wheat,** 1 regular | 14 |

| ▲ Power Foods | *PointsPlus*™ value |
|---|---|
| **#20 Pastrami & Swiss on White,** 1 regular | 14 |
| **#20 Reuben on Wheat,** 1 regular | 17 |
| **#20 Reuben on White,** 1 regular | 18 |
| **#43 Chipotle Chicken on Wheat,** 1 regular | 24 |
| **#43 Chipotle Chicken on White,** 1 regular | 24 |
| **#43 Chipotle Steak on Wheat,** 1 regular | 23 |
| **#43 Chipotle Steak on White,** 1 regular | 24 |
| **#56 Big Hahuna Chicken on White,** 1 regular | 17 |
| **#56 Big Kahuna Chicken on Wheat,** 1 regular | 17 |
| **#56 Big Kahuna Steak on Wheat,** 1 regular | 16 |
| **#56 Big Kahuna Steak on White,** 1 regular | 17 |

## CONDIMENTS

| | |
|---|---|
| **Mayonnaise for Mini Sandwich,** 1 serving | 4 |
| **Mayonnaise for Regular Sandwich or Tub,** 1 serving | 7 |
| **Oil for Mini Sandwich,** 1 serving | 4 |
| **Oil for Regular Sandwich or Tub,** 1 serving | 8 |
| **Sprinkles (Mayonnaise, Vinegar & Oil) for Regular Sandwich or Tub,** 1 serving | 15 |
| **Sprinklings (Mayonnaise, Vinegar & Oil) for Mini Sandwich,** 1 serving | 8 |

# JET'S PIZZA®

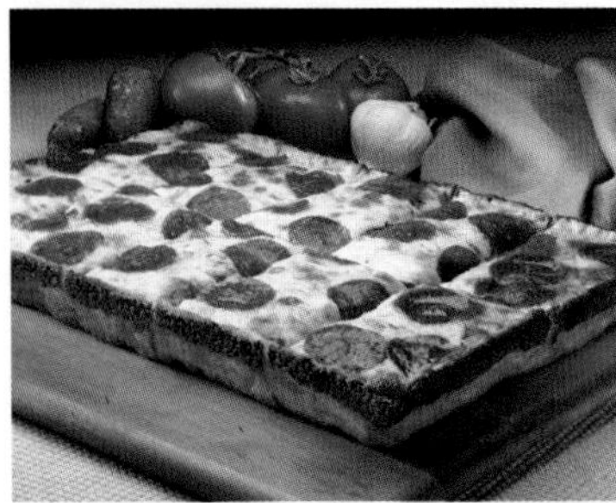

| ▲ Power Foods | *PointsPlus*™ value |
|---|---|
| **PIZZA** | |
| **Large 8 Corner Pizza,** 1/10 of the 14" | 12 |
| **Large Bold Fold Pizza,** 1/10 of the 14" | 8 |
| **Large Ham/Cheese Pizza,** 1/10 of the 14" | 8 |
| **Large Mild Pepper/Cheese Pizza,** 1/10 of the 14" | 8 |
| **Large Mushroom/Cheese Pizza,** 1/10 of the 14" | 8 |
| **Large Onion/Cheese Pizza,** 1/10 of the 14" | 8 |
| **Large Pineapple/Cheese Pizza,** 1/10 of the 14" | 8 |
| **Large Round Bacon & Cheese Pizza,** 1/10 of the 14" | 8 |
| **Large Round BBQ Chicken Pizza,** 1/10 of the 14" | 9 |
| **Large Round Cheese & Pepperoni Pizza,** 1/10 of the 14" | 11 |
| **Large Round Cheese Pizza,** 1/10 of the 14" | 8 |
| **Large Round Grilled Chicken Pizza,** 1/10 of the 14" | 8 |

| ▲ Power Foods | *PointsPlus*™ value |
|---|---|
| **Large Round Pepperoni, Mushroom, Sausage & Cheese Pizza,** 1/10 of the 14" | 10 |
| **Large Sausage/Cheese Pizza,** 1/10 of the 14" | 9 |
| **Large Square Cheese & Pepperoni Pizza,** 1/10 of the 14" | 14 |
| **Large Square Grilled Chicken Pizza,** 1/10 of the 14" | 10 |
| **Large Thin Cheese Pizza,** 1/10 of the 14" | 5 |
| **Large Thin Crust Cheese & Ham Pizza,** 1/10 of the 14" | 5 |
| **Large Thin Crust Cheese & Mushroom Pizza,** 1/10 of the 14" | 5 |
| **Large Thin Crust Cheese & Pepperoni Pizza,** 1/10 of the 14" | 5 |
| **Large Thin Crust Cheese, Ham, Mushroom Pizza,** 1/10 of the 14" | 5 |
| **Large Thin Crust Cheese/Pepperoni/Mushroom Pizza,** 1/10 of the 14" | 5 |
| **Large Thin Crust Mushroom, Cheeseless Pizza,** 1/10 of the 14" | 3 |
| **Medium Round Chicken Parmesan Pizza,** 1/8 of the 12" | 7 |
| **Small Round BBQ Chicken Pizza,** 1/6 of the 10" | 7 |
| **Small Round Cheeseless Pizza,** 1/6 of the 10" | 5 |
| **Small Round Veggie Pizza,** 1/6 of the 10" | 7 |
| **Small Square BBQ Chicken Pizza,** 1/6 of the 10" | 7 |
| **Small Thin BBQ Chicken Pizza,** 1/6 of the 10" | 5 |
| **Small Thin Cheese/Meat Pizza,** 1/6 of the 10" | 6 |

| ▲ Power Foods | *PointsPlus*™ value |
|---|---|
| **SUBS (8")** | |
| **Italian Sub with Fat Free Italian Dressing,** 1 | 16 |
| **Pizza Sub,** 1 | 22 |
| **Steak Sub with Fat Free Italian Dressing,** 1 | 18 |
| **Vegetarian Sub (no dressing),** 1 | 17 |
| **Vegetarian Sub (with fat free Italian dressing),** 1 | 17 |
| **Vegetarian Sub (with Italian dressing),** 1 | 21 |
| **JET'S BOATS** | |
| **Jet Boat,** 1 | 43 |
| **Steak/Cheese Deli Boat,** 1 | 45 |
| **Tuna Deli Boat,** 1 | 23 |
| **SALADS** | |
| **Personal Antipasto Salad (no dressing),** 1 | 7 |
| **Small Antipasto Salad (no dressing),** 1 | 14 |
| **Small Chicken Salad (no dressing),** 1 | 9 |
| **Small Garden Salad (no dressing),** 1 | 3 |
| **Small Tuna Salad,** 1 | 13 |
| **BREAD** | |
| **Large Jet Bread,** 1 serving | 6 |
| **Large Jet Bread with Bacon,** 1 serving | 6 |
| **Large Jet Bread with Pepperoni,** 1 serving | 6 |
| **Turbo Stix,** 1 serving | 4 |

# JOE'S CRAB SHACK

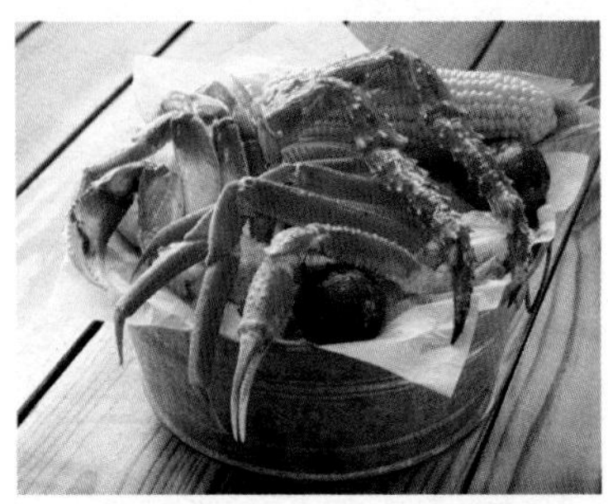

| ▲ Power Foods | ***PointsPlus™*** value |
|---|---|
| **APPETIZERS** | |
| **Bucket of Shrimp (12),** 1 serving | 0 |
| **SALADS** | |
| **Caesar Salad (without dressing),** 1 serving | 0 |
| **Chicken Caesar Salad (without dressing),** 1 serving | 11 |
| **Crab Cake Caesar Salad (without dressing),** 1 serving | 0 |
| **Shrimp Caesar Salad (without dressing),** 1 serving | 8 |

| ▲ Power Foods | ***PointsPlus™*** value |
|---|---|
| **ENTRÉES** | |
| **Blackened Tilapia without Sides,** 1 serving | 19 |
| **Crab Daddy Feast without Sides,** 1 serving | 14 |
| **Dungeness Crab without Sides,** 1 serving | 15 |
| **Grilled Malibu Shrimp without Sides,** 1 serving | 14 |
| **King Crab without Sides,** 1 serving | 14 |
| **Maui Mahi with Rice and Vegetable of the Day,** 1 serving | 14 |
| ▲ **Maui Mahi without Sides,** 1 serving | 7 |
| **Snow Crab without Sides,** 1 serving | 13 |
| **Wood Grilled Sunset Salmon without Sides,** 1 serving | 14 |
| **FLAVORING** | |
| **BBQ Crab Flavoring,** 1 serving | 0 |
| **Garlic Crab Flavoring,** 1 serving | 0 |
| **Spicy Boil Crab Flavoring,** 1 serving | 0 |

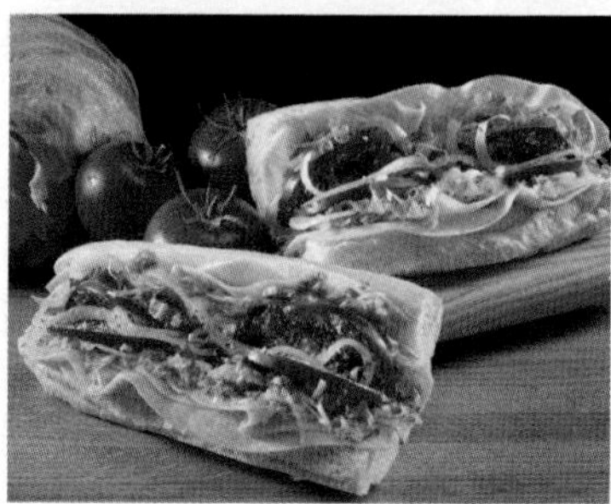

▲ Power Foods — *PointsPlus*™ value

## LOWER FAT CHOICES

|  | PointsPlus™ value |
|---|---|
| **Ham Sub on Wheat,** 1/2 | 5 |
| **Ham Sub on White,** 1/2 | 6 |
| **Roast Beef Sub on Wheat,** 1/2 | 6 |
| **Roast Beef Sub on White,** 1/2 | 6 |
| **Turkey Breast Sub on Wheat,** 1/2 | 6 |
| **Turkey Breast Sub on White,** 1/2 | 6 |

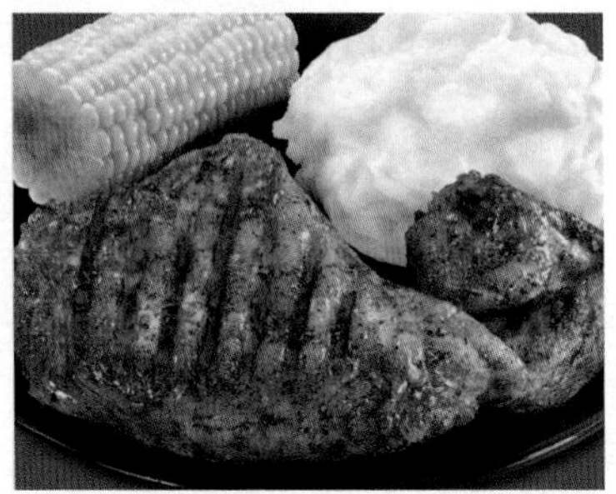

▲ Power Foods — *PointsPlus*™ value

## ORIGINAL RECIPE® CHICKEN

| Item | PointsPlus value |
|---|---|
| **Breast,** 1 (as served with skin) | 10 |
| ▲ **Breast (without skin or breading),** 1 | 3 |
| **Drumstick,** 1 (as served with skin) | 3 |
| **Thigh,** 1 (as served with skin) | 7 |
| **Whole Wing,** 1 (as served with skin) | 3 |

## EXTRA CRISPY™ CHICKEN

| Item | PointsPlus value |
|---|---|
| **Breast,** 1 (as served with skin) | 13 |
| **Drumstick,** 1 (as served with skin) | 4 |
| **Thigh,** 1 (as served with skin) | 10 |
| **Whole Wing,** 1 (as served with skin) | 4 |

## GRILLED CHICKEN

| Item | PointsPlus value |
|---|---|
| **Breast,** 1 breast | 4 |
| **Drumstick,** 1 drumstick | 2 |
| **Thigh,** 1 thigh | 4 |
| **Whole Wing,** 1 wing | 2 |

▲ Power Foods — *PointsPlus*™ value

## CRISPY STRIPS

| Item | PointsPlus value |
|---|---|
| **Crispy Strips®,** 3 | 10 |
| **Original Recipe® Strips,** 2 | 5 |
| **Original Recipe® Strips,** 3 | 8 |

## HOT & SPICY CHICKEN

| Item | PointsPlus value |
|---|---|
| **Breast,** 1 (as served with skin) | 12 |
| **Drumstick,** 1 (as served with skin) | 4 |
| **Thigh,** 1 (as served with skin) | 10 |
| **Whole Wing,** 1 (as served with skin) | 4 |

## POPCORN CHICKEN

| Item | PointsPlus value |
|---|---|
| **Popcorn Chicken,** 1 individual serving | 11 |
| **Popcorn Chicken,** 1 large serving | 15 |
| **Popcorn Chicken - Kids,** 1 serving | 8 |

## POT PIES & BOWLS

| Item | PointsPlus value |
|---|---|
| **Chicken and Biscuit Bowl,** 1 | 23 |
| **Chicken Pot Pie,** 1 | 19 |
| **Fiery Buffalo Hot Wings™ Snack Box,** 1 serving | 13 |
| **Honey BBQ Wings™ Snack Box,** 1 serving | 14 |
| **Hot Wings™ Snack Box,** 1 serving | 13 |
| **KFC Famous Bowls® - Mashed Potato with Gravy,** 1 serving | 18 |
| **KFC Famous Bowls® - Rice and Gravy,** 1 serving | 21 |
| **Popcorn Chicken Snack Box,** 1 serving | 18 |
| **Snack Bowl,** 1 | 8 |

| ▲ Power Foods | *PointsPlus*™ value |
|---|---|

## WINGS

| | |
|---|---|
| **Boneless Fiery Buffalo Wings,** 1 | 2 |
| **Boneless Honey BBQ Wings,** 1 | 2 |
| **Boneless Teriyaki Wings,** 1 | 2 |
| **Fiery Buffalo Hot Wings™,** 1 | 2 |
| **Fiery Buffalo Wings,** 1 | 2 |
| **Honey BBQ Hot Wings™,** 1 | 2 |
| **Honey BBQ Wings,** 1 | 2 |
| **Hot Wings®,** 1 | 2 |
| **Teriyaki Wings,** 1 | 2 |

## OTHER CHICKEN DISHES

| | |
|---|---|
| **Country Fried Steak with Peppered White Gravy,** 1 serving | 10 |
| **Country Fried Steak without Peppered White Gravy,** 1 serving | 10 |
| **KFC® Gizzards,** 1 serving | 5 |
| **KFC® Kentucky Nuggets®,** 1 | 1 |
| **KFC® Livers,** 1 serving | 5 |

## SANDWICHES & WRAPS

| | |
|---|---|
| **Chicken Little,** 1 | 5 |
| **Crispy Twister® with Crispy Strip,** 1 | 15 |
| **Crispy Twister® with Crispy Strip without Sauce,** 1 | 13 |
| **Crispy Twister® with Original Recipe® Strip without Sauce,** 1 | 11 |
| **Crispy Twister® with Original Strip,** 1 | 14 |
| **Double Crunch Sandwich with Crispy Strip,** 1 | 13 |
| **Double Crunch Sandwich with Crispy Strip without Sauce,** 1 | 10 |
| **Double Crunch Sandwich with Original Recipe® Strip without Sauce,** 1 | 9 |
| **Double Crunch™ Sandwich with Original Strip,** 1 | 12 |
| **Honey BBQ Sandwich,** 1 | 8 |
| **KFC Snacker® with Crispy Strip,** 1 | 8 |
| **KFC Snacker® with Crispy Strip without Sauce,** 1 | 7 |
| **KFC Snacker® with Crispy Strip, Buffalo,** 1 | 7 |
| **KFC Snacker® with Crispy Strip, Ultimate Cheese,** 1 | 7 |
| **KFC Snacker® with Original Recipe® Strip without Sauce,** 1 | 6 |
| **KFC Snacker® with Original Strip,** 1 | 7 |
| **KFC Snacker® with Original Strip, Buffalo,** 1 | 6 |
| **KFC Snacker® with Original Strip, Ultimate Cheese,** 1 | 7 |
| **KFC Snacker®, Fish,** 1 | 8 |
| **KFC Snacker®, Fish without Sauce,** 1 | 8 |
| **KFC Snacker®, Honey BBQ,** 1 | 5 |
| **Original Recipe® Filet Sandwich,** 1 | 12 |
| **Original Recipe® Filet Sandwich, without sauce,** 1 | 9 |
| **Oven Roasted Twister®, without Sauce,** 1 | 8 |
| **Tender Roast Twister®,** 1 | 12 |
| **Tender Roast Twister® without Sauce,** 1 | 9 |
| **Tender Roast® Sandwich,** 1 | 10 |
| **Tender Roast® Sandwich, without sauce,** 1 | 7 |
| **Toasted Wrap with Crispy Strip,** 1 | 9 |

*Sandwiches & Wraps (cont'd)*

| ▲ Power Foods | *PointsPlus™* value |
|---|---|
| **Toasted Wrap with Crispy Strip,** 1 | 9 |
| **Toasted Wrap with Crispy Strip without Sauce,** 1 | 8 |
| **Toasted Wrap with Original Recipe® Strip,** 1 | 9 |
| **Toasted Wrap with Original Recipe® Strip without Sauce,** 1 | 7 |
| **Toasted Wrap with Tender Roast® Fillet,** 1 | 8 |
| **Toasted Wrap with Tender Roast® Fillet without Sauce,** 1 | 7 |

## SALADS

| ▲ Power Foods | *PointsPlus™* value |
|---|---|
| **Caesar Side Salad without Dressing & Croutons,** 1 serving | 1 |
| **Crispy Chicken BLT Salad without Dressing,** 1 serving | 9 |
| **Crispy Chicken Caesar Salad without Dressing & Croutons,** 1 serving | 9 |
| ▲ **House Side Salad without Dressing,** 1 serving | 0 |
| **Original Recipe® Chicken BLT Salad without Dressing,** 1 | 8 |
| **Original Recipe® Chicken Caesar Salad without Dressing & Croutons,** 1 | 7 |
| **Parmesan Garlic Croutons Pouch,** 1 serving | 2 |
| **Roasted Chicken BLT Salad without Dressing,** 1 serving | 5 |
| **Roasted Chicken Caesar Salad without Dressing & Croutons,** 1 serving | 5 |

## SALAD DRESSINGS

| ▲ Power Foods | *PointsPlus™* value |
|---|---|
| **Heinz Buttermilk Ranch Dressing,** 1 serving | 4 |
| **Hidden Valley® The Original Ranch® Fat Free Dressing,** 1 serving | 1 |
| **KFC® Creamy Parmesan Caesar Dressing,** 1 serving | 7 |
| **Marzetti Light Italian Dressing,** 1 serving | 0 |

## SIDES

| ▲ Power Foods | *PointsPlus™* value |
|---|---|
| **BBQ Baked Beans,** 1 serving | 5 |
| **Biscuit,** 1 | 5 |
| **Cole Slaw,** 1 serving | 5 |
| ▲ **Corn on the Cob,** 1 (3") | 2 |
| ▲ **Corn on the Cob,** 1 (5 1/2") | 4 |
| ▲ **Green Beans,** 1 serving | 0 |
| **Jalapeno Peppers,** 1 serving | 0 |
| **KFC® Cornbread Muffin,** 1 | 6 |
| ▲ **KFC® Mean Greens®,** 1 serving | 0 |
| **KFC® Red Beans with Sausage and Rice,** 1 serving | 5 |
| **Macaroni & Cheese,** 1 serving | 5 |
| **Macaroni Salad,** 1 serving | 5 |
| **Mashed Potatoes with Gravy,** 1 serving | 3 |
| **Mashed Potatoes without Gravy,** 1 serving | 3 |
| **Potato Salad,** 1 serving | 5 |
| **Potato Wedges,** 1 serving | 7 |
| **Seasoned Rice,** 1 serving | 4 |
| ▲ **Sweet Kernel Corn,** 1 serving | 3 |
| **Three Bean Salad,** 1 serving | 2 |

▲ Power Foods — *PointsPlus*™ value

## DIPPING SAUCES

| Item | PointsPlus™ value |
| --- | --- |
| **Creamy Ranch Dipping Sauce,** 1 serving | 4 |
| **Fiery Buffalo Dipping Sauce,** 1 serving | 1 |
| **Garlic Parmesan Dipping Sauce,** 1 serving | 4 |
| **Honey BBQ Dipping Sauce,** 1 serving | 1 |
| **Honey Mustard Dipping Sauce,** 1 serving | 3 |
| **Sweet and Sour Dipping Sauce,** 1 serving | 1 |

## DESSERTS

| Item | PointsPlus™ value |
| --- | --- |
| **Apple Turnover,** 1 | 7 |
| **Café Valley Bakery® Chocolate Chip Cake,** 1 slice (6 slices per cake) | 8 |
| **Cookie Dough Pie,** 1 slice | 7 |
| **Dutch Apple Pie,** 1 slice | 9 |
| **Lemon Meringue Pie Slice,** 1 slice | 7 |
| **Little Bucket™ Chocolate Crème Parfait Cup,** 1 | 8 |
| **Little Bucket™ Lemon Crème Parfait Cup,** 1 | 11 |
| **Little Bucket™ Strawberry Shortcake Parfait Cup,** 1 | 6 |
| **Pecan Pie,** 1 slice | 11 |
| **Sara Lee® Sweet Potato Pie Slice,** 1 slice | 10 |
| **Sarah Lee® Apple Pie Slice,** 1 slice | 9 |
| **Sarah Lee® Pecan Pie Slice,** 1 slice | 13 |
| **Strawberry Cream Cheese,** 1 slice | 7 |
| **Sweet Life® Chocolate Chip Cookie,** 1 | 5 |
| **Sweet Life® Oatmeal Raisin Cookie,** 1 | 4 |
| **Sweet Life® Sugar Cookie,** 1 | 4 |
| **Teddy Grahams®, Graham Snacks, Cinnamon,** 1 serving | 2 |

# KOLACHE FACTORY

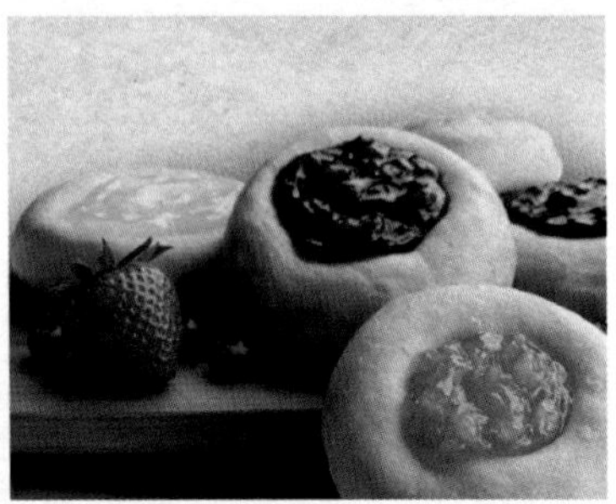

▲ Power Foods — *PointsPlus*™ value

## KOLACHES

|  | PointsPlus™ value |
|---|---|
| **Bacon & Cheese,** 1 serving | 7 |
| **Bacon, Egg & Cheese,** 1 serving | 10 |
| **BBQ Beef,** 1 serving | 6 |
| **Cream Cheese,** 1 serving | 6 |
| **Egg & Cheese,** 1 serving | 11 |
| **Fruit (average),** 1 serving | 5 |
| **Ham & Cheese,** 1 serving | 7 |
| **Italian Chicken,** 1 serving | 6 |
| **Jalapeno & Cheese,** 1 serving | 5 |
| **Pepperoni & Mushroom Pizza,** 1 | 8 |
| **Philly Cheese Steak,** 1 serving | 6 |
| **Pizza,** 1 serving | 5 |
| **Polish Sausage,** 1 serving | 13 |
| **Potato Egg & Cheese,** 1 serving | 9 |
| **Ranchero,** 1 serving | 9 |
| **Sausage,** 1 serving | 4 |
| **Sausage & Cheese,** 1 serving | 7 |
| **Sausage, Egg & Cheese,** 1 serving | 10 |
| **Spinach,** 1 serving | 8 |
| **Texas Hot Polish,** 1 serving | 12 |

▲ Power Foods — *PointsPlus*™ value

## SPECIALTIES

|  | PointsPlus™ value |
|---|---|
| **Cinnamon Raisin Nut Roll,** 1 | 11 |
| **Cinnamon Roll,** 1 serving | 8 |
| **Cinnamon Twist,** 1 serving | 16 |
| **Sticky Bun,** 1 serving | 17 |

## CROISSANTS

|  | PointsPlus™ value |
|---|---|
| **Ham & Cheese,** 1 serving | 17 |
| **Ham & Egg,** 1 serving | 17 |
| **Italian Chicken,** 1 serving | 15 |

# LA SALSA FRESH MEXICAN GRILL®

| ▲ Power Foods | *PointsPlus™* value |
|---|---|
| **APPETIZER** | |
| **Chips, Guacamole and Salsa,** 1 serving | 26 |
| **BURRITOS** | |
| **Bean & Cheese Burrito (Black Bean),** 1 | 15 |
| **Bean & Cheese Burrito (Pinto Bean),** 1 | 14 |
| **California Burrito (Steak with Black Beans),** 1 | 23 |
| **California Burrito (Steak with Pinto Beans),** 1 | 22 |
| **Californian Burrito (Chicken with Black Beans),** 1 | 22 |
| **Cheese & Chicken Burrito (Black Bean),** 1 | 19 |
| **Cheese & Chicken Burrito (Pinto Bean),** 1 | 18 |
| **Cheese & Steak Burrito (Black Bean),** 1 | 19 |
| **Cheese & Steak Burrito (Pinto Bean),** 1 | 18 |
| **Grande Burrito (Chicken with Black Beans),** 1 | 22 |
| **Grande Burrito (Steak with Black Beans),** 1 | 23 |
| **Grande Burrito (Steak with Pinto Beans),** 1 | 22 |
| **Los Cabos Grande Burrito (Shrimp),** 1 | 20 |
| **Three Pepper Fajita Burrito (Chicken),** 1 | 22 |
| **Three Pepper Fajita Burrito (Shrimp),** 1 | 20 |
| **Three Pepper Fajita Burrito (Steak),** 1 | 22 |

| ▲ Power Foods | *PointsPlus™* value |
|---|---|
| **TACOS** | |
| **Baja Grilled Fish Taco,** 1 taco shell | 10 |
| **Baja Grilled Fish Tacos,** 2 taco shells | 20 |
| **Baja Style Shrimp Taco,** 1 taco shell | 9 |
| **Baja Style Shrimp Tacos,** 2 taco shells | 17 |
| **Chicken Taquitos,** 1 basket | 23 |
| **Tacos La Salsa™ (Chicken),** 1 taco shell | 7 |
| **Tacos La Salsa™ (Chicken),** 2 taco shells | 14 |
| **Tacos La Salsa™ (Steak),** 2 taco shells | 14 |
| **Tacos La Salsa™ (Steak),** 1 taco shell | 7 |
| **QUESADILLAS** | |
| **Classic Quesadilla (Chicken),** 1 serving | 27 |
| **Classic Quesadilla (Steak),** 1 serving | 27 |
| **Classic Quesadilla,** 1 serving | 23 |
| **PLATTERS** | |
| **Cheese Enchilada Platter with Rice and Black Beans,** 1 platter | 24 |
| **Cheese Enchilada Platter with Rice and Pinto Beans,** 1 platter | 24 |
| **Enchilada (Chicken) Platter with Rice and Black Beans,** 1 platter | 20 |
| **Enchilada (Chicken) Platter with Rice and Pinto Beans,** 1 platter | 19 |
| **Enchilada (Steak) Platter with Rice and Black Beans,** 1 platter | 21 |
| **Enchilada (Steak) Platter with Rice and Pinto Beans,** 1 platter | 20 |
| **Three Pepper Fajita Platter (Chicken) with Rice and Beans,** 1 platter | 23 |

*Platters (cont'd)*

| ▲ Power Foods | *PointsPlus*™ value |
|---|---|
| **Three Pepper Fajita Platter (Steak) with Rice and Black Beans,** 1 platter | 24 |
| **Three Pepper Fajita Platter (Steak) with Rice and Pinto Beans,** 1 platter | 23 |
| **Two Soft Tacos (Chicken) Platter with Rice and Pinto Beans,** 1 platter | 19 |
| **Two Soft Tacos (Steak) Platter with Rice and Black Beans,** 1 platter | 20 |
| **Two Soft Tacos (Steak) Platter with Rice and Pinto Beans,** 1 platter | 20 |

## KID'S MEALS

| ▲ Power Foods | *PointsPlus*™ value |
|---|---|
| **Kids Platter, Cheese Quesadilla with Black Bean side,** 1 platter | 12 |
| **Kids Platter, Cheese Quesadilla with Pinto Bean side,** 1 platter | 12 |
| **Kids Platter, Cheese Quesadilla with Rice side,** 1 platter | 12 |
| **Kids Platter, Pinto Bean Burrito with Black Bean side,** 1 platter | 17 |
| **Kids Platter, Pinto Bean Burrito with Pinto Bean side,** 1 platter | 16 |
| **Kids Platter, Pinto Bean Burrito with Rice side,** 1 platter | 17 |

## SALSAS

| ▲ Power Foods | *PointsPlus*™ value |
|---|---|
| **Avocado Salsa,** 1 serving | 0 |
| **Habanero Salsa,** 1 serving | 0 |
| **Mango Salsa,** 1 serving | 0 |
| **Salsa Buena,** 1 serving | 0 |
| **Salsa Mexicana,** 1 serving | 0 |
| **Salsa Roja,** 1 serving | 0 |
| **Salsa Verde,** 1 serving | 0 |
| **Salsa, Roasted Tomato,** 1 serving | 0 |

## SIDES

| ▲ Power Foods | *PointsPlus*™ value |
|---|---|
| **1/2 Rice & 1/2 Black Beans,** 1 side serving | 8 |
| **1/2 Rice & 1/2 Pinto Beans,** 1 side serving | 7 |
| **Beans, Black,** 1 side serving | 6 |
| **Beans, Pinto,** 1 side serving | 5 |
| **Rice,** 1 side serving | 5 |
| **Tortilla Chips, Fried (served with meal),** 15 item | 5 |

# LEE'S FAMOUS RECIPE CHICKEN

| ▲ Power Foods | *PointsPlus™* value |
|---|---|
| **CHICKEN** | |
| **Crispy Plus Breast,** 1 | 13 |
| **Crispy Plus Drumstick,** 1 | 4 |
| **Crispy Plus Thigh,** 1 | 10 |
| **Crispy Plus Whole Wing,** 1 | 5 |
| **Famous Recipe Breast,** 1 | 9 |
| ▲ **Famous Recipe Breast without Skin/Breading,** 1 | 3 |
| **Famous Recipe Drumstick,** 1 | 4 |
| **Famous Recipe Thigh,** 1 | 10 |
| **Famous Recipe Whole Wing,** 1 | 4 |
| **Oven Roasted Breast,** 1 | 7 |
| **Oven Roasted Drumstick,** 1 | 3 |
| **Oven Roasted Thigh,** 1 | 6 |
| **Oven Roasted Whole Wing,** 1 | 4 |

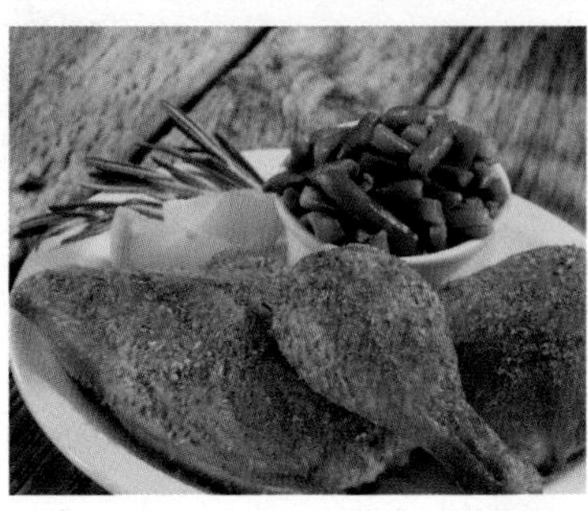

| ▲ Power Foods | *PointsPlus™* value |
|---|---|
| **HANDHELD CHICKEN** | |
| **Crispy Breast Strips,** 3 | 9 |
| **Jumbo Boneless Wings,** 6 pieces | 10 |
| **Oven Roasted Jumbo Boneless Breast Strips,** 3 | 4 |
| **POT PIE** | |
| **Chicken Pot Pie,** 1 serving | 23 |
| **SIDE ITEMS** | |
| **Baked Beans,** 1 serving | 5 |
| **Biscuit,** 1 | 5 |
| **Cole Slaw,** 1 serving | 5 |
| ▲ **Corn on the Cob,** 1 serving | 3 |
| ▲ **Green Beans,** 1 serving | 0 |
| **Macaroni & Cheese,** 1 serving | 4 |
| **Mashed Potatoes with Gravy,** 1 serving | 3 |
| **Potato Salad,** 1 serving | 5 |
| **Potato Wedges,** 1 serving | 6 |

# LITTLE CAESARS® PIZZA

| ▲ Power Foods | *PointsPlus™* value |
|---|---|
| **14" LARGE ROUND PIZZA** | |
| **Cheese,** 1 slice (1/8 of the pizza) | 7 |
| **Pepperoni Pizza,** 1 slice (1/8 of the pizza) | 8 |
| **LARGE DEEP DISH PIZZA** | |
| **Cheese Pizza,** 1 slice (1/8 of the pizza) | 9 |
| **Pepperoni Pizza,** 1 slice (1/8 of the pizza) | 10 |
| **SPECIALTY PIZZAS** | |
| **3 Meat Treat,** 1 slice (1/8 of the pizza) | 10 |
| **Ultimate Supreme,** 1 slice (1/8 of the pizza) | 8 |
| **Vegetarian Pizza,** 1 slice (1/8 of the pizza) | 8 |
| **BABY PAN! PAN!®** | |
| **Baby Pan!Pan!®, Cheese,** 1 slice | 9 |
| **Baby Pan!Pan!®, Pepperoni,** 1 slice | 10 |
| **FRESH & READY SALAD (WITHOUT DRESSING)** | |
| **Antipasto Salad,** 1 | 5 |
| **Caesar Salad,** 1 | 3 |
| ▲ **Garden Mixed Salad,** 1 | 0 |
| **Greek Salad,** 1 | 4 |
| **SALAD DRESSINGS** | |
| **Caesar Dressing,** 1 packet | 7 |
| **Fat Free Italian Dressing,** 1 packet | 1 |
| **Greek Dressing,** 1 packet | 7 |
| **Italian Dressing,** 1 packet | 6 |
| **Ranch Dressing,** 1 packet | 6 |

| ▲ Power Foods | *PointsPlus™* value |
|---|---|
| **APPETIZERS & SIDES** | |
| **Caesar Wings, Oven Roasted,** 1 | 1 |
| **Caesar Wings®, Barbecue,** 1 | 2 |
| **Caesar Wings®, Hot,** 1 | 1 |
| **Caesar Wings®, Mild,** 1 | 1 |
| **Crazy Bread®,** 1 stick | 3 |
| **Crazy Sauce®,** 1 container | 1 |
| **Little Caesars Italian Cheese Bread®,** 1 piece | 4 |
| **Little Caesars Pepperoni Cheese Bread® (10 piece),** 1 serving | 4 |

# LONG JOHN SILVER'S®

▲ Power Foods — *PointsPlus*™ value

## SIDES & STARTERS

| Item | *PointsPlus*™ value |
|---|---|
| **Breadstick,** 1 | 5 |
| **Broccoli Cheese Soup,** 1 bowl | 6 |
| **Coleslaw,** 1 serving | 5 |
| **Corn Cobbette (without butter oil),** 1 | 2 |
| **Corn Cobbette, with butter oil,** 1 | 4 |
| **Crumblies®,** 1 serving | 5 |
| **Fries,** 1 regular serving | 6 |
| **Hushpuppy,** 1 piece | 2 |
| **Lobster Stuffed Crab Cake,** 1 | 5 |
| **Rice,** 1 serving | 4 |
| ▲ **Vegetable Medley,** 1 serving | 1 |

## FISH, SEAFOOD & CHICKEN

| Item | *PointsPlus*™ value |
|---|---|
| **Alaskan Flounder,** 1 piece | 7 |
| ▲ **Baked Cod,** 1 piece | 3 |
| **Battered Fish,** 1 piece | 7 |
| **Battered Shrimp,** 3 pieces | 4 |
| **Breaded Clam Strips,** 1 snack box | 9 |
| **Buttered Lobster Bites,** 1 snack box | 6 |
| **Chicken Plank®,** 1 piece | 4 |
| ▲ **Grilled Pacific Salmon,** 2 fillets | 4 |
| ▲ **Grilled Tilapia,** 1 fillet | 3 |
| **Popcorn Shrimp,** 1 snack box | 7 |
| **Shrimp Scampi,** 8 pieces | 3 |

## SANDWICHES

| Item | *PointsPlus*™ value |
|---|---|
| **Chicken Sandwich,** 1 | 9 |
| **Fish Sandwich,** 1 | 13 |
| **Ultimate Fish Sandwich®,** 1 | 14 |

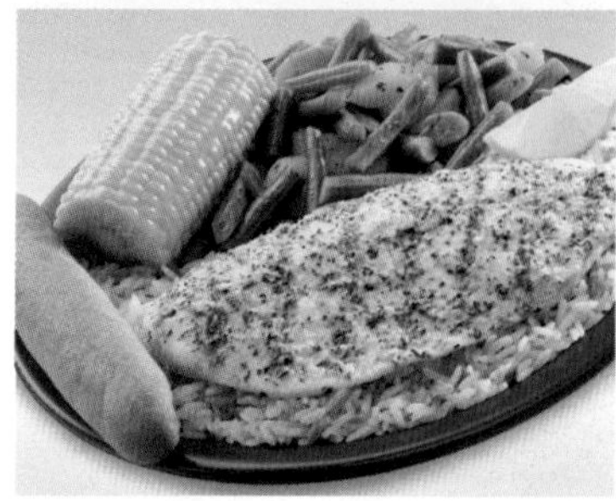

▲ Power Foods — *PointsPlus*™ value

## BOWLS & PLATES

| Item | *PointsPlus*™ value |
|---|---|
| **Salmon Bowl with Sauce,** 1 | 12 |
| **Salmon Bowl without Sauce,** 1 | 9 |
| **Shrimp Bowl with Sauce,** 1 | 10 |
| **Shrimp Bowl without Sauce,** 1 | 8 |
| **Smart Choice Salmon Plate,** 1 | 6 |
| **Smart Choice Shrimp Scampi Plate,** 1 | 6 |
| **Smart Choice Tilapia Plate,** 1 | 6 |

## DIPPING SAUCES

| Item | *PointsPlus*™ value |
|---|---|
| **Cocktail Sauce,** 1 oz | 1 |
| **Tartar Sauce,** 1 oz | 3 |

## CONDIMENTS

| Item | *PointsPlus*™ value |
|---|---|
| **Ginger Teriyaki Sauce,** 1 packet | 2 |
| **Louisiana Hot Sauce,** 1 tsp | 0 |
| **Malt Vinegar,** 1/2 oz | 0 |

## DESSERTS

| Item | *PointsPlus*™ value |
|---|---|
| **Chocolate Cream Pie,** 1 | 9 |
| **Pecan Pie,** 1 | 10 |
| **Pineapple Cream Pie,** 1 | 8 |

# MAID-RITE

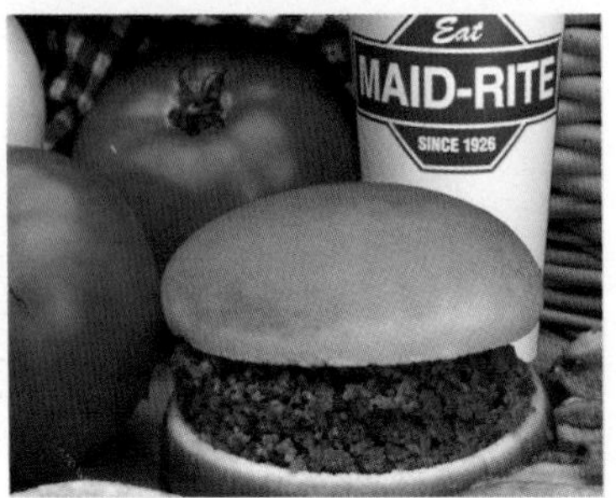


| ▲ Power Foods | *PointsPlus*™ value |
|---|---|

## SANDWICHES

| | |
|---|---|
| **Cheese-Rite Sandwich (without condiments),** 1 serving | 12 |
| **Chicken Sandwich (without condiments),** 1 serving | 10 |
| **Taco-Rite Sandwich,** 1 serving | 12 |
| **Value-Rite (without condiments),** 1 serving | 8 |

## WRAPS (INCLUDES CONDIMENTS)

| | |
|---|---|
| **Chicken Wrap,** 1 serving | 12 |
| **Maid-Rite Wrap,** 1 serving | 14 |

| ▲ Power Foods | *PointsPlus*™ value |
|---|---|

## SIDES

| | |
|---|---|
| **Baked Beans,** 1/2 cup | 4 |
| **Carb-Rite Cup (without condiments),** 1 serving | 9 |
| **Coleslaw,** 1/2 cup | 4 |
| **Maid-Rite Salad (without onions and pickles),** 1 serving | 12 |

## BEVERAGES

| | |
|---|---|
| **Diet Mountain Dew,** 1 serving | 0 |
| **Tropicana Pink Lemonade,** 1 serving | 7 |

| ▲ Power Foods | *PointsPlus*™ value |
|---|---|
| **LOWFAT FROZEN YOGURT** | |
| **Soft serve chocolate frozen yogurt, no sugar added,** 1 serving | 2 |
| **Soft serve nonfat classic vanilla frozen yogurt,** 1 serving | 3 |
| **Soft serve nonfat dark chocolate frozen yogurt,** 1 serving | 3 |
| **Soft serve nonfat french vanilla frozen yogurt,** 1 serving | 3 |
| **Soft serve nonfat Strawberry frozen yogurt,** 1 serving | 3 |
| **Soft serve vanilla frozen yogurt, no sugar added,** 1 serving | 2 |

# MAUI WOWI HAWAIIAN COFFEES & SMOOTHIES

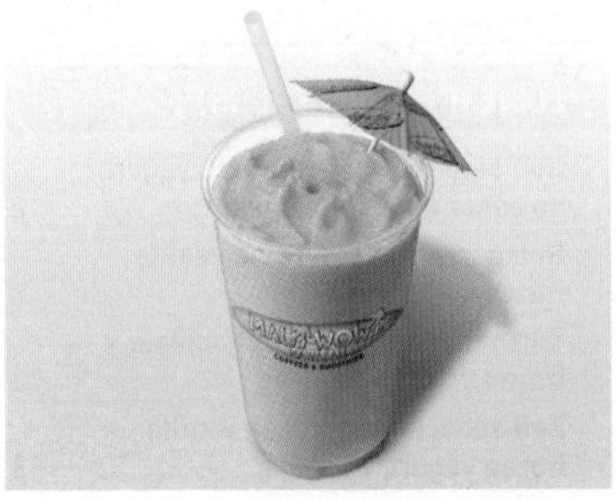

▲ Power Foods | *PointsPlus™* value

## SMOOTHIES

|  | PointsPlus™ value |
| --- | --- |
| **Banana Banana Smoothie,** 1 small serving | 5 |
| **Black Raspberry Banana Smoothie,** 1 small serving | 7 |
| **Cappuccino with Banana,** 1 small serving | 9 |
| **Cappuccino with Banana Smoothie,** 1 small serving | 7 |
| **Cappuccino without Banana Smoothie,** 1 small serving | 9 |
| **Kiwi Lemon Lime with Banana,** 1 small serving | 5 |
| **Kiwi Lemon Lime with Banana Smoothie,** 1 small serving | 3 |
| **Kiwi Lemon Lime without Banana Smoothie,** 1 small serving | 5 |
| **Mango Orange Banana Smoothie,** 1 small serving | 7 |
| **Passion Papaya Banana Smoothie,** 1 small serving | 6 |
| **Pina Colada with Banana,** 1 small serving | 6 |
| **Pina Colada with Banana Smoothie,** 1 small serving | 3 |
| **Pina Colada without Banana Smoothie,** 1 small serving | 6 |
| **Strawberry Banana Smoothie,** 1 small serving | 6 |

| ▲ Power Foods | *PointsPlus*™ value |
|---|---|
| **APPETIZERS** | |
| **Black Bean Roll-Ups,** 1 serving | 15 |
| **ENTRÉE SALADS** | |
| **Half Hula Bowl (with 2-oz of fat-free honey mustard dressing, without breadstick),** 1 serving | 9 |
| **Hula Bowl (with 3-oz of fat-free honey mustard dressing, without breadstick),** 1 serving | 15 |
| **SALAD DRESSINGS** | |
| **Fat Free French,** 2 Tbsp | 3 |
| **Fat Free Honey Mustard,** 2 Tbsp | 2 |
| **Italian,** 2 Tbsp | 3 |
| **Low-Fat Tex Mex,** 2 Tbsp | 0 |
| **Ranch,** 2 Tbsp | 3 |
| **SIDES** | |
| **Buttered Broccoli,** 1 serving | 3 |
| **Fruit Salad,** 1 serving | 2 |
| **Garlic Breadstick,** 1 | 4 |
| **BEVERAGES** | |
| **Fruit Smoothie,** 1 serving | 3 |

# MAZZIO'S ITALIAN EATERY®

| ▲ Power Foods | *PointsPlus™* value |
|---|---|

## STARTERS

| Item | PointsPlus value |
|---|---|
| **Artichoke Spinach Dip with Bread,** 1 serving | 7 |
| **Cheese Dippers (without sauce),** 3 slices (1/4 serving) | 11 |
| **Dip Sauce - BBQ,** 1 serving | 4 |
| **Dip Sauce - Bleu Cheese,** 1 serving | 9 |
| **Dip Sauce - Buffalo,** 1 serving | 0 |
| **Dip Sauce - Chocolate,** 1 serving | 5 |
| **Dip Sauce - Cool Ranch,** 1 serving | 10 |
| **Dip Sauce - Honey Mustard,** 1 serving | 7 |
| **Dip Sauce - Marinara,** 1 serving | 1 |
| **Dip Sauce - Picante,** 1 serving | 0 |
| **Dip Sauce - Southwestern Ranch,** 1 serving | 9 |
| **Dip Sauce - Vanilla,** 1 serving | 5 |
| **Dippin' Tostitos Chips,** 1 serving | 8 |
| **Meat Nachos (beef with jalapenos),** 1/2 order | 13 |
| **Meat Nachos (chicken with jalapenos),** 1/2 order | 12 |
| **Meat Nachos (sausage with jalapenos),** 1/2 order | 14 |
| **Pepperoni Quesapizza without Sauce,** 1 serving | 9 |
| **Toasted Ravioli without Sauce,** 1 serving | 3 |

## ORIGINAL CRUST PIZZA

| Item | PointsPlus value |
|---|---|
| **"Mazzio's Works" Pizza,** 1/8 of the medium pizza | 8 |
| **4 Meat,** 1/8 of the medium pizza | 8 |
| **California Alfredo Pizza,** 1/8 of the medium pizza | 8 |
| **Canadian Bacon,** 1/8 of the medium pizza | 6 |
| **Cheese Buster,** 1/8 of the medium pizza | 6 |
| **Cheese Pizza,** 1/8 of the medium pizza | 6 |
| **Chicken,** 1/8 of the medium pizza | 6 |
| **Chicken Club Pizza,** 1/8 of the medium pizza | 7 |
| **Combo Pizza,** 1/8 of the medium pizza | 7 |
| **Greek,** 1/8 of the medium pizza | 9 |
| **Hamburger,** 1/8 of the medium pizza | 7 |
| **Lucky 7,** 1/8 of the medium pizza | 7 |
| **Meatbuster® Pizza,** 1/8 of the medium pizza | 8 |
| **Mexican Pizza,** 1/8 of the medium pizza | 8 |
| **Pepperoni Pizza,** 1/8 of the medium pizza | 7 |
| **Sausage Pizza,** 1/8 of the medium pizza | 7 |
| **Supremebuster® Pizza,** 1/8 of the medium pizza | 7 |
| **Veggie,** 1/8 of the medium pizza | 6 |

## THIN CRUST PIZZA

| Item | PointsPlus value |
|---|---|
| **"Mazzio's Works" Pizza,** 1/8 of the medium pizza | 7 |
| **4 Meat,** 1/8 of the medium pizza | 7 |
| **California Alfredo Pizza,** 1/8 of the medium pizza | 6 |
| **Canadian Bacon,** 1/8 of the medium pizza | 5 |
| **Cheese Buster,** 1/8 of the medium pizza | 5 |
| **Cheese Pizza,** 1/8 of the medium pizza | 5 |
| **Chicken,** 1/8 of the medium pizza | 5 |
| **Chicken Club Pizza,** 1/8 of the medium pizza | 5 |
| **Combo Pizza,** 1/8 of the medium pizza | 6 |
| **Greek,** 1/8 of the medium pizza | 7 |
| **Hamburger,** 1/8 of the medium pizza | 6 |
| **Lucky 7,** 1/8 of the medium pizza | 5 |
| **Meatbuster® Pizza,** 1/8 of the medium pizza | 6 |
| **Mexican Pizza,** 1/8 of the medium pizza | 7 |

| ▲ Power Foods | *PointsPlus*™ value |
|---|---|
| **Pepperoni Pizza,** 1/8 of the medium pizza | 5 |
| **Sausage Pizza,** 1/8 of the medium pizza | 6 |
| **Supremebuster® Pizza,** 1/8 of the medium pizza | 5 |
| **Veggie,** 1/8 of the medium pizza | 5 |

## DEEP PAN PIZZA

| | |
|---|---|
| **"Mazzio's Works" Pizza,** 1/8 of the medium pizza | 11 |
| **4 Meat,** 1/8 of the medium pizza | 11 |
| **California Alfredo Pizza,** 1/8 of the medium pizza | 10 |
| **Canadian Bacon,** 1/8 of the medium pizza | 9 |
| **Cheese Buster,** 1/8 of the medium pizza | 9 |
| **Cheese Pizza,** 1/8 of the medium pizza | 9 |
| **Chicken,** 1/8 of the medium pizza | 9 |
| **Chicken Club Pizza,** 1/8 of the medium pizza | 9 |
| **Combo Pizza,** 1/8 of the medium pizza | 10 |
| **Greek,** 1/8 of the medium pizza | 11 |
| **Hamburger,** 1/8 of the medium pizza | 10 |
| **Lucky 7,** 1/8 of the medium pizza | 9 |
| **Meatbuster® Pizza,** 1/8 of the medium pizza | 10 |
| **Mexican Pizza,** 1/8 of the medium pizza | 11 |
| **Pepperoni Pizza,** 1/8 of the medium pizza | 9 |
| **Sausage Pizza,** 1/8 of the medium pizza | 10 |
| **Supremebuster® Pizza,** 1/8 of the medium pizza | 9 |
| **Veggie,** 1/8 of the medium pizza | 9 |

## FRENCH BREAD PIZZAS

| ▲ Power Foods | *PointsPlus*™ value |
|---|---|
| **Deli,** 1 serving | 13 |
| **Greek,** 1 serving | 17 |
| **Hawaiian,** 1 serving | 12 |
| **Pepperoni,** 1 serving | 13 |
| **Southwestern Chicken,** 1 serving | 14 |

## DIPPIN ZONE

| | |
|---|---|
| **Cheese Nachos (with jalapenos),** 1/2 order | 11 |

## PASTA CHOICES (WITHOUT BREAD)

| | |
|---|---|
| **Chicken Fried Chicken Alfredo,** 1 serving | 37 |
| **Chicken Parmesan,** 1 serving | 27 |
| **Chicken Spinach Artichoke Pasta,** 1 serving | 26 |
| **Fettuccine Alfredo,** 1 serving | 29 |
| **Greek Pasta,** 1 serving | 39 |
| **Lasagna Red & White,** 1 serving | 27 |
| **Lasagna with Alfredo,** 1 serving | 35 |
| **Lasagna with Marinara,** 1 serving | 18 |
| **Lasagna with Meat Sauce,** 1 serving | 25 |
| **Spaghetti with Marinara,** 1 serving | 17 |
| **Spaghetti with Marinara & 4 Meatballs,** 1 serving | 25 |
| **Spaghetti with Meat Sauce,** 1 serving | 21 |
| **Spaghetti with Meatballs (4) & Meat Sauce,** 1 serving | 30 |

## HOT TOASTED SANDWICHES (WITHOUT CHIPS OR PICKLE)

| | |
|---|---|
| **Chicken, Bacon & Swiss (Focaccia),** 1 | 28 |
| **Chicken, Bacon & Swiss (Hoagie),** 1 | 37 |
| **Ham & Cheddar (Focaccia),** 1 | 20 |
| **Mazzio's Sub (Focaccia),** 1 | 21 |
| **Turkey & Swiss (Focaccia),** 1 | 18 |
| **Tuscan Smash (Focaccia),** 1 | 17 |

# MAZZIO'S ITALIAN EATERY®

▲ Power Foods — *PointsPlus™* value

## SANDWICHES
(WITHOUT CHIPS, FRIES OR PICKLE)

|  | *PointsPlus™* value |
|---|---|
| **Ham & Cheddar (Hoagie),** 1 | 30 |
| **Mazzio's Sub (Hoagie),** 1 | 30 |
| **Turkey & Swiss (Hoagie),** 1 | 28 |
| **Tuscan Smash (Hoagie),** 1 | 26 |
| ▲ **Kosher Pickle Spear,** 1 | 0 |
| **Potato Chips (Lay's),** 1 serving | 4 |

## CALZONE RINGS & QUESAPIZZA

|  | *PointsPlus™* value |
|---|---|
| **Chicken Quesapizza without Sauce,** 1 serving | 8 |
| **Four Meat/Four Cheese Calzone without Sauce,** 1 serving | 7 |
| **Ham Bacon & Cheddar Calzone without Sauce,** 1 serving | 6 |
| **Pepperoni Calzone Ring®,** 1/10 of a calzone | 7 |

## FRIES

|  | *PointsPlus™* value |
|---|---|
| **Cheese Fries,** 1 serving | 11 |
| **Fries with Sandwich,** 1 serving | 15 |
| **Full Order Fries,** 1 serving | 7 |

## CHICKEN & RIBS

|  | *PointsPlus™* value |
|---|---|
| **Boneless Dippin' Chicken (10 count),** 1 serving | 3 |
| **Rib Dippers - Tossed with BBQ,** 1 serving | 12 |
| **Roasted & BBQ Tossed Wings (10 count),** 1 serving | 5 |
| **Wings of Fire (10 count) without Sauce,** 1 serving | 4 |

## BREAD

|  | *PointsPlus™* value |
|---|---|
| **Breadstick (without sauce),** 4 | 4 |
| **Cinnamon Sticks (without sauce),** 4 (1/4 serving) | 17 |
| **Garlic Cheese Toast (without sauce),** 1/4 order | 6 |
| **Garlic Toast (without sauce),** 1/4 order | 4 |

| ▲ Power Foods | *PointsPlus™* value |
|---|---|

## SANDWICHES

| | |
|---|---|
| **Hamburger,** 1 | 7 |
| **Cheeseburger,** 1 | 8 |
| **Double Cheeseburger,** 1 | 12 |
| **Quarter Pounder®,** 1 | 11 |
| **Quarter Pounder® with Cheese,** 1 | 13 |
| **Double Quarter Pounder® with Cheese,** 1 | 19 |
| **Big Mac®,** 1 | 14 |
| **Big Mac®, without Big Mac Sauce,** 1 | 12 |
| **Big N' Tasty®,** 1 | 12 |
| **Big N' Tasty® with Cheese,** 1 | 14 |
| **Big N' Tasty® with Cheese, without mayonnaise dressing,** 1 | 12 |
| **Big N' Tasty®, without mayonnaise dressing,** 1 | 11 |
| **Filet-O-Fish®,** 1 | 10 |
| **Filet-O-Fish®, without tartar sauce,** 1 | 8 |
| **McChicken®,** 1 | 10 |
| **McChicken®, without mayonnaise dressing,** 1 | 8 |
| **McDouble,** 1 | 10 |
| **McRib®,** 1 | 13 |
| **Premium Crispy Chicken Classic,** 1 | 14 |
| **Premium Crispy Chicken Classic, without mayonnaise dressing,** 1 | 12 |
| **Premium Crispy Chicken Club,** 1 | 17 |
| **Premium Crispy Chicken Club, without mayonnaise dressing,** 1 | 15 |
| **Premium Crispy Chicken Ranch BLT,** 1 | 15 |
| **Premium Crispy Chicken Ranch BLT, without ranch sauce,** 1 | 14 |
| **Premium Grilled Chicken Classic,** 1 | 11 |
| **Premium Grilled Chicken Classic, without mayonnaise dressing,** 1 | 9 |
| **Premium Grilled Chicken Club,** 1 | 13 |
| **Premium Grilled Chicken Club, without mayonnaise dressing,** 1 | 12 |
| **Premium Grilled Chicken Ranch BLT,** 1 | 12 |
| **Premium Grilled Chicken Ranch BLT Sandwich, without ranch sauce,** 1 | 11 |
| **Southern Style Crispy Chicken Sandwich,** 1 | 11 |
| **Chipotle BBQ Snack Wrap® (crispy),** 1 | 9 |
| **Chipotle BBQ Snack Wrap® (grilled),** 1 | 7 |
| **Honey Mustard Grilled Snack Wrap™ (grilled),** 1 | 7 |
| **Honey Mustard Snack Wrap™ (crispy),** 1 | 9 |
| **Ranch Grilled Snack Wrap™ (grilled),** 1 | 7 |
| **Ranch Snack Wrap™ (crispy),** 1 | 9 |

## FRENCH FRIES

| | |
|---|---|
| **French Fries,** 1 small serving | 6 |
| **French Fries,** 1 medium serving | 10 |
| **French Fries,** 1 large serving | 13 |

## CHICKEN MCNUGGETS®/ CHICKEN SELECTS®

| | |
|---|---|
| **Chicken Selects®,** 3 pieces | 11 |
| **Chicken McNuggets®,** 4 pieces | 5 |
| **Chicken McNuggets®,** 6 pieces | 7 |
| **Chicken McNuggets®,** 10 pieces | 13 |
| **Barbecue Sauce,** 1 package | 1 |
| **Creamy Ranch Sauce,** 1 package | 6 |
| **Honey Sauce,** 1 package | 1 |
| **Hot Mustard Sauce,** 1 package | 2 |

| ▲ Power Foods | PointsPlus™ value |
|---|---|
| **Southwestern Chipotle Barbeque Sauce,** 1 package | 2 |
| **Spicy Buffalo Sauce,** 1 package | 2 |
| **Sweet 'N Sour Sauce,** 1 package | 1 |
| **Tangy Honey Mustard Sauce,** 1 package | 2 |

## SALADS

| ▲ Power Foods | PointsPlus™ value |
|---|---|
| **Premium Bacon Ranch Salad (without chicken),** 1 serving | 3 |
| **Premium Bacon Ranch Salad with Crispy Chicken,** 1 serving | 10 |
| **Premium Bacon Ranch Salad with Grilled Chicken,** 1 serving | 6 |
| **Premium Caesar Salad (without chicken),** 1 serving | 2 |
| **Premium Caesar Salad with Crispy Chicken,** 1 serving | 9 |
| **Premium Caesar Salad with Grilled Chicken,** 1 serving | 5 |
| **Premium Southwest Salad (without chicken),** 1 serving | 3 |
| **Premium Southwest Salad with Crispy Chicken,** 1 serving | 11 |
| **Premium Southwest Salad with Grilled Chicken,** 1 serving | 8 |
| ▲ **Side Salad,** 1 serving | 0 |
| **Snack Size Fruit & Walnut Salad,** 1 package | 6 |
| **Butter Garlic Croutons,** 1 serving | 2 |

## SALAD DRESSINGS

| ▲ Power Foods | PointsPlus™ value |
|---|---|
| **Newman's Own® Creamy Caesar Dressing,** 1 serving | 5 |
| **Newman's Own® Creamy Southwest Dressing,** 1 serving | 3 |
| **Newman's Own® Low Fat Balsamic Vinaigrette Dressing,** 1 serving | 1 |
| **Newman's Own® Low Fat Family Recipe Italian Dressing,** 1 serving | 2 |
| **Newman's Own® Low Fat Sesame Ginger Dressing,** 1 serving | 2 |
| **Newman's Own® Ranch Dressing,** 1 serving | 5 |

## HAPPY MEALS

| ▲ Power Foods | PointsPlus™ value |
|---|---|
| **Happy Meals with Hamburger,** 1 box | 16 |
| **Happy Meals with Cheeseburger,** 1 box | 17 |
| **Happy Meals with Chicken McNuggets®,** 1 box | 14 |

## BREAKFAST

| ▲ Power Foods | PointsPlus™ value |
|---|---|
| **Bacon, Egg & Cheese Biscuit (regular size biscuit),** 1 | 11 |
| **Bacon, Egg & Cheese Biscuit (large size biscuit),** 1 | 14 |
| **Bacon, Egg & Cheese McGriddles®,** 1 | 11 |
| **Big Breakfast® (regular size biscuit),** 1 serving | 20 |
| **Big Breakfast® (large size biscuit),** 1 | 22 |
| **Biscuit - Regular Size,** 1 | 7 |
| **Biscuit - Large,** 1 | 9 |
| **Deluxe Breakfast (regular size biscuit, without syrup & margarine),** 1 serving | 29 |
| **Deluxe Breakfast (large size biscuit, without syrup & margarine,** 1 | 31 |
| **Egg McMuffin®,** 1 | 8 |
| **English Muffin,** 1 | 4 |
| **Hash Browns,** 1 serving | 4 |
| **Hotcake Syrup,** 1 package | 5 |
| **Hotcakes (without syrup, & margarine),** 1 serving | 9 |
| **Hotcakes and Sausage (without margarine & syrup),** 1 serving | 14 |

| ▲ Power Foods | *PointsPlus™* value |
|---|---|
| **McSkillet™ Burrito with Sausage,** 1 | 16 |
| **McSkillet™ Burrito with Steak,** 1 | 15 |
| **Sausage Biscuit (regular size biscuit),** 1 | 11 |
| **Sausage Biscuit (large size biscuit),** 1 | 13 |
| **Sausage Biscuit with Egg (regular size biscuit),** 1 | 14 |
| **Sausage Biscuit with Egg (large size biscuit),** 1 | 15 |
| **Sausage Burrito,** 1 | 8 |
| **Sausage McGriddles®,** 1 | 11 |
| **Sausage McMuffin®,** 1 | 10 |
| Sausage McMuffin® with Egg, 1 | 12 |
| **Sausage Patty,** 1 | 5 |
| **Sausage, Egg & Cheese McGriddles®,** 1 | 15 |
| **Scrambled Eggs,** 2 eggs | 4 |
| **Southern Style Chicken Biscuit (regular size biscuit),** 1 | 11 |
| **Southern Style Chicken Biscuit (large size biscuit),** 1 | 12 |
| **Whipped Margarine,** 1 pat | 1 |

## McCAFE COFFEES

| ▲ Power Foods | *PointsPlus™* value |
|---|---|
| **Cappuccino,** 1 small | 3 |
| **Cappuccino with Sugar Free Vanilla Syrup,** 1 small | 3 |
| **Caramel Cappuccino,** 1 small | 5 |
| **Caramel Latte,** 1 small | 6 |
| **Coffee,** 1 small serving | 0 |
| **Hazelnut Cappuccino,** 1 small | 5 |
| **Hazelnut Latte,** 1 small | 6 |
| **Hot Chocolate,** 1 small | 8 |
| **Hot Chocolate with Nonfat Milk,** 1 small | 7 |
| **Iced Caramel Latte,** 1 small | 4 |
| **Iced Coffee - Caramel,** 1 small | 4 |
| **Iced Coffee - Hazelnut,** 1 small | 4 |
| **Iced Coffee - Regular,** 1 small | 4 |
| **Iced Coffee - Vanilla,** 1 small | 4 |
| **Iced Coffee with Sugar Free Vanilla Syrup,** 1 small | 2 |
| **Iced Hazelnut Latte,** 1 small | 4 |
| **Iced Latte,** 1 small | 2 |
| **Iced Latte with Sugar Free Vanilla Syrup,** 1 small | 2 |
| **Iced Mocha,** 1 medium | 9 |
| **Iced Mocha with Nonfat Milk,** 1 medium | 7 |
| **Iced Nonfat Caramel Latte,** 1 small | 4 |
| **Iced Nonfat Hazelnut Latte,** 1 small | 4 |
| ▲ **Iced Nonfat Latte,** 1 small | 1 |
| ▲ **Iced Nonfat Latte with Sugar Free Vanilla Syrup,** 1 small | 2 |
| **Iced Nonfat Vanilla Latte,** 1 small | 4 |
| **Iced Vanilla Latte,** 1 small | 4 |
| **Latte,** 1 small | 4 |
| **Latte with Sugar Free Vanilla Syrup,** 1 small | 4 |
| **Mocha,** 1 small | 8 |
| **Mocha with Nonfat Milk,** 1 small | 6 |
| ▲ **Nonfat Cappuccino,** 1 small | 2 |
| **Nonfat Cappuccino with Sugar Free Vanilla Syrup,** 1 small | 2 |
| **Nonfat Caramel Cappuccino,** 1 small | 4 |
| **Nonfat Caramel Latte,** 1 small | 5 |
| **Nonfat Hazelnut Cappuccino,** 1 small | 4 |
| **Nonfat Hazelnut Latte,** 1 small | 5 |
| ▲ **Nonfat Latte,** 1 small | 2 |
| ▲ **Nonfat Latte with Sugar Free Vanilla Syrup,** 1 small | 3 |
| **Nonfat Vanilla Cappuccino,** 1 small | 4 |
| **Nonfat Vanilla Latte,** 1 small | 5 |
| **Vanilla Cappuccino,** 1 small | 5 |
| **Vanilla Latte,** 1 small | 6 |

# McDONALD'S®

| ▲ Power Foods | *PointsPlus*™ value |
|---|---|

## DESSERTS & SHAKES

| | |
|---|---|
| ▲ **Apple Dippers,** 1 serving | 0 |
| **Baked Hot Apple Pie,** 1 | 7 |
| **Chocolate Chip Cookie,** 1 | 4 |
| **Cinnamon Melts,** 4 oz | 12 |
| **Fruit 'n Yogurt Parfait,** 1 | 4 |
| **Fruit 'n Yogurt Parfait (without granola),** 1 | 4 |
| **Kiddie Cone,** 1 | 1 |
| **Low Fat Caramel Dip,** 1 serving | 2 |
| **McDonaldland® Cookies,** 2 oz | 7 |
| **McFlurry® with M&M'S® Candies,** 1 serving | 17 |
| **McFlurry® with Oreo® Cookies,** 1 serving | 15 |
| **Oatmeal Raisin Cookie,** 1 | 4 |
| **Peanuts (for sundaes),** 1 serving | 1 |
| **Sugar Cookie,** 1 | 4 |
| **Sundae - Hot Caramel,** 1 | 10 |
| **Vanilla Reduced Fat Ice Cream Cone,** 1 | 4 |
| **Chocolate Triple Thick® Shake,** 1 small | 12 |
| **Strawberry Triple Thick® Shake,** 1 small | 11 |
| **Vanilla Triple Thick® Shake,** 1 small | 11 |

| ▲ Power Foods | *PointsPlus*™ value |
|---|---|
| **BURGERS** | |
| **Super Burger,** 1 | 21 |
| **Super Cheeseburger,** 1 | 23 |
| **Super Bacon Cheeseburger,** 1 | 24 |
| **Super Bacon Cheeseburger (no cheese or mayonnaise),** 1 | 17 |
| **CHICKEN** | |
| **Chicken Tenders,** 3 | 14 |
| **Chicken Tenders Platter,** 1 serving | 36 |
| **Grilled Chicken Breast Platter,** 1 serving | 26 |
| **Grilled Chicken Sandwich,** 1 | 14 |
| **Grilled Chicken Sandwich (no mayonnaise),** 1 | 8 |
| **CHEESESTEAKS** | |
| **Cheesesteak - Classic,** 1 | 11 |
| **Cheesesteak - Original,** 1 | 11 |
| **Cheesesteak - Works,** 1 | 14 |
| **PITAS** | |
| **Chicken Pita,** 1 | 10 |
| **Gyros Pita,** 1 | 18 |
| **SUBS** (6", NO MAYONNAISE OR CHEESE) | |
| **Ham,** 1 | 7 |
| **Italian Deli,** 1 | 8 |
| **SUBS** (6", ORIGINAL RECIPES) | |
| **Ham and Cheese,** 1 | 12 |
| **Italian Deli,** 1 | 14 |
| **Meatball Sub,** 1 | 13 |
| **Tuna Sub,** 1 | 12 |
| **Turkey Sub,** 1 | 13 |

| ▲ Power Foods | *PointsPlus*™ value |
|---|---|
| **PLATTERS** | |
| **10 Krispy Wings (with fries, celery & blue cheese only),** 1 serving | 27 |
| **Chicken Breast Platter,** 1 serving | 19 |
| **Gyros Platter,** 1 serving | 38 |
| **SALADS** | |
| **Caesar Salad (includes dressing),** 1 | 12 |
| **Chicken Caesar Salad (includes dressing),** 1 | 16 |
| **Chicken Club Salad,** 1 | 12 |
| **Garden Salad,** 1 | 8 |
| **Greek Salad,** 1 | 7 |
| **SIDES** | |
| **Mozzarella Sticks,** 6 sticks | 20 |
| **Onion Rings,** 1 serving | 24 |
| **Spicy Fries,** 1 regular serving | 14 |
| **Spicy Fries,** 1 large serving | 28 |
| **ARTHUR TREACHER'S ITEMS** | |
| **Coleslaw,** 1 serving | 6 |
| **Fish Sandwich,** 1 | 12 |
| **Hush Puppy,** 2 | 7 |

# MIAMI SUBS PIZZA & GRILL

| ▲ Power Foods | ***PointsPlus™*** value |
|---|---|
| **NATHANS FAMOUS ITEMS** | |
| **Hot Dog Nuggets,** 6 | 10 |
| **Nathan's Famous Hot Dog,** 1 | 9 |
| **Nathan's French Fries,** 1 regular serving | 15 |
| **Nathan's French Fries,** 1 large serving | 21 |

| ▲ Power Foods | *PointsPlus*™ value |
|---|---|
| **MEAT, CHICKEN, FISH, TOFU** | |
| **Chicken,** 1 serving | 2 |
| ▲ **Grilled Tilapia,** 1 serving | 2 |
| ▲ **Ground Beef,** 1 serving | 2 |
| **Marinated Tofu,** 1 serving | 1 |
| ▲ **Pork,** 1 serving | 2 |
| ▲ **Steak,** 1 serving | 2 |

| ADDITIONAL SELECTIONS | |
|---|---|
| **Bacon,** 1 serving | 4 |
| ▲ **Black Beans,** 1 serving | 1 |
| **Black Olives,** 1 serving | 1 |
| **Chipotle Ranch,** 1 serving | 7 |
| **Grilled Veggies,** 1 serving | 1 |
| **Guacamole,** 1 serving | 1 |
| ▲ **Lettuce,** 1 serving for salad | 0 |
| **Pickled Jalapenos,** 1 serving | 1 |
| **Pico de Gallo,** 1 serving | 0 |
| ▲ **Pinto Beans,** 1 serving | 1 |
| **Queso,** 1 serving | 4 |
| **Rice,** 1 serving | 1 |
| **Shredded Cheese,** 1 serving | 3 |
| **Sour Cream,** 2 Tbsp | 2 |
| **Southwest Vinaigrette,** 1 serving | 5 |

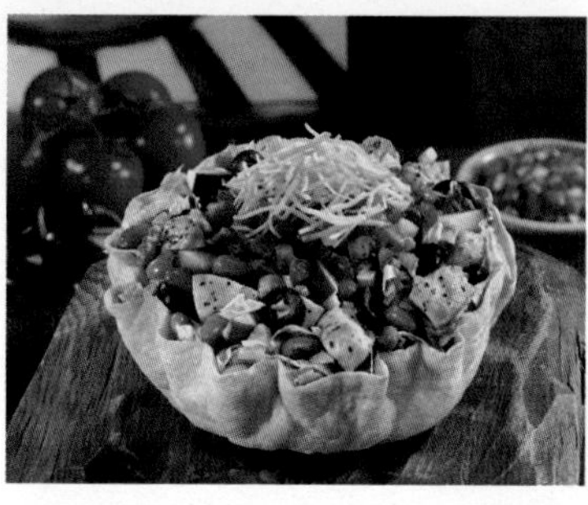

| ▲ Power Foods | *PointsPlus*™ value |
|---|---|
| **TORTILLAS** | |
| **6" Crispy Corn Tortilla,** 1 serving | 2 |
| **6" Flour Tortilla,** 1 serving | 2 |
| **8" Flour Tortilla,** 1 serving | 3 |
| **10" Flour Tortilla,** 1 serving | 5 |
| **10" Whole Grain Tortilla,** 1 serving | 5 |
| **12" Flour Tortilla,** 1 serving | 8 |
| **12" Whole Grain Tortilla,** 1 serving | 8 |

# MONICAL'S PIZZA®

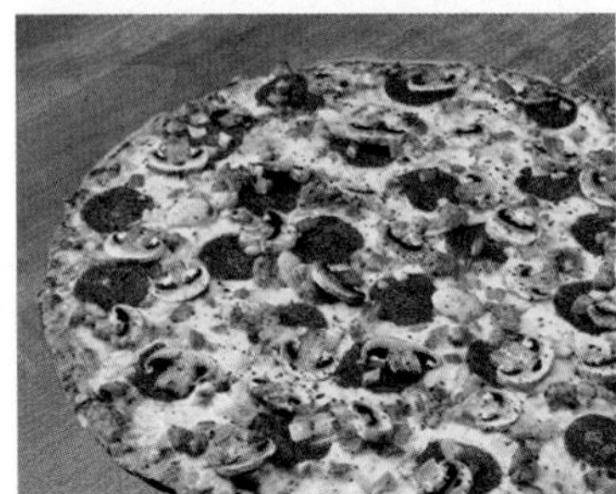

| ▲ Power Foods | *PointsPlus™* value |
|---|---|
| **STARTERS** | |
| **Breadsticks (plain),** 1 stick | 4 |
| **Cheddar Cheese,** 1 serving | 3 |
| **Hot Wings (without ranch),** 3 pieces | 5 |
| **Nacho Cheese,** 1 serving | 4 |
| **Pepperollies (without marinara),** 3 | 23 |
| **Plain Mild Cheddar Cheese Fries,** 1 pound | 30 |
| **Plain Mild Cheddar Cheese Fries (with toppings),** 1 pound | 34 |
| **Plain Nacho Cheese Fries,** 1 pound | 32 |
| **Plain Nacho Cheese Fries (with toppings),** 1 pound | 36 |
| **Tomato Sauce,** 1 serving | 2 |
| **POINT PIZZA** | |
| **Bacon,** 1/3 pizza | 25 |
| **BBQ Chicken,** 1/3 pizza | 23 |
| **Black Olive,** 1/3 pizza | 22 |
| **Cheese,** 1/3 pizza | 21 |
| **Green Olive,** 1/3 pizza | 23 |
| **Green Pepper,** 1/3 pizza | 21 |
| **Ham,** 1/3 pizza | 24 |
| **Hamburger,** 1/3 pizza | 24 |
| **Italian Hot Peppers,** 1/3 pizza | 21 |
| **Onion,** 1/3 pizza | 21 |
| **Pepperoni,** 1/3 pizza | 23 |
| **Premium Blend,** 1/3 pizza | 22 |
| **Red Pepper,** 1/3 pizza | 20 |
| **Sausage,** 1/3 pizza | 24 |
| **Spinach,** 1/3 pizza | 21 |
| **Steak,** 1/3 pizza | 22 |
| **GLUTEN FREE PIZZA** | |
| **Dough (whole crust),** 1 pizza | 17 |
| **Mozzarella Cheese,** 1 pizza | 10 |
| **Pizza Sauce,** 1 serving | 1 |
| **GLUTEN FREE PIZZA - SINGLE TOPPING PORTIONS** | |
| **Bacon,** 1 pizza | 6 |
| **Black Olives,** 1 pizza | 2 |
| **Colby Cheese,** 1 pizza | 2 |
| **Extra Cheese,** 1 pizza | 5 |
| **Garlic,** 1 pizza | 0 |
| **Green Olives,** 1 pizza | 3 |
| ▲ **Green Peppers,** 1 pizza | 0 |
| **Ham,** 1 pizza | 5 |
| **Hamburger,** 1 pizza | 4 |
| ▲ **Italian Hot Peppers,** 1 pizza | 0 |
| ▲ **Mushroom,** 1 pizza | 0 |
| ▲ **Onions/Red Onions,** 1 pizza | 0 |
| **Pepperoni,** 1 pizza | 4 |
| ▲ **Red Pepper,** 1 pizza | 0 |
| **Sausage,** 1 pizza | 4 |
| ▲ **Spinach,** 1 pizza | 0 |
| **Steak,** 1 pizza | 2 |
| ▲ **Tomatoes,** 1 pizza | 0 |

| ▲ Power Foods | PointsPlus™ value |
|---|---|
| **GLUTEN FREE PIZZA - SPECIALTY COMBINATIONS** | |
| **BBQ Chicken,** 1/2 pizza | 18 |
| **Delight,** 1/2 pizza | 21 |
| **Happy Heart,** 1/2 pizza | 14 |
| **Veggie,** 1/2 pizza | 18 |
| **MONICAL'S PIZZA® CRUST & SAUCE** | |
| **8" Pan Crust,** 1 individual serving | 14 |
| **8" Thin Crust,** 1 individual serving | 9 |
| **BBQ Sauce,** 1 serving | 1 |
| **Pan Pizza Sauce,** 1 serving | 1 |
| **Thin Pizza Sauce,** 1 serving | 0 |
| **MONICAL'S PIZZA® TOPPINGS** | |
| **BBQ Chicken,** 1 serving | 10 |
| **Cheese,** 1 serving | 5 |
| ▲ **Cheese Free,** 1 serving | 1 |
| **Delight,** 1 serving | 8 |
| **Deluxe,** 1 serving | 9 |
| **Happy Heart,** 1 serving | 4 |
| **Italian Special,** 1 serving | 8 |
| **Pepperoni,** 1 serving | 7 |
| **Sausage,** 1 serving | 6 |
| **PASTA** | |
| **Baked Ravioli,** 1 individual serving | 39 |
| **Garlic Stick,** 2 | 10 |
| **Lasagna,** 1 individual serving | 19 |
| **Meatballs,** 3 | 6 |
| **Spaghetti,** 1 individual serving | 12 |
| **Supreme (Premium blend),** 1 serving | 3 |
| **Tortellini,** 1 individual serving | 11 |

| ▲ Power Foods | PointsPlus™ value |
|---|---|
| **SANDWICHES (WITHOUT CHIPS)** | |
| **8" Bread,** 1 | 10 |
| **BBQ Chicken,** 1 sandwich | 26 |
| **Hot Sicilian,** 1 sandwich | 24 |
| **Italian Beef,** 1 sandwich | 15 |
| **Turkey,** 1 sandwich | 14 |
| **Side of Marinara Sauce,** 1 serving | 1 |
| **Side of Pepperoncinis,** 3 | 0 |
| **SAUCES & DIPS** | |
| **BBQ Sauce,** 1 serving | 2 |
| **Ranch,** 1 serving | 4 |
| **Red Hot Buffalo,** 1 serving | 1 |
| **SALADS** | |
| **Chef Salad,** 1 salad | 11 |
| **Individual Garden Salad,** 1 salad | 2 |
| **Pecan Grilled Chicken Salad,** 1 salad | 14 |
| **Southwest Chicken Salad,** 1 salad | 19 |
| **DRESSINGS** | |
| **1000 Island,** 2 Tbsp | 4 |
| **Creamy Italian,** 2 Tbsp | 3 |
| **Creamy Italian Lite,** 2 Tbsp | 1 |
| **Fat Free Vinaigrette,** 2 Tbsp | 1 |
| **Monical's® Sweet & Tart,** 2 Tbsp | 4 |
| **Ranch,** 2 Tbsp | 4 |

# MR. GOODCENTS® SUBS & PASTAS

| ▲ Power Foods | *PointsPlus™* value |
|---|---|
| **COLD SUB SANDWICH - 8"** | |
| **Centsable Sub™ on Wheat Bread,** 1/2 sandwich | 13 |
| **Centsable Sub™ on White Bread,** 1/2 sandwich | 13 |
| **Cheese Mix on Wheat Bread,** 1/2 sandwich | 16 |
| **Cheese Mix on White Bread,** 1/2 sandwich | 17 |
| **Ham & Cheese on White Bread,** 1/2 sandwich | 11 |
| **Ham and Cheese on Wheat Bread,** 1/2 sandwich | 11 |
| **Italian on Wheat Bread,** 1/2 sandwich | 17 |
| **Italian on White Bread,** 1/2 sandwich | 18 |
| **Mr. Goodcents Original™ on Wheat Bread,** 1/2 sandwich | 16 |
| **Mr. Goodcents Original™ on White Bread,** 1/2 sandwich | 13 |
| **Oven Roasted Chicken Breast on Wheat Bread,** 1/2 sandwich | 11 |
| **Oven Roasted Chicken Breast on White Bread,** 1/2 sandwich | 11 |
| **Penny Club™ on Wheat Bread,** 1/2 sandwich | 11 |
| **Penny Club™ on White Bread,** 1/2 sandwich | 11 |
| **Pepperoni and Cheese on Wheat Bread,** 1/2 sandwich | 21 |
| **Pepperoni and Cheese on White Bread,** 1/2 sandwich | 21 |
| **Roast Beef on Wheat Bread,** 1/2 sandwich | 11 |
| **Roast Beef on White Bread,** 1/2 sandwich | 11 |
| **Tuna Salad on Wheat Bread,** 1/2 sandwich | 14 |
| **Tuna Salad on White Bread,** 1/2 sandwich | 13 |
| **Turkey on Wheat Bread,** 1/2 sandwich | 11 |
| **Turkey on White Bread,** 1/2 sandwich | 11 |
| **Veggie on Wheat Bread,** 1/2 sandwich | 7 |
| **Veggie on White Bread,** 1/2 sandwich | 7 |
| **COLD SUB SANDWICH - 12"** | |
| **Centsable Sub™ on Wheat Bread,** 1 sandwich | 18 |
| **Centsable Sub™ on White Bread,** 1 sandwich | 19 |
| **Cheese Mix on Wheat Bread,** 1 sandwich | 22 |
| **Cheese Mix on White Bread,** 1 sandwich | 22 |
| **Ham and Cheese on Wheat Bread,** 1 sandwich | 14 |
| **Ham and Cheese on White Bread,** 1 sandwich | 14 |
| **Italian Sub on Wheat Bread,** 1 sandwich | 23 |
| **Italian Sub on White Bread,** 1 sandwich | 24 |
| **Mr. Goodcents Original™ on Wheat Bread,** 1 sandwich | 21 |
| **Mr. Goodcents Original™ on White Bread,** 1 sandwich | 21 |
| **Oven Roasted Chicken Breast on Wheat Bread,** 1 sandwich | 13 |
| **Oven Roasted Chicken Breast on White Bread,** 1 sandwich | 13 |
| **Penny Club™ on Wheat Bread,** 1 sandwich | 13 |

| ▲ Power Foods | *PointsPlus*™ value |
|---|---|
| **Penny Club™ on White Bread,** 1 sandwich | 13 |
| **Pepperoni and Cheese on Wheat Bread,** 1 sandwich | 26 |
| **Pepperoni and Cheese on White Bread,** 1 sandwich | 27 |
| **Roast Beef on Wheat Bread,** 1 sandwich | 13 |
| **Roast Beef on White Bread,** 1 sandwich | 13 |
| **Tuna Salad on Wheat Bread,** 1 sandwich | 19 |
| **Tuna Salad on White Bread,** 1 sandwich | 19 |
| **Turkey on Wheat Bread,** 1 sandwich | 13 |
| **Turkey on White Bread,** 1 sandwich | 13 |
| **Veggie on Wheat Bread,** 1 sandwich | 12 |
| **Veggie on White Bread,** 1 sandwich | 12 |

## HOT SUB SANDWICH - 8"

| | |
|---|---|
| **Chicken Bacon Ranch on Wheat Bread with Cheddar,** 1/2 sandwich | 18 |
| **Chicken Bacon Ranch on White Bread with Cheddar,** 1/2 sandwich | 18 |
| **Chicken Parmesan Sub on Wheat Bread with Mozzarella,** 1/2 sandwich | 14 |
| **Chicken Parmesan Sub on White Bread with Mozzarella,** 1/2 sandwich | 14 |
| **Meatball on Wheat Bread with Mozzarella,** 1/2 sandwich | 19 |
| **Meatball on White Bread with Mozzarella,** 1/2 sandwich | 19 |
| **Philly Jack 'n Cheese on Wheat,** 1/2 sandwich | 14 |
| **Philly Jack 'n Cheese on White,** 1/2 sandwich | 14 |

## DRESS OPTIONS

| ▲ Power Foods | *PointsPlus*™ value |
|---|---|
| **American Cheese,** 1 serving | 1 |
| **Bacon,** 3 slices | 2 |
| ▲ **Banana Peppers,** 1 serving | 0 |
| **Cheddar Cheese,** 1 serving | 2 |
| ▲ **Jalapenos,** 1 serving | 0 |
| **Mayonnaise,** 1 serving | 3 |
| **Mozzarella,** 1 serving | 1 |
| **Mustard,** 1 serving | 0 |
| **Olives,** 1 serving | 0 |
| **Pepper Jack,** 1 serving | 1 |
| ▲ **Pickles,** 1 serving | 0 |
| **Provolone,** 1 serving | 1 |
| **Ranch Dressing,** 1 serving | 3 |
| **Spicy Mustard,** 1 serving | 0 |
| **Spicy Ranch,** 1 serving | 3 |
| ▲ **Standard Dress, no oil,** 1 serving | 0 |
| **Swiss,** 1 serving | 1 |

## HOT PASTAS

| | |
|---|---|
| **Alfredo Sauce on Mostaccioli,** 1 serving | 34 |
| **Cheese Tortellini with Red Sauce,** 1 serving | 17 |
| **Chicken Alfredo on Mostaccioli,** 1 serving | 38 |
| **Chicken Parmesan on Mostaccioli,** 1 serving | 17 |
| **Garlic Bite,** 1 bite | 5 |
| **Red Sauce on Mostaccioli,** 1 serving | 13 |
| **Red Sauce on Mostaccioli with Meatball,** 1 serving | 19 |

# MR. GOODCENTS® SUBS & PASTAS

▲ Power Foods — *PointsPlus*™ value

## SALADS

|  | *PointsPlus*™ value |
|---|---|
| **Chef Salad,** 1 | 5 |
| **Garden Salad,** 1 | 2 |
| **Grilled Chicken Salad,** 1 | 6 |
| **Side Salad,** 1 | 1 |
| **Tuna Salad,** 1 | 9 |

## SOUPS

|  | *PointsPlus*™ value |
|---|---|
| **Broccoli Cheese Soup,** 1 serving | 10 |
| **Chicken Noodle Soup,** 1 serving | 3 |
| **Cream of Potato Soup,** 1 serving | 9 |

## SIDES

|  | *PointsPlus*™ value |
|---|---|
| **Bread Sticks,** 1 | 2 |
| **Meatballs,** 1 serving | 6 |
| **Pasta Salad,** 1 serving | 6 |
| **Potato Salad,** 1 | 5 |

## GOODCENTS SATISFIER

|  | *PointsPlus*™ value |
|---|---|
| **Centsable Sub™ Satisfier Bread,** 1 | 9 |
| **Cheese Mix Satisfier Bread,** 1 | 12 |
| **Ham and Cheese Satisfier Bread,** 1 | 7 |
| **Italian Sub Satisfier Bread,** 1 | 14 |
| **Mr. Goodcent Original™ Satisfier Bread,** 1 | 9 |
| **Oven Roasted Chicken Breast Satisfier Bread,** 1 | 6 |
| **Penny Club™ Satisfier Bread,** 1 | 6 |
| **Pepperoni and Satisfier Bread,** 1 | 17 |
| **Roast Beef Satisfier Bread,** 1 | 6 |
| **Tune Salad Satisfier Bread,** 1 | 9 |
| **Turkey Satisfier Bread,** 1 | 6 |
| **Veggie Sub Satisfier Bread,** 1 | 3 |

## BREAD

|  | *PointsPlus*™ value |
|---|---|
| **Mr. Goodcents Wheat Bread Half,** 1 | 7 |
| **Mr. Goodcents Wheat Footlong Bread,** 1 | 9 |
| **Mr. Goodcents White Bread Half,** 1 | 7 |
| **Mr. Goodcents White Footlong Bread,** 1 | 9 |

## DESSERTS

|  | *PointsPlus*™ value |
|---|---|
| **Baked Brownie,** 1 | 7 |
| **Giant Chocolate Chip Cookie,** 1 | 12 |
| **Giant Peanut Butter Cookie,** 1 | 9 |
| **Rich Chocolate Brownie,** 1 serving | 7 |

| ▲ Power Foods | *PointsPlus*™ value |
|---|---|
| **COOKIES** | |
| **Butter Toffee Cookie,** 1 | 8 |
| **Chewy Fudge Cookie,** 1 | 8 |
| **Chocolate Lovers Cookie,** 1 | 8 |
| **Cinnamon Sugar Cookie,** 1 | 8 |
| **Cranberry White Chunk Cookie,** 1 | 8 |
| **Debra's Special® (Oatmeal Raisin Walnut) Cookie,** 1 | 7 |
| **Frosted Lemon Cookie,** 1 | 10 |
| **Hand-Dipped Cookie, Chewy Fudge,** 1 | 12 |
| **Hand-Dipped Cookie, Peanut Butter,** 1 | 12 |
| **Milk Chocolate Chip Cookie,** 1 | 8 |
| **Milk Chocolate Chip with M&M,** 1 cookie | 9 |
| **Milk Chocolate Cookie Sandwich,** 1 | 23 |
| **Milk Chocolate Macadamia Cookie,** 1 | 8 |
| **Milk Chocolate Walnut Cookie,** 1 | 8 |
| **Oatmeal Peanut Butter Scotchy,** 1 cookie | 8 |
| **Peanut Butter Cookie,** 1 | 8 |
| **Peanut Butter with Milk Chocolate Chips Cookie,** 1 | 9 |
| **Pumpkin Harvest Cookie,** 1 | 7 |
| **Semi-Sweet Chocolate Chip Cookie,** 1 | 8 |
| **Semi-sweet Cookie Sandwich,** 1 | 23 |
| **Semi-Sweet Walnut Cookie,** 1 | 8 |
| **Sugar Butter Cookie,** 1 | 7 |
| **Sugar Butter with M&Ms Cookie,** 1 | 8 |
| **White Chunk Macadamia Cookie,** 1 | 8 |
| **COOKIE NIBBLER™** | |
| **Cinnamon Sugar Nibbler™,** 3 | 5 |
| **Debra's Special (Oatmeal Raisin Walnut) Nibbler™,** 3 | 4 |
| **Milk Chocolate Chip Nibbler™,** 3 | 5 |

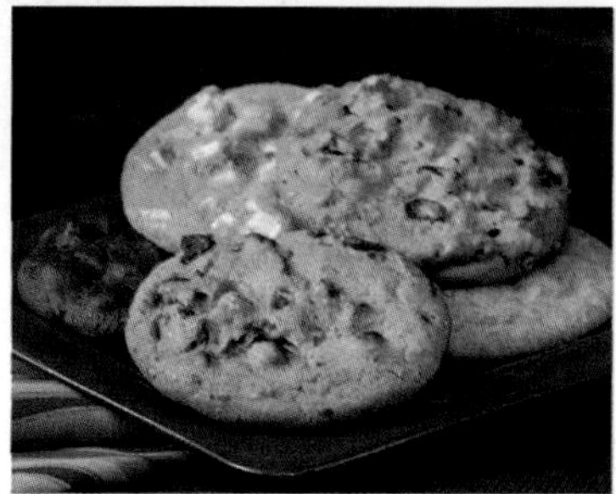

| ▲ Power Foods | *PointsPlus*™ value |
|---|---|
| **Milk Chocolate Walnut Nibbler™,** 3 | 5 |
| **Peanut Butter Nibbler™,** 3 | 5 |
| **Semi-Sweet Chocolate Chip Nibbler™,** 3 | 5 |
| **Sugar Butter with M&Ms Nibbler,** 3 | 4 |
| **White Chunk Macadamia Nibbler™,** 3 | 5 |
| **COOKIE CUPS** | |
| **Chewy Fudge,** 1 | 13 |
| **Peanut Butter,** 1 mini | 2 |
| **Semi-Sweet Chocolate Chip,** 1 mini | 2 |
| **COOKIE CAKES** | |
| **Big Cookie Cake,** 1/16 of a cookie | 13 |
| **Cookie Card,** 1/4 of the cookie | 14 |
| **Cookie Slice,** 1 slice | 19 |
| **Heart Cookie Cake,** 1/13 of the cookie | 12 |
| **DISNEY COOKIE/CAKES** | |
| **Cookie Cake - Piglet,** 1 serving | 11 |
| **Cookie Cake - Pooh,** 1 serving | 11 |
| **Cookie Cake - Tigger,** 1 serving | 11 |
| **Piglet Cookie,** 1 | 8 |
| **Pooh Cookie,** 1 | 10 |
| **Princess Cookie,** 1 | 7 |
| **Princess Cookie Cup,** 1 serving | 9 |

# MRS. FIELDS®

| ▲ Power Foods | *PointsPlus™* value |
|---|---|
| **BROWNIES & BAR** | |
| **Double Fudge Brownie,** 1 | 14 |
| **Frosted Fudge Brownie,** 1 | 14 |
| **Pecan Fudge Brownie,** 1 | 12 |
| **Rocky Mountain Mogul,** 1 | 18 |
| **Walnut Fudge Brownie,** 1 | 12 |
| **Peanut Butter Dream Bar,** 1 | 18 |
| **MUFFINS** | |
| **Blueberry,** 1 | 10 |
| **Chocolate,** 1 | 12 |
| **Chocolate Chip,** 1 | 12 |
| **Orange,** 1 | 10 |
| **Raspberry,** 1 mini | 2 |
| **BREEZER® SMOOTHIES** | |
| **Cappuccino Smoothie,** 1 | 17 |
| **Mango Smoothie,** 1 | 18 |
| **Piña-Colada Smoothie,** 1 | 19 |
| **SMOOTHIES & CHILLERS** | |
| **Cookies and Cream Chiller,** 1 | 33 |
| **Lemon Smoothie,** 1 | 19 |
| **Mocha Smoothie,** 1 | 17 |
| **Peach Smoothie,** 1 | 18 |
| **Peach Smoothie, Non-Dairy,** 1 | 14 |
| **Raspberry Smoothie,** 1 | 18 |
| **Raspberry Smoothie, Non-Dairy,** 1 | 14 |
| **Strawberry Banana Smoothie,** 1 | 18 |
| **Strawberry Banana Smoothie, Non-Dairy,** 1 | 14 |

| ▲ Power Foods | *PointsPlus™* value |
|---|---|

## ALL BEEF HOT DOGS

| Item | PointsPlus™ value |
|---|---|
| **Corn Dogs on a Stick,** 1 | 10 |
| **Hot Dog Nuggets,** 6 | 10 |
| **Nathan's Famous Beef Cheese Dog,** 1 | 9 |
| **Nathan's Famous Beef Chili Dog,** 1 | 11 |
| **Nathan's Famous Hot Dog,** 1 | 8 |

## BURGERS

| Item | PointsPlus™ value |
|---|---|
| **5 oz Burger with Cheese,** 1 | 19 |
| **Bacon Cheeseburger,** 1 | 21 |
| **Double Burger with Cheese,** 1 | 31 |
| **Super Cheeseburger,** 1 | 27 |

## CHEESESTEAKS

| Item | PointsPlus™ value |
|---|---|
| **Chicken Cheesesteak,** 1 | 16 |
| **Philly Cheesesteak,** 1 | 23 |
| **Philly Cheesesteak Supreme,** 1 | 24 |

## CHICKEN

| Item | PointsPlus™ value |
|---|---|
| **Chicken Tenders,** 3 | 14 |
| **Chicken Tender Platter,** 1 | 33 |
| **Chicken Wing Order with Bleu Cheese,** 5 wings | 18 |
| **Chicken Wing Order with Bleu Cheese,** 10 wings | 33 |
| **Chicken Wing Order with Bleu Cheese,** 20 wings | 67 |
| **Chicken Wing Order with Bleu Cheese & Fries,** 10 wings | 45 |
| **Grilled Chicken Breast Platter,** 1 serving | 22 |
| **Grilled Chicken Caesar Wrap,** 1 | 19 |
| **Grilled Chicken Club Sandwich,** 1 | 19 |
| **Grilled Chicken Sandwich,** 1 | 15 |
| **Grilled Chicken Santa Fe Wrap,** 1 | 23 |
| **Krispy Chicken Chipotle Club,** 1 | 23 |
| **Krispy Homestyle Chicken Sandwich,** 1 | 19 |
| **Original Krispy Chicken Sandwich,** 1 | 18 |

## SEAFOOD

| Item | PointsPlus™ value |
|---|---|
| **Breaded Clam & Chips,** 1 serving | 25 |
| **Breaded Clam Order,** 1 serving | 12 |
| **Fish & Chips Platter,** 1 serving | 44 |
| **Fish Sandwich,** 1 | 12 |
| **Seafood Sampler,** 1 serving | 55 |
| **Shrimp & Chips,** 1 serving | 40 |
| **Shrimp Boat,** 1 serving | 99 |

## SALADS

| Item | PointsPlus™ value |
|---|---|
| **Caesar Salad,** 1 | 11 |
| **Chicken Caesar Salad,** 1 | 14 |
| **Garden Salad,** 1 | 2 |
| **Krispy Chicken Salad,** 1 | 10 |

## SAUCES & DRESSINGS

| Item | PointsPlus™ value |
|---|---|
| **1000 Island Dressing,** 1 serving | 6 |
| **Barbeque Sauce,** 1 serving | 1 |
| **Garlic Sauce,** 1 serving | 2 |
| **Honey Mustard Dipping Sauce,** 1 serving | 5 |
| **Mayonnaise,** 1 serving | 3 |
| **Tartar Sauce,** 1 serving | 3 |
| **Tzatziki Sauce,** 1 serving | 2 |
| **Wing Sauce,** 2 Tbsp | 0 |

# NATHAN'S FAMOUS

| ▲ Power Foods | *PointsPlus™* value |
|---|---|
| **BREAD** | |
| **7" Pita Bread,** 1 serving | 6 |
| **Hoagie Roll,** 1 | 8 |
| **Hot Dog Roll,** 1 | 3 |
| **Hush Puppies,** 2 | 14 |
| **Kaiser Roll,** 1 | 5 |
| **FRENCH FRIES & ONION RINGS** | |
| **French Fries,** 1 medium serving | 11 |
| **Cheese French Fries - Super,** 1 serving | 29 |
| **Onion Rings,** 1 regular serving | 16 |
| **MISCELLANEOUS** | |
| **Aged Cheddar Cheese Sauce,** 1 serving | 3 |
| **Apple Pie,** 1 serving | 9 |
| **Chili with Beans,** 1 serving | 2 |
| **Cole Slaw,** 1 serving | 5 |
| ▲ **Corn on the Cob,** 1 | 4 |
| **Mozzarella Sticks,** 1 serving | 10 |
| **Nathan's Mustard,** 1 tsp | 0 |
| **Relish,** 1 serving | 0 |
| ▲ **Sauerkraut,** 1 serving | 0 |
| **Southwest Munchers,** 1 serving | 2 |
| **Swiss American Cheese,** 1 serving | 3 |
| **Yellow American Cheese,** 1 serving | 3 |
| **SOUPS** | |
| **Chicken Noodle Soup,** 1 serving | 5 |
| **Manhattan Clam Chowder,** 1 serving | 7 |
| **New England Clam Chowder,** 1 serving | 6 |

| ▲ Power Foods | *PointsPlus™* value |
|---|---|

## ASIAN SALADS

| | |
|---|---|
| **Chinese Chop Salad,** 1 regular | 6 |
| ▲ **Chinese Chop Salad (without dressing),** 1 regular | 3 |

## MEDITERRANEAN SALADS

| | |
|---|---|
| **The Med Salad,** 1 regular | 8 |
| **The Med Salad (without dressing),** 1 regular | 7 |

## AMERICAN SALADS

| | |
|---|---|
| **Caesar Salad,** 1 regular | 9 |
| **Caesar Salad, no dressing,** 1 regular | 4 |

## ASIAN SOUP

| | |
|---|---|
| **Thai Curry Soup,** 1 regular | 12 |

## MEDITERRANEAN SOUP

| | |
|---|---|
| **Tomato Bisque Soup,** 1 regular | 10 |

## ASIAN NOODLES

| | |
|---|---|
| **Bangkok Curry,** 1 regular | 13 |
| **Indonesian Peanut Saute,** 1 regular | 25 |
| **Japanese Pan Noodles,** 1 regular | 18 |
| **Pad Thai,** 1 regular | 18 |

## MEDITERRANEAN NOODLES

| | |
|---|---|
| **Pasta Fresca,** 1 regular | 20 |
| **Penne Rosa,** 1 regular | 21 |
| **Penne Rosa with Whole Grain Linguini,** 1 regular | 20 |

| ▲ Power Foods | *PointsPlus™* value |
|---|---|
| **Pesto Cavatappi,** 1 regular | 24 |
| **Pesto Cavatappi, no cream,** 1 small | 11 |
| **Whole Grain Tuscan Linguine,** 1 regular | 19 |
| **Whole Grain Tuscan Linguinie without Cream,** 1 regular | 16 |

## AMERICAN NOODLES

| | |
|---|---|
| **Buttered Noodles,** 1 regular | 16 |
| **Chicken Noodle Soup,** 1 regular | 7 |
| **House Marinara,** 1 regular | 17 |
| **House Marinara with Whole Grain Linguini,** 1 regular | 16 |
| **Mushroom Stroganoff,** 1 regular | 21 |
| **Spaghetti & Meatballs,** 1 regular serving | 24 |
| **Spaghetti with Marinara,** 1 regular serving | 17 |
| **Wisconsin Mac & Cheese,** 1 regular | 23 |

## SAMPLE TRIOS

| | |
|---|---|
| **Bangkok Curry TRIO with Organic Tofu and Tossed Green Salad with Balsamic Dressing,** 1 | 12 |

*Sample Trios (cont'd)*

| ▲ Power Foods | PointsPlus™ value |
|---|---|
| **Bangkok Curry TRIO with Organic Tofu and Tossed Green Side Salad with Fat Free Asian Dressing,** 1 | 11 |
| **Bangkok Curry TRIO with Chicken Breast & Caesar Side Salad,** 1 | 13 |
| **Bangkok Curry TRIO with Sauteed Shrimp and Tossed Green Side Salad with Fat Free Asian Dressing,** 1 | 8 |
| **Japanese Pan Noodles TRIO with Sauteed Shrimp and Tossed Green Side Salad with Fat Free Asian Dressing,** 1 | 10 |
| **Japanese Pan Noodles TRIO with Chicken Breast and Tossed Green Salad with Fat Free Asian Dressing,** 1 | 13 |
| **Japanese Pan TRIO with Organic Tofu and Tossed Green Side Salad and Fat Free Asian Dressing,** 1 | 13 |
| **Pad Thai TRIO with Organic Tofu & Tossed Green Side Salad with Asian Fat Free Dressing,** 1 | 14 |
| **Pad Thai TRIO with Sauteed Shrimp and Tossed Green Side Salad with Fat Free Asian Dressing,** 1 | 11 |
| **Pasta Fresca TRIO with Chicken Breast and Caesar Side Salad,** 1 | 17 |
| **Pasta Fresca TRIO with Sauteed Shrimp and Tossed Green Side Salad with Balsamic Dressing,** 1 | 13 |
| **Penne Rosa TRIO with Chicken Breast & Caesar Side Salad,** 1 | 17 |
| **Penne Rosa TRIO with Sauteed Shrimp and Tossed Green Side Salad with Balsamic Dressing,** 1 | 13 |
| **Pesto Cavatappi® TRIO (without cream) with Sauteed Shrimp and Tossed Green Side Salad with Balsamic Dressing,** 1 | 13 |
| **Pesto Cavatappi® TRIO with Chicken Breast and Tossed Green Side Salad with Balsamic Dressing,** 1 | 19 |
| **Pesto Cavatappi® TRIO Sauteed Shrimp, Tossed Green Side Salad with Balsamic Dressing,** 1 | 16 |

| ▲ Power Foods | PointsPlus™ value |
|---|---|
| **SIDES** | |
| **Braised Beef,** 1 serving | 5 |
| ▲ **Chicken Breast,** 1 serving | 3 |
| **Ciabatta Roll,** 1 | 4 |
| **Cucumber Tomato Salad,** 1 | 2 |
| **Flatbread,** 1 serving | 5 |
| **Meatballs,** 5 meatballs | 6 |
| **Parmesan Crusted Chicken Breast,** 1 serving | 4 |
| **Potstickers,** 3 | 5 |
| **Sauteed Beef,** 1 serving | 5 |
| **Sauteed Shrimp,** 1 serving | 1 |
| **Sauteed Tofu,** 1 serving | 5 |
| **Tossed Green Salad (without dressing),** 1 serving | 2 |
| **Tossed Green Salad with Fat Free Asian,** 1 serving | 1 |
| **Tossed Green Side Salad,** 1 salad | 2 |
| **Tossed Green Side Salad with Fat Free Asian Dressing,** 1 salad | 1 |
| **ADD-ONS - CHEESE** | |
| **Extra Cheddar Jack Cheese,** 1 serving | 5 |
| **Extra Feta Cheese,** 1 serving | 2 |
| **Extra Parmesan Cheese,** 1 serving | 3 |
| **ADD-ONS - FRESH VEGGIE** | |
| ▲ **Extra Broccoli,** 1 serving | 0 |
| ▲ **Extra Carrots,** 1 serving | 0 |
| ▲ **Extra Cucumbers,** 1 serving | 0 |
| **Extra Kalamata Olives,** 1 serving | 1 |
| ▲ **Extra Mushrooms,** 1 serving | 0 |
| ▲ **Extra Red Onions,** 1 serving | 0 |
| ▲ **Extra Red Pepper,** 1 serving | 0 |
| ▲ **Extra Shiitake Mushrooms,** 1 serving | 0 |
| ▲ **Extra Spinach,** 1 serving | 0 |
| ▲ **Extra Tomatoes,** 1 serving | 0 |

| ▲ Power Foods | *PointsPlus*™ value |
|---|---|

## ADD-ONS - PROTEIN

| | |
|---|---|
| **Marinated Chicken Breast,** 1 | 3 |
| **Parmesan Chicken Breast,** 1 serving | 4 |
| ▲ **Shrimp, cooked,** 1 serving | 1 |
| **Tofu, cooked,** 1 serving | 5 |

## DRESSINGS

| | |
|---|---|
| **Balsamic Vinaigrette, as served,** 1 serving | 3 |
| **Caesar, as served,** 1 serving | 5 |
| **Fat Free Asian, as served,** 1 serving | 0 |
| **Mediterranean, as served,** 1 serving | 1 |
| **Sesame Soy, as served,** 1 serving | 3 |

## DESSERTS

| | |
|---|---|
| **Chocolate Chunk Puddin Cookie,** 1 | 10 |
| **Rice Krispy Treat,** 1 | 15 |
| **Snickerdoodle Cookie,** 1 | 9 |

# OLD CHICAGO

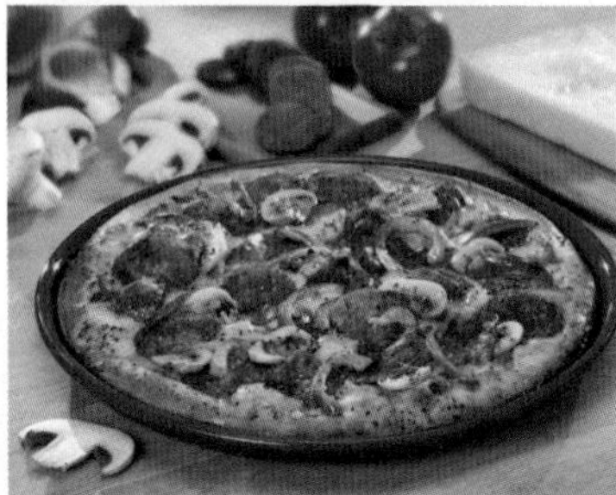

▲ Power Foods — *PointsPlus™* value

## STARTER

|  | *PointsPlus™* value |
|---|---|
| **Extra Hot Buffalo Wings,** 1 serving (4 servings per plate) | 10 |
| **Hot Buffalo Wings,** 1 serving (4 servings per plate) | 10 |
| **Italian Nachos,** 1 serving (4 servings per plate) | 9 |
| **Italian Nachos, Half,** 1 serving (4 servings per plate) | 5 |
| **Jerk Wings,** 1 serving (4 servings per plate) | 9 |
| **Nachos Grande,** 1 serving (4 servings per plate) | 14 |
| **Nachos Grande, Half,** 1 serving (4 servings per plate) | 7 |
| **Nachos Grande, with Chicken,** 1 serving (4 servings per plate) | 15 |
| **Nachos Grande, with Chicken, Half,** 1 serving (4 servings per plate) | 8 |
| **Original Buffalo Wings,** 1 serving (4 servings per plate) | 10 |

▲ Power Foods — *PointsPlus™* value

## PIZZA

|  | *PointsPlus™* value |
|---|---|
| **Cheese Only, Chicago Style, Individual,** 1 slice | 9 |
| **Cheese Only, Chicago Style, Medium,** 1 slice | 12 |
| **Cheese Only, Chicago Style, Large,** 1 slice | 12 |
| **Cheese Only, Deep Dish, Medium,** 1 slice | 12 |
| **Cheese Only, Deep Dish, Large,** 1 slice | 12 |
| **Cheese Only, Express, Chicago Style,** 1 slice | 4 |
| **Cheese Only, Express, Thin Crust,** 1 slice | 4 |
| **Cheese Only, Thin Crust, 14",** 1 slice | 6 |
| **Cheese Only, Thin Crust, Individual,** 1 slice | 6 |
| **Chicago Seven Pizza, Chicago Style, Individual,** 1 slice | 11 |
| **Chicago Seven Pizza, Chicago Style, Medium,** 1 slice | 14 |
| **Chicago Seven Pizza, Chicago Style, Large,** 1 slice | 15 |
| **Chicago Seven Pizza, Deep Dish, Medium,** 1 slice | 13 |
| **Chicago Seven Pizza, Deep Dish, Large,** 1 slice | 15 |
| **Chicago Seven Pizza, Thin Crust, 14",** 1 slice | 9 |
| **Chicago Seven Pizza, Thin Crust, Individual,** 1 slice | 8 |
| **Classic Chicago Style Pizza, Chicago Style, Individual,** 1 slice | 12 |
| **Classic Chicago Style Pizza, Chicago Style, Medium,** 1 slice | 14 |
| **Classic Chicago Style Pizza, Chicago Style, Large,** 1 slice | 15 |

| ▲ Power Foods | *PointsPlus™* value |
|---|---|
| **Classic Chicago Style Pizza, Deep Dish, Medium,** 1 slice | 13 |
| **Classic Chicago Style Pizza, Deep Dish, Large,** 1 slice | 14 |
| **Classic Chicago Style Pizza, Thin Crust, 14",** 1 slice | 9 |
| **Classic Chicago Style Pizza, Thin Crust, Individual,** 1 slice | 8 |
| **Double Deckeroni Pizza, Chicago Style, Individual,** 1 slice | 13 |
| **Double Deckeroni Pizza, Chicago Style, Medium,** 1 slice | 15 |
| **Double Deckeroni Pizza, Chicago Style, Large,** 1 slice | 17 |
| **Double Deckeroni Pizza, Deep Dish, Medium,** 1 slice | 15 |
| **Double Deckeroni Pizza, Deep Dish, Large,** 1 slice | 16 |
| **Double Deckeroni Pizza, Thin Crust, 14",** 1 slice | 11 |
| **Double Deckeroni Pizza, Thin Crust, Individual,** 1 slice | 9 |
| **Hawaiian Pizza, Chicago Style, Individual,** 1 slice | 10 |
| **Hawaiian Pizza, Chicago Style, Medium,** 1 slice | 13 |
| **Hawaiian Pizza, Chicago Style, Large,** 1 slice | 14 |
| **Hawaiian Pizza, Deep Dish, Medium,** 1 slice | 13 |
| **Hawaiian Pizza, Deep Dish, Large,** 1 slice | 14 |
| **Hawaiian Pizza, Thin Crust, 14",** 1 slice | 8 |
| **Hawaiian Pizza, Thin Crust, Individual,** 1 slice | 7 |
| **Meat Me Pizza, Chicago Style, Individual,** 1 slice | 13 |
| **Meat Me Pizza, Chicago Style, Medium,** 1 slice | 16 |

| ▲ Power Foods | *PointsPlus™* value |
|---|---|
| **Meat Me Pizza, Chicago Style, Large,** 1 slice | 17 |
| **Meat Me Pizza, Deep Dish, Medium,** 1 slice | 16 |
| **Meat Me Pizza, Deep Dish, Large,** 1 slice | 17 |
| **Meat Me Pizza, Thin Crust, 14",** 1 slice | 12 |
| **Meat Me Pizza, Thin Crust, Individual,** 1 slice | 10 |
| **Thai Pie, Chicago Style, Individual,** 1 slice | 11 |
| **Thai Pie, Chicago Style, Medium,** 1 slice | 14 |
| **Thai Pie, Chicago Style, Large,** 1 slice | 15 |
| **Thai Pie, Deep Dish, Medium,** 1 slice | 13 |
| **Thai Pie, Deep Dish, Large,** 1 slice | 14 |
| **Thai Pie, Thin Crust, 14",** 1 slice | 8 |
| **Thai Pie, Thin Crust, Individual,** 1 slice | 7 |
| **Vegetarian 7 Pizza, Chicago Style, Medium,** 1 slice | 13 |
| **Vegetarian 7 Pizza, Chicago Style, Individual,** 1 slice | 10 |
| **Vegetarian 7 Pizza, Chicago Style, Large,** 1 slice | 13 |
| **Vegetarian 7 Pizza, Deep Dish, Medium,** 1 slice | 12 |
| **Vegetarian 7 Pizza, Deep Dish, Large,** 1 slice | 13 |
| **Vegetarian 7 Pizza, Thin Crust, 14",** 1 slice | 7 |
| **Vegetarian 7 Pizza, Thin Crust, Individual,** 1 slice | 6 |

# OLD CHICAGO

| ▲ Power Foods | *PointsPlus*™ value |
|---|---|
| **CALZONE** | |
| **Cheese Calzone,** 1 | 25 |
| **Meat Me Calzone,** 1 | 42 |
| **Spinach Artichoke Calzone,** 1 | 29 |
| **The Famous Chicago Seven Calzone,** 1 | 33 |
| **SANDWICH** | |
| **Classic Club Sandwich (no side),** 1 sandwich | 22 |
| **Classic Italian Melt (no side),** 1 sandwich | 28 |
| **Grilled Chicken Wrap (no side),** 1 sandwich | 15 |
| **Grilled Chicken Wrap, Half (no side),** 1 sandwich | 7 |
| **SALAD** | |
| **Antipasto Salad,** 1 salad | 9 |
| **Caesar Salad,** 1 salad | 8 |
| **Classic Caesar Salad,** 1 salad | 23 |
| **Grilled Chicken Caesar Salad (with bread),** 1 salad | 27 |
| **Grilled Chicken Caesar Salad, Half (with bread),** 1 salad | 16 |
| **House Salad,** 1 salad | 3 |
| **SIDE** | |
| **Coleslaw,** 1 serving | 5 |
| **French Fries,** 1 serving | 8 |
| **BREAD** | |
| **Garlic Bread,** 1 slice | 4 |

| ▲ Power Foods | *PointsPlus*™ value |
|---|---|

## DINNER ENTRÉES

| | |
|---|---|
| **Capellini Pomodoro,** 1 serving | 21 |
| **Cheese Ravioli with Marinara Sauce,** 1 serving | 17 |
| **Cheese Ravioli with Meat Sauce,** 1 serving | 20 |
| **Chicken Marsala,** 1 serving | 19 |
| **Eggplant Parmigiana,** 1 serving | 25 |
| **Herb-Grilled Salmon,** 1 serving | 13 |
| **Lasagna Classico,** 1 serving | 21 |
| **Linguine alla Marinara,** 1 serving | 11 |
| **Mixed Grill,** 1 serving | 19 |
| **Parmesan Crusted Tilapia,** 1 serving | 15 |
| **Ravioli di Portobello,** 1 serving | 17 |
| **Seafood Portofino,** 1 serving | 20 |
| **Shrimp & Asparagus Risotto,** 1 serving | 15 |
| **Shrimp Primavera,** 1 serving | 18 |
| **Spaghetti with Meat Sauce,** 1 serving | 18 |
| **Steak Toscano,** 1 serving | 22 |
| **Stuffed Chicken Marsala,** 1 serving | 22 |
| **Venetian Apricot Chicken,** 1 serving | 9 |

## LUNCH ENTRÉES

| | |
|---|---|
| **Capellini Pomodoro,** 1 serving | 12 |
| **Cheese Ravioli with Marinara Sauce,** 1 serving | 14 |
| **Cheese Ravioli with Meat Sauce,** 1 serving | 15 |
| **Chicken Parmigiana,** 1 serving | 14 |
| **Eggplant Parmigiana,** 1 serving | 16 |
| **Grilled Chicken Spiedini,** 1 serving | 11 |

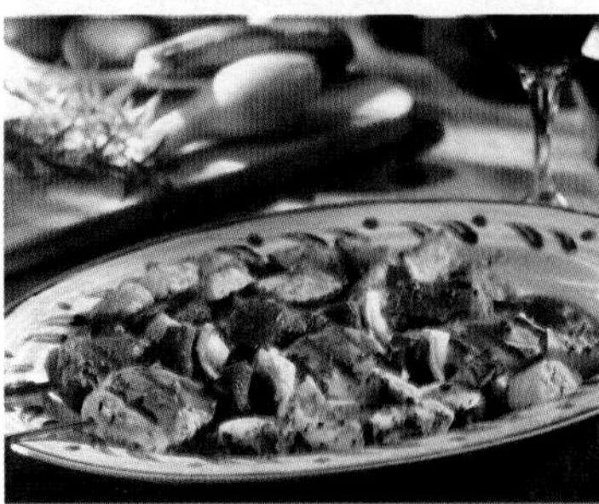

| ▲ Power Foods | *PointsPlus*™ value |
|---|---|
| **Lasagna Classico,** 1 serving | 15 |
| **Linguine alla Marinara,** 1 serving | 8 |
| **Ravioli di Portobello,** 1 serving | 12 |
| **Shrimp Primavera,** 1 serving | 14 |
| **Spaghetti with Meat Sauce,** 1 serving | 14 |
| **Venetian Apricot Chicken,** 1 serving | 6 |

## OTHER

| | |
|---|---|
| **Breadstick (with garlic-butter),** 1 serving | 4 |
| **Chicken & Gnocchi,** 1 serving | 7 |
| **Garden-Fresh Salad (without dressing),** 1 serving | 3 |
| **Italian Salad Dressing,** 1 serving | 5 |
| **Low Fat Italian Salad Dressing,** 1 serving | 2 |
| **Marinara Dipping Sauce,** 1 serving | 2 |
| **Minestrone,** 1 serving | 2 |
| **Mussels di Napoli,** 1 serving | 5 |
| **Pasta e Fagioli,** 1 serving | 3 |
| **Zuppa Toscana,** 1 serving | 4 |

# ON THE BORDER

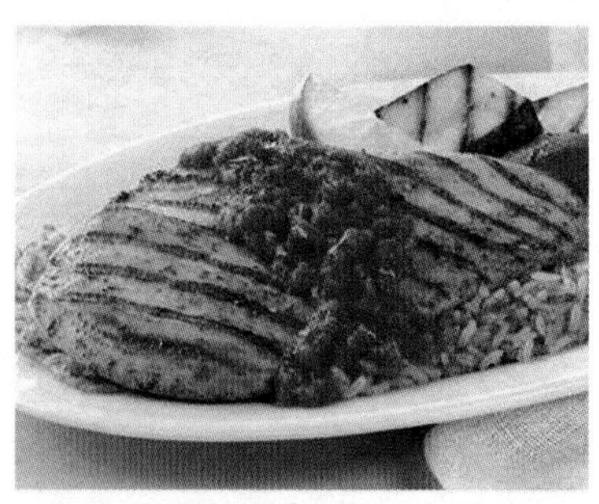

▲ Power Foods — *PointsPlus™* value

## BORDER LUNCH FAVORITES
(WITH RICE, WITHOUT BEANS)

| Item | *PointsPlus™* value |
|---|---|
| **Border's Best Lunch Chicken Fajitas - w/o Tortillas and Condiments,** 1 serving | 11 |
| **Mesquite-Grilled Fajitas - Chicken,** 1 serving | 11 |

## CREATE YOUR OWN COMBO
(WITHOUT RICE OR BEANS)

| Item | *PointsPlus™* value |
|---|---|
| **Crispy Taco - Chicken,** 1 each | 6 |
| **Enchilada - Beef with Chili Con Carne,** 1 each | 7 |
| **Enchilada - Chicken with Sour Cream Sauce,** 1 each | 6 |

## FRESH GRILL

| Item | *PointsPlus™* value |
|---|---|
| **Chicken Salsa Fresca with Mexican Rice and Grilled Veggies,** 1 serving | 12 |
| **Jalapeno-BBQ Salmon with Black Beans and Grilled Veggies,** 1 serving | 13 |

▲ Power Foods — *PointsPlus™* value

## KID'S MENU

| Item | *PointsPlus™* value |
|---|---|
| **Grilled Chicken (no sides),** 1 serving | 2 |
| **Grilled Chicken Sandwich (no sides),** 1 serving | 9 |

## SOUPS & SALADS

| Item | *PointsPlus™* value |
|---|---|
| **Chicken Tortilla Soup,** 1 cup | 9 |
| **Chicken Tortilla Soup,** 1 bowl | 13 |
| **Citrus Chipotle Chicken Salad with Mango Citrus Vinaigrette,** 1 serving | 7 |
| **Side - House Salad (no dressing),** 1 serving | 5 |

## SALAD DRESSINGS & SAUCES

| Item | *PointsPlus™* value |
|---|---|
| **Fat-free Balsamic Vinaigrette,** 2 oz | 1 |
| **Fat-free Mango Citrus Vinaigrette,** 1 serving | 1 |

## SIDE ITEMS & EXTRAS

| Item | *PointsPlus™* value |
|---|---|
| **Side - Black Beans w/ Cheese,** 1 serving | 3 |
| **Side - Mexican Rice,** 1 serving | 7 |
| **Side - Vegetables - Grilled,** 1 serving | 2 |

## DESSERTS

| Item | *PointsPlus™* value |
|---|---|
| **Sopapillas - Two w/ Chocolate Syrup,** 1 serving | 15 |
| **Sopapillas - Two w/ Honey,** 1 serving | 17 |

| ▲ Power Foods | *PointsPlus*™ value |
|---|---|
| **JULIUS® FRUIT DRINKS** | |
| **Bananarilla®,** 1 small | 9 |
| **Blackberry,** 1 small | 8 |
| **Lemon Julius®,** 1 small | 6 |
| **Orange Julius®,** 1 small | 4 |
| **Orange Passion Julius®,** 1 small | 4 |
| **Peach Julius®,** 1 small | 4 |
| **Pina Colada,** 1 small | 7 |
| **Pineapple Julius®,** 1 small | 3 |
| **Pomegranate Julius®,** 1 small | 4 |
| **Raspberry,** 1 small | 8 |
| **Raspberry Julius®,** 1 small | 6 |
| **Strawberry Banana,** 1 small | 8 |
| **Strawberry Julius®,** 1 small | 5 |
| **Strawberry Lemonade Julius®,** 1 small | 6 |
| **Tripleberry®,** 1 small | 9 |
| **Tropical,** 1 small | 9 |
| **Tropical Sunlight™,** 1 | 6 |
| **JULIUS® PREMIUM FRUIT SMOOTHIES** | |
| **3-Berry Blast,** 1 | 12 |
| **Berry Banana Squeeze,** 1 | 7 |
| **Berry Lemon Lively,** 1 | 11 |
| **Blackberry Storm,** 1 | 18 |
| **Blackberry Toner,** 1 | 11 |
| **Blueberrathon,** 1 | 9 |
| **Blueberry Burst,** 1 | 10 |
| **Cocoa Latte Swirl,** 1 | 26 |
| **Mango Passion,** 1 | 10 |
| **Orange Swirl™,** 1 | 14 |
| **Peaches and Cream,** 1 | 10 |
| **Pomegranate & berries,** 1 | 10 |
| **Raspberry Crème,** 1 | 17 |
| **Raspberry Crush,** 1 | 10 |
| **Strawberry Sensation,** 1 | 11 |
| **Strawberry Xtreme,** 1 | 10 |
| **Tart 'N' Berry™,** 1 | 11 |
| **Tropi-Colada,** 1 | 14 |
| **Tropical Tango,** 1 | 10 |
| **Wild Blue Twist,** 1 | 11 |
| **ADD A BANANA** | |
| ▲ **Banana,** 1 | 0 |
| **JULIUS® LIGHT PREMIUM FRUIT SMOOTHIES** | |
| **Berry-Pom Twilight™,** 1 | 6 |
| **Strawberry Delight™,** 1 | 6 |
| **JULIUS® OTHER BEVERAGES** | |
| **Cool Cappuccino,** 1 small | 8 |
| **Cool Mocha,** 1 small | 11 |
| **Eggnog,** 1 small | 7 |
| **DRINKS** | |
| **Barq's®,** 1 small | 5 |
| **Bottled Water,** 1 serving | 0 |
| **Coca-Cola®,** 1 small | 5 |
| **Coffee,** 12 fl oz | 0 |
| **Diet Coca-Cola®,** 1 small | 0 |
| **Diet Pepsi®,** 1 small | 0 |
| **Dr. Pepper®,** 1 small | 5 |
| **Milk, whole,** 8 fl oz | 4 |
| **Mountain Dew®,** 1 small | 6 |
| **Mug®,** 1 small | 5 |
| **Orange Juice,** 12 fl oz | 4 |
| **Pepsi®,** 1 small | 5 |
| **Sierra Mist®,** 1 small | 5 |
| **Sprite®,** 1 small | 5 |

# ORANGE JULIUS®

| ▲ Power Foods | *PointsPlus*™ value |
|---|---|
| **JULIUS® HOT DOGS** | |
| **Bacon Cheese Dog,** 1 | 13 |
| **Cheese Dog,** 1 | 12 |
| **Chicago Dog,** 1 | 11 |
| **Chili Melt Dog,** 1 | 13 |
| **Chili Slaw Dog,** 1 | 12 |
| **Pepperoni Cheese Dog,** 1 | 12 |
| **Relish Dog,** 1 | 11 |
| **Reuben Dog,** 1 | 14 |
| **Sauerkraut Dog,** 1 | 11 |
| **Southwest Chili Dog,** 1 | 13 |
| **Triple Cheese Dog,** 1 | 15 |
| **JULIUS® PITAS** | |
| **Chicken Caesar Pita,** 1 | 12 |
| **Chicken Fajita Pita,** 1 | 7 |
| **Garden Veggie Pita,** 1 | 13 |
| **Santa Fe Grilled Chicken Pita,** 1 | 12 |
| **Steak Fajita Pita,** 1 | 11 |
| **Turkey Club Pita,** 1 | 12 |
| **JULIUS® OTHER FOOD** | |
| **Nachos - Small,** 1 serving | 8 |
| **Nachos - Large,** 1 serving | 15 |
| **Salted Pretzel,** 1 | 4 |
| **NUTRITION BOOSTS** | |
| **Fiber Plus,** 1 serving | 0 |
| **Heart Health,** 1 serving | 0 |
| **Joint Care,** 1 serving | 1 |
| **Protein,** 1 serving | 2 |

▲ Power Foods — *PointsPlus*™ value

## AUSSIE-TIZERS® TO SHARE

| Item | PointsPlus™ value |
|---|---|
| **Alice Springs Chicken Quesadilla®,** 1 regular serving | 14 |
| **Aussie Cheese Fries,** 1 small serving | 11 |
| **Aussie Cheese Fries,** 1 regular serving | 10 |
| **Bloomin Onion,** 1/6 of the onion | 7 |
| **Gold Coast Coconut Shrimp,** 1 serving | 4 |
| **Kookaburra Wings® (hot),** 1 serving | 15 |
| **Kookaburra Wings® (medium),** 1 serving | 14 |
| **Kookaburra Wings® (mild),** 1 serving | 14 |
| **Seared Ahi Tuna,** 1 small serving | 4 |
| **Seared Ahi Tuna,** 1 regular serving | 3 |

## BURGERS & SANDWICHES

| Item | PointsPlus™ value |
|---|---|
| **Bacon Cheese Burger,** 1 burger | 30 |
| **Grilled Chicken and Swiss Sandwich,** 1 sandwich | 18 |
| **Roasted Filet Sandwich,** 1 sandwich | 19 |
| **The Bloomin' Burger®,** 1 burger | 31 |
| **The Outbacker Burger,** 1 burger | 20 |

## JOEY MENU

| Item | PointsPlus™ value |
|---|---|
| **Boomerang Cheese Burger,** 1 sandwich | 11 |
| **Grilled Cheese-A-Roo,** 1 sandwich | 11 |
| **Joey Grilled Chicken on the Barbie,** 1 entrée order | 5 |
| **Joey Sirloin,** 1 entrée order | 6 |
| **Junior Ribs,** 1 entrée order | 17 |
| **Kookaburra Chicken Fingers,** 1 entrée order | 18 |
| **Mac A Roo 'N Cheese,** 1 serving | 11 |
| **Spotted Dog Sundae,** 1 serving | 35 |
| **Spotted Dog Sundae (with chocolate sauce),** 1 serving | 35 |

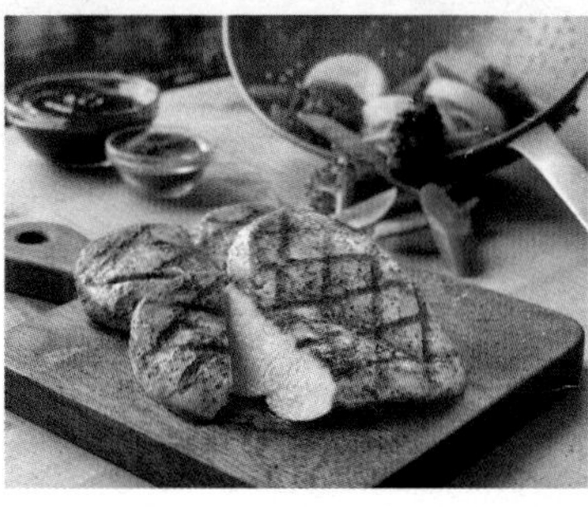

▲ Power Foods — *PointsPlus*™ value

## OUTBACK FAVORITES

| Item | PointsPlus™ value |
|---|---|
| **Alice Springs Chicken®,** 1 entrée order | 35 |
| **Baby Back Ribs - Full Rack,** 1 entrée order | 54 |
| **Back Back Ribs,** 1 entrée order | 28 |
| **Filet with Wild Mushroom Sauce,** 1 entrée order | 9 |
| **Grilled Chicken on the Barbie,** 1 entrée order | 11 |
| **New Zealand Rack of Lamb,** 1 entrée order | 35 |
| **No Rules Parmesan Pasta,** 1 meal | 37 |
| **Sweet Glazed Roasted Pork Tenderloin,** 1 entrée order | 9 |

## SIGNATURE STEAKS

| Item | PointsPlus™ value |
|---|---|
| **New York Strip,** 1 steak (14 oz) | 18 |
| **New York Strip,** 1 steak (8 oz) | 10 |
| **Outback Special®,** 1 steak (12 oz) | 14 |
| **Outback Special®,** 1 steak (6 oz) | 8 |
| **Outback Special®,** 1 steak (9 oz) | 11 |
| **Prime Rib,** 1 steak (8 oz) | 14 |
| **Prime Rib,** 1 steak (12 oz) | 21 |
| **Prime Rib,** 1 steak (16 oz) | 28 |

*Signature Steaks (cont'd)*

| ▲ Power Foods | PointsPlus™ value |
|---|---|
| **Ribeye,** 1 steak (10 oz) | 24 |
| **Ribeye,** 1 steak (14 oz) | 32 |
| **Teriyaki Marinated Sirlion,** 1 steak (9 oz) | 10 |
| **The Melbourne,** 1 steak (20 oz) | 25 |
| **Victoria's Fillet®,** 1 steak (9 oz) | 19 |

## PERFECT COMBINATIONS

| ▲ Power Foods | PointsPlus™ value |
|---|---|
| **Filet and Shrimp Scampi (without sides),** 1 entrée order | 16 |
| **Outback Special® and Grilled Shrimp on the Barbie,** 1 entrée order (12 oz steak) | 18 |
| **Outback Special® and Grilled Shrimp on the Barbie (without sides),** 1 entrée order (9 oz steak) | 16 |
| **Ribs and Alice Springs Chicken® (without sides),** 1 entrée order | 34 |
| **Teriyaki Filet Medallions (without sides),** 1 entrée order | 12 |

## STRAIGHT FROM THE SEA

| ▲ Power Foods | PointsPlus™ value |
|---|---|
| **Atlantic Salmon,** 1 entrée order | 16 |
| **Fresh Tilapia with Pure Lumb Crab Meat,** 1 entrée order | 13 |
| **Lobster Tails (without sides),** 1 entrée order | 17 |
| **Shrimp En Fuego Fettucine,** 1 entrée order | 31 |

## ADD ON MATES

| ▲ Power Foods | PointsPlus™ value |
|---|---|
| **Grilled Scallops,** 1 serving | 6 |
| **Lobster and Mushroom Topping,** 1 serving | 11 |
| **Lobster Tail,** 1 serving | 15 |
| **Sauteed Mushroom,** 1 serving | 3 |
| **Shrimp Scampi,** 1 serving | 8 |
| **Three Grilled Shrimp,** 1 serving | 4 |

## SOUPS & SALADS

| ▲ Power Foods | PointsPlus™ value |
|---|---|
| **Chicken Caesar Salad,** 1 salad | 28 |
| **Classic Roasted Filet Wedge Salad,** 1 salad | 14 |
| **Queensland Salad,** 1 salad | 29 |
| **Shrimp Caesar Salad,** 1 salad | 19 |
| **Walkabout Soup® of the Day - Baked Potato,** 1 bowl | 21 |
| **Walkabout Soup® of the Day - Baked Potato,** 1 cup | 15 |
| **Walkabout Soup® of the Day - Broccoli,** 1 cup | 8 |
| **Walkabout Soup® of the Day - Broccoli,** 1 bowl | 11 |
| **Walkabout Soup® of the Day - Onion,** 1 bowl | 12 |
| **Walkabout Soup® of the Day - Onion,** 1 cup | 8 |

## FRESH MADE SIDES

| ▲ Power Foods | PointsPlus™ value |
|---|---|
| **Aussie Fries,** 1 serving | 10 |
| **Blue Cheese Pecan Chopped Salad,** 1 salad | 14 |
| **Caesar Salad,** 1 salad | 9 |
| **Classic Blue Cheese Wedge Salad,** 1 salad | 10 |
| **Dressed Baked Potato (no toppings),** 1 potato | 8 |
| **Fresh Seasonal Veggies,** 1 serving | 1 |
| **Fresh Steamed Green Beans,** 1 serving | 0 |
| **Garlic Mashed Potatoes,** 1 serving | 10 |
| **House Salad (no dressing),** 1 salad | 6 |
| **House Salad (with oil & vinegar),** 1 salad | 10 |
| **Potato Boats,** 1 serving | 4 |
| **Potato Wedges,** 1 serving | 7 |
| **Side Bread and Butter,** 1 serving | 2 |
| **Sweet Potato,** 1 potato | 11 |

Power Foods | *PointsPlus*™ value

## IRRESISTIBLE DESSERTS

| | |
|---|---|
| **Carrot Cake,** 1/4 of the dessert | 3 |
| **Chocolate Thunder From Down Under®,** 1 slice | 14 |
| **Chocolate Thunder From Down Under® Sample,** 1 slice | 28 |
| **Classic Cheesecake,** 1/4 of the dessert | 5 |
| **Classic Cheesecake Sample,**1 slice | 28 |
| **Nutter Butter® Peanut Butter Pie Sample,** 1 slice | 25 |
| **Sweet Adventure Sampler Trio™,** 1 slice | 17 |

# PAPA GINO'S®

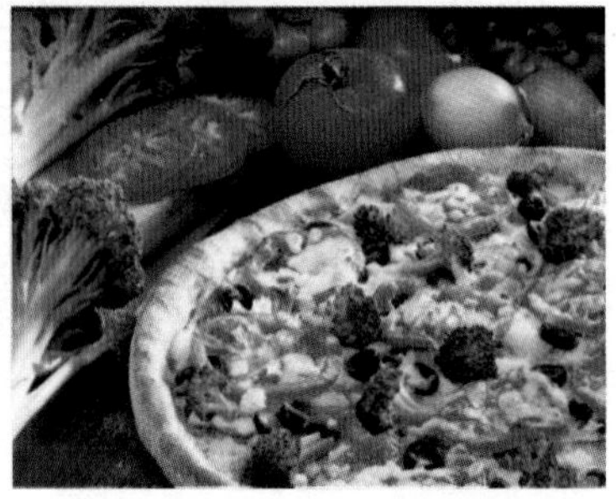

| ▲ Power Foods | *PointsPlus*™ value |
|---|---|

## APPETIZERS & SNACKS

| | |
|---|---|
| **BBQ Chicken Tenders,** 1 serving | 13 |
| **Buffalo Chicken Tender,** 1/2 small serving | 5 |
| **Cheese Breadsticks,** 1/2 small serving | 71 |
| **Cheese Garlic Bread,** 1/4 large serving | 6 |
| **Chicken Tender,** 1/2 small serving | 5 |
| **Cinnamon Stick Icing,** 1/2 small serving | 6 |
| **Cinnamon Sticks,** 1/2 small serving | 8 |
| **French Fries,** 1/2 small serving | 10 |
| **Marinara Dipping Sauce,** 1/2 small serving | 2 |
| **Mozzarella Sticks,** 1/2 small serving | 10 |

## THIN CRUST PIZZA

| | |
|---|---|
| **BBQ Chicken Pizza,** 1/8 of the 14" large pizza | 7 |
| **Buffalo Chicken Pizza,** 1/8 of the 14" large pizza | 6 |
| **Cheese Pizza,** 1/8 of the 14" large pizza | 6 |
| **Chicken Pepper Pizza,** 1/8 of the 14" large pizza | 7 |
| **Garlic Chicken Pizza,** 1/8 of the 14" large pizza | 8 |

| ▲ Power Foods | *PointsPlus*™ value |
|---|---|
| **Meat Combo Pizza,** 1/8 of the 14" large pizza | 9 |
| **PapaRoni Pizza,** 1/8 of the 14" large pizza | 9 |
| **Pepperoni Pizza,** 1/8 of the 14" large pizza | 7 |
| **Super Veggie Pizza,** 1/8 of the 14" large pizza | 6 |
| **The Works Pizza,** 1/8 of the 14" large pizza | 8 |

## THICK CRUST PIZZA

| | |
|---|---|
| **BBQ Chicken,** 1/8 of the 14" large pizza | 12 |
| **Buffalo Chicken,** 1/8 of the 14" large pizza | 11 |
| **Cheese,** 1/8 of the 14" large pizza | 9 |
| **Chicken Pepper,** 1/8 of the 14" large pizza | 12 |
| **Garlic Chicken,** 1/8 of the 14" large pizza | 10 |
| **Meat Combo,** 1/8 of the 14" large pizza | 14 |
| **PapaRoni,** 1/8 of the 14" large pizza | 11 |
| **Pepperoni,** 1/8 of the 14" large pizza | 12 |
| **Super Veggie,** 1/8 of the 14" large pizza | 11 |
| **Works,** 1/8 of the 14" large pizza | 11 |

## RUSTIC PIZZA

| | |
|---|---|
| **BBQ Chicken,** 1/12 of the pizza | 6 |
| **Buffalo Chicken,** 1/12 of the pizza | 6 |
| **Cheese,** 1/12 of the pizza | 5 |
| **Chicken Pepper,** 1/12 of the pizza | 6 |
| **Garlic Chicken,** 1/12 of the pizza | 7 |
| **Meat Combo,** 1/12 of the pizza | 8 |
| **PapaRoni,** 1/12 of the pizza | 7 |
| **Pepperoni,** 1/12 of the pizza | 7 |
| **Super Veggie,** 1/12 of the pizza | 6 |
| **Works,** 1/12 of the pizza | 7 |

| ▲ Power Foods | *PointsPlus*™ value |
|---|---|

## PIZZA SLICES (PER SLICE)

| | |
|---|---|
| **Cheese,** 1 slice | 8 |
| **Pepperoni,** 1 slice | 10 |

## PASTA

| | |
|---|---|
| **Papa Platter-Penne,** 1 serving | 26 |
| **Papa Platter-Spaghetti,** 1 serving | 26 |
| **Pasta Trio Plate,** 1 serving | 26 |
| **Penne,** 1 entrée portion | 17 |
| **Penne Alfredo,** 1 entrée portion | 24 |
| **Penne Alfredo Chicken Broccoli,** 1 entrée portion | 31 |
| **Ravioli,** 1 entrée portion | 16 |
| **Single Breadsticks,** 1 serving | 5 |
| **Spaghetti,** 1 entrée portion | 17 |
| **Spaghetti & Meatballs,** 1 entrée portion | 23 |
| **Spaghetti Alfredo,** 1 serving | 24 |
| **Spaghetti Alfredo Chicken Broccoli,** 1 serving | 27 |
| **Spaghetti Chicken Parmesan,** 1 entrée portion | 28 |
| **Trio Plate,** 1 entrée portion | 26 |

## BREADS & TOPPINGS

| | |
|---|---|
| **Bacon,** 1 serving | 2 |
| **Black Olives,** 1 serving | 0 |
| ▲ **Broccoli,** 1 serving | 0 |
| **Capicola,** 1 serving | 0 |
| **Extra Cheese,** 1 serving | 1 |
| ▲ **Extra Hot Peppers,** 3/4 oz | 0 |
| ▲ **Green Pepper,** 1 serving | 0 |
| **Hamburger,** 1 serving | 1 |
| **Mayonnaise,** 2 Tbsp | 6 |
| ▲ **Mushrooms,** 1 oz | 0 |
| ▲ **Onions,** 1 serving | 0 |
| **Pepperoni,** 1 serving | 1 |
| ▲ **Pickles,** 1 serving | 0 |
| **Pocket,** 1 | 8 |
| **Processed American Cheese,** 1 oz | 3 |
| **Provolone Cheese,** 1 oz | 3 |
| **Sausage,** 1 serving | 2 |
| **Single Breadstick,** 1 | 6 |
| ▲ **Sliced Tomato,** 1 serving | 0 |
| **Sub Roll,** 1 small | 8 |
| ▲ **Sweet Green Peppers,** 1 serving | 0 |

## SUBS & SANDWICHES

| | |
|---|---|
| **BLT,** 1 large | 29 |
| **Chicken Cutlet,** 1 large | 24 |
| **Chicken Parmesan,** 1 large | 29 |
| **Hot Dog with Roll,** 1 small | 11 |
| **Italian,** 1 small | 24 |
| **Italian,** 1 large | 33 |
| **Lobster Roll,** 1 small | 15 |
| **Meatball,** 1 small | 19 |
| **Meatball,** 1 large | 31 |
| **Meatball Parmesan,** 1 small | 22 |
| **Meatball Parmesan,** 1 large | 37 |
| **Seafood Salad,** 1 small | 18 |
| **Seafood Salad,** 1 large | 25 |
| **Steak,** 1 small | 16 |
| **Steak,** 1 large | 25 |
| **Steak & Cheese,** 1 small | 19 |
| **Steak & Cheese,** 1 large | 32 |
| **Super Steak,** 1 small | 20 |
| **Super Steak,** 1 large | 34 |
| **Tuna,** 1 small | 20 |
| **Tuna,** 1 large | 30 |
| **Turkey,** 1 small | 12 |
| **Turkey,** 1 large | 17 |
| **Turkey Club,** 1 small | 17 |
| **Turkey Club,** 1 large | 24 |
| **Vegetarian,** 1 large | 18 |

▲ Power Foods — *PointsPlus*™ value

## SUB PANINIS

| Item | PointsPlus™ value |
|---|---|
| **Basil Chicken,** 1 | 29 |
| **Eggplant,** 1 | 23 |
| **Italian Deli,** 1 | 28 |
| **Sausage & Pepper,** 1 | 31 |

## KIDZ MENU

| Item | PointsPlus™ value |
|---|---|
| **Cheese Slice,** 1 serving | 8 |
| **Chicken Tender Meal,** 1 serving | 13 |
| **Hot Dog Meal,** 1 serving | 12 |
| **Penne,** 1 serving | 9 |
| **Pepperoni Slice,** 1 serving | 10 |
| **Spaghetti & Meatballs,** 1 serving | 12 |

## SALADS

| Item | PointsPlus™ value |
|---|---|
| **Buffalo Chicken Tender Salad,** 1 entrée order | 9 |
| **Caesar Salad,** 1 entrée order | 5 |
| **Caesar Salad,** 1 side order | 2 |
| **Chicken Bacon Cheddar Salad,** 1 entrée order | 12 |
| **Chicken Caesar Salad,** 1 entrée order | 8 |
| **Chicken Tender Salad,** 1 entrée order | 7 |
| **Garden Salad,** 1 side order | 2 |
| **Garden Salad,** 1 entrée order | 5 |
| **Single Breadsticks,** 1 | 5 |

## SALAD DRESSINGS

| Item | PointsPlus™ value |
|---|---|
| **Balsamic,** 1 | 6 |
| **Bleu Cheese,** 1 serving | 4 |
| **Caesar,** 1 serving | 12 |
| **Fat Free Honey Dijon,** 1 serving | 1 |
| **Honey Mustard,** 1 serving | 4 |
| **Olive Oil Vinaigrette,** 1 serving | 5 |
| **Ranch,** 1 serving | 8 |

## SIDES

| Item | PointsPlus™ value |
|---|---|
| **Meatballs,** 2 meatballs | 7 |
| **Penne,** 1 side order | 9 |
| **Penne Alfredo,** 1 side order | 12 |
| **Spaghetti,** 1 side order | 9 |
| **Spaghetti Alfredo,** 1 side order | 12 |

| ▲ Power Foods | *PointsPlus*™ value |
|---|---|

## THIN CRUST PIZZA

| | |
|---|---|
| **BBQ Chicken & Bacon Pizza,** 1/8 of the 14" large pizza | 7 |
| **Chicken Bacon Ranch Pizza,** 1/8 of the 14" large pizza | 7 |
| **Chicken Bacon Ranch Pizza,** 1/8 of the 14" large pizza | 7 |
| **Garden Fresh Pizza,** 1/8 of the 14" large pizza | 6 |
| **Hawaiian BBQ Chicken Pizza,** 1/8 of the 14" large pizza | 8 |
| **Italian Meats Trio Pizza,** 1/8 of the 14" large pizza | 7 |
| **Papa's White Pizza,** 1/8 of the 14" large pizza | 6 |
| **Sicilian Classic Pizza,** 1/8 of the 14" large pizza | 7 |
| **Smokehouse Bacon & Ham Pizza,** 1/8 of the 14" large pizza | 7 |
| **Spicy Italian Pizza,** 1/8 of the 14" large pizza | 7 |
| **Spinach Alfredo Chicken Tomato Pizza,** 1/8 of the 14" large pizza | 7 |
| **Spinach Alfredo Pizza,** 1/8 of the 14" large pizza | 6 |
| **The Meats Pizza,** 1/8 of the 14" large pizza | 8 |
| **The Works Pizza,** 1/8 of the 14" large pizza | 7 |
| **Tuscan Six Cheese Pizza,** 1/8 of the 14" large pizza | 7 |

## WHOLE WHEAT CRUST PIZZA

| | |
|---|---|
| **BBQ Chicken & Bacon Pizza,** 1/8 of the 14" large pizza | 9 |
| **Chicken Bacon Ranch Pizza,** 1/8 of the 14" large pizza | 9 |
| **Garden Fresh Pizza,** 1/8 of the 14" large pizza | 7 |
| **Hawaiian BBQ Chicken Pizza,** 1/8 of the 14" large pizza | 9 |
| **Italian Meats Trio Pizza,** 1/8 of the 14" large pizza | 8 |
| **Papa's White Pizza,** 1/8 of the 14" large pizza | 7 |
| **Sicilian Classic Pizza,** 1/8 of the 14" large pizza | 8 |
| **Smokehouse Bacon & Ham Pizza,** 1/8 of the 14" large pizza | 8 |
| **Spicy Italian Pizza,** 1/8 of the 14" large pizza | 8 |
| **Spinach Alfredo Chicken Tomato Pizza,** 1/8 of the 14" large pizza | 8 |
| **Spinach Alfredo Pizza,** 1/8 of the 14" large pizza | 7 |
| **The Meats Pizza,** 1/8 of the 14" large pizza | 9 |
| **The Works Pizza,** 1/8 of the 14" large pizza | 8 |
| **Tuscan Six Cheese Pizza,** 1/8 of the 14" large pizza | 8 |

## ORIGINAL CRUST PIZZA

| | |
|---|---|
| **BBQ Chicken Pizza,** 1/8 of the 14" large pizza | 9 |
| **BBQ Chicken & Bacon Pizza,** 1/6 of the 10" small pizza | 6 |
| **BBQ Chicken & Bacon Pizza,** 1/8 of the 12" medium pizza | 6 |
| **BBQ Chicken & Bacon Pizza,** 1/8 of the 14" large pizza | 9 |
| **BBQ Chicken & Bacon Pizza,** 1/10 of the 16" extra-large pizza | 9 |
| **Chicken Bacon Ranch Pizza,** 1/6 of the 10" small pizza | 6 |
| **Chicken Bacon Ranch Pizza,** 1/8 of the 12" medium pizza | 6 |
| **Chicken Bacon Ranch Pizza,** 1/8 of the 14" large pizza | 9 |

*Original Crust Pizza (cont'd)*

| ▲ Power Foods | *PointsPlus*™ value |
|---|---|
| **Chicken Bacon Ranch Pizza,** 1/10 of the 16" extra-large pizza | 10 |
| **Garden Fresh Pizza,** 1/6 of the 10" small pizza | 5 |
| **Garden Fresh Pizza,** 1/8 of the 12" medium pizza | 5 |
| **Garden Fresh Pizza,** 1/8 of the 14" large pizza | 7 |
| **Garden Fresh Pizza,** 1/10 of the 16" extra-large pizza | 8 |
| **Hawaiian BBQ Chicken Pizza,** 1/6 of the 10" small pizza | 6 |
| **Hawaiian BBQ Chicken Pizza,** 1/8 of the 12" medium pizza | 7 |
| **Hawaiian BBQ Chicken Pizza,** 1/8 of the 14" large pizza | 9 |
| **Hawaiian BBQ Chicken Pizza,** 1/10 of the 16" extra-large pizza | 10 |
| **Italian Meats Trio Pizza,** 1/6 of the 10" small pizza | 4 |
| **Italian Meats Trio Pizza,** 1/8 of the 12" medium pizza | 6 |
| **Italian Meats Trio Pizza,** 1/8 of the 14" large pizza | 8 |
| **Italian Meats Trio Pizza,** 1/10 of the 16" extra-large pizza | 9 |
| **Papa's White Pizza,** 1/6 of the 10" small pizza | 5 |
| **Papa's White Pizza,** 1/8 of the 12" medium pizza | 6 |
| **Papa's White Pizza,** 1/8 of the 14" large pizza | 8 |
| **Papa's White Pizza,** 1/10 of the 16" extra-large pizza | 8 |
| **Pepperoni Pizza,** 1/8 of the 14" large pizza | 9 |
| **Sicilian Classic Pizza,** 1/6 of the 10" small pizza | 6 |
| **Sicilian Classic Pizza,** 1/8 of the 12" medium pizza | 6 |
| **Sicilian Classic Pizza,** 1/8 of the 14" large pizza | 9 |

| ▲ Power Foods | *PointsPlus*™ value |
|---|---|
| **Sicilian Classic Pizza,** 1/10 of the 16" extra-large pizza | 9 |
| **Smokehouse Bacon & Ham Pizza,** 1/6 of the 10" small pizza | 6 |
| **Smokehouse Bacon & Ham Pizza,** 1/8 of the 12" medium pizza | 6 |
| **Smokehouse Bacon & Ham Pizza,** 1/8 of the 14" large pizza | 9 |
| **Smokehouse Bacon & Ham Pizza,** 1/10 of the 16" extra-large pizza | 9 |
| **Spicy Italian Pizza,** 1/6 of the 10" small pizza | 5 |
| **Spicy Italian Pizza,** 1/8 of the 12" medium pizza | 6 |
| **Spicy Italian Pizza,** 1/8 of the 14" large pizza | 8 |
| **Spicy Italian Pizza,** 1/10 of the 16" extra-large pizza | 9 |
| **Spinach Alfredo Chicken Tomato Pizza,** 1/6 of the 10" small pizza | 6 |
| **Spinach Alfredo Chicken Tomato Pizza,** 1/8 of the 12" medium pizza | 6 |
| **Spinach Alfredo Chicken Tomato Pizza,** 1/8 of the 14" large pizza | 8 |
| **Spinach Alfredo Chicken Tomato Pizza,** 1/10 of the 16" extra-large pizza | 9 |
| **Spinach Alfredo Pizza,** 1/6 of the 10" small pizza | 5 |
| **Spinach Alfredo Pizza,** 1/8 of the 12" medium pizza | 6 |
| **Spinach Alfredo Pizza,** 1/8 of the 14" large pizza | 8 |
| **Spinach Alfredo Pizza,** 1/10 of the 16" extra-large pizza | 8 |
| **The Meats Pizza,** 1/6 of the 10" small pizza | 6 |
| **The Meats Pizza,** 1/8 of the 12" medium pizza | 7 |
| **The Meats Pizza,** 1/8 of the 14" large pizza | 10 |
| **The Meats Pizza,** 1/10 of the 16" extra-large pizza | 10 |

| ▲ Power Foods | PointsPlus™ value |
|---|---|
| **The Works Pizza,** 1/6 of the 10" small pizza | 5 |
| **The Works Pizza,** 1/8 of the 12" medium pizza | 6 |
| **The Works Pizza,** 1/8 of the 14" large pizza | 8 |
| **The Works Pizza,** 1/10 of the 16" extra-large pizza | 9 |
| **Tuscan Six Cheese Pizza,** 1/6 of the 10" small pizza | 6 |
| **Tuscan Six Cheese Pizza,** 1/8 of the 12" medium pizza | 6 |
| **Tuscan Six Cheese Pizza,** 1/8 of the 14" large pizza | 9 |
| **Tuscan Six Cheese Pizza,** 1/10 of the 16" extra-large pizza | 9 |

## PAN CRUST PIZZA

| ▲ Power Foods | PointsPlus™ value |
|---|---|
| **BBQ Chicken & Bacon Pizza,** 1/8 of the 12" medium pizza | 12 |
| **Chicken Bacon Ranch Pizza,** 1/8 of the 12" medium pizza | 12 |
| **Garden Fresh Pizza,** 1/8 of the 12" medium pizza | 10 |
| **Hawaiian BBQ Chicken Pizza,** 1/8 of the 12" medium pizza | 12 |
| **Italian Meats Trio Pizza,** 1/8 of the 12" medium pizza | 11 |
| **Papa's White Pizza,** 1/8 of the 12" medium pizza | 10 |
| **Sicilian Classic Pizza,** 1/8 of the 12" medium pizza | 11 |
| **Smokehouse Bacon & Ham Pizza,** 1/8 of the 12" medium pizza | 11 |
| **Spicy Italian Pizza,** 1/8 of the 12" medium pizza | 11 |
| **Spinach Alfredo Chicken Tomato Pizza,** 1/8 of the 12" medium pizza | 11 |
| **Spinach Alfredo Pizza,** 1/8 of the 12" medium pizza | 10 |
| **The Meats Pizza,** 1/8 of the 12" medium pizza | 12 |
| **The Works Pizza,** 1/8 of the 12" medium pizza | 11 |
| **Tuscan Six Cheese Pizza,** 1/8 of the 12" medium pizza | 11 |

## SIDES

| | |
|---|---|
| **BBQ Wings,** 2 | 4 |
| **Buffalo Wings,** 2 | 4 |
| **Chickenstrips,** 2 | 4 |

## BREADSTICKS & CHEESE STICKS

| | |
|---|---|
| **Breadstick,** 2 | 8 |
| **Cheesesticks,** 4 | 10 |
| **Garlic Parmesan Breadstick,** 2 | 9 |
| **Whole Wheat Breadsticks,** 2 | 7 |

## DIPPING SAUCES

| | |
|---|---|
| **Barbeque Sauce,** 1 container | 1 |
| **Blue Cheese,** 1 container | 4 |
| **Buffalo Sauce,** 1 container | 0 |
| **Cheese Dipping Sauce,** 1 container | 1 |
| **Honey Mustard,** 1 container | 4 |
| **Pizza Sauce,** 1 container | 1 |
| **Ranch Sauce,** 1 container | 3 |
| **Special Garlic Dipping Sauce,** 1 container | 4 |

## DESSERTS

| | |
|---|---|
| **Apple Twist Sweetreat,** 2 slice | 10 |
| **Chocolate Pastry Delights,** 1 | 5 |
| **Cinna Swirl Sweetreat,** 2 slice | 12 |
| **Cinnamon Sweetsticks,** 4 | 15 |

# PAPA MURPHY'S® TAKE 'N' BAKE PIZZA

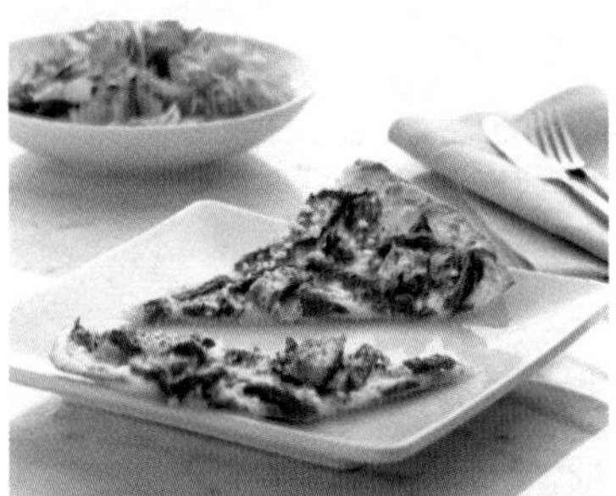

▲ Power Foods — *PointsPlus*™ value

## APPETIZERS

|  | *PointsPlus*™ value |
|---|---|
| **Cheesy Bread (without sauce),** 2 slices | 6 |
| **Marinara Sauce,** 1 cup | 0 |

## FAMILY SIZE ORIGINAL CRUST PIZZA

|  | *PointsPlus*™ value |
|---|---|
| **All meat,** 1/12 of the pizza | 10 |
| **Barbecue Chicken,** 1/12 of the pizza | 9 |
| **Cheese Pizza,** 1/12 of the pizza | 7 |
| **Cowboy**™, 1/12 of the pizza | 10 |
| **Gourmet Chicken Garlic,** 1/12 of the pizza | 9 |
| **Gourmet Classic Italian,** 1/12 of the pizza | 9 |
| **Gourmet Vegetarian,** 1/12 of the pizza | 8 |
| **Hawaiian Pizza,** 1/12 of the pizza | 8 |
| **Herb Chicken Mediterranean,** 1/12 of the pizza | 9 |
| **Murphy's Combination Pizza,** 1/12 of the pizza | 10 |
| **Papa-Roni,** 1/12 of the pizza | 9 |
| **Papa's Favorite,** 1/12 of the pizza | 10 |
| **Pepperoni,** 1/12 of the pizza | 9 |
| **Rancher,** 1/12 of the pizza | 9 |
| **Specialty of the House,** 1/12 of the pizza | 9 |
| **Taco Grande,** 1/12 of the pizza | 9 |
| **Veggie Combo,** 1/12 of the pizza | 8 |
| **Veggie Mediterranean,** 1/12 of the pizza | 8 |

## THIN CRUST DeLITE® PIZZA

|  | *PointsPlus*™ value |
|---|---|
| **All Meat,** 1/10 of the pizza | 5 |
| **Barbecue Chicken,** 1/10 of the pizza | 5 |
| **Cheese,** 1/10 of the pizza | 4 |
| **Chicken Bacon Artichoke,** 1/10 of the pizza | 5 |
| **Cowboy**™, 1/10 of the pizza | 5 |
| **Gourmet Chicken Bacon Artichoke deLITE®,** 1/10 of the large pizza | 5 |
| **Gourmet Chicken Garlic,** 1/10 of the pizza | 5 |
| **Gourmet Classic Italian,** 1/10 of the pizza | 5 |
| **Gourmet Vegetarian,** 1/10 of the pizza | 4 |
| **Hawaiian,** 1/10 of the pizza | 4 |
| **Herb Chicken Mediterranean,** 1/10 of the pizza | 5 |
| **Murphy's Combination**™, 1/10 of the pizza | 6 |
| **Papa's All Meat deLITE®,** 1/10 of the large pizza | 5 |
| **Papa's Favorite®,** 1/10 of the pizza | 6 |
| **Pepperoni,** 1/10 of the pizza | 5 |
| **Rancher**™, 1/10 of the pizza | 5 |
| **Specialty of the House,** 1/10 of the pizza | 5 |
| **Taco Grande,** 1/10 of the pizza | 5 |
| **Vegetarian Combo,** 1/10 of the pizza | 4 |
| **Veggie,** 1/10 of the pizza | 4 |
| **Veggie Mediterranean,** 1/10 of the pizza | 4 |

| ▲ Power Foods | *PointsPlus*™ value |
|---|---|
| **STUFFED PIZZA** | |
| **5-Meat,** 1/16 of a family size pizza | 10 |
| **Big Murphy®,** 1/16 of a family size pizza | 10 |
| **Chicago Style,** 1/16 of a family size pizza | 10 |
| **Chicken and Bacon,** 1/16 of a family size pizza | 10 |
| **SIGNATURE SALADS (WITHOUT DRESSING OR CROUTONS)** | |
| **Caesar,** 1/2 salad | 1 |
| **Chicken Caesar,** 1/2 salad | 3 |
| **Club,** 1/2 salad | 4 |
| **Garden,** 1/2 salad | 3 |
| **Italian,** 1/2 salad | 4 |
| **Crouton,** 1 packet | 2 |
| **SALAD DRESSING** | |
| **Buttermilk Ranch,** 1/2 packet | 4 |
| **Caesar,** 1/2 packet | 4 |
| **Low Calorie Italian,** 1/2 packet | 0 |
| **DESSERTS** | |
| **Apple Dessert Pizza,** 1/8 of the pizza | 6 |
| **Cherry Dessert Pizza,** 1/8 of the pizza | 6 |
| **Chocolate Chip Cookie Dough,** 2 oz | 7 |
| **Cinnamon Wheel (without frosting),** 1/8 of the cinnamon wheel | 7 |
| **Cookie Dough with Hershey's Chocolate Chips,** 1/16 of the tub | 3 |
| **Cream Cheese Frosting,** 1/8 of the cup of cream cheese frosting | 1 |

# PETRO'S® CHILI & CHIPS

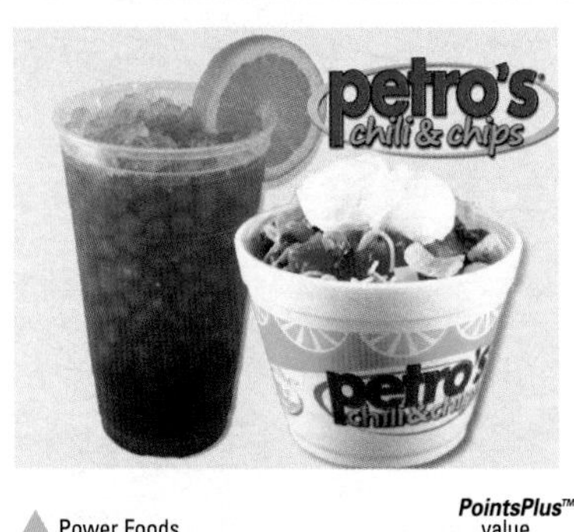


| ▲ Power Foods | *PointsPlus*™ value |
|---|---|
| **SMALL PETRO®** | |
| **Chicken,** 1 serving | 12 |
| **Original,** 1 serving | 14 |
| **Veggie,** 1 serving | 14 |
| **MEDIUM PETRO®** | |
| **Chicken,** 1 serving | 18 |
| **Original,** 1 serving | 20 |
| **Veggie,** 1 serving | 20 |
| **LARGE PETRO®** | |
| **Chicken,** 1 serving | 26 |
| **Original,** 1 serving | 29 |
| **Veggie,** 1 serving | 30 |
| **PEE WEE PETRO®** | |
| **Chicken,** 1 serving | 7 |
| **Original,** 1 serving | 8 |
| **Veggie,** 1 serving | 8 |
| **LITE PETRO®** | |
| **Small,** 1 serving | 10 |
| **Medium,** 1 serving | 14 |
| **Large,** 1 serving | 20 |

| ▲ Power Foods | *PointsPlus*™ value |
|---|---|
| **PASTA PETRO®** | |
| **Small,** 1 serving | 11 |
| **Medium,** 1 serving | 16 |
| **Large,** 1 serving | 22 |
| **LITE PASTA PETRO®** | |
| **Small,** 1 serving | 8 |
| **Medium,** 1 serving | 12 |
| **Large,** 1 serving | 17 |
| **PETRO SALADS** | |
| **Grilled Chicken,** 1 salad | 19 |
| **Original,** 1 salad | 16 |
| **GARDEN SALADS** | |
| **Small,** 1 serving | 1 |
| **Large,** 1 serving | 2 |
| **HOT DOGS** | |
| **Chili,** 1 serving | 8 |
| **Chili/Cheese,** 1 serving | 9 |
| **Loaded,** 1 serving | 9 |
| **Plain,** 1 serving | 7 |
| **Slaw,** 1 serving | 7 |
| **BAKED POTATOES** | |
| **#1 Lite,** 1 serving | 9 |
| **#2 Butter & Sour Cream,** 1 serving | 13 |
| **#3 Loaded,** 1 serving | 18 |
| **#4 Loaded with Chili,** 1 serving | 21 |
| **#5 Broccoli 3 Cheese,** 1 serving | 17 |
| **TOSTITOS™ CHIPS** | |
| **Loaded Tostitos™/Ultimate Nachos,** 1 serving | 25 |

| ▲ Power Foods | *PointsPlus™* value |
|---|---|

## ENTRÉES

|  | *PointsPlus™* value |
|---|---|
| **Angus Chop House Beef Steak,** 1 serving | 4 |
| **Beef Roast,** 1 serving | 17 |
| **Beef, Corned,** 1 serving | 13 |
| **Beef, Steak, Ribeye,** 1 | 24 |
| **Beef, Steak, Swiss,** 1 serving | 12 |
| **Beef, Stew, Chuck Wagon,** 1 serving | 7 |
| **Beef, Stroganoff,** 1 serving | 13 |
| **Braised Beef & Noodles,** 1 serving | 12 |
| **Cheese Enchiladas,** 1 serving | 13 |
| **Chicken & Almonds,** 1 serving | 10 |
| **Chicken Cacciatore,** 1 serving | 25 |
| **Chicken Etouffee, Louisiana,** 1 serving | 10 |
| **Chicken Livers, Fried,** 1 serving | 17 |
| **Chicken Pie,** 1 serving | 14 |
| **Chicken Stewed and Dumplings,** 1 serving | 8 |
| **Chicken Teriyaki with Polynesian Rice,** 1 serving | 16 |
| **Chicken Tetrazzini,** 1 serving | 10 |
| **Chicken, Baked Cajun, Boneless Breast,** 1 serving | 11 |
| **Chicken, Baked Cajun, Halves,** 1 serving | 42 |
| **Chicken, Baked Italian, Boneless Breast,** 1 serving | 15 |
| **Chicken, Boneless Breast, Blackened with Vegetables,** 1 serving | 14 |
| **Chicken, Breast Sesame Glaze with Asian Fried Rice,** 1 serving | 13 |
| **Chicken, Breast, Coconut Breaded,** 1 serving | 12 |
| **Chicken, Broiled,** 1 serving | 33 |
| **Chicken, Caribbean, Halves,** 1 serving | 32 |
| **Chicken, Fried,** 2 pieces | 21 |

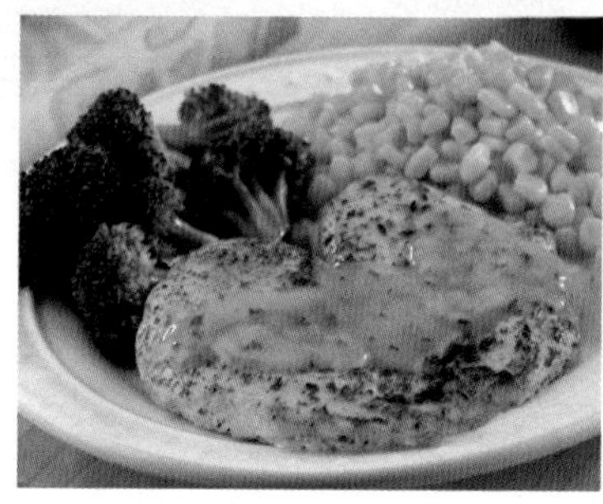

| ▲ Power Foods | *PointsPlus™* value |
|---|---|
| **Chicken, Fried Chicken Breast,** 1 serving | 19 |
| **Chicken, Half, Buffalo,** 1 serving | 48 |
| **Chicken, Italian Baked, (Quarters),** 1 serving | 26 |
| **Chicken, Italian Baked, Halves,** 1 serving | 34 |
| **Chicken, Jambalaya, Chicken,** 1 serving | 10 |
| **Chicken, Lemon Pepper, Halves,** 1 serving | 33 |
| **Chicken, Rotisserie-Herb Style (Halves),** 1 half | 31 |
| **Chicken, Southwestern Chicken Breast with Yellow Rice,** 1 serving | 19 |
| **Chicken, Spanish,** 1 serving | 12 |
| **Chicken, Spicy Cajun,** 1 1/4 cups | 16 |
| **Chicken, Sweet & Sour with Fried Rice,** 1 serving | 19 |
| **Chicken, Tenders Fried, Kids,** 1 serving | 12 |
| **Chimichangas (Chicken),** 1 serving | 13 |
| **Crawfish Etouffee, Louisiana,** 1 serving | 10 |
| **Crawfish, Fried,** 1 serving | 4 |
| **Fish, Baked (4 oz),** 1 serving | 8 |
| **Fish, Cajun Baked,** 1 serving | 7 |

Entrées (cont'd)

| ▲ Power Foods | *PointsPlus*™ value |
|---|---|
| **Fish, Fried,** 1 serving | 9 |
| **Fish, Salmon Pattie,** 1 serving | 6 |
| **Fish, Southern Fried,** 1 serving | 9 |
| **Fish, Southern Fried Catfish,** 1 serving | 10 |
| **Fish, Tilapia with Shrimp Cream Sauce,** 1 serving | 5 |
| **Fish, Tilapia, Blackened with Grilled,** 1 serving | 12 |
| **Fish, Tilapia, Cajun Baked,** 1 serving | 7 |
| **Fish, Tilapia, Mediterranean,** 1 serving | 3 |
| **Fish, Tilapia, Parmesan Crusted,** 1 serving | 7 |
| **Fish, Tilapia, Stuffed,** 1 serving | 9 |
| **Ham, Pit-Style Smoked,** 1 serving | 6 |
| **Italian Meat Sauce & Spaghetti,** 1 serving | 14 |
| **Liver, Beef, Fried with Onion Sauce,** 1 serving | 13 |
| **Liver, Broiled & Grilled Onions,** 1 serving | 8 |
| **Meat Loaf, Baked,** 1 serving | 12 |
| **Pasta, Macaroni and Cheese, Baked,** 1 serving | 7 |
| **Pork, Chop, Baked & Escalloped Potatoes,** 1 serving | 27 |
| **Pork, Chop, Blackened with Fettuccine Alfredo,** 1 serving | 11 |
| **Pork, Chop, Smothered,** 1 serving | 20 |
| **Pork, Chop, Southwest Style with Mexican Rice,** 1 serving | 13 |
| **Pork, Sausage, Smoked, Red Beans & Rice,** 1 serving | 17 |
| **Pork, Sweet and Sour with Rice,** 1 serving | 16 |
| **Shrimp Creole and Rice,** 1 serving | 9 |
| **Shrimp Scampi and Fettuccini,** 1 serving | 12 |
| **Shrimp, Blackened, Fettuccine,** 1 serving | 21 |
| **Shrimp, Diablo,** 1 serving | 8 |
| **Shrimp, Etouffee, Louisiana,** 1 serving | 13 |
| **Shrimp, Fried,** 1 serving | 2 |
| **Shrimp, New Orleans Style Sauteed, Large,** 1 serving | 18 |
| **Turkey and Dressing,** 1 serving | 9 |
| **Turkey Breast, Carved,** 1 serving | 6 |

## SALADS

| ▲ Power Foods | *PointsPlus*™ value |
|---|---|
| **Fruit, Ambrosia, Southern,** 1 serving | 5 |
| **Fruit, Dixie Land Fruit Salad,** 1 serving | 5 |
| **Fruit, Peaches, Sliced,** 1 serving | 5 |
| **Fruit, Strawberry and Banana, Fresh,** 1 serving | 6 |
| **Gelatin, Plain,** 1 serving | 3 |
| **Pasta, Rotini Salad, Italian,** 1 serving | 5 |
| **Salad, Broccoli,** 1 serving | 4 |
| **Salad, Broccoli Madeline,** 1 serving | 7 |
| **Salad, Caesar,** 1 serving | 4 |
| **Salad, Carrot and Raisin,** 1 serving | 5 |
| **Salad, Carrot and Raisin,** 1 large serving | 7 |
| **Salad, Coleslaw with Cream,** 1 serving | 3 |
| **Salad, Coleslaw, Cream Slaw,** 1 serving | 3 |
| **Salad, Italian Bowl,** 1 serving | 3 |
| **Salad, Neptune,** 1 serving | 7 |
| **Salad, Pasta with Seasoning,** 1 serving | 7 |
| **Salad, Pea,** 1 serving | 5 |
| **Salad, Piccadilly Club,** 1 serving | 18 |
| **Salad, Piccadilly Fruit,** 1 serving | 2 |
| **Salad, Potato,** 1 serving | 4 |

| ▲ Power Foods | *PointsPlus*™ value |
|---|---|
| **Salad, Southwest Fiesta Chicken,** 1 serving | 9 |
| **Salad, Spinach, Tossed,** 1 serving | 2 |
| ▲ **Salad, Spring Salad Bowl,** 1 serving | 0 |
| ▲ **Salad, Tomato (Cherry), Cucumber,** 1 serving | 0 |

## SIDES

| ▲ Power Foods | *PointsPlus*™ value |
|---|---|
| **Broccoli and Rice, Au Gratin,** 1 serving | 5 |
| **Dressing, Beef-Rice,** 1 serving | 5 |
| **Dressing, Corn Bread,** 1 serving | 4 |
| **Gravy, Brown,** 1 serving | 1 |
| **Mushrooms, Marinated,** 1 serving | 6 |
| **Onions, Caramelized,** 1 serving | 2 |
| **Potatoes, New, Roasted,** 1 serving | 6 |
| **Rice, Fried, Asian,** 1 serving | 8 |
| **Rice, Mexican Style, Fried,** 1 serving | 5 |
| **Rice, Polynesian,** 1 serving | 6 |
| **Rice, Steamed,** 1 serving | 3 |
| **Rice, Yellow, Spanish,** 1 serving | 3 |
| ▲ **Watermelon,** 1 serving | 0 |

## VEGETABLES

| ▲ Power Foods | *PointsPlus*™ value |
|---|---|
| **Beans, Baby Lima,** 1 serving | 4 |
| **Beans, Black Beans and Rice,** 1 serving | 2 |
| ▲ **Beans, Green,** 1 serving | 0 |
| **Beets, Spiced,** 1 serving | 4 |
| **Bell Pepper, Stuffed,** 1 serving | 9 |
| **Broccoli, Florets,** 1 serving | 2 |
| **Cabbage, Buttered, Steamed,** 1 serving | 2 |
| **Carrot Souffle,** 1 serving | 11 |
| **Carrots, Baby, Buttered,** 1 serving | 2 |
| **Cauliflower, Fresh Whole with Cheese,** 1 serving | 1 |
| **Corn,** 1 serving | 4 |
| **Green Bean Supreme,** 1 serving | 3 |
| ▲ **Greens, with Diced Turnips,** 1 serving | 1 |
| **Harvard Beets,** 1 serving | 5 |
| **Okra, Breaded,** 1 serving | 6 |
| **Okra, Buttered,** 1 serving | 2 |
| **Okra, Smothered,** 1 serving | 3 |
| **Peas, Black-Eyed,** 1 serving | 2 |
| ▲ **Pinto,** 1 serving | 4 |
| **Potato, Baked,** 1 | 14 |
| **Potatoes, Candied Sweet,** 1 serving | 11 |
| **Potatoes, French Fried,** 1 serving | 8 |
| **Potatoes, Hash Browns,** 1 serving | 8 |
| **Potatoes, Mashed, Idahoan,** 1 serving | 3 |
| **Potatoes, New, Boiled,** 1 serving | 5 |
| **Potatoes, Roasted Garlic, Mashed,** 1 serving | 3 |
| **Potatoes, Twice Baked Casserole,** 1 serving | 4 |
| **Squash, Mixed, Yellow and Zucchini,** 1 serving | 3 |
| **Squash, Yellow, Baked, French Style,** 1 serving | 3 |

## SOUP

| ▲ Power Foods | *PointsPlus*™ value |
|---|---|
| **Gumbo, Chicken and Sausage,** 1 serving | 7 |
| **Gumbo, Seafood,** 1 serving | 5 |
| **Soup, Broccoli, Cream,** 1 serving | 4 |
| **Soup, Chicken-Rice,** 1 serving | 2 |
| **Soup, Shrimp and Corn,** 1 serving | 6 |
| **Soup, Tomato-Macaroni,** 1 serving | 3 |
| **Soup, Vegetable,** 1 serving | 1 |

# PICCADILLY CAFETERIA

▲ Power Foods — *PointsPlus*™ value

## BREAD & ROLLS

|  | *PointsPlus*™ value |
|---|---|
| **Bread, Garlic,** 1 slice | 6 |
| **Bread, Mexican Corn Bread,** 1 | 6 |
| **Bread, Spoon Bread, Virginia,** 1 serving | 5 |
| **Corn Sticks,** 1 | 4 |
| **Cornbread,** 1 serving | 6 |
| **Hush Puppies,** 1 | 5 |
| **Muffins, Banana Nut,** 1 serving | 5 |
| **Muffins, Raisin-Bran,** 1 | 7 |
| **Rolls, Dough,** 1 | 6 |
| **Rolls, Sticky Cinnamon,** 1 serving | 9 |
| **Rolls, Whole Wheat,** 1 | 6 |

## DESSERT

|  | *PointsPlus*™ value |
|---|---|
| **Apple Piccadilly,** 1 serving | 17 |
| **Cake, Black Forest,** 1 slice | 8 |
| **Cake, Cheesecake,** 1 serving | 13 |
| **Cake, Chocolate,** 1 slice | 23 |
| **Cake, Cupcakes,** 1 | 5 |
| **Cake, Italian Cream,** 1 slice | 22 |
| **Cake, Italian Delight,** 1 slice | 23 |
| **Cake, Red Velvet, from layers,** 1 slice | 23 |
| **Cake, Southern Sweet,** 1 serving | 14 |
| **Cobbler, Blackberry,** 1 serving | 11 |
| **Cobbler, Cherry,** 1 serving | 7 |
| **Cobbler, Peach,** 1 serving | 10 |
| **Custard, Caramel (flan),** 1 serving | 11 |
| **Custard, Cup,** 1 serving | 6 |
| **Dumpling, Apple,** 1 serving | 13 |
| **Pie, Buttermilk Chess,** 1 slice | 16 |
| **Pie, Chocolate Cream,** 1 slice | 10 |
| **Pie, Coconut, Cream,** 1 slice | 12 |
| **Pie, Custard,** 1 slice | 9 |
| **Pie, Lemon Icebox,** 1 slice | 14 |
| **Pie, Mississippi Mud,** 1 slice | 12 |
| **Pie, Peanut Butter, Chocolate Satin,** 1 slice | 23 |
| **Pie, Pecan,** 1 slice | 17 |
| **Pie, Pumpkin,** 1 serving | 8 |
| **Pie, Sweet Potato,** 1 slice | 12 |
| **Pudding, Bread with Lemon Sauce or Rum,** 1 serving | 12 |
| **Pudding, Chocolate,** 1 serving | 6 |
| **Pudding, Vanilla,** 1 serving | 7 |
| **Shortcake, Strawberry, Mary Ann, Cake Style,** 1 serving | 8 |

# PICKERMAN'S SOUP AND SANDWICHES

▲ Power Foods — *PointsPlus*™ value

## SANDWICHES
(INCLUDES BREAD, MEAT & VEGETABLE)

| | *PointsPlus*™ value |
|---|---|
| **BBQ,** 1 | 12 |
| **B.L.T.,** 1 | 10 |
| **Caesar Salad,** 1 | 17 |
| **Chicken,** 1 | 8 |
| **Chicken Caesar,** 1 | 18 |
| **Classic Club,** 1 | 11 |
| **Garden Salad,** 1 | 10 |
| **Greek Salad,** 1 | 11 |
| **Ham & Swiss,** 1 | 10 |
| **Meatball,** 1 | 17 |
| **Numero Uno,** 1 | 11 |
| **Roast Beef,** 1 | 9 |
| **That's Italian,** 1 | 11 |
| **Tuna,** 1 | 11 |
| **Turkey,** 1 | 9 |
| **Veggie,** 1 | 8 |

## SOUP

| | *PointsPlus*™ value |
|---|---|
| **5 Star Mushroom,** 1 serving | 3 |
| **Asiago Cheese Bisque,** 1 serving | 6 |
| **Beef Noodle,** 1 serving | 2 |
| **Black Bean,** 1 serving | 4 |
| **Black Forest Lentil,** 1 serving | 3 |
| **Broccoli Cheddar,** 1 serving | 6 |
| **Cauliflower Cheddar,** 1 serving | 5 |
| **Chicken Gumbo,** 1 serving | 3 |
| **Chicken Noodle,** 1 serving | 3 |
| **Chicken with Rice,** 1 serving | 5 |
| **Clam Chowder,** 1 serving | 5 |
| **Country Bean,** 1 serving | 3 |
| **Country Potato,** 1 serving | 4 |
| **Country Vegetable,** 1 serving | 2 |
| **French Onion,** 1 serving | 2 |
| **Loaded Baked Potato,** 1 serving | 6 |
| **Minestrone,** 1 serving | 2 |
| **Pickerman's Stew,** 1 serving | 5 |
| **Potato Cheddar,** 1 serving | 6 |
| **Potato Cream Cheese,** 1 serving | 5 |
| **Roasted Garlic Tomato,** 1 serving | 5 |
| **Santa Fe Tortilla,** 1 serving | 3 |
| **Southwest Roasted Corn,** 1 serving | 3 |
| **Spring Asparagus,** 1 serving | 4 |
| **Texas Chili,** 1 serving | 5 |
| **Tomato Basil,** 1 serving | 1 |
| **Vegetable Beef Barley,** 1 serving | 3 |
| **Vegetarian Chili,** 1 serving | 4 |
| **White Chicken Chili,** 1 serving | 4 |
| **Wisconsin Cheese,** 1 serving | 5 |

# PIZZA HUT®

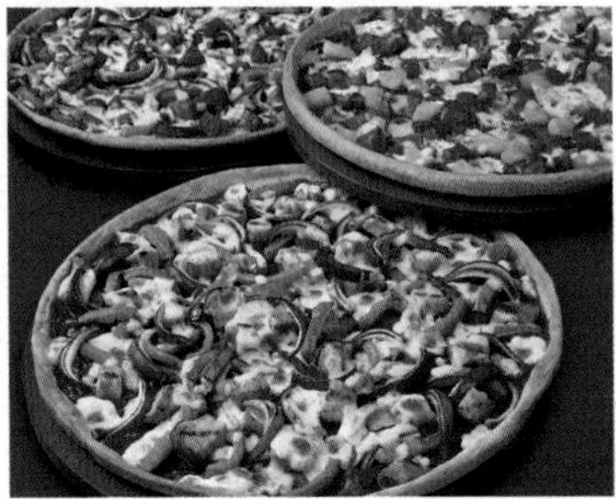

| ▲ Power Foods | *PointsPlus™* value |
|---|---|

## APPETIZERS & BREAD

| | |
|---|---|
| **Bread Sticks,** 1 each | 4 |
| **Cheese Breadsticks,** 1 each | 5 |
| **Hot Wings,** 2 pieces | 3 |
| **Mild Wings,** 2 pieces | 3 |
| **Wing Blue Cheese Dipping Sauce,** 1 1/2 oz | 6 |
| **Wing Ranch Dipping Sauce,** 1 1/2 oz | 6 |

## FIT 'N DELICIOUS® PIZZA

| | |
|---|---|
| **Chicken, Mushroom & Jalapeño Pizza,** 1/8 of the 12" medium pizza | 4 |
| **Chicken, Mushroom & Jalapeño Pizza,** 1/8 of the 14" large pizza | 6 |
| **Chicken, Red Onion and Green Pepper Pizza,** 1/8 of the 12" medium pizza | 5 |
| **Chicken, Red Onion and Green Pepper Pizza,** 1/8 of the 14" large pizza | 6 |
| **Diced Red Tomato, Mushroom and Jalapeño Pizza,** 1/8 of the 12" medium pizza | 4 |
| **Diced Red Tomato, Mushroom and Jalapeño Pizza,** 1/8 of the 14" large pizza | 5 |
| **Green Pepper, Red Onion & Diced Red Tomato Pizza,** 1/8 of the 12" medium pizza | 4 |

| ▲ Power Foods | *PointsPlus™* value |
|---|---|
| **Green Pepper, Red Onion & Diced Red Tomato Pizza,** 1/8 of the 14" large pizza | 5 |
| **Ham, Pineapple and Diced Red Tomato Pizza,** 1/8 of the 12" medium pizza | 4 |
| **Ham, Pineapple and Diced Red Tomato Pizza,** 1/8 of the 14" large pizza | 6 |
| **Ham, Red Onion and Mushroom Pizza,** 1/8 of the 12" medium pizza | 4 |
| **Ham, Red Onion and Mushroom Pizza,** 1/8 of the 14" large pizza | 6 |

## THIN 'N CRISPY® PIZZA

| | |
|---|---|
| **All Natural Italian Sausage & Red Onion Pizza,** 1/8 of the 12" medium pizza | 6 |
| **All Natural Pepperoni Pizza,** 1/8 of the 12" medium pizza | 5 |
| **All Natural Pepperoni & Mushroom,** 1/8 of the 14" large pizza | 7 |
| **Cheese Only Pizza,** 1/8 of the 12" medium pizza | 5 |
| **Meat Lover's® Pizza,** 1/8 of the 12" medium pizza | 8 |
| **Pepperoni & Mushroom Pizza,** 1/8 of the 12" medium pizza | 5 |
| **Pepperoni & Mushroom Pizza,** 1/8 of the 14" large pizza | 7 |
| **Quartered Ham & Pineapple Pizza,** 1/8 of the 12" medium pizza | 5 |
| **Supreme Pizza,** 1/8 of the 12" medium pizza | 6 |
| **Veggie Lover's® Pizza,** 1/8 of the 12" medium pizza | 5 |

## HAND-TOSSED STYLE PIZZA

| | |
|---|---|
| **All Natural Italian Sausage & Red Onion Pizza,** 1/8 of the 12" medium pizza | 6 |

| ▲ Power Foods | *PointsPlus™* value |
|---|---|
| **All Natural Pepperoni Pizza,** 1/8 of the 12" medium pizza | 6 |
| **All Natural Pepperoni & Mushroom,** 1/8 of the 12" medium pizza | 6 |
| **All Natural Pepperoni & Mushroom,** 1/8 of the 14" large pizza | 8 |
| **Cheese Only Pizza,** 1/8 of the 12" medium pizza | 6 |
| **Meat Lover's® Pizza,** 1/8 of the 12" medium pizza | 8 |
| **Pepperoni & Mushroom Pizza,** 1/8 of the 12" medium pizza | 6 |
| **Pepperoni & Mushroom Pizza,** 1/8 of the 14" large pizza | 9 |
| **Quartered Ham & Pineapple Pizza,** 1/8 of the 12" medium pizza | 5 |
| **Supreme Pizza,** 1/8 of the 12" medium pizza | 7 |
| **Veggie Lover's® Pizza,** 1/8 of the 12" medium pizza | 5 |

## PAN PIZZA

| ▲ Power Foods | *PointsPlus™* value |
|---|---|
| **All Natural Italian Sausage & Red Onion,** 1/8 of the 12" medium pizza | 7 |
| **All Natural Italian Sausage & Red Onion,** 1/8 of the 14" large pizza | 10 |
| **All Natural Pepperoni Pizza,** 1/8 of the 12" medium pizza | 6 |
| **All Natural Pepperoni & Mushroom,** 1/8 of the 14" large pizza | 9 |
| **All Natural Pepperoni & Mushroom,** 1/8 of the 12" medium pizza | 6 |
| **Cheese Only Pizza,** 1/8 of the 12" medium pizza | 6 |
| **Italian Sausage & Red Onion,** 1/8 of the 14" large pizza | 8 |
| **Italian Sausage & Red Onion,** 1/8 of the 12" medium pizza | 11 |
| **Meat Lover's® Pizza,** 1/8 of the 12" medium pizza | 9 |
| **Pepperoni & Mushroom Pizza,** 1/8 of the 12" medium pizza | 7 |
| **Pepperoni & Mushroom Pizza,** 1/8 of the 14" large pizza | 10 |
| **Quartered Ham & Pineapple Pizza,** 1/8 of the 12" medium pizza | 6 |
| **Supreme Pizza,** 1/8 of the 12" medium pizza | 7 |
| **Veggie Lover's® Pizza,** 1/8 of the 12" medium pizza | 6 |

## PERSONAL PAN PIZZA®

| ▲ Power Foods | *PointsPlus™* value |
|---|---|
| **All Natural Italian Sausage & Red Onion,** 1 whole | 19 |
| **All Natural Pepperoni Pizza,** 1 whole | 18 |
| **All Natural Pepperoni & Mushroom Pizza,** 1 whole | 16 |
| **Cheese Only Pizza,** 1 whole | 17 |
| **Meat Lover's® Pizza,** 1 whole | 24 |
| **Quartered Ham & Pineapple Pizza,** 1 whole | 16 |
| **Supreme Pizza,** 1 whole | 20 |
| **Veggie Lover's® Pizza,** 1 whole | 15 |

## STUFFED CRUST PIZZA

| ▲ Power Foods | *PointsPlus™* value |
|---|---|
| **All Natural Italian Sausage & Red Onion Pizza,** 1/8 of the 14" large pizza | 10 |
| **All Natural Pepperoni Pizza,** 1/8 of the 14" large pizza | 10 |
| **All Natural Pepperoni & Mushroom Pizza,** 1/8 of the 14" large pizza | 9 |
| **Cheese Only Pizza,** 1/8 of the 14" large pizza | 9 |
| **Meat Lover's® Pizza,** 1/8 of the 14" large pizza | 13 |
| **Quartered Ham & Pineapple Pizza,** 1/8 of the 14" large pizza | 9 |
| **Supreme Pizza,** 1/8 of the 14" large pizza | 11 |
| **Veggie Lover's® Pizza,** 1/8 of the 14" large pizza | 9 |

# PIZZA HUT®

| ▲ Power Foods | *PointsPlus™* value |
|---|---|
| **XL FULL HOUSE PIZZA™** | |
| **Cheese Only Pizza,** 1 slice | 7 |
| **Italian Sausage & Red Onion Pizza,** 1 slice | 8 |
| **Meat Lover's®,** 1 slice | 10 |
| **Pepperoni Pizza,** 1 slice | 8 |
| **Pepperoni & Mushroom Pizza,** 1 slice | 7 |
| **Quartered Ham & Pineapple,** 1 slice | 7 |
| **Supreme Pizza,** 1 slice | 8 |
| **Veggie Lover's®,** 1 slice | 7 |
| **TUSCANI PASTA** | |
| **Bacon Mac N Cheese,** 1/4 order | 13 |
| **Chicken Alfredo,** 1/4 order | 17 |
| **Lasagna,** 1/4 order | 15 |
| **Meaty Marinara,** 1/4 serving | 13 |
| **SALAD DRESSINGS & DIPPING SAUCES** | |
| **French Dressing,** 2 Tbsp | 4 |
| **Italian Dressing,** 2 Tbsp | 4 |
| **Lite Italian Dressing,** 2 Tbsp | 2 |
| **Lite Ranch Dressing,** 2 Tbsp | 2 |
| **Ranch Dressing,** 2 Tbsp | 3 |
| **Thousand Island Dressing,** 2 Tbsp | 3 |
| **Bread Stick Dipping Sauce,** 3 oz | 1 |
| **DESSERTS** | |
| **Apple Dessert Pizza,** 1 slice | 7 |
| **Cherry Dessert Pizza,** 1 slice | 7 |
| **Cinnamon Sticks,** 2 pieces | 5 |
| **White Icing Dipping Cup,** 2 oz | 5 |

| ▲ Power Foods | *PointsPlus*™ value |
|---|---|

## PEOPLE PLEASERS

| | |
|---|---|
| **Chicken Wings (no sauce),** 4 pieces | 5 |
| **Garlic Bread,** 1 slice | 5 |
| **Lasagna,** 1 serving | 15 |

## PIZZA

| | |
|---|---|
| **Bruschetta (herbed olive oil, dried sweet tomatoes, prepared with garlic & onion),** 1 medium slice | 5 |
| **Cheese,** 1 medium slice | 5 |
| **Hawaiian (Smoked Ham, Pineapple),** 1 medium slice | 5 |
| **Pepperoni,** 1 medium slice | 5 |
| **Pepperoni, Mushrooms, Green Peppers,** 1 medium slice | 5 |
| **Super Gourmet (Sun Dried Tomatoes, Grilled Chicken, Roasted Red Peppers, Feta Cheese),** 1 medium slice | 6 |
| **Veggie (Mushrooms, Green Peppers, Onions),** 1 medium slice | 5 |
| **Whole Wheat Chicken alla Biana (Herbed Olive Oil, Grilled Chicken, Roasted Red Peppers, Parmigiano Cheese),** 1 medium slice | 5 |
| **Whole Wheat Thin Crust (Broccoli, Red Pepper, Artichokes),** 1 medium slice | 3 |

# PLANET SMOOTHIE®

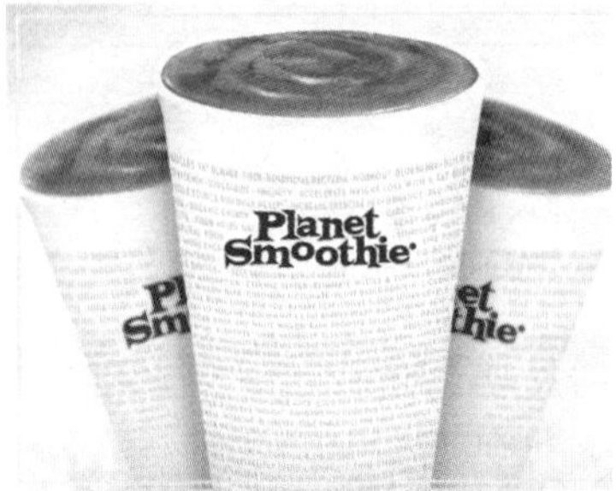


▲ Power Foods — *PointsPlus™* value

## ENERGY & COFFEE SMOOTHIES (22 FL OZ)

| | |
|---|---|
| **Berry Bada-Bing,** 1 | 10 |
| **Chocolate Elvis,** 1 | 12 |
| **Choctane,** 1 | 7 |
| **Frozen Goat,** 1 | 6 |
| **Grape Ape,** 1 | 6 |
| **Java the Nut,** 1 | 13 |
| **Love Ya Latte,** 1 | 9 |
| **Road Runner,** 1 | 8 |
| **Spazz,** 1 | 7 |

## PROTEIN SMOOTHIES (22 FL OZ)

| | |
|---|---|
| **Big Bang (Protein Blast),** 1 | 9 |
| **Big Bang (Workout Blast),** 1 | 9 |
| **Cherry Low Carb,** 1 | 4 |
| **Chocolate Chimp (Protein Blast),** 1 | 5 |
| **Chocolate Chimp (Workout Blast),** 1 | 5 |
| **Chocolate Low Carb,** 1 | 4 |
| **Merlin's Mix (Pineapple),** 1 | 8 |
| **Merlin's Mix (Strawberry),** 1 | 11 |
| **Merlin's Mix (Strawberry/ Banana),** 1 | 10 |
| **Mr. Mongo - Chocolate (Protein Blast),** 1 | 8 |
| **Mr. Mongo - Chocolate (Workout Blast),** 1 | 7 |
| **Mr. Mongo - Strawberry (Protein Blast),** 1 | 10 |

▲ Power Foods — *PointsPlus™* value

| | |
|---|---|
| **Mr. Mongo - Strawberry (Workout Blast),** 1 | 9 |
| **Pina Colada Low Carb,** 1 | 4 |
| **Pineapple Low Carb,** 1 | 4 |

## WEIGHT LOSS SMOOTHIES (22 FL OZ)

| | |
|---|---|
| **Billy Bob Banana,** 1 | 7 |
| **Leapin' Lizard,** 1 | 7 |
| **Lunar Lemonade - Raspberry,** 1 | 7 |
| **Lunar Lemonade - Strawberry,** 1 | 7 |
| **Mediterranean Monster,** 1 | 7 |
| **Rasmanian Devil,** 1 | 7 |
| **Two Piece Bikini-Chocolate,** 1 | 6 |
| **Two Piece Bikini-Strawberry,** 1 | 8 |

## WELLNESS & COOL BLENDED SMOOTHIES (22 FL OZ)

| | |
|---|---|
| **Acai,** 1 | 10 |
| **Acai Bowl,** 1 | 10 |
| **Earth Quaker,** 1 | 13 |
| **Hangover Over,** 1 | 9 |
| **PB & J,** 1 | 20 |
| **Screamsicle,** 1 | 8 |
| **Shag-A-Delic,** 1 | 8 |
| **The Last Mango,** 1 | 9 |
| **Thelma & Louise,** 1 | 7 |
| **Twigs & Berries,** 1 | 8 |
| **Vinnie Del Rocco,** 1 | 10 |
| **Werewolf - Strawberry,** 1 | 7 |
| **Yo' Adriane,** 1 | 9 |
| **Zeus Juice,** 1 | 7 |

## KID'S SMOOTHIES (12 FL OZ)

| | |
|---|---|
| **Bonzai Berry,** 1 | 6 |
| **Captain Kid,** 1 | 5 |
| **Peanut Butter Dream,** 1 | 8 |
| **Plain Jane,** 1 | 4 |
| **Purple Primate,** 1 | 4 |
| **Strawberry Shortcake,** 1 | 4 |
| **Twig Junior,** 1 | 5 |

▲ Power Foods — *PointsPlus*™ value

## GRILLED CHICKEN

|  | PointsPlus™ value |
|---|---|
| **1/4 Chicken Dark Meat,** 1 serving | 7 |
| **1/4 Chicken Dark Meat, without skin,** 1 serving | 5 |
| **1/4 Chicken White Meat,** 1 serving | 9 |
| **1/4 Chicken White Meat, without skin,** 1 serving | 6 |
| **1/2 Chicken,** 1 serving | 16 |
| ▲ **Boneless Chicken Breast,** 2 breasts | 6 |
| **Caribbean Wings,** 2 wings | 1 |

## REGULAR TROPICHOPS®

|  | PointsPlus™ value |
|---|---|
| **Chicken Tropichop® with White Rice & Black Beans,** 1 serving | 14 |
| **Chicken TropiChop® with Yellow Rice,** 1 serving | 9 |
| **Roast Pork Tropichop® with White Rice & Black Beans,** 1 serving | 18 |
| **Roast Pork TropiChop® with Yellow Rice,** 1 serving | 13 |
| **Ropa Vieja TropiChop® (shredded beef),** 1 serving | 16 |
| **Vegetarian TropiChop®,** 1 serving | 15 |

## LARGE TROPICHOPS®

|  | PointsPlus™ value |
|---|---|
| **Chicken Tropichop® Max with White Rice & Black Beans,** 1 serving | 29 |
| **Chicken Tropichop® with Yellow Rice & Vegetables,** 1 serving | 22 |
| **Roast Pork Tropichop® with White Rice & Black Beans,** 1 serving | 34 |
| **Roast Pork Tropichop® with Yellow Rice & Vegetables,** 1 serving | 27 |
| **Ropa Vieja TropiChop® (shredded beef),** 1 large serving | 30 |
| **Vegetarian TropiChop ®,** 1 serving | 25 |

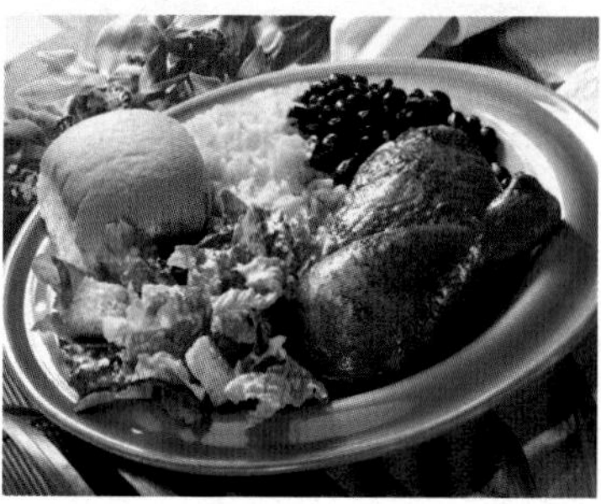

▲ Power Foods — *PointsPlus*™ value

## A-LA-CARTE

|  | PointsPlus™ value |
|---|---|
| **Chicken Fajita with Fixings,** 1 serving | 18 |
| ▲ **Churrasco Steak,** 1 serving | 4 |
| **Pork Ribs - 1/4 Rack Ribs,** 1 serving | 5 |
| **Pork Ribs - 1/2 Rack Ribs,** 1 serving | 11 |
| **Roast Pork Tropical,** 1 serving | 10 |
| **Roasted Pork with grilled Onions,** 1 serving | 11 |
| **Shrimp Skewer,** 1 serving | 2 |
| **Steak Fajita with Fixings,** 1 serving | 17 |

## SIDE DISHES

|  | PointsPlus™ value |
|---|---|
| **Balsamic Tomatos,** 1 combo side | 3 |
| ▲ **Black Beans,** 1 serving | 3 |
| **Black Beans and White Rice,** 1 serving | 8 |
| **Black Beans with Yellow Rice,** 1 serving | 7 |
| **Boiled Yuca with Mojo Sauce,** 1 combo side | 8 |
| ▲ **Broccoli & Carrots,** 1 regular serving | 0 |
| ▲ **Broccoli & Carrots,** 1 side serving | 0 |
| **Corn,** 1 combo side | 3 |
| **Curly Fries,** 1 combo side | 8 |
| **Dinner Roll,** 1 | 2 |

# POLLO TROPICAL®

*Side Dishes (cont'd)*

| ▲ Power Foods | *PointsPlus™* value |
|---|---|
| **Flour Tortilla,** 1 | 3 |
| **Macaroni & Cheese Combo,** 1 combo side | 5 |
| **Red Beans,** 1 side serving | 3 |
| **Red Beans and White Rice,** 1 serving | 8 |
| **Red Beans and Yellow Rice,** 1 serving | 7 |
| **White Rice,** 1 side serving | 5 |
| **White Rice and Black Beans,** 1 combo side | 8 |
| **Yellow Rice,** 1 combo side | 4 |

## TROPICAL FAVORITES

| ▲ Power Foods | *PointsPlus™* value |
|---|---|
| **Sweet Plantain - 7 pieces (sandwich),** 1 serving | 12 |
| **Sweet Plantains - 5 pieces (combo),** 1 combo side | 9 |
| **Yuca Fries®,** 1 serving | 13 |

## WRAPS & SANDWICHES

| ▲ Power Foods | *PointsPlus™* value |
|---|---|
| **Chicken Caesar Wrap,** 1 wrap | 10 |
| **Chicken Chipotle Sandwich,** 1 sandwich | 12 |
| **Classic Chicken Sandwich,** 1 sandwich | 12 |
| **Cuban Wrap,** 1 wrap | 11 |
| **Grilled Chicken Wrap,** 1 | 19 |
| **Guava Pork BBQ Sandwich,** 1 sandwich | 12 |
| **Roast Pork Wrap,** 1 | 20 |

## SOUP & SALADS

| ▲ Power Foods | *PointsPlus™* value |
|---|---|
| **Caribbean Chicken Soup,** 1 small | 3 |
| **Caesar Salad,** 1 combo side | 4 |
| **Caesar Salad (side),** 1 serving | 6 |
| **Chicken Caesar Salad,** 1 | 19 |
| **Caribbean Cobb Chicken Salad,** 1 serving | 23 |

## VALUE MEALS (WITH BLACK BEANS, WHITE RICE & DINNER ROLL)

| ▲ Power Foods | *PointsPlus™* value |
|---|---|
| **1/4 Chicken (Dark),** 1 serving | 7 |
| **1/4 Chicken (White),** 1 serving | 9 |
| **1/2 Chicken,** 1 serving | 16 |
| **Caribbean Ribs,** 1 serving | 13 |
| **Chicken (Dark) & Rib,** 1 serving | 15 |
| **Chicken (White) & Rib,** 1 serving | 17 |
| **Chicken Wings,** 1 serving | 10 |
| **Churrasco Steak,** 1 serving | 6 |
| **Roast Pork Tropical,** 1 serving | 11 |

## VALUE MEAL SIDES

| ▲ Power Foods | *PointsPlus™* value |
|---|---|
| **Black Beans and White Rice,** 1 serving | 13 |
| **Black Beans and Yellow Rice,** 1 serving | 10 |
| **Red Beans and White Rice,** 1 serving | 12 |
| **Red Beans and Yellow Rice,** 1 serving | 10 |

## KIDS MEAL

| ▲ Power Foods | *PointsPlus™* value |
|---|---|
| **Chicken (dark) Kids Meal,** 1 serving | 17 |
| **Chicken (white) Kids Meal,** 1 serving | 19 |
| **Chicken Breast Kids Meal,** 1 serving | 13 |

## CONDIMENTS & SAUCES

| ▲ Power Foods | *PointsPlus™* value |
|---|---|
| **Barbeque Sauce,** 1 serving | 1 |
| **Caesar Dressing,** 1 serving | 8 |
| **Chimichurri Sauce,** 1 serving | 3 |
| **Curry Mustard Sauce,** 1 serving | 4 |
| ▲ **Fresh Salsa,** 1 serving | 0 |
| **Guacamole,** 1 serving | 1 |
| **Guava Barbeque Sauce,** 1 serving | 1 |
| **Mojo Sauce,** 1 serving | 2 |

| ▲ Power Foods | *PointsPlus™* value |
|---|---|
| ▲ **Salsa Fuego,** 1 serving | 0 |
| **Shredded Cheese Blend,** 1 serving | 2 |
| **Sour Cream,** 1 serving | 2 |

## TROPICAL CHILLERS®

| | |
|---|---|
| **Mango Cream Smoothie,** 1 | 9 |
| **Mango Fruit Only,** 1 | 8 |
| **Pina Colada Cream Smoothie,** 1 | 10 |
| **Pina Colada Fruit Only,** 1 | 9 |
| **Strawberry Cream Smoothie,** 1 | 9 |
| **Strawberry Fruit Only,** 1 | 8 |

## DESSERTS

| | |
|---|---|
| **Flan,** 1 serving | 6 |
| **Guava Cheesecake,** 1 slice | 9 |
| **Key Lime Pie,** 1 slice | 10 |
| **Tres Leches,** 1 serving | 11 |

# PORT OF SUBS®

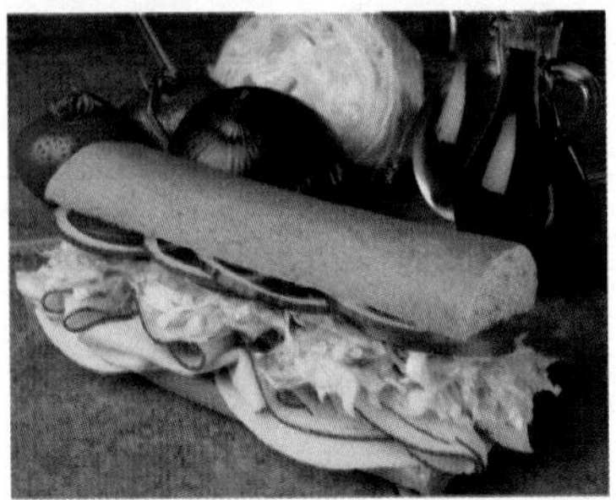

▲ Power Foods — *PointsPlus*™ value

## COLD SUBMARINE SANDWICHES
(5" WHITE OR WHEAT BREAD, WITH LETTUCE, TOMATO, PURPLE ONION, OIL, VINEGAR, & SPICES)

|  | *PointsPlus*™ value |
|---|---|
| **Bacon, Lettuce & Tomato,** 1 sub | 11 |
| **Cheese Combo (Provolone, Smokey Cheddar & Swiss),** 1 sub | 13 |
| **Ham, American,** 1 sub | 12 |
| **Ham, Salami, Capicolla, Pepperoni, Provolone,** 1 sub | 14 |
| **Ham, Salami, Provolone,** 1 sub | 12 |
| **Ham, Turkey,** 1 sub | 8 |
| **Ham, Turkey, Provolone,** 1 sub | 11 |
| **Peppered Pastrami,** 1 sub | 7 |
| **Peppered Pastrami, Swiss,** 1 sub | 11 |
| **Roast Beef,** 1 sub | 8 |
| **Roast Beef, Provolone,** 1 sub | 10 |
| **Roast Beef, Turkey,** 1 sub | 8 |
| **Roast Beef, Turkey, Provolone,** 1 sub | 11 |
| **Roasted Chicken Breast,** 1 sub | 8 |
| **Roasted Chicken Breast, Provolone,** 1 sub | 11 |
| **Salami, Pepperoni, Provolone,** 1 sub | 14 |
| **Salami, Provolone,** 1 sub | 13 |
| **Salami, Turkey, Provolone,** 1 sub | 12 |
| **Smoked Ham,** 1 sub | 7 |
| **Smoked Ham, Swiss,** 1 sub | 11 |
| **Smoked Ham, Turkey, Smokey Cheddar,** 1 sub | 11 |
| **Smoked Ham-Turkey,** 1 sub | 8 |
| **Tuna (without cheese),** 1 sub | 11 |
| **Turkey,** 1 sub | 8 |
| **Turkey, Provolone,** 1 sub | 11 |
| **Vegetarian (no cheese, olives/avocado),** 1 sub | 6 |
| **Vegetarian (without cheese, includes avocado & olives),** 1 sub | 9 |

## HOT SUBMARINE SANDWICHES
(5" SUBS WITH CHEESE INCLUDED)

|  | *PointsPlus*™ value |
|---|---|
| **BBQ Pulled Pork Griller on Ciabatta Bread,** 1 small | 20 |
| **Grilled Chicken Griller on Ciabatta Bread,** 1 small | 13 |
| **Hot Pastrami Griller on Ciabatta Bread,** 1 small | 14 |
| **Italian Griller on Ciabatta Bread,** 1 small | 14 |
| **NY Steak & Cheese Griller on Ciabatta Bread,** 1 small | 15 |

## WRAPS (SERVED ON 12" TORTILLA)

|  | *PointsPlus*™ value |
|---|---|
| **Chicken Caesar,** 1 | 16 |
| **Hot Grilled Chicken & Smokey Cheddar,** 1 | 12 |
| **Tortilla Only,** 1 | 5 |
| **Turkey & Bacon Ranch,** 1 | 16 |

| ▲ Power Foods | *PointsPlus™* value |
|---|---|

## PRETZELS

| | |
|---|---|
| **Caramel Nut,** 1 | 10 |
| **Cinnamon Sugar,** 1 | 10 |
| **Garlic Pretzel,** 1 | 9 |
| **Iced Cinnamon Swirl,** 1 | 12 |
| **Original,** 1 | 9 |
| **Parmesan,** 1 | 10 |
| **Plain Pretzel,** 1 | 8 |
| **Pretzel - Ranch,** 1 | 9 |

## SAUCES

| | |
|---|---|
| **Caramel,** 1 1/2 oz | 4 |
| **Cheddar Cheese,** 1 1/2 oz | 2 |
| **Cream Cheese,** 1 1/2 oz | 6 |
| **Cream Cheese Icing,** 1 1/2 oz | 6 |
| **Ketchup,** 2 packets | 0 |
| **Mustard,** 2 packets | 0 |
| **Nacho Cheese,** 1 1/2 oz | 2 |
| **Pizza Sauce,** 1 1/2 oz | 2 |

## PRETZEL DOG

| | |
|---|---|
| **Pretzel Dog,** 1 | 12 |

| ▲ Power Foods | *PointsPlus™* value |
|---|---|

## DAIRY SMOOTHIES

| | |
|---|---|
| **Coffee,** 1 | 18 |
| **Mocha,** 1 | 17 |
| **Peach,** 1 | 18 |
| **Raspberry,** 1 | 18 |
| **Strawberry Banana,** 1 | 18 |

## NON-DAIRY SMOOTHIES

| | |
|---|---|
| **Peach,** 1 | 14 |
| **Raspberry,** 1 | 14 |
| **Strawberry Banana,** 1 | 14 |

## BITES

| | |
|---|---|
| **Bites,** 1 small serving | 13 |
| **Bites,** 1 medium serving | 16 |
| **Bites,** 1/2 large serving | 14 |
| **Bites - Cinnamon Sugar,** 1 serving | 14 |

# PRETZELMAKER

| ▲ Power Foods | *PointsPlus*™ value |
|---|---|
| **PRETZELS** | |
| **Caramel Nut,** 1 | 10 |
| **Cinnamon Sugar,** 1 | 12 |
| **Garlic,** 1 | 9 |
| **Iced Cinnamon Swirl,** 1 | 12 |
| **Original,** 1 | 9 |
| **Parmesan,** 1 | 10 |
| **Plain,** 1 | 8 |
| **Ranch,** 1 | 9 |
| **SAUCES** | |
| **Caramel,** 1 1/2 oz | 4 |
| **Cheddar Cheese,** 1 1/2 oz | 2 |
| **Cream Cheese,** 1 1/2 oz | 6 |
| **Cream Cheese Icing,** 1 1/2 oz | 6 |
| **Ketchup,** 2 packets | 0 |
| **Mustard,** 2 packets | 0 |
| **Nacho Cheese,** 1 1/2 oz | 2 |
| **Pizza Sauce,** 1 1/2 oz | 2 |
| **PRETZEL DOG** | |
| **Pretzel Dog,** 1 | 12 |

| ▲ Power Foods | *PointsPlus*™ value |
|---|---|
| **DAIRY SMOOTHIES** | |
| **Coffee,** 1 | 18 |
| **Mocha,** 1 | 17 |
| **Peach,** 1 | 18 |
| **Raspberry,** 1 | 18 |
| **Strawberry Banana,** 1 | 18 |
| **NON-DAIRY SMOOTHIES** | |
| **Peach,** 1 | 14 |
| **Raspberry,** 1 | 14 |
| **Strawberry Banana,** 1 | 14 |
| **BITES** | |
| **Bites,** 1 small serving | 13 |
| **Bites,** 1 medium serving | 16 |
| **Bites,** 1/2 large serving | 14 |
| **Bites - Cinnamon Sugar,** 1 serving | 14 |

| ▲ Power Foods | *PointsPlus™* value |
|---|---|
| **ALL NATURAL FROZEN YOGURT** | |
| **Original,** 1/2 cup | 2 |
| **Green Tea,** 1/2 cup | 2 |
| **Pomegranate,** 1/2 cup | 3 |
| **Tangomonium™,** 1/2 cup | 2 |

# RITTERS FROZEN CUSTARD

| ▲ Power Foods | *PointsPlus*™ value |
| --- | --- |
| **FROZEN CUSTARD** | |
| **Ritter's Original Frozen Custard (Base Mix),** 1/2 cup | 5 |
| **Ritter's Lite™ Frozen Custard Low-Fat, No Sugar Added,** 1/2 cup | 3 |
| **No Sugar Added, Low-Fat Chocolate Topping,** 1 fl oz | 3 |

| ▲ Power Foods | *PointsPlus*™ value |
|---|---|
| **BLACK FOREST HAM & ROAST PORK SANDWICHES** | |
| **BarBQ Pork Melt on Wheat,** 1 small | 7 |
| **BarBQ Pork Melt on White,** 1 small | 8 |
| **Italian Classic on Wheat,** 1 small | 5 |
| **Italian Classic on White,** 1 small | 8 |
| **Key West Cuban Mix on Wheat,** 1 small | 8 |
| **Key West Cuban Mix on White,** 1 small | 9 |
| **Peachtree Melt on Wheat,** 1 small | 7 |
| **Peachtree Melt on White,** 1 small | 7 |
| **Porky's Nightmare on Wheat,** 1 small | 8 |
| **Porky's Nightmare on White,** 1 small | 8 |
| **Southside Club on Wheat,** 1 small | 10 |
| **Southside Club on White,** 1 small | 10 |
| **CHICKEN SANDWICHES** | |
| **Basil Cashew Chicken on Wheat,** 1 small | 7 |
| **Basil Cashew Chicken on White,** 1 small | 7 |
| **Buffalo Chicken Melt on Wheat,** 1 small | 8 |
| **Buffalo Chicken Melt on White,** 1 small | 9 |
| **Catalina Chicken Salad on Wheat,** 1 small | 7 |
| **Catalina Chicken Salad on White,** 1 small | 8 |
| **Chicken Caesar on Wheat,** 1 small | 7 |
| **Chicken Caesar on White,** 1 small | 7 |
| **Chicken Cordon Bleu on Wheat,** 1 small | 8 |
| **Chicken Cordon Bleu on White,** 1 small | 8 |
| **Chicken Fajita on Wheat,** 1 small | 8 |
| **Chicken Fajita on White,** 1 small | 8 |

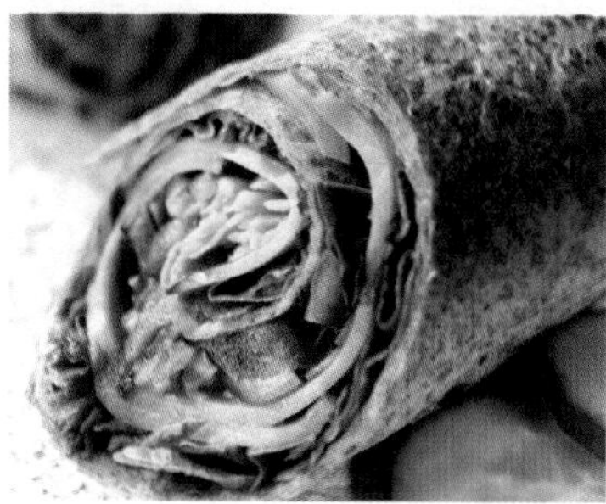

| ▲ Power Foods | *PointsPlus*™ value |
|---|---|
| **Chicken Popper on Wheat,** 1 small | 7 |
| **Chicken Popper on White,** 1 small | 7 |
| **Cobb Salad on Wheat,** 1 small | 7 |
| **Cobb Salad on White,** 1 small | 7 |
| **Delhi Chicken on Wheat,** 1 small | 8 |
| **Delhi Chicken on White,** 1 small | 8 |
| **Hickory Chicken on Wheat,** 1 small | 7 |
| **Hickory Chicken on White,** 1 small | 8 |
| **Oriental Chicken on Wheat,** 1 small | 6 |
| **Oriental Chicken on White,** 1 small | 6 |
| **Pesto Chicken on Wheat,** 1 small | 10 |
| **Pesto Chicken on White,** 1 small | 11 |
| **Santa Fe Chicken on Wheat,** 1 small | 8 |
| **Santa Fe Chicken on White,** 1 small | 8 |
| **TUNA SALAD SANDWICHES** | |
| **Classic Tuna Melt on Wheat,** 1 small | 9 |
| **Classic Tuna Melt on White,** 1 small | 9 |
| **Texas Tuna Melt on White,** 1 small | 8 |
| **Texas Tuna on Wheat,** 1 small | 7 |
| **Thai Hot Tuna on Wheat,** 1 small | 7 |
| **Thai Hot Tuna on White,** 1 small | 8 |
| **Tuna Luau on Wheat,** 1 small | 8 |
| **Tuna Luau on White,** 1 small | 9 |

# ROLY POLY SANDWICHES

| ▲ Power Foods | *PointsPlus*™ value |
|---|---|
| **SLICED STEAK & ROAST BEEF SANDWICHES** | |
| **Chipotle Cheesesteak on Wheat,** 1 small | 9 |
| **Chipotle Cheesesteak on White,** 1 small | 10 |
| **Pepper Steak on Wheat,** 1 small | 7 |
| **Pepper Steak on White,** 1 small | 7 |
| **Philly Melt on Wheat,** 1 small | 7 |
| **Philly Melt on White,** 1 small | 7 |
| **Ranch Roast on Wheat,** 1 small | 8 |
| **Ranch Roast on White,** 1 small | 8 |
| **Russian Beef on Wheat,** 1 small | 7 |
| **Russian Beef on White,** 1 small | 7 |
| **Santa Fe Steak on Wheat,** 1 small | 8 |
| **Santa Fe Steak on White,** 1 small | 9 |
| **Steak Fajita on Wheat,** 1 small | 8 |
| **Steak Fajita on White,** 1 small | 9 |
| **TURKEY & SMOKED TURKEY SANDWICHES** | |
| **California Turkey on Wheat,** 1 small | 9 |
| **California Turkey on White,** 1 small | 9 |
| **Hickory Cristo on Wheat,** 1 small | 7 |
| **Hickory Cristo on White,** 1 small | 7 |
| **Hot Honey on Wheat,** 1 small | 7 |
| **Hot Honey on White,** 1 small | 7 |
| **Italian Turkey on Wheat,** 1 small | 8 |
| **Italian Turkey on White,** 1 small | 8 |
| **Pesto Turkey Club on Wheat,** 1 small | 10 |
| **Pesto Turkey Club on White,** 1 small | 11 |
| **Smokehouse Turkey on Wheat,** 1 small | 7 |
| **Smokehouse Turkey on White,** 1 small | 8 |
| **Thanksgiving on Wheat,** 1 small | 7 |
| **Thanksgiving on White,** 1 small | 7 |
| **Turkey Applejack on Wheat,** 1 small | 8 |
| **Turkey Applejack on White,** 1 small | 8 |
| **Tuscan Turkey on Wheat,** 1 small | 6 |
| **Tuscan Turkey on White,** 1 small | 6 |
| **Wild Turkey on Wheat,** 1 small | 7 |
| **Wild Turkey on White,** 1 small | 8 |
| **VEGGIE & CHEESE SANDWICHES** | |
| **California Hummer on Wheat,** 1 small | 7 |
| **California Hummer on White,** 1 small | 7 |
| **French Twist on Wheat,** 1 small | 6 |
| **French Twist on White,** 1 small | 7 |
| **Italian Veggie on Wheat,** 1 small | 6 |
| **Italian Veggie on White,** 1 small | 6 |
| **Monster Veggie on Wheat,** 1 small | 6 |
| **Monster Veggie on White,** 1 small | 6 |
| **Nut & Honey on Wheat,** 1 small | 9 |
| **Nut & Honey on White,** 1 small | 9 |
| **Spinach Stuffer on Wheat,** 1 small | 6 |
| **Spinach Stuffer on White,** 1 small | 6 |
| **Ultimate Veggie on Wheat,** 1 small | 4 |
| **Ultimate Veggie on White,** 1 small | 5 |
| **Veggie Fajita on Wheat,** 1 small | 6 |
| **Veggie Fajita on White,** 1 small | 6 |
| **SPECIALS** | |
| **Alpine Chicken Melt on Wheat,** 1 small | 11 |
| **Alpine Chicken Melt on White,** 1 small | 11 |
| **Buffalo Chicken Melt on Low-Carb,** 1 small | 7 |
| **Buffalo Chicken Melt on Wheat,** 1 small | 8 |
| **Buffalo Chicken Melt on White,** 1 small | 9 |
| **Cajun Chicken Melt on Low-Carb,** 1 small | 8 |
| **Cajun Chicken Melt on Wheat,** 1 small | 10 |

| ▲ Power Foods | *PointsPlus™* value |
|---|---|
| **Cajun Chicken Melt on White,** 1 small | 10 |
| **Cajun Club on Low-Carb,** 1 small | 8 |
| **Cajun Club on Wheat,** 1 small | 9 |
| **Cajun Club on White,** 1 small | 10 |
| **Caribbean Mix on Low-Carb,** 1 small | 11 |
| **Caribbean Mix on Wheat,** 1 small | 12 |
| **Caribbean Mix on White,** 1 small | 11 |
| **Carnita Chicken on Low-Carb,** 1 small | 8 |
| **Carnita Chicken on Wheat,** 1 small | 9 |
| **Carnita Chicken on White,** 1 small | 10 |
| **Carnita Steak on Low-Carb,** 1 small | 8 |
| **Carnita Steak on Wheat,** 1 small | 10 |
| **Carnita Steak on White,** 1 small | 10 |
| **Carolina Shrimp Melt on Low-Carb,** 1 small | 6 |
| **Carolina Shrimp Melt on Wheat,** 1 small | 7 |
| **Carolina Shrimp Melt on White,** 1 small | 8 |
| **Cherry Pecan Chicken Club on Low-Carb,** 1 small | 15 |
| **Cherry Pecan Chicken Club on Wheat,** 1 small | 17 |
| **Cherry Pecan Chicken Club on White,** 1 small | 17 |
| **Chicken Bruschetta on Low-Carb,** 1 small | 7 |
| **Chicken Bruschetta on Wheat,** 1 small | 8 |
| **Chicken Bruschetta on White,** 1 small | 9 |
| **Chicken Pizza on Low-Carb,** 1 small | 9 |
| **Chicken Pizza on Wheat,** 1 small | 10 |
| **Chicken Pizza on White,** 1 small | 11 |
| **Chipotle Cheesesteak on Low-Carb,** 1 small | 8 |
| **Chipotle Cheesesteak on Wheat,** 1 small | 9 |

| ▲ Power Foods | *PointsPlus™* value |
|---|---|
| **Chipotle Cheesesteak on White,** 1 small | 10 |
| **Chipotle Chicken on Low-Carb,** 1 small | 9 |
| **Chipotle Chicken on Wheat,** 1 small | 10 |
| **Chipotle Chicken on White,** 1 small | 11 |
| **Coney Island Melt on Low-Carb,** 1 small | 11 |
| **Coney Island Melt on Wheat,** 1 small | 12 |
| **Coney Island Melt on White,** 1 small | 13 |
| **Extreme Veggie on Wheat,** 1 small | 7 |
| **Extreme Veggie on White,** 1 small | 7 |
| **Grand Central on Low-Carb,** 1 small | 9 |
| **Grand Central on Wheat,** 1 small | 10 |
| **Grand Central on White,** 1 small | 11 |
| **Holiday Meltdown on Low-Carb,** 1 small | 9 |
| **Holiday Meltdown on Wheat,** 1 small | 10 |
| **Holiday Meltdown on White,** 1 small | 11 |
| **Huevos Rancheros on Low-Carb,** 1 small | 8 |
| **Huevos Rancheros on Wheat,** 1 small | 9 |
| **Huevos Rancheros on White,** 1 small | 10 |
| **Longhorn Melt on Low-Carb,** 1 small | 9 |
| **Longhorn Melt on Wheat,** 1 small | 11 |
| **Longhorn Melt on White,** 1 small | 11 |
| **Monster Fajita on Low-Carb,** 1 small | 8 |
| **Monster Fajita on Wheat,** 1 small | 10 |
| **Monster Fajita on White,** 1 small | 10 |
| **Monterey Chicken on Low-Carb,** 1 small | 9 |
| **Monterey Chicken on Wheat,** 1 small | 11 |
| **Monterey Chicken on White,** 1 small | 11 |
| **Moroccan Tofu on Low-Carb,** 1 small | 5 |
| **Moroccan Tofu on Wheat,** 1 small | 6 |

*Specials (cont'd)*

| ▲ Power Foods | *PointsPlus™* value |
|---|---|
| **Moroccan Tofu on White,** 1 small | 7 |
| **Nantucket Lobster on Wheat,** 1 small | 9 |
| **Nantucket Lobster on White,** 1 small | 9 |
| **New Orleans Melt on Low-Carb,** 1 small | 6 |
| **New Orleans Melt on Wheat,** 1 small | 7 |
| **New Orleans Melt on White,** 1 small | 8 |
| **New Yorker on Low-Carb,** 1 small | 7 |
| **New Yorker on Wheat,** 1 small | 8 |
| **New Yorker on White,** 1 small | 8 |
| **Orange County Smoked Turkey on Low-Carb,** 1 small | 12 |
| **Orange County Smoked Turkey on Wheat,** 1 small | 13 |
| **Orange County Smoked Turkey on White,** 1 small | 14 |
| **Palm Beach Tuna on Low-Carb,** 1 small | 7 |
| **Palm Beach Tuna on Wheat,** 1 small | 8 |
| **Palm Beach Tuna on White,** 1 small | 9 |
| **Pesto Chicken on Low-Carb,** 1 small | 9 |
| **Pesto Chicken on Wheat,** 1 small | 10 |
| **Pesto Chicken on White,** 1 small | 11 |
| **Pesto Club on Low-Carb,** 1 small | 8 |
| **Pesto Club on Wheat,** 1 small | 10 |
| **Pesto Club on White,** 1 small | 10 |
| **Ranchero Chicken on Low-Carb,** 1 small | 8 |
| **Ranchero Chicken on Wheat,** 1 small | 9 |
| **Ranchero Chicken on White,** 1 small | 10 |
| **Ranchero Steak on Low-Carb,** 1 small | 8 |
| **Ranchero Steak on Wheat,** 1 small | 9 |
| **Ranchero Steak on White,** 1 small | 10 |
| **Roly Poly Pounder on Low-Carb,** 1 small | 10 |
| **Roly Poly Pounder on Wheat,** 1 small | 11 |
| **Roly Poly Pounder on White,** 1 small | 12 |
| **Roly Polynesian on Low-Carb,** 1 small | 9 |

| ▲ Power Foods | *PointsPlus™* value |
|---|---|
| **Roly Polynesian on Wheat,** 1 small | 10 |
| **Roly Polynesian on White,** 1 small | 10 |
| **Roly Reuben on Low-Carb,** 1 small | 8 |
| **Roly Reuben on Wheat,** 1 small | 9 |
| **Roly Reuben on White,** 1 small | 10 |
| **Roma Chicken on Low-Carb,** 1 small | 7 |
| **Roma Chicken on Wheat,** 1 small | 8 |
| **Roma Chicken on White,** 1 small | 9 |
| **Shrimp Club on Low-Carb,** 1 small | 8 |
| **Shrimp Club on Wheat,** 1 small | 9 |
| **Shrimp Club on White,** 1 small | 9 |
| **Steak & Bearnaise on Low-Carb,** 1 small | 8 |
| **Steak & Bearnaise on Wheat,** 1 small | 9 |
| **Steak & Bearnaise on White,** 1 small | 10 |
| **Teriyaki Tuna on Low-Carb,** 1 small | 10 |
| **Teriyaki Tuna on Wheat,** 1 small | 11 |
| **Teriyaki Tuna on White,** 1 small | 12 |
| **Thai Peanut Chicken on Low-Carb,** 1 small | 8 |
| **Thai Peanut Chicken on Wheat,** 1 small | 10 |
| **Thai Peanut Chicken on White,** 1 small | 10 |
| **Thai Peanut Tofu on Low-Carb,** 1 small | 5 |
| **Thai Peanut Tofu on Wheat,** 1 small | 6 |
| **Thai Peanut Tofu on White,** 1 small | 7 |
| **Tofu Tahini on Low-Carb,** 1 small | 5 |
| **Tofu Tahini on Wheat,** 1 small | 6 |
| **Tofu Tahini on White,** 1 small | 7 |
| **Tuna Club on Low-Carb,** 1 small | 9 |
| **Tuna Club on Wheat,** 1 small | 11 |
| **Tuna Club on White,** 1 small | 11 |
| **Turkey Saga on Low-Carb,** 1 small | 8 |
| **Turkey Saga on Wheat,** 1 small | 9 |
| **Turkey Saga on White,** 1 small | 10 |
| **Westport Club on Wheat,** 1 small | 10 |
| **Westport Club on White,** 1 small | 11 |

| ▲ Power Foods | *PointsPlus*™ value |
|---|---|
| **SALADS** (WITHOUT DRESSING) | |
| **Alpine Chef,** 1 | 11 |
| **Chipotle Caesar,** 1 | 15 |
| **Cobb Salad,** 1 | 14 |
| **Greek Salad,** 1 | 6 |
| **Las Olas Salad,** 1 | 8 |
| **Spa Salad,** 1 | 7 |
| **Walnut Spinach,** 1 | 14 |
| **SAUCES & DRESSINGS** | |
| **Asian Tahini Dressing,** 1 Tbsp | 2 |
| **Balsamic Vinegar Dressing,** 1 Tbsp | 2 |
| **BBQ Ranch Dressing,** 1 Tbsp | 2 |
| **Blue Cheese Dressing,** 1 Tbsp | 2 |
| **Caesar Dressing,** 1 Tbsp | 3 |
| **Chipotle Ranch Dressing,** 1 Tbsp | 2 |
| **Creamy Italian Dressing,** 1 Tbsp | 1 |
| **Dill Dressing,** 1 Tbsp | 3 |
| **Fat Free Apple Ranch Dressing,** 1 Tbsp | 1 |
| **Fat Free Horsey Ranch Dressing,** 1 Tbsp | 1 |
| **Fat Free Ranch Dressing,** 1 Tbsp | 0 |
| **Fat Free Sundried Tomato Basil Dressing,** 1 Tbsp | 1 |
| **Honey Mustard Dressing,** 1 Tbsp | 2 |
| **Lite Dill Dressing,** 1 Tbsp | 0 |
| **Lower Fat Blue Cheese Dressing,** 1 Tbsp | 1 |
| **Oriental Sesame Dressing,** 1 Tbsp | 0 |
| **Ranch Dressing,** 1 Tbsp | 1 |
| **Basil Mayonnaise,** 1 Tbsp | 2 |
| **Cranberry Honey Mustard,** 1 Tbsp | 1 |

| ▲ Power Foods | *PointsPlus*™ value |
|---|---|
| **Curry Sauce,** 1 Tbsp | 3 |
| **Dill Horseradish Sauce,** 1 Tbsp | 1 |
| **Fajita Sauce,** 1 Tbsp | 2 |
| **Fat Free Creole Sauce,** 1 Tbsp | 0 |
| **Fat Free Curried Mayonnaise,** 1 Tbsp | 0 |
| **Honey Mustard Relish,** 1 Tbsp | 2 |
| **Horsey (horseradish) Sauce,** 1 Tbsp | 3 |
| **Peach Salsa,** 1 Tbsp | 0 |
| **Peaches & Pepper Relish,** 1 Tbsp | 2 |
| **Pesto Mayonnaise,** 1 Tbsp | 3 |
| **Roasted Red Pepper Hummus,** 1 Tbsp | 2 |
| **Roasted Red Pepper Mayonnaise,** 1 Tbsp | 1 |
| **Spicy Cajun Mayonnaise,** 1 Tbsp | 1 |
| **Tarragon Mayonnaise,** 1 Tbsp | 3 |
| **CLASSIC SOUPS** | |
| **Baja Chicken Enchilada,** 1 serving | 6 |
| **Broccoli Cheddar,** 1 serving | 4 |
| **Chili,** 1 serving | 4 |
| **Clam Chowder,** 1 serving | 3 |
| **Corn & Green Chili Bisque,** 1 serving | 4 |
| **Garden Vegetable,** 1 serving | 1 |
| **Harvest Mushroom Bisque,** 1 serving | 3 |
| **Loaded Baked Potato,** 1 serving | 5 |
| **Mexican Style Chicken Tortilla,** 1 serving | 3 |
| **Old Fashioned Chicken Noodle,** 1 serving | 2 |
| **Roasted Garlic Tomato,** 1 serving | 4 |
| **Seafood Bisque,** 1 serving | 6 |
| **Spring Asparagus,** 1 serving | 4 |

# ROLY POLY SANDWICHES

| ▲ Power Foods | PointsPlus™ value |
|---|---|
| **EGG ROLYS** | |
| **All American Egg Roly on Low-Carb,** 1 small | 11 |
| **All American Egg Roly on Wheat,** 1 small | 12 |
| **All American Egg Roly on White,** 1 small | 13 |
| **Christo Melt on Low-Carb,** 1 small | 7 |
| **Christo Melt on Wheat,** 1 small | 9 |
| **Christo Melt on White,** 1 small | 9 |
| **Steak and Eggs on Low-Carb,** 1 small | 7 |
| **Steak and Eggs on Wheat,** 1 small | 9 |
| **Steak and Eggs on White,** 1 small | 9 |
| **Veggie Scramble Egg Roly on Low-Carb,** 1 small | 7 |
| **Veggie Scramble Egg Roly on Wheat,** 1 small | 8 |
| **Veggie Scramble Egg Roly on White,** 1 small | 9 |
| **Western Egg Roly on Low-Carb,** 1 small | 7 |
| **Western Egg Roly on Wheat,** 1 small | 9 |
| **Western Egg Roly on White,** 1 small | 9 |
| **KIDS ITEMS** | |
| **Cheese Dog on Low-Carb,** 1 | 6 |
| **Cheese Dog on Wheat,** 1 | 7 |
| **Cheese Dog on White,** 1 | 8 |
| **Chicken Melt on on Low-Carb,** 1 | 4 |
| **Chicken Melt on Wheat,** 1 | 5 |
| **Chicken Melt on White,** 1 | 6 |
| **Grilled Cheese on Low-Carb,** 1 | 4 |
| **Grilled Cheese on Wheat,** 1 | 6 |
| **Grilled Cheese on White,** 1 | 6 |
| **Meat and Cheese on Low-Carb,** 1 | 4 |
| **Meat and Cheese on Wheat,** 1 | 5 |
| **Meat and Cheese on White,** 1 | 6 |
| **Peanut Butter and Jelly on Low-Carb,** 1 | 6 |
| **Peanut Butter and Jelly on Wheat,** 1 | 7 |
| **Peanut Butter and Jelly on White,** 1 | 8 |
| **SWEETS** | |
| **Apple Strudel,** 1 serving | 11 |
| **Chocolate Cheese Cake,** 1 serving | 13 |
| **Fruit Melt,** 1 serving | 8 |
| **Peach Granola,** 1 serving | 13 |
| **Rock N Roll Sweet Roly,** 1 serving | 13 |

▲ Power Foods — *PointsPlus™* value

## ANTIPASTI

| Item | PointsPlus™ value |
|---|---|
| **Crab-Stuffed Mushrooms,** 1 serving | 8 |
| **Fresh Mozzarella Fritti,** 1 serving | 18 |
| **Mozzarella Alla Caprese,** 1 serving | 9 |
| **Roasted Vegetables,** 1 serving | 8 |
| **Tomato Bruschetta,** 1 serving | 14 |

## AMORE DE LA GRILL

| Item | PointsPlus™ value |
|---|---|
| **Chicken Portobello (includes sides),** 1 serving | 27 |
| **Grilled Salmon, Teriyaki (includes sides),** 1 serving | 32 |
| **Honey Balsamic Chicken (includes sides),** 1 serving | 31 |
| **Pollo Magro "Skinny Chicken",** 1 serving | 8 |
| **Simple Salmon (includes sides),** 1 serving | 17 |

## MEDITERRANEAN GRILL

| Item | PointsPlus™ value |
|---|---|
| **Aged Beef Tenderloin Spiedini,** 1 serving | 10 |
| **Center-Cut Lamb Spiedini,** 1 serving | 13 |
| **Grilled Chicken Spiedini,** 1 serving | 8 |
| **Jumbo Shrimp Spiedini,** 1 serving | 5 |

## CLASSICO

| Item | PointsPlus™ value |
|---|---|
| **Chicken Cannelloni,** 1 serving | 15 |
| **Spaghetti Bolognese,** 1 serving | 15 |

## HANDCRAFTED PASTA

| Item | PointsPlus™ value |
|---|---|
| **Capellini Pomodoro,** 1 serving | 10 |
| **Lobster Ravioli,** 1 serving | 14 |
| **Pollo Caprese,** 1 serving | 14 |
| **Seafood Linguine,** 1 serving | 17 |
| **Shrimp Portofino,** 1 serving | 15 |

## BRICK OVEN PIZZA

| Item | PointsPlus™ value |
|---|---|
| **BBQ Chicken Pizza,** 1/2 pizza | 25 |

## NEAPOLITAN PIZZA

| Item | PointsPlus™ value |
|---|---|
| **Pepperoni,** 1 pizza | 24 |
| **Prosciutto e Arugula,** 1 pizza | 23 |
| **Roasted Vegetali,** 1 pizza | 21 |

## KID'S MEAL & SIDE

| Item | PointsPlus™ value |
|---|---|
| **Spaghetti & Meatball (Red Sauce),** 1 serving | 6 |
| ▲ **Steamed Broccoli,** 1 serving | 0 |

## SALADS

| Item | PointsPlus™ value |
|---|---|
| **Caesar della Casa (House) with Dressing,** 1 | 7 |
| **Caesar della Casa (House) without Dressing,** 1 | 3 |
| **Chicken Caesar without Dressing,** 1 | 11 |
| **Chicken Florentine Salad (without dressing),** 1 | 13 |
| **Chicken Florentine with Dressing,** 1 | 23 |
| **Garden della Casa (House) with Dressing,** 1 | 6 |

*Salads (cont'd)*

| ▲ Power Foods | *PointsPlus*™ value |
|---|---|
| **Garden della Casa (House) without Dressing,** 1 | 3 |
| **Insalata Blu with Chicken & Dressing,** 1 | 19 |
| **Insalata Blu with Chicken without Dressing,** 1 | 14 |
| **Insalata Blu with Dressing,** 1 | 16 |
| **Insalata Blu without Dressing,** 1 | 11 |
| **Scallops & Spinach Salad,** 1 serving | 8 |
| **Warm Spinach Salad,** 1 serving | 9 |

## DRESSINGS

| | |
|---|---|
| **Balsamic Vinaigrette Dressing,** 1 fl oz | 3 |
| **Fat-Free Creamy Italian Dressing,** 1 fl oz | 0 |
| **Low-fat Caesar Dressing,** 1 fl oz | 1 |
| **Pizzaiola Sauce,** 1 fl oz | 1 |
| **Roasted Garlic Lemon Vinaigrette Dressing,** 1 fl oz | 5 |

## DESSERTS

| | |
|---|---|
| **Italian Sorbetto with Biscotti,** 1 serving | 6 |
| **Simple Lemon Pound Cake,** 1 serving | 7 |

▲ Power Foods — *PointsPlus*™ value

## ORIGINAL CRUST PIZZA

|  | PointsPlus™ value |
|---|---|
| **Cheese,** 1/12 of a large pizza | 6 |
| **Chicken & Garlic Gourmet™,** 1/12 of a large pizza | 7 |
| **Chicken Smokehouse,** 1/12 of a large pizza | 7 |
| **Gourmet Veggie™,** 1/12 of a large pizza | 6 |
| **Guinevere's Garden Delight®,** 1/12 of a large pizza | 6 |
| **Hawaiian,** 1/12 of a large pizza | 6 |
| **Italian Garlic Supreme™,** 1/12 of a large pizza | 7 |
| **King Arthur's Supreme®,** 1/12 of a large pizza | 7 |
| **Maui Zaui™ Pizza (Polynesian sauce),** 1/12 of a large pizza | 7 |
| **Maui Zaui™ Pizza (with zesty red sauce),** 1/12 of a large pizza | 6 |
| **Montague's All Meat Marvel®,** 1/12 of a large pizza | 8 |
| **Pepperoni,** 1/12 of a large pizza | 6 |
| **Smokehouse Combo,** 1/12 of a large pizza | 7 |
| **Ulti-Meat,** 1/12 of a large pizza | 8 |
| **Wombo Combo,** 1/12 of a large pizza | 7 |

## PAN CRUST PIZZA

|  | PointsPlus™ value |
|---|---|
| **Cheese,** 1/12 of a large pizza | 8 |
| **Chicken & Garlic Gourmet™,** 1/12 of a large pizza | 9 |
| **Chicken Smokehouse,** 1/12 of a large pizza | 9 |
| **Gourmet Veggie™,** 1/12 of a large pizza | 8 |
| **Guinevere's Garden Delight®,** 1/12 of a large pizza | 8 |
| **Hawaiian,** 1/12 of a large pizza | 8 |

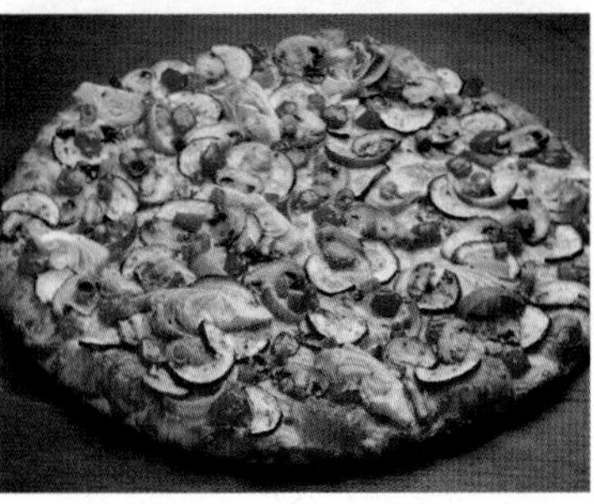

▲ Power Foods — *PointsPlus*™ value

|  | PointsPlus™ value |
|---|---|
| **Italian Garlic Supreme™,** 1/12 of a large pizza | 10 |
| **King Arthur's Supreme®,** 1/12 of a large pizza | 9 |
| **Maui Zaui™ Pizza (Polynesian sauce),** 1/12 of a large pizza | 9 |
| **Maui Zaui™ Pizza (with zesty red sauce),** 1/12 of a large pizza | 9 |
| **Montague's All Meat Marvel®,** 1/12 of a large pizza | 9 |
| **Pepperoni,** 1/12 of a large pizza | 9 |
| **Smokehouse Combo,** 1/12 of a large pizza | 10 |
| **Ulti-Meat,** 1/12 of a large pizza | 10 |
| **Wombo Combo,** 1/12 of a large pizza | 9 |

## SKINNY CRUST PIZZA

|  | PointsPlus™ value |
|---|---|
| **Cheese,** 1/12 of a large pizza | 5 |
| **Chicken & Garlic Gourmet™,** 1/12 of a large pizza | 6 |
| **Chicken Smokehouse,** 1/12 of a large pizza | 6 |
| **Gourmet Veggie™,** 1/12 of a large pizza | 5 |
| **Guinevere's Garden Delight®,** 1/12 of a large pizza | 5 |
| **Hawaiian,** 1/12 of a large pizza | 5 |

*Skinny Crust Pizza (cont'd)*

| ▲ Power Foods | *PointsPlus*™ value |
|---|---|
| **Italian Garlic Supreme™,** 1/12 of a large pizza | 6 |
| **King Arthur's Supreme®,** 1/12 of a large pizza | 6 |
| **Maui Zaui™ (Polynesian Sauce),** 1/12 of a large pizza | 6 |
| **Maui Zaui™ (Zesty Red Sauce),** 1/12 of a large pizza | 6 |
| **Montague's All Meat Marvel®,** 1/12 of a large pizza | 7 |
| **Pepperoni,** 1/12 of a large pizza | 6 |
| **Smokehouse Combo,** 1/12 of a large pizza | 7 |
| **Ulti-Meat,** 1/12 of a large pizza | 7 |
| **Wombo Combo,** 1/12 of a large pizza | 6 |

▲ Power Foods — *PointsPlus*™ value

## BURRITOS (CHIPS NOT INCLUDED)

|  | PointsPlus™ value |
|---|---|
| **Baja Grill Burrito Chicken,** 1 | 16 |
| **Baja Grill Burrito Steak,** 1 | 18 |
| **Bean & Cheese Burrito,** 1 | 18 |
| **Big Burrito Especial Chicken,** 1 | 22 |
| **Big Burrito Especial Steak,** 1 | 23 |
| **Carnitas Rajas Burrito,** 1 | 21 |
| **Fish Burrito,** 1 | 20 |
| **Grilled Mesquite Shrimp Burrito,** 1 | 19 |
| **Grilled Veggie Burrito,** 1 | 17 |
| **HealthMex® Chicken Burrito,** 1 | 14 |
| **HealthMex® Mahi Mahi Burrito,** 1 | 14 |
| **Mahi Mahi Burrito,** 1 | 19 |

## TACOS

|  | PointsPlus™ value |
|---|---|
| **Carnitas Rajas Taco,** 1 | 6 |
| **Fish Taco Especial,** 1 | 9 |
| **Grilled Chicken Taco,** 1 | 7 |
| **Grilled Mahi Mahi Taco,** 1 | 8 |
| **Grilled Mesquite Shrimp Taco,** 1 | 6 |
| **Grilled Steak Taco,** 1 | 6 |
| **HealthMex Mahi Mahi Taco,** 1 | 5 |
| **HealthMex® Chicken Taco,** 1 | 5 |
| **World Famous Fish Taco,** 1 serving | 9 |

## STREET TACOS (MADE WITH CORN TORTILLAS)

|  | PointsPlus™ value |
|---|---|
| **Carnitas,** 1 | 3 |
| **Chicken,** 1 | 3 |
| **Steak,** 1 | 3 |

## GRILLED GOURMET TACOS (MADE WITH CORN TORTILLAS)

|  | PointsPlus™ value |
|---|---|
| **Garlic Herb Shrimp,** 1 | 10 |
| **Grilled Chicken,** 1 | 10 |
| **Grilled Portobello & Poblano,** 1 | 9 |
| **Sirloin Steak,** 1 | 11 |

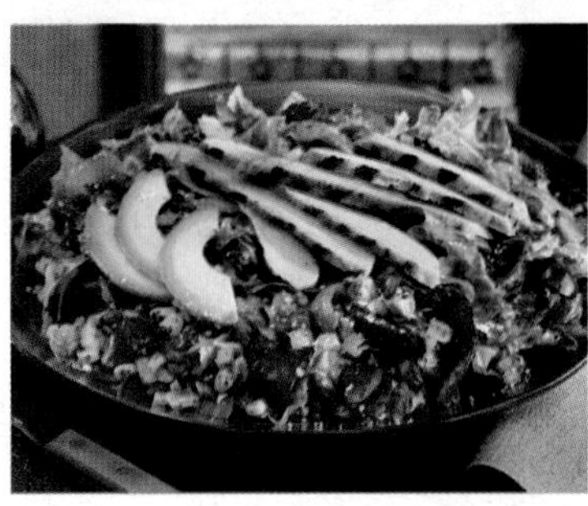

▲ Power Foods — *PointsPlus*™ value

## WRAPSALADAS (DRESSING NOT INCLUDED)

|  | PointsPlus™ value |
|---|---|
| **Chicken Chipotle Ranch Wrapsalada,** 1 | 14 |
| **Chicken Chopped Wrapsalada,** 1 | 17 |
| **Chicken Fiesta Wrapsalada,** 1 | 14 |
| **Chicken Tropical,** 1 | 12 |

## ENCHILADA PLATES (2 ENCHILADAS, CHIPS, RICE & BLACK BEANS)

|  | PointsPlus™ value |
|---|---|
| **Carnitas,** 1 serving | 33 |
| **Cheese,** 1 serving | 30 |
| **Chicken,** 1 serving | 33 |

## OTHER FAVORITES

|  | PointsPlus™ value |
|---|---|
| **Cheese Quesadilla,** 1 serving | 23 |
| **Chicken Quesadilla,** 1 serving | 25 |
| **Chicken Taquitos (3),** 1 serving | 7 |
| **Nachos Grande,** 1 serving | 34 |
| **Nachos Grande Chicken,** 1 serving | 37 |
| **Nachos Grande Steak,** 1 serving | 38 |
| **Steak Quesadilla,** 1 serving | 26 |

## SIDES

|  | PointsPlus™ value |
|---|---|
| ▲ **Black Beans,** 1 small serving | 3 |
| ▲ **Black Beans,** 1 large serving | 9 |

*Sides (cont'd)*

| ▲ Power Foods | *PointsPlus*™ value |
|---|---|
| **Brownie,** 1 | 12 |
| **Chips,** 1 regular serving | 6 |
| **Chips,** 1 large serving | 15 |
| **Churro,** 1 serving | 5 |
| **Guacamole,** 1 small serving | 5 |
| **Guacamole & Chips,** 1 serving | 21 |
| **Make it a Plate (pinto beans & chips),** 1 serving | 9 |
| ▲ **Pinto Beans,** 1 regular serving | 3 |
| ▲ **Pinto Beans,** 1 large serving | 12 |
| **Rice,** 1 regular serving | 3 |
| **Rice,** 1 large serving | 11 |

## SALADS & BOWLS (DRESSING NOT INCLUDED)

| | |
|---|---|
| **Chicken Chipotle Ranch Salad,** 1 | 8 |
| **Chicken Chopped Salad,** 1 | 10 |
| **Chicken Fiesta Salad,** 1 | 8 |
| **Chicken Grilled Grande Bowl,** 1 | 14 |
| **Chicken Tropical Salad,** 1 | 5 |

## DRESSINGS

| | |
|---|---|
| **Chipotle Dressing,** 2 oz | 4 |
| **Chipotle Ranch Dressing,** 2 oz | 6 |
| **Creamy Mandarin Dressing,** 2 oz | 5 |
| **Roasted Tomato Tomatillo Dressing,** 2 oz | 3 |

## SALSAS & SAUCES

| | |
|---|---|
| **Chipotle White Sauce,** 1 oz | 4 |
| ▲ **Roasted Chipotle,** 1 serving | 0 |
| ▲ **Salsa Picante,** 1 serving | 0 |
| ▲ **Salsa Regular,** 1 serving | 0 |
| ▲ **Salsa Verde,** 1 serving | 0 |
| **White Sauce,** 1 oz | 4 |

| ▲ Power Foods | *PointsPlus*™ value |
|---|---|

## KID'S MEALS

| | |
|---|---|
| **Add Mini Churro,** 1 serving | 2 |
| **Bean & Cheese Burrito,** 1 serving | 14 |
| **Chicken Taquitos (2),** 1 serving | 5 |
| **Kid's Cheese Quesadilla,** 1 serving | 10 |

| ▲ Power Foods | *PointsPlus*™ value |
|---|---|
| **WRAPS** | |
| **Buffalo Chicken Wrap,** 1 wrap | 13 |
| **Chicken Caesar Wrap,** 1 wrap | 10 |
| **Chicken Fajita Wrap,** 1 wrap | 12 |
| **Chicken Verona Wrap,** 1 wrap | 13 |
| **Chipotle Chicken Wrap,** 1 wrap | 11 |
| **Classic BLT Wrap,** 1 wrap | 15 |
| **Classic Ham & Swiss Wrap,** 1 wrap | 16 |
| **Garden Turkey Wrap,** 1 | 9 |
| **Hummus Wrap,** 1 wrap | 9 |
| **Pacific Chicken Wrap,** 1 wrap | 13 |
| **Pesto Turkey Wrap,** 1 wrap | 13 |
| **Roast Beef Club Wrap,** 1 wrap | 14 |
| **Spicy Roast Beef Wrap,** 1 wrap | 12 |
| **Sweet & Spicy Chicken Wrap,** 1 wrap | 12 |
| **Turkey & Bacon Wrap,** 1 wrap | 12 |
| **Turkey Basil Club Wrap,** 1 wrap | 15 |
| **Veggie Wrap,** 1 wrap | 9 |
| **PANINIS** | |
| **All American Omelet Panini,** 1 | 10 |
| **Buffalo,** 1 | 17 |
| **Chicken Delicato,** 1 | 15 |
| **Provolone & Veggie,** 1 | 12 |
| **South of the Border,** 1 | 9 |
| **Spinach Ham & Swiss Panini,** 1 | 13 |
| **Turkey & Mozzarella Panini,** 1 | 14 |
| **Tuscan Chicken Panini,** 1 | 16 |
| **Western Omelet Panini,** 1 | 9 |

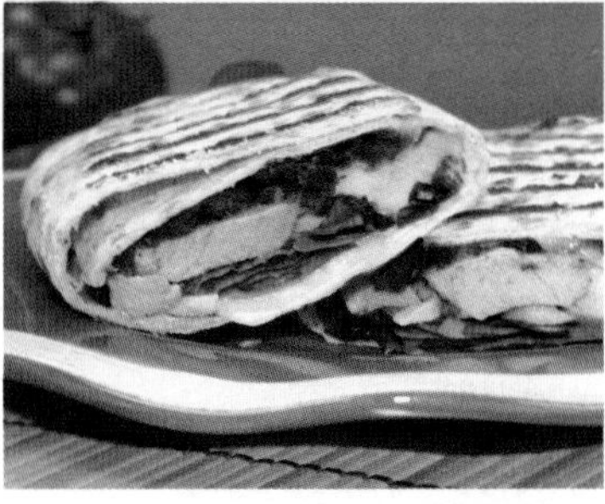

| ▲ Power Foods | *PointsPlus*™ value |
|---|---|
| **QUESADILLAS** | |
| **Barbecue Quesadilla,** 1 | 16 |
| **California Quesadilla,** 1 | 11 |
| **Cheese Quesadilla,** 1 | 11 |
| **Chicken Fajita Quesadilla,** 1 | 10 |
| **Mediterranean Quesadilla,** 1 | 13 |
| **Southwestern Quesadilla,** 1 | 15 |
| **RICE BOWLS** | |
| **Black Beans & Rice Bowl,** 1 | 18 |
| **Cheddar Chicken & Broccoli Bowl,** 1 | 20 |
| **Chicken Fajita Bowl,** 1 | 16 |
| **GRILLED FLAT BREAD** | |
| **Aloha,** 1 serving | 16 |
| **Brazillian Chicken,** 1 serving | 15 |
| **Cheese,** 1 serving | 11 |
| **Margherita,** 1 serving | 15 |
| **Pesto Chicken,** 1 serving | 18 |
| **Spinach & Bacon,** 1 serving | 20 |
| **Vegetarian,** 1 serving | 14 |

# SANDELLA'S

| ▲ Power Foods | *PointsPlus™* value |
|---|---|
| **SALADS** | |
| **Aloha Salad,** 1 serving | 11 |
| **Aloha Salad, without bread,** 1 serving | 9 |
| **Caesar Salad,** 1 serving | 5 |
| **Caesar Salad, without bread,** 1 serving | 3 |
| **Greek Salad,** 1 serving | 7 |
| **Greek Salad, without bread,** 1 serving | 5 |
| **Mozzarella Salad,** 1 serving | 14 |
| **Mozzarella Salad, without bread,** 1 serving | 12 |
| **Tomato & Cucumber Salad,** 1 serving | 13 |
| **Tomato & Cucumber Salad, without bread,** 1 serving | 11 |

| ▲ Power Foods | *PointsPlus™* value |
|---|---|
| **OVEN-TOASTED SANDWICHES** | |
| **Angus Corned Beef,** 1 small | 10 |
| **BLT,** 1 small | 10 |
| **Chicken & Pesto,** 1 small | 10 |
| **Chipotle Chicken,** 1 small | 10 |
| **Dijon Shaved Chicken,** 1 small | 8 |
| **Fresh Veggie,** 1 small | 9 |
| **Grilled Chicken Breast,** 1 small | 12 |
| **Santa Fe Chicken,** 1 small | 11 |
| **Smoked Turkey Breast Sandwich,** 1 small | 9 |
| **The Original™,** 1 small | 15 |
| **Turkey & Guacamole,** 1 small | 9 |

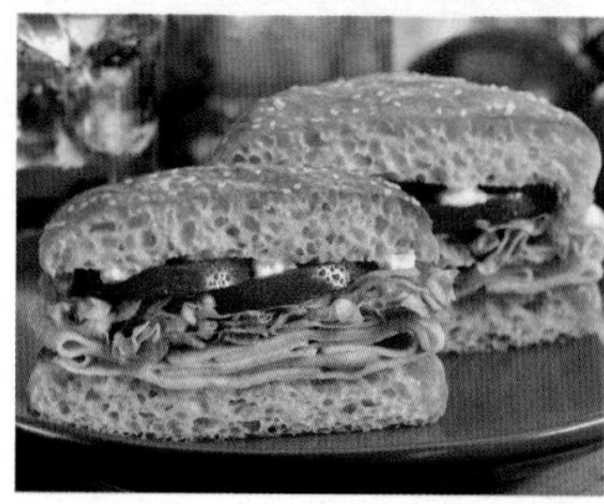

| ▲ Power Foods | *PointsPlus™* value |
|---|---|
| **FRESHLY BAKED PIZZAS** | |
| **Baby Spinach Salad Pizza,** 1 whole | 12 |
| **FRESH SALADS** (WITHOUT DRESSING, CROUTONS, OR CHOW MEIN NOODLES) | |
| **Baby Spinach & Feta Cheese Salad,** 1 | 3 |
| **Caesar Salad,** 1 | 3 |
| **Chicken Salad,** 1 | 10 |
| **Garden Salad,** 1 | 2 |
| **Greek Salad,** 1 | 4 |
| **Grilled Chicken Caesar Salad,** 1 | 8 |
| **Ham & Turkey Chef's Salad,** 1 | 7 |
| **Side Garden Salad,** 1 | 1 |
| **Smoked Turkey Chef Salad,** 1 | 8 |

# SIZZLER®

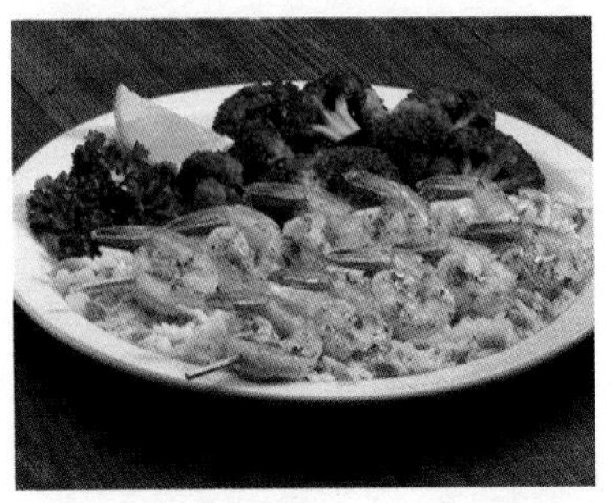

▲ Power Foods — *PointsPlus™* value

## BURGERS & SANDWICHES

|  | *PointsPlus™* value |
|---|---|
| **Sizzler Burger,** 1 burger (1/3 pound) | 16 |

## CLASSIC STEAKS

|  | *PointsPlus™* value |
|---|---|
| **6 oz,** 1 steak | 6 |
| **8 oz,** 1 steak | 8 |

## SIZZLIN' STEAKS

|  | *PointsPlus™* value |
|---|---|
| ▲ **Classic 6.25 oz. USDA Choice Sizzler Steak (without sizzling veggies, choice of starch & cheese toast),** 1 serving | 7 |
| **Ribeye Steak (without choice of starch & cheese toast),** 1 serving | 28 |

## STEAK COMBOS

|  | *PointsPlus™* value |
|---|---|
| **Steak & Grilled Shrimp Skewers with Sizzling Veggies (without choice of starch, melted margarine & cheese toast),** 1 serving | 8 |
| **Steak & Hibachi Grilled Chicken (without choice of starch & cheese toast),** 1 serving | 12 |
| **Steak & Lemon Herb Chicken (without choice of starch, cheese toast and melted margarine),** 1 serving | 12 |
| **Steak & Lobster Tail (without choice of starch, cheese toast and melted margarine),** 1 serving | 12 |

## CHICKEN

|  | *PointsPlus™* value |
|---|---|
| **Hibachi Chicken (single),** 1 serving | 5 |
| **Hibachi Chicken (double),** 1 serving | 10 |
| **5 oz Hibachi Grilled Chicken (without sizzling veggies, choice of starch & cheese toast),** 1 serving | 11 |
| **5 oz Lemon Herb Grilled Chicken (without sizzling veggies, choice of starch & cheese toast),** 1 serving | 11 |
| **Lemon Herb Chicken (single),** 1 serving | 5 |
| **Lemon Herb Chicken (double),** 1 serving | 11 |

## SEAFOOD

|  | *PointsPlus™* value |
|---|---|
| ▲ **Grilled Salmon (without sizzling veggies, choice of starch & cheese toast),** 1 serving | 9 |
| **Grilled Salmon, served on Rice Pilaf,** 1 serving | 14 |
| **Grilled Shrimp Skewers,** 1 serving | 14 |
| ▲ **Grilled Shrimp Skewers (without sizzling vegetables, choice of starch & cheese toast),** 2 skewers | 5 |

## SIDES

|  | *PointsPlus™* value |
|---|---|
| **Baked Potato,** 1 potato | 7 |
| ▲ **Broccoli,** 1 serving | 0 |

| ▲ Power Foods | *PointsPlus™* value |
|---|---|
| **SMOOTHIES** (20 FL OZ) | |
| **Acai Adventure®**, 1 | 11 |
| **Acai Adventure® (without turbinado)**, 1 | 10 |
| **Activator® - Chocolate (without turbinado)**, 1 | 8 |
| **Activator® - Strawberry (without turbinado)**, 1 | 12 |
| **Activator® - Vanilla (without turbinado)**, 1 | 8 |
| **Angel Food™ (without turbinado)**, 1 | 7 |
| **Banana Berry Treat®**, 1 | 9 |
| **Banana Berry Treat® (without turbinado)**, 1 | 8 |
| **Banana Boat® (without turbinado)**, 1 | 12 |
| **Banana Boat™**, 1 | 15 |
| **Berry Punch**, 1 | 10 |
| **Blackberry Dream™ (without turbinado)**, 1 | 7 |
| **Blueberry Heaven®**, 1 | 9 |
| **Caribbean Way® (without turbinado)**, 1 | 8 |
| **Carribean Way®**, 1 | 10 |
| **Celestial Cherry High™**, 1 | 9 |
| **Celestial Cherry High™ (without turbinado)**, 1 | 6 |
| **Cherry Picker®**, 1 | 11 |
| **Cherry Picker® (without turbinado)**, 1 | 10 |
| **Chocolate Shredder**, 1 | 8 |
| **Coconut Surprise® (without turbinado)**, 1 | 7 |
| **Coconut Surprise™**, 1 | 12 |
| **Coffee Smoothie Caramel**, 1 | 9 |
| **Coffee Smoothie Caramel (without turbinado)**, 1 | 6 |
| **Coffee Smoothie Mocha (without turbinado)**, 1 | 4 |

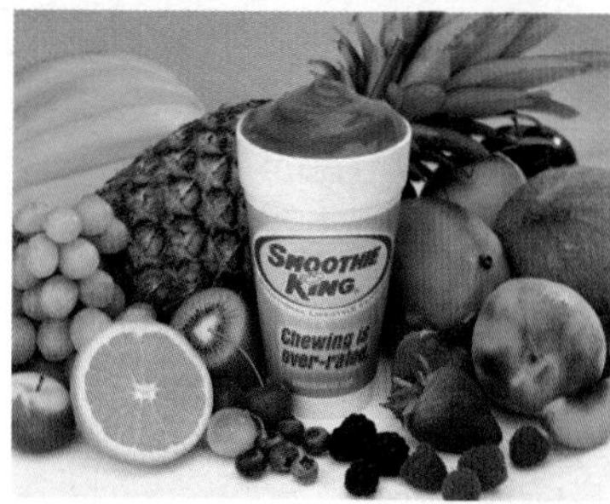


| ▲ Power Foods | *PointsPlus™* value |
|---|---|
| **Coffee Smoothie Vanilla**, 1 | 9 |
| **Coffee Smoothie Vanilla (without turbinado)**, 1 | 7 |
| **Cranberry Cooler™**, 1 | 13 |
| **Cranberry Cooler™ (without turbinado)**, 1 | 10 |
| **Cranberry Supreme®**, 1 | 14 |
| **Cranberry Supreme® (without turbinado)**, 1 | 12 |
| **Fruit Fusion**, 1 | 9 |
| **Go Goji**, 1 | 11 |
| **Go Goji (without turbinado)**, 1 | 9 |
| **Grape Expectations®**, 1 | 10 |
| **Grape Expectations II™**, 1 | 14 |
| **Grape Expectations® (without turbinado)**, 1 | 8 |
| **Grape ExpectationsII™ (without turbinado)**, 1 | 12 |
| **Green Tea Tango**, 1 | 7 |
| **Green Tea Tango (without turbinado)**, 1 | 5 |
| **Hearty Apple®**, 1 | 10 |
| **High Protein - Almond Mocha**, 1 | 9 |
| **High Protein - Almond Mocha (without turbinado)**, 1 | 7 |
| **High Protein - Banana**, 1 | 8 |
| **High Protein - Chocolate**, 1 | 9 |

*Smoothies, 20 oz (cont'd)*

| ▲ Power Foods | PointsPlus™ value |
|---|---|
| High Protein - Chocolate (without turbinado), 1 | 7 |
| High Protein - Lemon, 1 | 9 |
| High Protein - Pineapple, 1 | 8 |
| Immune Builder®, 1 | 10 |
| Immune Builder® (without turbinado), 1 | 7 |
| Instant Vigor™, 1 | 9 |
| Instant Vigor™ (without turbinado), 1 | 8 |
| Island Impact®, 1 | 8 |
| Island Treat®, 1 | 9 |
| Island Treat® (without turbinado), 1 | 6 |
| Kiwi Island Treat®, 1 | 13 |
| Kiwi Island Treat® (without turbinado), 1 | 11 |
| Lemon Twist® Banana, 1 | 9 |
| Lemon Twist® Banana (without turbinado), 1 | 7 |
| Lemon Twist® Strawberry, 1 | 11 |
| Lemon Twist® Strawberry (without turbinado), 1 | 9 |
| Light & Fluffy®, 1 | 10 |
| Light & Fluffy® (without turbinado), 1 | 8 |
| Malt, 1 | 20 |
| Malt (without turbinado), 1 | 18 |
| MangoFest™, 1 | 8 |
| Mangosteen Madness, 1 | 10 |
| Mangosteen Madness (without turbinado), 1 | 8 |
| Mo'cuccino™ Mocha, 1 | 12 |
| Mo'cuccino Caramel™, 1 | 15 |
| Mo'cuccino Caramel™ (without turbinado), 1 | 10 |
| Mo'cuccino Vanilla™, 1 | 14 |
| Mo'cuccino Vanilla™ (without turbinado), 1 | 9 |
| Mo'cuccino™ Mocha (without turbinado), 1 | 7 |

| ▲ Power Foods | PointsPlus™ value |
|---|---|
| Muscle Punch Plus™, 1 | 9 |
| Muscle Punch Plus™ (without turbinado), 1 | 7 |
| Muscle Punch®, 1 | 9 |
| Muscle Punch® (without turbinado), 1 | 7 |
| Orange Ka-Bam®, 1 | 13 |
| Orange Ka-Bam® (without turbinado), 1 | 10 |
| Passion Passport®, 1 | 10 |
| Passion Passport® (without turbinado), 1 | 8 |
| Peach Slice Plus®, 1 | 12 |
| Peach Slice Plus® (without turbinado), 1 | 9 |
| Peach Slice™, 1 | 8 |
| Peach Slice™ (without turbinado), 1 | 6 |
| Peanut Power Plus™ Grape, 1 | 20 |
| Peanut Power Plus™ Grape (without turbinado), 1 | 15 |
| Peanut Power Plus™ Strawberry, 1 | 19 |
| Peanut Power Plus™ Strawberry (without turbinado), 1 | 14 |
| Peanut Power®, 1 | 15 |
| Peanut Power® (without turbinado), 1 | 10 |
| Pep Upper, 1 | 11 |
| Pep Upper (without turbinado), 1 | 9 |
| Pina Colada Island®, 1 | 15 |
| Pina Colada Island® (without turbinado), 1 | 10 |
| Pineapple Pleasure®, 1 | 7 |
| Pineapple Pleasure® (without turbinado), 1 | 5 |
| Pineapple Surf®, 1 | 12 |
| Pineapple Surf® (without turbinado), 1 | 9 |
| Pomegranate Punch, 1 | 12 |

| ▲ Power Foods | *PointsPlus™* value |
|---|---|
| Pomegranate Punch (without turbinado), 1 | 11 |
| Power Punch Plus®, 1 | 13 |
| Power Punch Plus® (without turbinado), 1 | 10 |
| Power Punch®, 1 | 11 |
| Power Punch® (without turbinado), 1 | 9 |
| Raspberry Collider, 1 | 9 |
| Raspberry Sunrise™, 1 | 10 |
| Raspberry Sunrise™ (without turbinado), 1 | 8 |
| Shake, 1 | 20 |
| Shake (without turbinado), 1 | 18 |
| Slim & Trim™ - Chocolate (without turbinado), 1 | 5 |
| Slim & Trim™ - Chocolate, 1 | 8 |
| Slim & Trim™ - Orange-Vanilla, 1 | 6 |
| Slim & Trim™ - Strawberry, 1 | 10 |
| Slim & Trim™ - Strawberry (without turbinado), 1 | 7 |
| Slim & Trim™ - Vanilla, 1 | 6 |
| Slim & Trim™ - Vanilla (without turbinado), 1 | 4 |
| Strawberry Kiwi Breeze®, 1 | 10 |
| Strawberry Shredder™, 1 | 9 |
| Strawberry X-Treme®, 1 | 10 |
| Super Punch Plus®, 1 | 12 |
| Super Punch™, 1 | 11 |
| The Activator® - Chocolate, 1 | 11 |
| The Activator® - Strawberry, 1 | 14 |
| The Activator® - Vanilla, 1 | 11 |
| The Hulk™ - Chocolate, 1 | 24 |
| The Hulk™ - Chocolate (without turbinado), 1 | 22 |
| The Hulk™ - Strawberry, 1 | 28 |
| The Hulk™ - Strawberry (without turbinado), 1 | 25 |

| ▲ Power Foods | *PointsPlus™* value |
|---|---|
| The Hulk™ - Vanilla, 1 | 24 |
| The Hulk™ - Vanilla (without turbinado), 1 | 22 |
| Vanilla Shredder, 1 | 7 |
| Yerba Mate - Mixed Berry (without turbinado), 1 | 8 |
| Yogurt D-Lite®, 1 | 9 |
| Yogurt D-Lite® (without turbinado), 1 | 6 |
| Youth Fountain™, 1 | 7 |
| Youth Fountain™ (without turbinado), 1 | 4 |

## LOW CARB SMOOTHIES (20 FL OZ)

| | |
|---|---|
| Banana, 1 | 7 |
| Chocolate, 1 | 7 |
| Strawberry, 1 | 7 |
| Vanilla, 1 | 7 |

## STAY HEALTHY (20 FL OZ)

| | |
|---|---|
| Yerba Mate - Mango, 1 | 10 |
| Yerba Mate - Mixed Berry, 1 | 11 |
| Yerba Mate - Pomengranate, 1 | 10 |

## TRIM DOWN (20 FL OZ)

| | |
|---|---|
| Angel Food™, 1 | 9 |
| Blackberry Dream™, 1 | 10 |

## KIDS KUPS (12 FL OZ)

| | |
|---|---|
| Choc-A-Laka™, 1 | 7 |
| CW, Jr.™, 1 | 7 |
| Gimme-Grape™, 1 | 7 |
| Lil Angel™, 1 | 6 |
| Smarti Tarti™, 1 | 5 |
| Berry Interesting™, 1 | 7 |

# SONIC®, AMERICA'S DRIVE-IN®

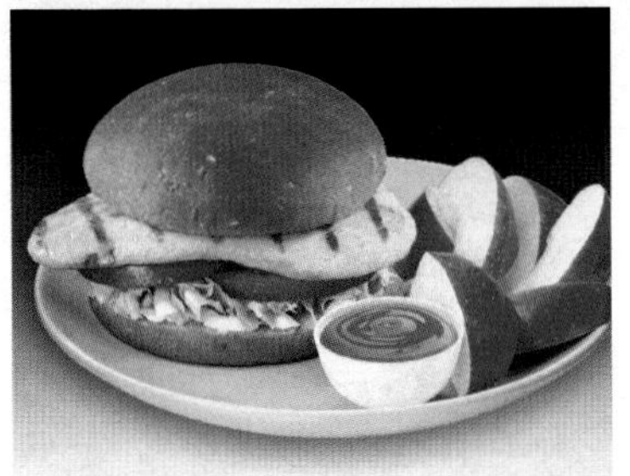

| ▲ Power Foods | *PointsPlus™* value |
|---|---|
| **BURGERS** | |
| **Bacon Cheeseburger,** 1 | 18 |
| **Chili Cheeseburger,** 1 | 18 |
| **Hickory Cheeseburger,** 1 | 17 |
| **Jalapeno Burger,** 1 | 14 |
| **Jalapeno Cheeseburger,** 1 | 16 |
| **Jr. Bacon Cheeseburger,** 1 | 11 |
| **Jr. Burger,** 1 | 8 |
| **Jr. Cheeseburger,** 1 | 10 |
| **Jr. Deluxe Burger,** 1 | 9 |
| **Jr. Double Cheeseburger,** 1 | 15 |
| **SONIC® Bacon Cheeseburger,** 1 | 21 |
| **SONIC® Bacon Cheeseburger with Mayonnaise,** 1 sandwich | 21 |
| **SONIC® Burger with Ketchup,** 1 | 15 |
| **SONIC® Burger with Mayonnaise,** 1 | 17 |
| **SONIC® Burger with Mustard,** 1 | 15 |
| **SONIC® Cheeseburger with Ketchup,** 1 | 17 |
| **SONIC® Cheeseburger with Mayonnaise,** 1 | 19 |
| **SONIC® Cheeseburger with Mustard,** 1 | 16 |
| **SuperSONIC® Cheeseburger with Ketchup,** 1 | 24 |
| **SuperSONIC® Cheeseburger with Mayonnaise,** 1 | 27 |

| ▲ Power Foods | *PointsPlus™* value |
|---|---|
| **SuperSONIC® Cheeseburger with Mustard,** 1 | 24 |
| **SuperSONIC® Jalapeno Cheeseburger,** 1 | 24 |
| **CHICKEN** | |
| **Breaded Chicken Sandwich,** 1 | 15 |
| **Chicken Strip Dinner,** 4 strips | 25 |
| **Crispy Chicken Bacon Ranch,** 1 sandwich | 16 |
| **Crispy Chicken Sandwich,** 1 sandwich | 15 |
| **Grilled Chicken Bacon Ranch,** 1 sandwich | 12 |
| **Grilled Chicken Sandwich,** 1 | 11 |
| **Honey Mustard Sauce,** 1 serving | 3 |
| **Jumbo Popcorn Chicken®,** 1 small | 10 |
| **Jumbo Popcorn Chicken®,** 1 large | 15 |
| **CONEYS** | |
| **Corn Dog,** 1 | 6 |
| **Ex-Long Chili Cheese Coney,** 1 | 18 |
| **Extra-Long Cheese Coney,** 1 | 18 |
| **Regular Coney,** 1 | 11 |
| **EVERYDAY VALUE MENU** | |
| **Chicken Strip Sandwich,** 1 sandwich | 11 |
| **French Fries,** 1 small | 5 |
| **Jr. Breakfast Burrito,** 1 | 9 |
| **Jr. FRITOS® Chili Cheese Wrap,** 1 | 9 |
| **Tater Tots,** 1 small | 6 |
| **TOASTER® SANDWICHES** | |
| **BLT,** 1 | 14 |
| **Chicken Club,** 1 | 20 |
| **Country Fried Steak,** 1 | 18 |
| **Fish Sandwich,** 1 sandwich | 17 |

# SONIC®, AMERICA'S DRIVE-IN®

▲ Power Foods — *PointsPlus*™ value

## UPGRADES

| Item | *PointsPlus*™ value |
|---|---|
| **Bacon,** 1 serving | 2 |
| **Cheese,** 1 serving | 2 |
| **Chili,** 1 serving | 1 |
| ▲ **Jalapeno,** 1 serving | 0 |

## WRAPS

| Item | *PointsPlus*™ value |
|---|---|
| **Chicken Strip Wrap,** 1 | 13 |
| **Crispy Chicken,** 1 | 13 |
| **Fritos® Chili Cheese,** 1 | 19 |
| **Fritos® Chili Cheese Wrap,** 1 | 18 |
| **Grilled Chicken,** 1 | 10 |

## KIDS' MEAL

| Item | *PointsPlus*™ value |
|---|---|
| **Apple Slices,** 1 serving | 1 |
| **Apple Slices with Fat-Free Caramel Dipping Sauce,** 1 serving | 3 |
| **Chicken Strips,** 2 strips | 5 |
| **Corn Dog,** 1 | 6 |
| ▲ **Fresh Banana,** 1 | 0 |
| **Grilled Cheese,** 1 | 10 |
| **Jr. Burger,** 1 | 8 |
| **Jr. Cheeseburger,** 1 Wacky Pack® | 10 |
| **Milk (1%),** 1 container | 3 |
| **Milk Chocolate (1%),** 1 container | 4 |

## ADD-ONS

| Item | *PointsPlus*™ value |
|---|---|
| ▲ **Green Chilies,** 1 serving | 0 |
| ▲ **Grilled Onions,** 1 serving | 0 |
| **Slaw,** 1 serving | 1 |

## SNACKS & SIDES

| Item | *PointsPlus*™ value |
|---|---|
| **Ched 'R' Bites®,** 12 bites | 7 |
| **Ched 'R' Peppers®,** 4 pieces | 9 |
| **French Fries,** 1 small serving | 5 |
| **French Fries with Cheese,** 1 small serving | 7 |
| **French Fries with Chili & Cheese,** 1 small serving | 8 |
| **Fritos® Chili Pie,** 1 medium | 13 |
| **Fritos® Chili Pie,** 1 large | 26 |
| **Mozzarella Sticks,** 5 | 12 |
| **Onion Rings,** 1 medium serving | 12 |
| **Tater Tots,** 1 small serving | 3 |
| **Tater Tots with Cheese,** 1 small serving | 5 |
| **Tater Tots with Chili & Cheese,** 1 small serving | 6 |
| **Tater Tots with Chili & Cheese,** 1 regular serving | 9 |

## SALADS

| Item | *PointsPlus*™ value |
|---|---|
| **Crispy Chicken,** 1 salad | 9 |
| **Grilled Chicken,** 1 salad | 6 |
| **JUMBO POPCORN CHICKEN® Salad,** 1 salad | 13 |
| **Santa Fe Grilled Chicken Salad,** 1 salad | 9 |

## HIDDEN VALLEY RANCH DRESSINGS

| Item | *PointsPlus*™ value |
|---|---|
| **Fat Free Italian,** 1 serving | 1 |
| **Honey Mustard,** 1 serving | 5 |
| **Light Ranch Dressing,** 1 serving | 3 |
| **Original Ranch Dressing,** 1 serving | 5 |
| **Thousand Island,** 1 serving | 6 |

## OTHER SALAD DRESSING

| Item | *PointsPlus*™ value |
|---|---|
| **Southwest Ranch,** 1 serving | 4 |

# SONIC®, AMERICA'S DRIVE-IN®

## CONDIMENTS

| ▲ Power Foods | *PointsPlus™* value |
|---|---|
| **BBQ Sauce,** 1 serving | 1 |
| **French Fry Sauce,** 1 serving | 1 |
| **Grape Jelly,** 1 serving | 1 |
| **Ketchup,** 1 serving | 0 |
| **Marinara Sauce,** 1 serving | 0 |
| **Mayonnaise,** 1 serving | 2 |
| **Mustard,** 1 serving | 0 |
| **Picante Sauce,** 1 serving | 0 |
| **Ranch Sauce,** 1 serving | 4 |
| **Strawberry Jam,** 1 serving | 1 |

## BREAKFAST FOODS

| ▲ Power Foods | *PointsPlus™* value |
|---|---|
| **Breakfast Burritos - Bacon, Egg & Cheese,** 1 | 13 |
| **Breakfast Burritos - Ham, Egg & Cheese,** 1 | 12 |
| **Breakfast Burritos - Sausage, Egg & Cheese,** 1 | 14 |
| **BREAKFAST TOASTER® Bacon, Egg & Cheese,** 1 | 14 |
| **BREAKFAST TOASTER® Ham, Egg & Cheese,** 1 | 13 |
| **BREAKFAST TOASTER® Sausage, Egg & Cheese,** 1 | 17 |
| **CroisSONIC Breakfast Sandwich - Bacon,** 1 sandwich | 14 |
| **CroisSONIC™ Breakfast Sandwich - Sausage,** 1 sandwich | 17 |
| **French Toast Sticks,** 4 sticks | 14 |
| **Sausage Biscuit dippers™ with Gravy,** 3 | 19 |
| **Steak and Egg Breakfast Burrito,** 1 | 16 |
| **SuperSonic® Breakfast Burrito,** 1 | 16 |
| **Syrup,** 1 serving | 1 |

## DESSERTS

| ▲ Power Foods | *PointsPlus™* value |
|---|---|
| **Banana Fudge,** 1 | 12 |
| **Banana Split,** 1 | 11 |
| **Hot Fudge Cake Sundae,** 1 | 13 |
| **Jr. Banana Split,** 1 | 5 |

## CONES & DISHES

| ▲ Power Foods | *PointsPlus™* value |
|---|---|
| **Vanilla Cone,** 1 | 5 |
| **Vanilla Dish,** 1 serving | 6 |

## SINGLE TOPPING SUNDAES

| ▲ Power Foods | *PointsPlus™* value |
|---|---|
| **Caramel Sundae,** 1 | 11 |
| **Chocolate Sundae,** 1 | 11 |
| **Hot Fudge Sundae,** 1 | 12 |
| **Jr. Butterfinger® Sundae,** 1 | 5 |
| **Jr. M&M's® Sundae,** 1 | 5 |
| **Jr. Oreo® Sundae,** 1 | 4 |
| **Jr. Reese's® Sundae,** 1 | 4 |
| **Peanut Butter Sundae,** 1 | 14 |
| **Peanut Butter Fudge Sundae,** 1 | 13 |
| **Pineapple Sundae,** 1 | 10 |
| **Strawberry Sundae,** 1 | 10 |
| **Nuts Add-On,** 1 serving | 1 |

## MALTS

| ▲ Power Foods | *PointsPlus™* value |
|---|---|
| **Banana Malt,** 1 regular | 13 |
| **Caramel Malt,** 1 regular | 15 |
| **Chocolate Malt,** 1 regular | 15 |
| **Hot Fudge Malt,** 1 regular | 16 |
| **Pineapple Malt,** 1 regular | 14 |
| **Strawberry Malt,** 1 regular | 14 |
| **Vanilla Malt,** 1 regular | 13 |

▲ Power Foods — *PointsPlus*™ value

## SHAKES

|  | PointsPlus™ value |
|---|---|
| **Banana Shake,** 1 regular | 13 |
| **Caramel Shake,** 1 regular | 14 |
| **Chocolate Shake,** 1 regular | 14 |
| **Hot Fudge Shake,** 1 regular | 15 |
| **Peanut Butter Fudge Shake,** 1 regular | 17 |
| **Peanut Butter Shake,** 1 regular | 18 |
| **Pineapple Shake,** 1 regular | 13 |
| **Strawberry Shake,** 1 regular | 14 |
| **Vanilla Shake,** 1 regular | 13 |

## CREAM PIE SHAKES

|  | PointsPlus™ value |
|---|---|
| **Banana Cream,** 1 regular | 16 |
| **Chocolate Cream,** 1 regular | 18 |
| **Coconut Cream,** 1 regular | 16 |
| **Strawberry Cream,** 1 regular | 17 |

## SONIC BLAST®

|  | PointsPlus™ value |
|---|---|
| **Butterfinger®,** 1 regular | 16 |
| **M&M®,** 1 regular | 16 |
| **Oreo®,** 1 regular | 15 |
| **Reese's® Peanut Butter Cups,** 1 regular | 15 |

## REAL FRUIT SLUSHES

|  | PointsPlus™ value |
|---|---|
| **Lemon,** 1 Wacky Pack® | 5 |
| **Lemon-Berry,** 1 Wacky Pack® | 5 |
| **Lime,** 1 Wacky Pack® | 5 |
| **Minute Maid® Cranberry Juice,** 1 Wacky Pack® | 5 |
| **Strawberry,** 1 Wacky Pack® | 5 |

▲ Power Foods — *PointsPlus*™ value

## CREAMSLUSH® TREAT

|  | PointsPlus™ value |
|---|---|
| **Blue Coconut,** 1 regular | 12 |
| **Cherry,** 1 regular | 12 |
| **Grape,** 1 regular | 12 |
| **Lemon,** 1 regular | 12 |
| **Lemon-Berry,** 1 regular | 13 |
| **Lime,** 1 regular | 12 |
| **Orange,** 1 regular | 12 |
| **Strawberry,** 1 regular | 13 |
| **Watermelon,** 1 regular | 12 |

## FLOATS/BLENDED FLOATS

|  | PointsPlus™ value |
|---|---|
| **Banana Fudge Sundae,** 1 serving | 12 |
| **Barq's® Root Beer,** 1 regular | 8 |
| **Coca-Cola®,** 1 regular | 8 |
| **Diet Coke®,** 1 regular | 6 |
| **Diet Dr. Pepper®,** 1 regular | 6 |
| **Dr Pepper®,** 1 regular | 9 |
| **Dr. Pepper® Float,** 1 regular | 8 |
| **Junior Banana Split,** 1 serving | 5 |
| **Sprite Zero®,** 1 regular | 6 |
| **Sprite®,** 1 regular | 8 |

## FRUIT SMOOTHIES

|  | PointsPlus™ value |
|---|---|
| **Strawberry,** 1 regular | 13 |
| **Strawberry,** 1 large | 18 |
| **Strawberry-Banana,** 1 large | 16 |
| **Tropical,** 1 regular | 13 |
| **Tropical,** 1 large | 16 |

## JUICE SLUSHES

|  | PointsPlus™ value |
|---|---|
| **Minute Maid® Apple Juice Slush,** 1 Wacky Pack® | 5 |
| **Minute Maid® Cranberry Juice Slush,** 1 Wacky Pack® | 5 |

| ▲ Power Foods | *PointsPlus™* value |
|---|---|
| **FAMOUS SLUSHES** | |
| **Blue Coconut,** 1 Wacky Pack® | 5 |
| **Bubble Gum,** 1 Wacky Pack® | 5 |
| **Cherry,** 1 Wacky Pack® | 5 |
| **Grape,** 1 Wacky Pack® | 5 |
| **Green Apple,** 1 Wacky Pack® | 5 |
| **Orange,** 1 Wacky Pack® | 5 |
| **Watermelon,** 1 Wacky Pack® | 5 |
| **LIMEADES** | |
| **Cherry,** 1 Wacky Pack® | 4 |
| **Cherry,** 1 medium | 6 |
| **Cherry,** 1 large | 10 |
| **Limeade,** 1 Wacky Pack® | 3 |
| **Limeade,** 1 medium | 5 |
| **Limeade,** 1 large | 8 |
| **Lo-Cal Diet Cherry,** 1 Wacky Pack® | 0 |
| **Lo-Cal Diet Limeade,** 1 Wacky Pack® | 0 |
| **Minute Maid® Apple Juice Limeade,** 1 Wacky Pack® | 4 |
| **Minute Maid® Cranberry,** 1 Wacky Pack® | 4 |
| **Strawberry,** 1 Wacky Pack® | 4 |
| **Strawberry,** 1 medium | 7 |
| **Strawberry,** 1 large | 10 |
| **CHILLERS** | |
| **Java Chiller, Caramel,** 1 regular | 15 |
| **Java Chiller, Caramel/Hazelnut,** 1 regular | 14 |
| **Java Chiller, Chocolate,** 1 regular | 15 |
| **Java Chiller, Chocolate/Hazelnut,** 1 regular | 15 |
| **Java Chiller, Hazelnut,** 1 regular | 15 |
| **Mocha Chip Java Chiller (limited time only),** 14 oz | 19 |

| ▲ Power Foods | *PointsPlus™* value |
|---|---|
| **OCEAN WATER®** | |
| **Ocean Water®,** 1 medium | 6 |
| **Ocean Water®,** 1 large | 9 |
| **POWERADE® DRINKS & SLUSHES** | |
| **POWERADE® Mountain Blast®,** 1 Wacky Pack® | 2 |
| **POWERADE® Mountain Blast® Slush,** 1 Wacky Pack® | 5 |
| **COFFEE & COFFEE DRINKS** | |
| **Hot Latte, Caramel,** 1 regular | 6 |
| **Hot Latte, Caramel/Hazelnut,** 1 regular | 6 |
| **Hot Latte, Caramel/Mocha,** 1 regular | 6 |
| **Hot Latte, Hazelnut,** 1 regular | 5 |
| **Hot Latte, Hazelnut/Mocha,** 1 regular | 6 |
| **Hot Latte, Mocha,** 1 regular | 5 |
| **Iced Latte, Mocha,** 1 regular | 7 |
| **Iced Latte, Mocha/Caramel,** 1 regular | 7 |
| **Iced Latte, Mocha/Hazelnut,** 1 regular | 7 |
| **Java Chiller, Hazelnut/Mocha,** 1 regular | 15 |
| **Java Chiller, Mocha,** 1 regular | 15 |
| **Java Chiller, Mocha/Caramel,** 1 regular | 15 |
| **PREMIUM ROAST COFFEES** | |
| **Coffee,** 1 regular | 0 |
| **Iced Latte, Caramel,** 1 regular | 7 |
| **Iced Latte, Caramel/Hazelnut,** 1 regular | 7 |
| **Iced Latte, Chocolate,** 1 regular | 7 |
| **Iced Latte, Chocolate/Caramel,** 1 regular | 7 |
| **Iced Latte, Chocolate/Hazelnut,** 1 regular | 7 |
| **Iced Latte, Hazelnut,** 1 regular | 7 |

| ▲ Power Foods | *PointsPlus™* value |
|---|---|

## HOT CHOCOLATE

| | |
|---|---|
| **Hot Chocolate,** 1 regular | 3 |

## ADD-IN FLAVOR & TOPPINGS

| | |
|---|---|
| **Apple Juice,** 1 Wacky Pack® | 0 |
| **Blue Coconut,** 1 Wacky Pack® | 1 |
| **Bubble Gum,** 1 Wacky Pack® | 1 |
| **Caramel Topping,** 1 Wacky Pack® | 1 |
| **Cherry,** 1 Wacky Pack® | 1 |
| **Chocolate Topping,** 1 Wacky Pack® | 1 |
| **Cranberry Juice,** 1 Wacky Pack® | 1 |
| **Fresh Lemon,** 1 Wacky Pack® | 0 |
| **Fresh Lime,** 1 Wacky Pack® | 0 |
| **Grape,** 1 Wacky Pack® | 1 |
| **Green Apple,** 1 Wacky Pack® | 1 |
| **Hi-C®,** 1 Wacky Pack® | 1 |
| **Lo-Cal Diet Cherry,** 1 Wacky Pack® | 0 |
| **Minute Maid® Apple Juice,** 1 Wacky Pack® | 0 |
| **Minute Maid® Cranberry Juice,** 1 Wacky Pack® | 1 |
| **Orange,** 1 Wacky Pack® | 1 |
| **Pineapple Topping,** 1 Wacky Pack® | 1 |
| **POWERADE®,** 1 Wacky Pack® | 1 |
| **Strawberry Topping,** 1 Wacky Pack® | 1 |
| **Vanilla,** 1 Wacky Pack® | 1 |
| **Watermelon,** 1 Wacky Pack® | 1 |

## ICED TEA

| | |
|---|---|
| **Cranberry Iced Tea,** 1 Wacky Pack® | 1 |
| **Diet Green Iced Tea,** 1 Wacky Pack® | 0 |
| **Iced Tea,** 1 Wacky Pack® | 0 |
| **Sweet Iced Tea,** 1 Wacky Pack® | 3 |

| ▲ Power Foods | *PointsPlus™* value |
|---|---|

## SOFT DRINKS

| | |
|---|---|
| **Barq's® Root Beer,** 1 Wacky Pack® | 4 |
| **Diet Dr. Pepper®,** 1 Wacky Pack® | 0 |
| **Diet-Coke®,** 1 Wacky Pack® | 0 |
| **Dr. Pepper®,** 1 Wacky Pack® | 3 |
| **Fanta® Orange,** 1 Wacky Pack® | 4 |
| **Hi-C® Fruit Punch,** 1 Wacky Pack® | 3 |
| **Minute Maid® Light Lemonade,** 1 Wacky Pack® | 0 |
| **Minute Maid® Strawberry Soda,** 1 Wacky Pack® | 4 |
| **Sprite Zero®,** 1 Wacky Pack® | 0 |
| **Sprite®,** 1 Wacky Pack® | 3 |

## MINUTE MAID® JUICES

| | |
|---|---|
| **Apple,** 1 Wacky Pack® | 3 |
| **Cranberry,** 1 Wacky Pack® | 4 |
| **Orange,** 1 Wacky Pack® | 3 |

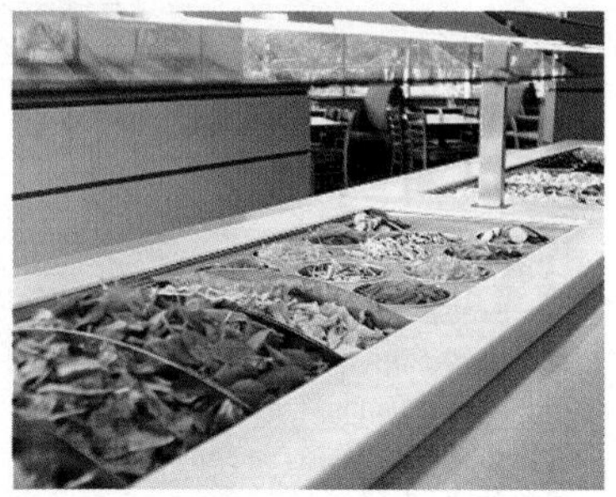

▲ Power Foods — *PointsPlus™* value

## FEATURED SALAD

|  | PointsPlus™ value |
|---|---|
| **Apple Walnut Salad,** 1 cup | 4 |
| **Asian Chicken Salad,** 1 cup | 2 |
| **Asian Shrimp Salad,** 1 cup | 3 |
| **Buffalo Chicken Salad,** 1 cup | 2 |
| **Capri Salad,** 1 cup | 1 |
| **Chicago Chopped Salad,** 1 cup | 3 |
| **Chicken Caesar Salad,** 1 cup | 3 |
| **Chicken Salsa Caesar Salad,** 1 cup | 2 |
| **Cobb Salad,** 1 cup | 3 |
| **Green Goddess Crab Salad,** 1 cup | 2 |
| **Italian Antipasto Salad,** 1 cup | 2 |
| **Marinated Tomato Salad,** 1 cup | 2 |
| **Salmon Medley Salad,** 1 cup | 2 |
| **Shrimp and Crab Louie,** 1 cup | 3 |
| **Shrimp Caesar Salad,** 1 cup | 2 |
| **Southwest Chicken Chipotle,** 1 cup | 2 |

## SIGNATURE SALAD

|  | PointsPlus™ value |
|---|---|
| **Broccoli Coleslaw,** 1/3 cup | 2 |
| **California Chicken Salad,** 1/3 cup | 2 |
| **Chickpea Salad,** 1/3 cup | 3 |
| **Edamame Bean Salad,** 1/3 cup | 0 |
| **Fettucini Pasta Salad,** 1/3 cup | 3 |
| **Fisherman's Kettle Shrimp & Crab Salad,** 1/3 cup | 3 |
| **Gazpacho Salad,** 1/3 cup | 1 |
| **Marinated Mushrooms,** 1/3 cup | 2 |
| **Marinated Oriental Cucumber Salad,** 1/3 cup | 0 |
| **Mustard Potato Salad,** 1/3 cup | 2 |
| **Paco's Taco Salad,** 1/3 cup | 3 |
| **Pasta de Garden,** 1/3 cup | 2 |
| **Pasta Primavera Salad,** 1/3 cup | 1 |
| **Red Potato Salad,** 1/3 cup | 1 |
| **Rice Florentine Salad,** 1/3 cup | 2 |
| **Roasted Mushrooms & Artichokes with Feta Cheese,** 1/3 cup | 1 |
| **Roasted Vegetables,** 1/3 cup | 1 |
| **Salad of the Sea,** 1/3 cup | 1 |
| **Santa Fe Corn Salad,** 1/3 cup | 2 |
| **Sweet Garden Slaw,** 1/3 cup | 1 |
| **Thai Chicken Pasta Salad,** 1/3 cup | 3 |
| **Tropical Tuxedo Salad,** 1/3 cup | 2 |
| **Tuna Fish Salad,** 1/3 cup | 2 |
| **Tuna Skroodle Pasta Salad,** 1/3 cup | 4 |

## SALAD BAR TOPPING

|  | PointsPlus™ value |
|---|---|
| **Bacon Bits, Imitation,** 2 Tbsp | 1 |
| ▲ **Beets,** 1/4 cup | 0 |
| ▲ **Broccoli Florettes,** 2 pieces | 0 |
| ▲ **Carrots, shredded,** 1/4 cup | 0 |
| ▲ **Cauliflower Florettes,** 2 pieces | 0 |
| ▲ **Celery, sliced,** 1/4 cup | 0 |
| **Cheddar, imitation, shredded,** 1/4 cup | 2 |
| ▲ **Cucumbers, sliced,** 1/4 cup | 0 |
| ▲ **Dark Red Kidney Beans,** 1/4 cup | 2 |
| ▲ **Eggs,** 1/4 cup | 2 |
| ▲ **Garbanzo Beans,** 1/4 cup | 1 |
| ▲ **Green Bell Peppers,** 1/4 cup | 0 |

| ▲ Power Foods | *PointsPlus*™ value |
|---|---|
| **Green Olives, sliced,** 1/4 cup | 1 |
| ▲ **Iceberg Lettuce,** 1 cup | 0 |
| ▲ **Jalapenos, Nacho Slice,** 1/4 cup | 0 |
| ▲ **Jicama,** 1/4 cup | 0 |
| ▲ **Mushrooms, sliced,** 1/4 cup | 0 |
| ▲ **Peas,** 1/4 cup | 0 |
| **Pepperoncini, whole,** 1 | 0 |
| **Pepperoni,** 4 slices | 0 |
| ▲ **Radishes, sliced,** 1/4 cup | 0 |
| ▲ **Red Onions,** 3 rings | 0 |
| ▲ **Roma Tomatoes,** 1/4 cup | 0 |
| ▲ **Romaine Lettuce,** 1 cup | 0 |
| ▲ **Spinach,** 1 cup | 0 |
| **Turkey Ham,** 1/4 cup | 0 |
| ▲ **Zucchini, sliced,** 1/4 cup | 0 |

## DRESSINGS

| ▲ Power Foods | *PointsPlus*™ value |
|---|---|
| **Balsamic Vinegar Dressing,** 1 oz | 2 |
| **Bleu Cheese Dressing,** 2 oz | 6 |
| **Caesar Dressing,** 2 oz | 9 |
| **Chipotle Ranch Dressing,** 2 oz | 8 |
| **Cranberry Vinaigrette,** 2 oz | 3 |
| **French Dressing, Fat Free,** 2 oz | 2 |
| **Green Goddess,** 2 oz | 7 |
| **Honey Mustard,** 2 oz | 7 |
| **House Vinaigrette,** 2 oz | 6 |
| **Italian Dressing with Cheese, Fat Free,** 2 oz | 1 |
| **Mayonnaise,** 2 Tbsp | 6 |
| **Olive Oil,** 1 oz | 7 |
| **Peppercorn Ranch Dressing,** 2 oz | 6 |
| **Ranch Dressing,** 2 oz | 6 |
| **Ranch Dressing, Reduced Calorie,** 2 oz | 3 |
| **Tangy Oriental,** 2 oz | 4 |
| **Thousand Island,** 2 oz | 8 |

## HOT BAR

| ▲ Power Foods | *PointsPlus*™ value |
|---|---|
| **Bacon Bits, Real,** 2 Tbsp | 2 |
| **Chili Potato Topping,** 1 serving | 2 |
| **Colby, Shredded,** 2 oz | 3 |
| **Crackers, Gold, Waverly,** 1 package | 1 |
| **Flour Tortilla,** 1 | 2 |
| **Jalapeno Cheese Sauce,** 2 oz | 1 |
| **Melba Toast,** 1 package | 1 |
| **Parmesan,** 1 Tbsp | 1 |
| ▲ **Potato Baked, Plain,** 1 | 5 |
| **Red Pepper, Crushed,** 1/4 tsp | 0 |
| **Rice, White, prepared,** 1/3 cup | 2 |
| **Romano,** 1 Tbsp | 1 |
| **Saltine Crackers,** 1 package | 1 |
| **Southwestern Beans with Roasted Corn,** 1/3 cup | 1 |
| **Southwestern Quesadilla,** 1 slice | 2 |
| **Spanish Rice,** 1/3 cup | 2 |

## HOT PASTA

| ▲ Power Foods | *PointsPlus*™ value |
|---|---|
| **Alfredo Sauce for Pasta Bar,** 1 1/2 Tbsp | 1 |
| **Basil Pesto for Pasta Bar,** 1 Tbsp | 1 |
| **Bowtie for Pasta Bar,** 1/2 cup | 3 |
| **Marinara for Pasta Bar,** 1 1/2 Tbsp | 0 |
| **Meaty Marinara,** 1 1/2 Tbsp | 1 |
| **Spaghetti,** 1/2 cup | 3 |
| **Tortellini,** 1/2 cup | 4 |

## PIZZA

| ▲ Power Foods | *PointsPlus*™ value |
|---|---|
| **Cheese Pizza,** 1 slice | 2 |
| **Garden Pizza,** 1 slice | 2 |
| **Pepperoni Pizza,** 1 slice | 2 |
| **Sausage Pizza,** 1 slice | 2 |

| ▲ Power Foods | *PointsPlus*™ value |
|---|---|
| **SOUP** | |
| **Adobe Rice and Chicken,** 1 bowl | 3 |
| **Alaskan Salmon Chowder,** 1 bowl | 2 |
| **Beef Mushroom Barley,** 1 bowl | 2 |
| **Beef Noodle,** 1 bowl | 2 |
| **Beef Shellini,** 1 bowl | 2 |
| **Beef Stroganoff,** 1 bowl | 3 |
| **Black Bean Soup,** 1 bowl | 3 |
| **Broccoli Cheese Soup,** 1 bowl | 2 |
| **Cajun Gumbo Soup,** 1 bowl | 3 |
| **Cauliflower Cheese Soup,** 1 bowl | 2 |
| **Cheddar Chicken Broccoli Stew,** 1 bowl | 4 |
| **Cherokee Joe's Cornbread Soup,** 1 bowl | 2 |
| **Chicken Creole,** 1 bowl | 3 |
| **Chicken Enchilada Soup,** 1 bowl | 5 |
| **Chicken Gumbo Soup,** 1 bowl | 2 |
| **Chicken Mushroom Barley,** 1 bowl | 2 |
| **Chicken Noodle,** 1 bowl | 2 |
| **Chicken Tetrazini Soup,** 1 bowl | 3 |
| **Chicken Tortilla Soup,** 1 bowl | 2 |
| **Cream of Asparagus Soup,** 1 bowl | 3 |
| **Cream of Broccoli Soup,** 1 bowl | 2 |
| **Cream of Cauliflower Soup,** 1 bowl | 2 |
| **Cream of Chicken Soup,** 1 bowl | 3 |
| **Cream of Mushroom Soup,** 1 bowl | 2 |
| **Cream of Spinach Soup,** 1 bowl | 2 |
| **Holiday Harvest,** 1 bowl | 2 |
| **Hungarian Mushroom Soup,** 1 bowl | 3 |
| **Long Island Seafood Stew,** 1 bowl | 2 |
| **Macaroni Cheese Soup,** 1 bowl | 4 |
| **Mama Mia Chicken,** 1 bowl | 2 |
| **Meatball Fazuli,** 1 bowl | 5 |
| **Mexican Corn Cheddar Soup,** 1 bowl | 2 |

| ▲ Power Foods | *PointsPlus*™ value |
|---|---|
| **Minestrone,** 1 bowl | 2 |
| **Mr. B's Hot & Sour Chicken,** 1 bowl | 1 |
| **Mushroom Barley,** 1 bowl | 2 |
| **Mushroom Cheese Soup,** 1 bowl | 2 |
| **New England Clam Chowder,** 1 bowl | 2 |
| **Old Fashioned Chicken Stew,** 1 bowl | 3 |
| **Pasta e Fagioli,** 1 bowl | 2 |
| **Pasta Tortellini,** 1 bowl | 3 |
| **Potato Corn Chowder Soup,** 1 bowl | 3 |
| **Potato Leek Soup,** 1 bowl | 2 |
| **Pumpkin Bisque,** 1 bowl | 2 |
| **Red Beans, Rice & Sausage,** 1 bowl | 2 |
| **Red French Onion (with crouton),** 1 bowl | 2 |
| **Red French Onion (without crouton),** 1 bowl | 1 |
| **Santa Fe Chicken Soup,** 1 bowl | 3 |
| **Seafood Bisque,** 1 bowl | 3 |
| **Seafood Gumbo,** 1 bowl | 3 |
| **Shrimp Creole,** 1 bowl | 2 |
| **Southwest Chicken,** 1 bowl | 2 |
| **Southwest Chili,** 1 bowl | 2 |
| **Spicy Meatballs with Rice,** 1 bowl | 3 |
| **Tomato Basil,** 1 bowl | 2 |
| **Twice Baked Potato Soup,** 1 bowl | 3 |
| **Vegan Split Pea,** 1 bowl | 2 |
| **Vegetable Beef,** 1 bowl | 2 |
| **Vegetable Beef Soup with Beef Tips,** 1 bowl | 2 |
| **Vegetable Cheese Soup,** 1 bowl | 2 |
| **Vegetable Lentil,** 1 bowl | 2 |
| **Vegetarian Butter Bean,** 1 bowl | 2 |
| **Vegetarian Vegetable,** 1 bowl | 1 |
| **White Bean Chicken Chili Stew,** 1 bowl | 2 |
| **White Seafood Stew,** 1 bowl | 3 |
| **Zucchini Chicken,** 1 bowl | 2 |

▲ Power Foods

| | *PointsPlus*™ value |
|---|---|
| **BREAD** | |
| **Blueberry Bread,** 1 square | 4 |
| **Bread, Cheese Drop Biscuit,** 1 | 2 |
| **Breadstick, Garlic,** 1 | 3 |
| **Cornbread,** 1 square | 5 |
| **Gingerbread,** 1 square | 5 |
| **DESSERT** | |
| **Banana Pudding,** 1/2 cup | 5 |
| **Caramel Dessert Topping,** 1 Tbsp | 1 |
| **Chocolate Pudding,** 1/2 cup | 5 |
| **Chocolate Syrup,** 1 Tbsp | 1 |
| **Cottage Cheese, Lowfat,** 1/2 cup | 2 |
| **Oreo Crumbles,** 1 Tbsp | 1 |
| **Peaches,** 1/2 cup | 2 |
| **Pineapple Tidbits,** 1/4 cup | 2 |
| **Pineapple Topping,** 1 Tbsp | 1 |
| **Rainbow Sprinkles,** 1 Tbsp | 1 |
| **Soft serve Ice Cream Cone, Chocolate,** 1 | 3 |
| **Soft Serve Ice Cream Cone, Vanilla,** 1 | 3 |
| **Sponge Cake, Yellow,** 4 pieces | 2 |
| **Strawberry Parfait,** 1/2 cup | 3 |
| **Vanilla Wafers,** 4 | 2 |
| **Whipped Topping,** 1/2 cup | 3 |
| **DRINKS** | |
| **Green Tea,** 1 serving | 0 |
| **Lemonade, Mango Premium,** 1 | 6 |
| **Lemonade, Premium,** 1 | 5 |
| **Lemonade, Raspberry Premium,** 1 | 6 |
| **Lemonade, Strawberry Premium,** 1 | 6 |
| **Mango Smoothie,** 1 tall | 7 |
| **Peach Smoothie,** 1 tall | 7 |
| **Raspberry Smoothie,** 1 tall | 7 |
| **Strawberry Smoothie,** 1 tall | 7 |

# SOUPLANTATION®

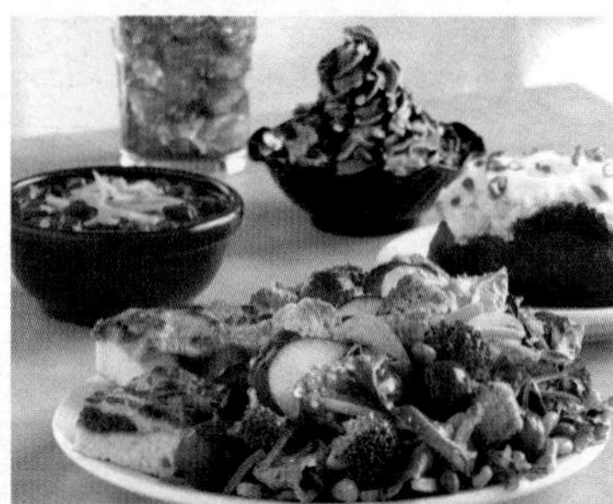

| ▲ Power Foods | *PointsPlus*™ value |
|---|---|
| **FRESH TOSSED SALADS** | |
| **Azteca Taco with Turkey Salad,** 1 cup | 3 |
| **Bartlett Pear & Caramelized Walnut Salad (Veterarian),** 1 cup | 5 |
| **BBQ Julienne Chopped Salad with Chicken,** 1 cup | 6 |
| **BBQ Smokehouse with Bacon & Peanuts,** 1 cup | 8 |
| **Buffalo Chicken,** 1 cup | 5 |
| **Caesar Salad Asiago (Non-Vegetarian),** 1 cup | 7 |
| **California Cobb with Bacon Salad,** 1 cup | 5 |
| **Cambay Curry with Almonds & Coconut (Vegetarian),** 1 cup | 6 |
| **Cape Cod Spinach with Walnuts & Bacon,** 1 cup | 4 |
| **Cherry Chipotle Spinach (Vegetarian),** 1 cup | 4 |
| **Chicken Tortilla Salad,** 1 cup | 5 |
| **Classic Antipasto (Tossed Salad),** 1 cup | 8 |
| **Classic Greek Salad (Vegetarian),** 1 cup | 3 |
| **Club Blue BLT with Bacon,** 1 cup | 7 |
| **Country French Salad with Bacon,** 1 cup | 6 |

| ▲ Power Foods | *PointsPlus*™ value |
|---|---|
| **Crunchy Island Pineapple (Vegetarian),** 1 cup | 4 |
| **Field of Greens: Sweet Maple (Vegetarian),** 1 cup | 5 |
| **Fields of Greens: Citrus Vinaigrette (Vegan),** 1 cup | 4 |
| **Green Chile Ranch with Spicy Tortilla Chips (Vegetarian),** 1 cup | 7 |
| **Honey Minted Fruit Toss (Vegetarian),** 1 cup | 0 |
| **Mandarin Spinach Salad with Caramelized Walnuts (Vegan),** 1 cup | 4 |
| **Monterey Blue Salad with Peanuts (Vegetarian),** 1 cup | 7 |
| **Outrageous Orange with Cashews (Vegetarian),** 1 cup | 6 |
| **Ranch House BLT Salad with Turkey & Bacon,** 1 cup | 5 |
| **Roasted Vegetables Salad with Feta & Olives (Vegetarian),** 1 cup | 5 |
| **San Marino Spinach with Pumpkin Seeds & Cranberries (Vegetarian),** 1 cup | 5 |
| **Sedona Green Chile & Chipotle (Non-Vegetarian),** 1 cup | 6 |
| **Smoked Turkey & Spinach Salad with Almonds,** 1 cup | 5 |
| **Sonoma Spinach Salad with Honey Dijon Vinaigrette (Vegetarian),** 1 cup | 6 |
| **Spiced Pecan & Roasted Vegetable with Bacon,** 1 cup | 5 |
| **Spinach Gorgonzola with Spiced Pecans and Bacon,** 1 cup | 6 |
| **Strawberry Fields with Caramelized Walnuts (Vegan),** 1 cup | 4 |
| **Summer Lemon with Spiced Pecans (Vegetarian),** 1 cup | 6 |
| **Sweet Tomato, Mozzarella & Basil Salad (Vegetarian),** 1 cup | 3 |
| **Thai Peanut & Red Pepper (Vegan),** 1 cup | 6 |

| ▲ Power Foods | PointsPlus™ value |
|---|---|
| **Thai Udon & Peanut (Vegan),** 1 cup | 6 |
| **Traditional Spinach Salad with Bacon,** 1 cup | 5 |
| **Won Ton Chicken Happiness,** 1 cup | 4 |

## SIGNATURE PREPARED SALADS

| ▲ Power Foods | PointsPlus™ value |
|---|---|
| **Ambrosia with Coconut (Vegetarian),** 1/2 cup | 6 |
| **Artichoke Rice Salad (Vegetarian),** 1/2 cup | 5 |
| **Aunt Doris' Red Pepper Slaw (Fat-free, Vegan),** 1/2 cup | 2 |
| **Baja Bean & Cilantro Salad (Low-fat, Vegan),** 1/2 cup | 4 |
| **BBQ Potato Salad (Vegetarian),** 1/2 cup | 5 |
| **Carrot Raisin Salad (Low-fat, Vegetarian),** 1/2 cup | 3 |
| **Chinese Krab Salad,** 1/2 cup | 4 |
| **Citrus Noodles Salad with Snow Peas (Vegetarian),** 1/2 cup | 4 |
| **Dijon Potato Salad with Garlic Dill Vinaigrette (Vegan),** 1/2 cup | 4 |
| **Field Corn & Very Wild Rice Vegetarian,** 1/2 cup | 5 |
| **Greek Couscous Salad with Feta Cheese and Pinenuts (Vegetarian),** 1/2 cup | 5 |
| **Italian White Bean Salad (Vegan),** 1/2 cup | 4 |
| **Jalapeño Potato Salad (Vegetarian),** 1/2 cup | 5 |
| **Joan's Broccoli Madness Salad (Non-Vegetarian),** 1/2 cup | 5 |
| **Lemon Rice with Cashews (Vegan),** 1/2 cup | 4 |
| **Mandarin Noodles Salad with Broccoli (Low-fat, Vegan),** 1/2 cup | 4 |
| **Mandarin Shells Salad with Almonds (Low-fat, Vegan),** 1/2 cup | 3 |
| **Old Fashioned Macaroni Salad with Ham,** 1/2 cup | 6 |
| **Oriental Ginger Slaw with Krab (Low-fat),** 1/2 cup | 2 |
| **Penne Pasta Salad with Chicken in a Citrus Vinaigrette (Low-fat),** 1/2 cup | 3 |
| **Pesto Pasta Salad (Vegetarian),** 1/2 cup | 5 |
| **Picnic Potato Salad (Vegetarian),** 1/2 cup | 5 |
| **Pineapple Coconut Slaw (Vegetarian),** 1/2 cup | 4 |
| **Poppyseed Coleslaw (Vegetarian),** 1/2 cup | 3 |
| **Red Potato & Tomato (Vegetarian),** 1/2 cup | 5 |
| **Roasted Potato Salad with Chipotle Chile Vinaigrette (Vegan),** 1/2 cup | 3 |
| **San Francisco Herb Rice (Non-Vegetarian),** 1/2 cup | 5 |
| **Shrimp & Seafood Shells Salad,** 1/2 cup | 6 |
| **Smoky Ham & Cheddar Broccoli Slaw,** 1/2 cup | 7 |
| **Southern Dill Potato Salad (Low-fat, Vegetarian),** 1/2 cup | 3 |
| **Southwestern Rice & Beans Salad (Low-fat, Vegetarian),** 1/2 cup | 2 |
| **Spicy Cajun Shells (Vegetarian),** 1/2 cup | 8 |
| **Spicy Southwestern Pasta Salad (Low-fat, Vegan),** 1/2 cup | 3 |
| **Summer Barley Salad with Black Beans (Low-fat, Vegan),** 1/2 cup | 3 |
| **Sweet & Sour Broccoli Slaw (Low-fat, Vegan),** 1/2 cup | 4 |
| **Sweet Marinated Vegetables (Fat-free, Vegan),** 1/2 cup | 2 |
| **Tabouli (Vegan),** 1/2 cup | 5 |
| **Thai Citrus & Brown Rice (Vegan),** 1/2 cup | 6 |

*Signature Prepared Salads (cont'd)*

| ▲ Power Foods | PointsPlus™ value |
|---|---|
| **Thai Noodle Salad with Chicken & Peanut Sauce,** 1/2 cup | 5 |
| **Three Bean Marinade Salad (Vegan),** 1/2 cup | 5 |
| **Tomato Cucumber Marinade Salad (Vegan),** 1/2 cup | 2 |
| **Tuna Tarragon Salad,** 1/2 cup | 7 |
| **Turkey Chutney Pasta Salad,** 1/2 cup | 6 |
| **Wheat Berry & Curry (Vegetarian),** 1/2 cup | 5 |
| **Whole Grain Fiesta Couscous (Vegetarian),** 1/2 cup | 7 |
| **Wild Rice & Chicken Salad,** 1/2 cup | 8 |
| **Zesty Tortellini Salad (Vegetarian),** 1/2 cup | 6 |

## SALAD DRESSINGS & CROUTONS

| ▲ Power Foods | PointsPlus™ value |
|---|---|
| **Avocado Ranch Dressing,** 2 Tbsp | 4 |
| **Bacon Dressing,** 2 Tbsp | 4 |
| **Balsamic Vinaigrette (Non-Vegan),** 2 Tbsp | 5 |
| **Basil Vinaigrette,** 2 Tbsp | 4 |
| **BBQ Vinaigrette,** 2 Tbsp | 2 |
| **Blue Cheese Dressing,** 2 Tbsp | 4 |
| **Citrus Vinaigrette,** 2 Tbsp | 4 |
| **Cranberry Orange Vinaigrette (Low-fat),** 2 Tbsp | 2 |
| **Creamy Italian Dressing,** 2 Tbsp | 3 |
| **Cucumber Dressing (Reduced Calorie),** 2 Tbsp | 2 |
| **Fat Free Honey Mustard Dressing,** 2 Tbsp | 1 |
| **Fat Free Italian Dressing,** 2 Tbsp | 1 |
| **Fat Free Ranch Dressing,** 2 Tbsp | 0 |
| **Garlic Parmesan Seasoned Croutons,** 5 pieces | 2 |
| **Green Chili Ranch Dressing,** 2 Tbsp | 4 |
| **Honey Lime Cilantro Vinaigrette,** 2 Tbsp | 3 |
| **Honey Mint Lemonade Dressing,** 2 Tbsp | 4 |
| **Honey Mustard Dressing,** 2 Tbsp | 4 |
| **Italian Vinaigrette with Basil & Romano Cheese,** 2 Tbsp | 4 |
| **Kahlena French Dressing,** 2 Tbsp | 3 |
| **Monterey Blue Salad Dressing,** 2 Tbsp | 3 |
| **Parmesan Pepper Cream Dressing,** 2 Tbsp | 4 |
| **Pineapple Vinaigrette,** 2 Tbsp | 3 |
| **Ranch Dressing,** 2 Tbsp | 4 |
| **Roasted Garlic Dressing,** 2 Tbsp | 3 |
| **Smoky BBQ Vinaigrette,** 2 Tbsp | 3 |
| **Spicy Buffalo Ranch Dressing,** 2 Tbsp | 4 |
| **Spicy Southwest Chipotle,** 2 Tbsp | 5 |
| **Strawberry Balsamic Vinaigrette,** 2 Tbsp | 4 |
| **Sweet Maple Dressing,** 2 Tbsp | 5 |
| **Thousand Island Dressing,** 2 Tbsp | 3 |
| **Warm Bacon Dressing,** 2 Tbsp | 3 |
| **Chow Mein Noodles,** 1/4 cup | 2 |
| **Plain Croutons,** 5 pieces | 1 |
| **Tomato Basil Croutons,** 5 pieces | 2 |

## SOUP & CHILI

| ▲ Power Foods | PointsPlus™ value |
|---|---|
| **8 Vegetable Chicken Stew,** 1 cup | 4 |
| **Albondigas Locas (A Meatball Soup),** 1 cup | 5 |
| **Asian Ginger Broth (Low-fat, Vegetarian),** 1 cup | 0 |
| **Beef & Barley Stew,** 1 cup | 5 |
| **Better Than Mom's Beef Stew,** 1 cup | 7 |
| **Big Chunk Chicken Noodle (Low-fat),** 1 cup | 4 |
| **Border Black Bean & Chorizo,** 1 cup | 6 |
| **Broccoli Cheese (Vegetarian),** 1 cup | 7 |
| **Canadian Cheese with Smoked Ham,** 1 cup | 10 |

| ▲ Power Foods | PointsPlus™ value |
|---|---|
| **Cheese Stuffed Cappelletti Soup (Non-Vegetarian),** 1 cup | 7 |
| **Chesapeake Corn Chowder (Non-Vegetarian),** 1 cup | 8 |
| **Chicken & Rice,** 1 cup | 4 |
| **Chicken Fajitas & Black Bean Soup,** 1 cup | 7 |
| **Chicken Pot Pie Stew,** 1 cup | 8 |
| **Chicken Tortilla Soup with Jalapeño Chiles & Tomatoes (Low-fat),** 1 cup | 2 |
| **Chili Cheeseburger,** 1 cup | 7 |
| **Chunky Potato Cheese Soup with Thyme (Vegetarian),** 1 cup | 6 |
| **Classical French Onion Soup (Non-Vegetarian),** 1 cup | 4 |
| **Classical Minestrone Soup (Low-fat, Vegan),** 1 cup | 3 |
| **Classical Shrimp Bisque,** 1 cup | 6 |
| **Continental Lentil & Spinach (Low-fat, Vegetarian),** 1 cup | 3 |
| **Corned Beef & Cabbage,** 1 cup | 4 |
| **Country Corn & Red Potato Chowder (Non-Vegetarian),** 1 cup | 6 |
| **Cream of Broccoli Soup (Vegetarian),** 1 cup | 7 |
| **Cream of Chicken Soup,** 1 cup | 8 |
| **Cream of Mushroom Soup (Non-Vegetarian),** 1 cup | 8 |
| **Cream of Rosemary Potato (Non-vegetarian),** 1 cup | 9 |
| **Creamy Herbed Turkey Soup,** 1 cup | 9 |
| **Creamy Vegetable Chowder (Vegetarian),** 1 cup | 7 |
| **Curried Yellow Split Pea (Low-fat, Vegetarian),** 1 cup | 5 |
| **Deep Kettle House Chili (Low-fat),** 1 cup | 4 |
| **Deep Kettle House Chili with 33% more meat!,** 1 cup | 6 |
| **Deep Kettle House Chili with 50% More Meat!,** 1 cup | 7 |

| ▲ Power Foods | PointsPlus™ value |
|---|---|
| **El Paso Lime & Chicken Soup,** 1 cup | 4 |
| **Field of Creams - Cauliflower with Proud to be American Cheese (Vegetarian),** 1 cup | 8 |
| **Field of Creams - Sweet Tomato Basil (Vegetarian),** 1 cup | 6 |
| **Fire Roasted Green Chile & Corn Chowder with Bacon,** 1 cup | 7 |
| **Garden Fresh Vegetable Soup (Low-fat, Vegetarian),** 1 cup | 3 |
| **Garden of Eatin' (Low-fat/Vegetarian),** 1 cup | 3 |
| **Golden Yam Bisque (Vegetarian),** 1 cup | 5 |
| **Green Chile Stew with Pork,** 1 cup | 4 |
| **Irish Potato Leek Soup (Vegetarian),** 1 cup | 7 |
| **Lemon Chicken Orzo,** 1 cup | 6 |
| **Loaded Baked Potato & Cheese with Bacon,** 1 cup | 8 |
| **Longhorn Beef Chili,** 1 cup | 5 |
| **Marvelous Minestrone Soup with Bacon,** 1 cup | 6 |
| **Minestrone with Italian Sausage,** 1 cup | 5 |
| **Moroccan Garbanzo & Lentil Bean (Low-fat, Vegetarian),** 1 cup | 5 |
| **Mulligatawny Soup (Non-Vegetarian),** 1 cup | 6 |
| **Neighbor Joe's Gumbo (Non-Vegetarian),** 1 cup | 5 |
| **New Mexican Corn Tortilla with Chicken,** 1 cup | 5 |
| **New Orleans Jambalaya (Non-Vegetarian),** 1 cup | 6 |
| **Old Fashion Vegetable Soup (Low-fat/Vegetarian),** 1 cup | 2 |
| **Pinto Bean & Basil Barley (Low-fat, Vegetarian),** 1 cup | 4 |
| **Posole Soup with Pork,** 1 cup | 3 |
| **Potato Tomato & Spinach (Low-fat, Vegetarian),** 1 cup | 4 |

*Soup & Chili (cont'd)*

| ▲ Power Foods | *PointsPlus™* value |
|---|---|
| **Ratatouille Provencale (Fat-free, Vegan),** 1 cup | 3 |
| **Roasted Mushroom with Sage (Non-Vegetarian),** 1 cup | 9 |
| **Rustic Tuscan Stew (Low-fat, Non-Vegetarian),** 1 cup | 3 |
| **Santa Fe Black Bean Chili (Low-fat/Vegan),** 1 cup | 4 |
| **Savory Turkey Harvest,** 1 cup | 6 |
| **Smoky Pinto & Brown Rice (Low-fat, Vegetarian),** 1 cup | 4 |
| **Southwest Tomato Cream (Vegetarian),** 1 cup | 3 |
| **Southwest Tomato Cream Soup (Vegetarian),** 1 cup | 3 |
| **Southwest Turkey Chowder with Bacon,** 1 cup | 7 |
| **Spicy Sausage & Pasta Soup,** 1 cup | 8 |
| **Split Pea & Potato Barley (Low-fat, Vegetarian),** 1 cup | 4 |
| **Split Pea Soup with Ham,** 1 cup | 7 |
| **Sweet Tomato Onion Soup (Low-fat/Vegan),** 1 cup | 2 |
| **Texas Red Chili (Non-Vegetarian),** 1 cup | 5 |
| **Three-Bean Turkey Chili (Low-fat),** 1 cup | 4 |
| **Tomato Chipotle Bisque (Non-Vegetarian),** 1 cup | 7 |
| **Tomato Parmesan & Vegetables (Low-fat/Vegetarian),** 1 cup | 3 |
| **Turkey Cassoulet with Bacon,** 1 cup | 6 |
| **Turkey Vegetable Soup,** 1 cup | 5 |
| **U.S. Senate Bean with Smoked Ham,** 1 cup | 4 |
| **Vegetable Medley Soup (Low-fat/Vegetarian),** 1 cup | 2 |
| **Vegetarian Harvest Soup (Vegan),** 1 cup | 5 |
| **White Bean & Lime Chicken Chili,** 1 cup | 5 |
| **X-treme Spice Vegetable Chili with Energy Boost (Low-fat, Vegetarian),** 1 cup | 2 |
| **Yankee Clipper Clam Chowder with Bacon,** 1 cup | 9 |

## HOT TOSSED PASTAS/ KITCHEN FAVORITES

| ▲ Power Foods | *PointsPlus™* value |
|---|---|
| **4-Cheese Alfredo (Vegetarian),** 1 cup | 10 |
| **Arizona Marinara (Vegetarian),** 1 cup | 9 |
| **Broccoli Alfredo with Basil (Vegetarian),** 1 cup | 10 |
| **Bruschetta (Vegetarian),** 1 cup | 6 |
| **Carbonara Pasta with Bacon,** 1 cup | 8 |
| **Chicken Tetrazzini,** 1 cup | 13 |
| **Cilantro Lime Pesto (Vegetarian),** 1 cup | 10 |
| **Creamy Bruschetta (Vegetarian),** 1 cup | 10 |
| **Creamy Herb Chicken,** 1 cup | 8 |
| **Curried Pineapple & Ginger (Low-fat, Non-vegetarian),** 1 cup | 5 |
| **Fettuccine Alfredo (Vegerarian),** 1 cup | 9 |
| **Fire-Roasted Tomato & Basil Alfredo (Vegetarian),** 1 cup | 10 |
| **Garden Vegetable with Italian Sausage,** 1 cup | 8 |
| **Garden Vegetable with Meatballs,** 1 cup | 8 |
| **Greek Mediterranean (Vegetarian),** 1 cup | 8 |
| **Hand-Crafted Mexican Beans (Low-fat, Vegan),** 1 cup | 6 |
| **Italian Sausage with Red Pepper Puree,** 1 cup | 7 |
| **Italian Vegetable Beef,** 1 cup | 8 |
| **Lemon Cream with Capers (Non-vegetarian),** 1 cup | 11 |

| ▲ Power Foods | *PointsPlus*™ value |
|---|---|
| **Linguini with Clam Sauce,** 1 cup | 10 |
| **Macaroni & Cheese (Vegetarian),** 1 cup | 9 |
| **Nutty Mushroom (Vegetarian),** 1 cup | 11 |
| **Oriental Noodle & Green Bean (Low-fat, Vegan),** 1 cup | 6 |
| **Pasta Florentine (Vegetarian),** 1 cup | 10 |
| **Penne Arrabbiatta (Vegetarian),** 1 cup | 9 |
| **Ragin Cajun with Andouille Sausage,** 1 cup | 10 |
| **Roasted Eggplant Marinara (Vegetarian),** 1 cup | 9 |
| **Roasted Mushroom Alfredo with Rosemary (Vegetarian),** 1 cup | 10 |
| ▲ **Salsa de Lupe (fat-free, Vegan),** 1/4 cup | 0 |
| **Sauteed Balsamic Vegetables (Vegan),** 1/2 cup | 3 |
| **Smoked Salmon & Dill,** 1 cup | 10 |
| **Smoky BBQ Baked Beans (Low-fat, Non-vegetarian),** 1 cup | 8 |
| **Spicy Italian Sausage & Peppers,** 1 cup | 9 |
| **Steamed Vegetables with Lemon Herb Butter (Vegetarian),** 1/2 cup | 3 |
| **Stuffing (Non-vegetarian),** 1/2 cup | 6 |
| **Tomato Spinach Whole Wheat (Vegetarian),** 1 cup | 7 |
| **Tuscany Sausage with Capers & Olives,** 1 cup | 6 |
| **Vegetable Ragu (Vegetarian),** 1 cup | 7 |
| **Vegetarian Marinara with Basil (Vegetarian),** 1 cup | 6 |
| **Walnut Pesto (Vegetarian),** 1 cup | 8 |

## FRESH BAKED MUFFINS & BREADS

| ▲ Power Foods | *PointsPlus*™ value |
|---|---|
| **Apple Cinnamon Bran Muffin (96% fat free),** 1 | 3 |
| **Apple Raisin Muffin,** 1 | 4 |
| **Banana Nut Muffin,** 1 | 4 |
| **Bruschetta Focaccia,** 1 piece | 4 |
| **Buttermilk Cornbread (Low-fat),** 1 piece | 4 |
| **Cappuccino Chip Muffin,** 1 | 5 |
| **Caribbean Key Lime Muffin,** 1 | 5 |
| **Carrot Pineapple Muffin with Oat Bran,** 1 | 4 |
| **Cherry Nut Muffin,** 1 | 4 |
| **Chipotle Lime Butter,** 1 Tbsp | 3 |
| **Chocolate Brownie Muffin,** 1 | 5 |
| **Chocolate Chip Muffin,** 1 | 5 |
| **Country Blackberry Muffin,** 1 | 5 |
| **Cranberry Orange Bran Muffin (96% Fat-free),** 1 | 3 |
| **Fruit Medley Bran Muffin (96% Fat-free),** 1 | 3 |
| **Garlic Asiago Focaccia,** 1 piece | 4 |
| **Georgia Peach Poppyseed Muffin,** 1 | 4 |
| **Indian Grain Bread (Low-fat),** 1 piece | 5 |
| **Lemon Vanilla Butter,** 1 Tbsp | 2 |
| **Maple Walnut Muffin,** 1 | 6 |
| **Old World Greek Focaccia,** 1 piece | 5 |
| **Pauline's Apple Walnut Cake,** 1 piece | 6 |
| **Pesto & Sun-dried Tomato Focaccia,** 1 piece | 5 |
| **Pumpkin Raisin Muffin,** 1 | 4 |
| **Quattro Formaggio Focaccia,** 1 piece | 4 |
| **Ragin Cajun Vegetable Focaccia (Vegetarian),** 1 piece | 4 |
| **Roasted Potato Focaccia,** 1 piece | 4 |
| **Sauteed Vegetable Focaccia,** 1 piece | 5 |
| **Sourdough Bread (Low-fat),** 1 piece | 4 |
| **Southwest Chipotle Focaccia,** 1 piece | 4 |
| **Spiced Pumpkin Muffin with Cranberries,** 1 piece | 5 |
| **Strawberry Buttermilk Muffin,** 1 | 4 |
| **Sweet Cherry Butter,** 1 Tbsp | 2 |
| **Sweet Orange & Cranberry Muffin,** 1 | 5 |

*Fresh Baked Muffins & Breads (cont'd)*

| ▲ Power Foods | PointsPlus™ value |
|---|---|
| **Sweet Strawberry Butter,** 1 Tbsp | 2 |
| **Taffy Apple Muffin,** 1 | 4 |
| **Tangy Lemon Muffin,** 1 | 4 |
| **Thai Chicken Focaccia with Peanuts,** 1 piece | 5 |
| **Wildly Blue Blueberry Muffin,** 1 piece | 4 |
| **Zucchini Nut Muffin,** 1 | 4 |

## MORNING MENU/BREAKFAST

| ▲ Power Foods | PointsPlus™ value |
|---|---|
| **Blueberry Sauce/Blueberry Stir-in,** 2 Tbsp | 2 |
| **Granola Topping,** 2 Tbsp | 3 |
| ▲ **Homemade Oatmeal (plain),** 3/4 cup | 3 |
| **Mediterranean Sunrise Pasta,** 1 cup | 6 |
| **Potatoes O'Brien,** 1/2 cup | 4 |
| **Scrambled Eggs,** 1/2 cup | 3 |
| **Sticky Granola Clusters with Almonds,** 1/4 cup | 7 |
| **Strawberry Sauce/Strawberry Stir-in,** 2 Tbsp | 1 |
| **Tom's Country Gravy,** 2 Tbsp | 2 |
| **Warm Marion Blackberry Sauce,** 1/4 cup | 2 |

## DESSERTS

| ▲ Power Foods | PointsPlus™ value |
|---|---|
| **Apple Cobbler,** 1/2 cup | 10 |
| **Apple Medley (Fat-free),** 1/2 cup | 2 |
| **Banana Pudding,** 1/2 cup | 4 |
| **Banana Royale (Fat-free),** 1/2 cup | 2 |
| **Butterscotch Pudding (Low-fat),** 1/2 cup | 4 |
| **Candy Sprinkles (Low-fat),** 1 Tbsp | 2 |
| **Caramel Apple Cobbler,** 1/2 cup | 11 |
| **Caramel Syrup,** 2 Tbsp | 4 |
| **Cherry Apple Cobbler,** 1/2 cup | 9 |
| **Chocolate Chip Cookie,** 1 small | 2 |
| **Chocolate Frozen Yogurt (Fat-free),** 1/2 cup | 3 |
| **Chocolate Lava Cake,** 1/2 cup | 9 |
| **Chocolate Pudding (Low-fat),** 1/2 cup | 4 |
| **Chocolate Pudding (Low-fat) (No Sugar Added),** 1/2 cup | 3 |
| **Chocolate Syrup,** 2 Tbsp | 3 |
| **Cranberry Apple Cobbler,** 1/2 cup | 9 |
| **Cran-Raspberry Gelatin (Fat-free),** 1/2 cup | 3 |
| **Gelatin (Fat-free),** 1/2 cup | 2 |
| **Gelatin (Sugar Free, Fat-free),** 1/2 cup | 0 |
| **Granola Topping,** 2 Tbsp | 3 |
| **Green Tea Mousse,** 1/2 cup | 5 |
| **Hot Lemon Lava Cake,** 1/2 cup | 8 |
| **Nutty Waldorf Salad (Low-fat),** 1/2 cup | 2 |
| **Oatmeal Raisin Cookie,** 1 small | 3 |
| **Pineapple Gelatin (Fat-free),** 1/2 cup | 3 |
| **Pineapple Upside-down Cake,** 1/2 cup | 7 |
| **Raspberry Apple Cobbler,** 1/2 cup | 10 |
| **Rice Pudding (Low-fat),** 1/2 cup | 3 |
| **Shortcake,** 1 cake | 6 |
| **Sugar-free Cherry Chocolate Mousse,** 1/2 cube | 1 |
| **Sugar-free Chocolate Mousse,** 1/2 cup | 1 |
| **Sugar-free Lemon Mousse,** 1/2 cup | 1 |
| **Sugar-free Raspberry Mousse,** 1/2 cup | 1 |
| **Sugar-free Strawberry Mousse,** 1/2 cup | 1 |
| **Tapioca Pudding (Low-fat),** 1/2 cup | 4 |
| **Vanilla Pudding,** 1/2 cup | 4 |
| **Vanilla Soft Serve (Reduced-fat),** 1/2 cup | 4 |
| **Warm Carrot Cake with Cream Cheese Lava,** 1/2 cup | 8 |

| ▲ Power Foods | *PointsPlus*™ value |
|---|---|
| **ESPRESSO** | |
| **Espresso Doppio,** 1 serving | 0 |
| **Espresso Solo,** 1 serving | 0 |
| **CAFFÈ LATTE** | |
| **Caffè Latte, made with 2% milk,** 1 tall | 4 |
| ▲ **Caffè Latte, made with nonfat milk,** 1 tall | 3 |
| ▲ **Caffè Latte, made with soymilk,** 1 tall | 4 |
| **Syrup Flavored Latte, made with 2% milk,** 1 tall | 5 |
| **Syrup Flavored Latte, made with nonfat milk,** 1 grande | 5 |
| **Syrup Flavored Latte, made with soy milk,** 1 tall | 5 |
| **Vanilla Latte, made with 2% milk,** 1 short | 3 |
| ▲ **Vanilla Latte, made with nonfat milk,** 1 short | 3 |
| ▲ **Vanilla Latte, made with soymilk,** 1 short | 3 |
| **CAFFÈ MOCHA** | |
| **Caffè Mocha, made with 2% milk,** 1 tall | 6 |
| **Caffè Mocha, made with 2% milk and whipped cream,** 1 tall | 8 |
| **Caffè Mocha, made with nonfat milk,** 1 grande | 6 |
| **Caffè Mocha, made with nonfat milk and whipped cream,** 1 tall | 7 |
| **Caffè Mocha, made with soy milk, with whipped cream,** 1 tall | 7 |
| **Caffè Mocha, made with soymilk,** 1 tall | 6 |

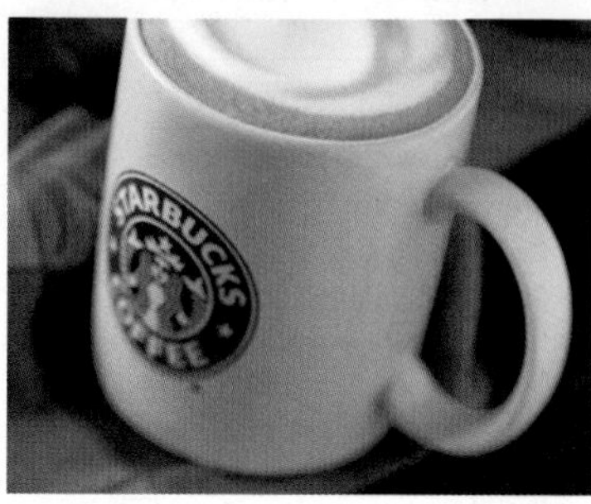


| ▲ Power Foods | *PointsPlus*™ value |
|---|---|
| **CAPPUCCINO** | |
| **Cappuccino, made with 2% milk,** 1 tall | 2 |
| ▲ **Cappuccino, made with nonfat milk,** 1 tall | 1 |
| ▲ **Cappuccino, made with soymilk,** 1 tall | 3 |
| **SIGNATURE ESPRESSO DRINKS** | |
| **Caramel Macchiato, made with 2% milk,** 1 tall | 5 |
| **Caramel Macchiato, made with nonfat milk,** 1 grande | 5 |
| **Caramel Macchiato, made with soymilk,** 1 tall | 5 |
| **Espresso Chocolate Truffle, made with nonfat milk,** 1 short | 5 |
| **White Chocolate Mocha, made with 2% milk,** 1 short | 5 |
| **White Chocolate Mocha, made with nonfat milk,** 1 short | 5 |
| **White Chocolate Mocha, made with soymilk,** 1 short | 5 |

# STARBUCKS COFFEE

| ▲ Power Foods | PointsPlus™ value |
|---|---|
| **OTHER HOT DRINKS (WITHOUT WHIPPED CREAM)** | |
| **Brewed Coffee,** 1 grande | 0 |
| **Caffé Americano,** 1 grande | 0 |
| **Caramel Apple Spice,** 1 short | 4 |
| **Hot Chocolate, made with 2% milk,** 1 short | 5 |
| **Hot Chocolate, made with nonfat milk,** 1 short | 4 |
| **Hot Chocolate, made with soymilk,** 1 short | 4 |
| **Signature Hot Chocolate, made with nonfat milk,** 1 short | 5 |
| **FRAPPUCCINO® BLENDED COFFEE** | |
| **Caramel Frappuccino® Blended Coffee, with whipped cream,** 1 tall | 8 |
| **Caramel, without whipped cream,** 1 grande | 7 |
| **Coffee,** 1 grande | 6 |
| **Mocha Frappuccino® Blended Coffee, with whipped cream,** 1 tall | 8 |
| **Mocha, without whipped cream,** 1 grande | 7 |
| **Strawberries & Cream Frappuccino® Blended Crème (with whip),** 1 tall | 10 |
| **Vanilla Bean Frappuccino® Blended Crème (with whip),** 1 tall | 9 |
| **FRAPPUCCINO® BLENDED CRÈME** | |
| **Double Chocolaty Chip, without whipped cream,** 1 tall | 8 |
| **Strawberries & Cream, without whipped cream,** 1 tall | 7 |
| **Vanilla Bean, without whipped cream,** 1 tall | 7 |

| ▲ Power Foods | PointsPlus™ value |
|---|---|
| **FRAPPUCCINO® LIGHT BLENDED COFFEE** | |
| **Caramel,** 1 grande | 4 |
| **Coffee,** 1 grande | 3 |
| **Mocha,** 1 grande | 4 |
| **ICED CAFFÈ** | |
| **Iced Caffe Con Leche, made with 2% milk,** 1 tall | 2 |
| **Iced Caffe Con Leche, made with nonfat milk,** 1 tall | 2 |
| **Iced Caffe Con Leche, made with soy milk,** 1 tall | 2 |
| **Iced Caffe Latte, made with 2% milk,** 1 tall | 3 |
| ▲ **Iced Caffe Latte, made with nonfat milk,** 1 tall | 2 |
| ▲ **Iced Caffe Latte, made with soy milk,** 1 tall | 2 |
| ▲ **Iced Skinny Cinnamon Dolce Latte,** 1 grande | 2 |
| **Iced Sugar Free Syrup Flavored Latte, made with 2% milk,** 1 tall | 2 |
| ▲ **Iced Sugar Free Syrup Flavored Latte, made with nonfat milk,** 1 tall | 2 |
| ▲ **Iced Sugar Free Syrup Flavored Latte, made with soy milk,** 1 tall | 2 |
| **Iced Syrup Flavored Latte, made with 2% milk,** 1 tall | 4 |
| **Iced Syrup Flavored Latte, made with nonfat milk,** 1 tall | 3 |
| **Iced Syrup Flavored Latte, made with soy milk,** 1 tall | 4 |
| **Sugar Free Syrup Flavored Latte, made with 2% milk,** 1 tall | 4 |
| ▲ **Sugar Free Syrup Flavored Latte, made with nonfat milk,** 1 tall | 2 |
| ▲ **Sugar Free Syrup Flavored Latte, made with soy milk,** 1 tall | 3 |

| ▲ Power Foods | *PointsPlus*™ value |
|---|---|
| **SKINNY LATTE** | |
| ▲ **Skinny Caramel Latte,** 1 grande | 3 |
| ▲ **Skinny Cinnamon Dolce Latte,** 1 grande | 3 |
| ▲ **Skinny Hazelnut Latte,** 1 grande | 3 |
| ▲ **Skinny Latte (any flavor),** 1 short | 2 |
| ▲ **Skinny Vanilla Latte,** 1 grande | 3 |
| **SHAKEN ICED BEVERAGES** | |
| **Iced Brewed Coffee, made with 2% milk,** 1 tall | 2 |
| ▲ **Iced Brewed Coffee, made with nonfat milk,** 1 tall | 2 |
| **Iced Brewed Coffee, made with soymilk,** 1 tall | 2 |
| **Iced Brewed Coffee, with classic syrup,** 1 tall | 2 |
| **Tazo® Shaken Iced Tea Lemonade, with classic syrup,** 1 tall | 3 |
| **Tazo® Shaken Iced Tea, with classic syrup,** 1 tall | 2 |
| **TAZO® TEA DRINKS** | |
| **Tazo® Chai Tea Latte, made with 2% milk,** 1 tall | 5 |
| **Tazo® Chai Tea Latte, made with nonfat milk,** 1 tall | 4 |
| **Tazo® Chai Tea Latte, made with soymilk,** 1 tall | 5 |
| **Tazo® Full Leaf Red Tea Latte, made with 2% milk (Awake™ or Earl Grey),** 1 short | 3 |
| **Tazo® Full Leaf Red Tea Latte, made with nonfat milk (Awake™ or Earl Grey),** 1 short | 2 |
| **Tazo® Full Leaf Red Tea Latte, made with soymilk (Awake™ or Earl Grey),** 1 short | 3 |
| **Tazo® Full Leaf Tea Latte, made with 2% milk (Awake™ or Earl Grey),** 1 short | 3 |
| **Tazo® Full Leaf Tea Latte, made with nonfat milk (Awake™ or Earl Grey),** 1 short | 2 |
| **Tazo® Full Leaf Tea Latte, made with soymilk (Awake™ or Earl Grey),** 1 short | 3 |
| **Tazo® Green Tea Latte, made with 2% milk,** 1 tall | 7 |
| **Tazo® Green Tea Latte, made with nonfat milk,** 1 tall | 5 |
| **Tazo® Green Tea Latte, made with soymilk,** 1 tall | 5 |
| **THINGS TO ADD OR LEAVE OUT** | |
| **Caramel Drizzle,** 1 serving | 0 |
| **Chocolate Drizzle,** 1 serving | 0 |
| **Espresso Shot,** 1 serving | 0 |
| **Flavored Sugar-Free Syrup,** 1 pump | 0 |
| **Flavored Syrup,** 1 pump | 1 |
| **Matcha Green Tea Powder,** 1 scoop | 1 |
| **Mocha Syrup,** 1 pump | 1 |
| **Protein & Fiber Powder,** 1 scoop | 1 |
| **Sweetened Whipped Cream, cold,** 1 tall | 2 |
| **Sweetened Whipped Cream, hot,** 1 short | 1 |
| **VIVANNO™ SMOOTHIES** | |
| **Banana Chocolate, made with 2% milk,** 1 grande | 8 |
| **Banana Chocolate, made with nonfat milk,** 1 grande | 7 |
| **Banana Chocolate, made with soymilk,** 1 grande | 7 |
| **Orange Mango Banana, made with 2% milk,** 1 grande | 7 |

*Vivanno™ Smoothies (cont'd)*

| Power Foods | PointsPlus™ value |
|---|---|
| **Orange Mango Banana, made with nonfat milk,** 1 grande | 7 |
| **Orange Mango Banana, made with soymilk,** 1 grande | 7 |
| **Strawberry Banana, made with 2% milk,** 1 grande | 7 |
| **Strawberry Banana, made with nonfat milk,** 1 grande | 7 |
| **Strawberry Banana, made with soymilk,** 1 grande | 7 |

## FOOD AT STARBUCKS

| Power Foods | PointsPlus™ value |
|---|---|
| **Ham, Egg Frittata, Cheddar Cheese on Artisan Roll,** 1 sandwich | 10 |
| **Morning Bun,** 1 pastry | 9 |
| **Perfect Oatmeal,** 1 serving | 3 |
| **Perfect Oatmeal Topping - Brown Sugar,** 1 serving | 1 |
| **Perfect Oatmeal Topping - Dried Fruit,** 1 serving | 3 |
| **Perfect Oatmeal Topping - Nut Medley,** 1 serving | 3 |
| **Petite Vanilla Bean Scone,** 1 scone | 4 |
| **Reduced Fat Turkey Bacon, Cholesterol Free Egg White, Reduced-Fat White Cheddar Breakfast Sandwich,** 1 sandwich | 9 |
| **Reduced Fat Very Berry Coffee Cake,** 1 slice | 9 |
| **Spinach, Roasted Tomato, Feta & Egg White Wrap,** 1 wrap | 7 |

## OVEN-TOASTED BREAKFAST ITEMS

| Power Foods | PointsPlus™ value |
|---|---|
| **Bacon, Gouda Cheese, Egg Frittata on Artisan Roll,** 1 serving | 10 |
| **Classic Sausage, Egg & Aged Cheddar Breakfast Sandwich,** 1 sandwich | 14 |

## BROWNIES, COOKIES & BARS

| Power Foods | PointsPlus™ value |
|---|---|
| **Blueberry Oat Bar with Organic Blueberries,** 1 bar | 6 |
| **Chocolate Chunk Cookie,** 1 cookie | 10 |
| **Double Chocolate Brownie,** 1 brownie | 11 |
| **Marshmallow Dream Bar,** 1 bar | 6 |
| **Outrageous Oatmeal Cookie,** 1 cookie | 10 |
| **Rich Toffee Pecan Bar,** 1 bar | 9 |
| **Starbucks® Indulgent Cookie,** 1 cookie | 9 |

## CROISSANTS, BAGELS & BREADS

| Power Foods | PointsPlus™ value |
|---|---|
| **Asiago Bagel,** 1 bagel | 8 |
| **Butter Croissant,** 1 | 8 |
| **Chocolate Croissant,** 1 | 8 |
| **Chonga Bagel,** 1 | 8 |
| **Hawaiian Bagel,** 1 | 10 |
| **Multigrain Bagel,** 1 | 10 |
| **Plain Bagel,** 1 | 8 |

## DOUGHNUTS, SWEET ROLLS & DANISHES

| Power Foods | PointsPlus™ value |
|---|---|
| **Apple Fritter,** 1 | 12 |
| **Cheese Danish,** 1 | 11 |
| **Chocolate Old Fashioned Doughnut,** 1 doughnut | 12 |
| **Classic Glazed Old Fashioned Doughnut,** 1 doughnut | 12 |
| **Double Iced Cinnamon Roll,** 1 roll | 13 |

## LOAVES & COFFEE CAKES

| Power Foods | PointsPlus™ value |
|---|---|
| **Banana Bread,** 1 slice | 13 |
| **Marble Loaf,** 1 slice | 10 |

| ▲ Power Foods | *PointsPlus™* value |
|---|---|
| **Pumpkin Bread,** 1 slice | 11 |
| **Reduced Fat Banana Chocolate Chip Coffee Cake,** 1 slice | 11 |
| **Reduced Fat Cinnamon Swirl Coffee Cake,** 1 slice | 9 |
| **Starbucks® Classic Coffee Cake,** 1 slice | 12 |

## MUFFINS & SCONES

| | |
|---|---|
| **Apple Bran Muffin with Omega-3s,** 1 muffin | 9 |
| **Blueberry Muffin,** 1 | 9 |
| **Blueberry Scone,** 1 scone | 13 |
| **Blueberry Streusel Muffin,** 1 muffin | 9 |
| **Cranberry Orange Scone,** 1 scone | 12 |
| **Low Fat Red Raspberry Muffin,** 1 muffin | 9 |
| **Maple Oat Pecan Scone,** 1 scone | 13 |
| **Pumpkin Scone,** 1 scone | 13 |
| **Zucchini Walnut Muffin,** 1 muffin | 13 |

# SUBWAY® RESTAURANTS

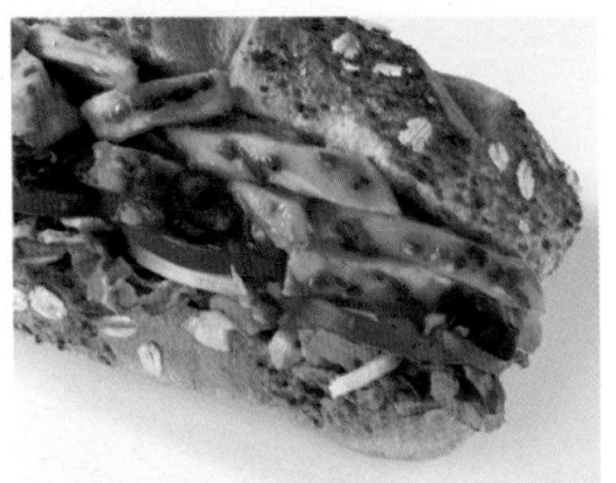

| ▲ Power Foods | *PointsPlus™* value |
|---|---|
| **6" SUBS** (LIMITED TIME OFFER/REGIONAL SUBS) | |
| **Barbecue Chicken,** 1 | 8 |
| **Barbecue Rib Patty,** 1 | 11 |
| **Buffalo Chicken (with regular ranch dressing),** 1 | 11 |
| **Chicken Pizziola (includes cheese),** 1 | 12 |
| **Low fat Buffalo Chicken (with light ranch),** 1 | 10 |
| **Pastrami, Big (includes cheese),** 1 | 15 |
| **Subway Seafood Sensation® (includes cheese),** 1 | 12 |
| **Turkey Bacon Avocado (includes cheese),** 1 | 11 |
| **Tuscan Chicken (includes cheese),** 1 | 10 |
| **Veggie Pattie,** 1 | 9 |
| **6" SANDWICHES** (ON 9-GRAIN WHEAT BREAD WITH CHEESE & FRESH VEGETABLES) | |
| **Big Philly Cheesesteak,** 1 | 13 |
| **BLT,** 1 | 9 |
| **Chicken & Bacon Ranch,** 1 | 15 |
| **Cold Cut Combo,** 1 | 11 |
| **Italian B.M.T.®,** 1 | 12 |
| **Meatball Marinara,** 1 | 15 |
| **Spicy Italian,** 1 | 14 |

| ▲ Power Foods | *PointsPlus™* value |
|---|---|
| **Subway Melt®,** 1 | 10 |
| **The Feast,** 1 | 14 |
| **Tuna,** 1 | 14 |
| **6" LOW FAT SANDWICHES WITH 6 GRAMS OF FAT OR LESS** | |
| **Black Forest Ham,** 1 | 8 |
| **Oven Roasted Chicken Breast,** 1 | 8 |
| **Roast Beef,** 1 | 8 |
| **Subway Club®,** 1 | 8 |
| **Sweet Onion Chicken Teriyaki,** 1 | 10 |
| **Turkey Breast,** 1 | 7 |
| **Turkey Breast & Black Forest Ham,** 1 | 7 |
| **Veggie Delite®,** 1 | 6 |
| **LOW FAT FOOTLONG SANDWICHES** | |
| **Black Forest Ham,** 1 | 15 |
| **Oven Roasted Chicken,** 1 | 16 |
| **Roast Beef,** 1 | 16 |
| **Subway Club®,** 1 | 17 |
| **Sweet Onion Chicken Teriyaki,** 1 | 19 |
| **Turkey Breast,** 1 | 14 |
| **Turkey Breast & Black Forest Ham,** 1 | 15 |
| **Veggie Delite®,** 1 | 12 |
| **FLATBREAD SANDWICHES WITH 8 GRAM OF FAT OR LESS** (ON 9-GRAIN WHEAT BREAD WITH CHEESE & FRESH VEGETABLES) | |
| **Black Forest Ham,** 1 | 8 |
| **Oven Roasted Chicken,** 1 | 9 |
| **Roast Beef,** 1 | 9 |
| **Subway Club®,** 1 | 9 |
| **Sweet Onion Chicken Teriyaki,** 1 | 10 |
| **Turkey Breast,** 1 | 8 |
| **Turkey Breast and Black Forest Ham,** 1 | 8 |
| **Veggie Delite®,** 1 | 7 |

▲ Power Foods — *PointsPlus™* value

## 6" BREADS

| Item | *PointsPlus™* value |
|---|---|
| **9-Grain Wheat Bread,** 1 | 5 |
| **Flatbread,** 1 | 6 |
| **Hearty Italian,** 1 | 6 |
| **Honey Oat,** 1 | 7 |
| **Italian (White),** 1 | 5 |
| **Italian Herbs & Cheese,** 1 | 6 |
| **Mini Italian,** 1 | 4 |
| **Mini Wheat,** 1 | 4 |
| **Monterey Cheddar,** 1 | 6 |
| **Parmesan Oregano,** 1 | 6 |
| **Roasted Garlic,** 1 | 6 |
| **Wheat,** 1 | 5 |
| **Wrap,** 1 | 8 |

## CHEESE
(AMOUNT ON 6" SUB, FLATBREAD OR SALAD)

| Item | *PointsPlus™* value |
|---|---|
| **American, Processed,** 1 serving | 1 |
| **Monterey Cheddar, Shredded,** 1 serving | 2 |
| **Natural Cheddar,** 1 serving | 2 |
| **Pepperjack,** 1 serving | 1 |
| **Provolone,** 1 serving | 1 |
| **Swiss,** 1 serving | 2 |

## INDIVIDUAL MEATS
(AMOUNT ON 6" SUB OR SALAD)

| Item | *PointsPlus™* value |
|---|---|
| **Chicken Patty, Roasted,** 1 patty | 2 |
| **Ham,** 1 serving | 2 |
| **Seafood Sensation,** 1 serving | 5 |
| **Steak (no cheese),** 1 | 3 |
| **Subway Club®,** 1 serving | 2 |
| **Tuna,** 1 serving | 7 |
| ▲ **Turkey Breast,** 1 serving | 1 |
| **Veggie Patty,** 1 patty | 4 |

## KIDS PAK® SANDWICHES

| Item | *PointsPlus™* value |
|---|---|
| **Black Forest Ham,** 1 | 5 |
| **Roast Beef,** 1 | 5 |
| **Turkey Breast,** 1 | 5 |
| **Veggie Delite®,** 1 | 4 |

## VEGETABLES

| Item | *PointsPlus™* value |
|---|---|
| ▲ **Banana Peppers,** 3 rings | 0 |
| ▲ **Cucumbers,** 3 slices | 0 |
| ▲ **Green Peppers,** 3 strips | 0 |
| ▲ **Jalapeno Peppers,** 3 pieces | 0 |
| ▲ **Lettuce,** 1 serving | 0 |
| **Olives,** 3 pieces | 0 |
| ▲ **Onions,** 1 serving | 0 |
| **Pickles,** 3 chips | 0 |
| ▲ **Tomatoes,** 3 slices | 0 |

## SANDWICH CONDIMENTS

| Item | *PointsPlus™* value |
|---|---|
| **Bacon,** 2 strips | 1 |
| **Chipotle Southwest Sauce,** 1 serving | 3 |
| **Honey Mustard Sauce Fat Free,** 1 1/2 Tbsp | 1 |
| **Light Mayonnaise,** 1 Tbsp | 1 |
| **Mayonnaise,** 1 Tbsp | 3 |
| **Mustard Yellow or Deli Brown,** 2 tsp | 0 |
| **Olive Oil Blend,** 1 tsp | 1 |
| **Ranch Dressing,** 1 packet | 3 |
| **Red Wine Vinaigrette, Fat Free,** 1 packet | 1 |
| **Sweet Onion Sauce, Fat Free,** 1 serving | 1 |
| **Vinegar,** 1 tsp | 0 |

# SUBWAY® RESTAURANTS

| ▲ Power Foods | *PointsPlus™* value |
|---|---|
| **8" PIZZA** | |
| **Cheese,** 1 pizza | 19 |
| **Cheese & Veggies,** 1 pizza | 20 |
| **Pepperoni,** 1 pizza | 22 |
| **Sausage,** 1 pizza | 23 |
| **SOUP** | |
| **Chicken & Dumpling,** 1 bowl | 4 |
| **Chicken Tortilla,** 1 bowl | 2 |
| **Chili Con Carne,** 1 bowl | 8 |
| **Chipotle Chicken Corn Chowder,** 1 bowl | 4 |
| **Cream of Potato with Bacon,** 1 bowl | 6 |
| **Fire-Roasted Tomato Orzo,** 1 bowl | 3 |
| **Golden Broccoli & Cheese,** 1 bowl | 5 |
| **Minestrone,** 1 bowl | 2 |
| **New England Style Clam Chowder,** 1 bowl | 4 |
| **Roasted Chicken Noodle,** 1 bowl | 2 |
| **Rosemary Chicken and Dumpling,** 1 bowl | 2 |
| **Spanish Style Chicken & Rice with Pork,** 1 bowl | 3 |
| **Tomato Garden Vegetable with Rotini,** 1 bowl | 2 |
| **Vegetable Beef,** 1 bowl | 3 |
| **BREAKFAST** (6" 9-GRAIN BREAD WITH REGULAR EGG) | |
| **Black Forest Ham & Cheese,** 1 sandwich | 12 |
| **Double Bacon & Cheese,** 1 sandwich | 14 |
| **Egg & Cheese,** 1 sandwich | 11 |
| **Mega,** 1 sandwich | 19 |
| **Sausage & Cheese,** 1 sandwich | 18 |
| **Steak & Cheese,** 1 sandwich | 13 |
| **Western & Cheese,** 1 sandwich | 12 |

| ▲ Power Foods | *PointsPlus™* value |
|---|---|
| **BREAKFAST** (ENGLISH MUFFIN WITH REGULAR EGG) | |
| **Black Forest Ham & Cheese,** 1 sandwich | 5 |
| **Cheese,** 1 sandwich | 4 |
| **Double Bacon & Cheese,** 1 sandwich | 6 |
| **Mega,** 1 sandwich | 8 |
| **Sausage,** 1 sandwich | 8 |
| **Steak & Cheese,** 1 sandwich | 5 |
| **Western with Cheese,** 1 sandwich | 5 |
| **BREAKFAST** (FLATBREAD SANDWICHES WITH REGULAR EGG) | |
| **Black Forest Ham & Cheese,** 1 sandwich | 13 |
| **Double Bacon & Cheese,** 1 sandwich | 15 |
| **Egg & Cheese,** 1 sandwich | 12 |
| **Mega,** 1 sandwich | 20 |
| **Sausage & Cheese,** 1 sandwich | 19 |
| **Steak & Cheese,** 1 sandwich | 14 |
| **Western & Cheese,** 1 sandwich | 13 |
| **BREAKFAST SIDE** | |
| **Hash Browns,** 4 pieces | 4 |
| **SALADS WITH 6 GRAMS OF FAT OR LESS** | |
| ▲ **Black Forest Ham,** 1 salad | 3 |
| ▲ **Oven Roasted Chicken Breast,** 1 salad | 3 |
| ▲ **Roast Beef,** 1 salad | 4 |
| ▲ **Subway Club®,** 1 salad | 4 |
| **Sweet Onion Chicken Teriyaki,** 1 salad | 5 |
| ▲ **Turkey Breast & Ham,** 1 salad | 3 |
| ▲ **Veggie Delite®,** 1 salad | 1 |

▲ Power Foods — *PointsPlus*™ value

## SALAD DRESSINGS

| Item | PointsPlus value |
|---|---|
| **Fat Free Italian,** 1 packet | 1 |
| **Ranch Dressing,** 1 packet | 8 |

## CHIPS

| Item | PointsPlus value |
|---|---|
| **Baked Lay's®,** 1 bag | 3 |
| **Baked Lay's® Sour Cream & Onion,** 1 bag | 4 |
| **Doritos Nacho,** 1 bag | 7 |
| **Lay® Classic,** 1 bag | 6 |
| **Sunchips Harvest Cheddar,** 1 bag | 6 |

## COOKIES & DESSERTS

| Item | PointsPlus value |
|---|---|
| **Apple Pie,** 1 pie | 7 |
| ▲ **Apple Slices,** 1 package | 0 |
| **Chocolate Chip,** 1 cookie | 6 |
| **Chocolate Chunk,** 1 cookie | 6 |
| **Double Chocolate Chip,** 1 cookie | 6 |
| **M&M®,** 1 cookie | 6 |
| **Oatmeal Raisin,** 1 cookie | 6 |
| **Peanut Butter,** 1 cookie | 6 |
| **Sugar,** 1 cookie | 6 |
| **White Chip Macadamia Nut,** 1 cookie | 6 |
| ▲ **Yogurt Dannon® Light & Fit®,** 1 container | 2 |

# SWEET TOMATOES®

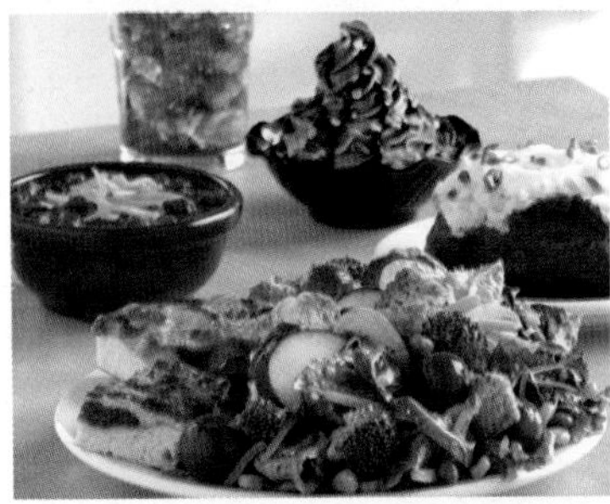

| ▲ Power Foods | *PointsPlus™* value |
|---|---|
| **FRESH TOSSED SALADS** | |
| **Azteca Taco with Turkey Salad,** 1 cup | 3 |
| **Bartlett Pear & Caramelized Walnut Salad (Vegetarian),** 1 cup | 5 |
| **BBQ Julienne Chopped Salad with Chicken (Vegetarian),** 1 cup | 6 |
| **Buffalo Chicken,** 1 cup | 5 |
| **Caesar Salad Asiago (Non-Vegetarian),** 1 cup | 7 |
| **California Cobb Salad with Bacon,** 1 cup | 5 |
| **Cambay Curry with Almonds & Coconut (Vegetarian),** 1 cup | 6 |
| **Cape Cod Spinach with Walnuts & Bacon,** 1 cup | 4 |
| **Cherry Chipotle Spinach (Vegetarian),** 1 cup | 4 |
| **Chicken Tortilla Salad,** 1 cup | 5 |
| **Classic Greek Salad (Vegetarian),** 1 cup | 3 |
| **Club Blue BLT with Bacon,** 1 cup | 7 |
| **Country French Salad with Bacon,** 1 cup | 6 |
| **Crunchy Island Pineapple (Vegetarian),** 1 cup | 4 |

| ▲ Power Foods | *PointsPlus™* value |
|---|---|
| **Field of Greens: Citrus Vinaigrette (Vegan),** 1 cup | 4 |
| **Field of Greens: Sweet Maple (Vegetarian),** 1 cup | 5 |
| **Honey Minted Fruit Toss (Vegetarian),** 1 cup | 0 |
| **Mandarin Spinach Salad with Caramelized Walnuts (Vegan),** 1 cup | 4 |
| **Monterey Blue Salad with Peanuts (Vegetarian),** 1 cup | 7 |
| **Outrageous Orange with Cashews (Vegetarian),** 1 cup | 6 |
| **Ragin' Cajun Salad with Chicken,** 1 cup | 6 |
| **Ranch House BLT Salad with Turkey & Bacon,** 1 cup | 5 |
| **Roasted Vegetables Salad with Feta & Olives (Vegetarian),** 1 cup | 5 |
| **Sedona Green Chile & Chipotle (Non-Vegetarian),** 1 cup | 6 |
| **Smoked Turkey & Spinach Salad with Almonds,** 1 cup | 5 |
| **Sonoma Spinach Salad with Honey Dijon Vinaigrette (Vegetarian),** 1 cup | 6 |
| **Spiced Pecan & Roasted Vegetable with Bacon,** 1 cup | 5 |
| **Spinach Gorgonzola with Spiced Pecans and Bacon,** 1 cup | 6 |
| **Strawberry Fields with Caramelized Walnuts (Vegan),** 1 cup | 4 |
| **Summer Lemon with Spiced Pecans (Vegetarian),** 1 cup | 6 |
| **Sweet Tomato, Mozzarella & Basil Salad (Vegetarian),** 1 cup | 3 |
| **Thai Peanut & Red Pepper (Vegan),** 1 cup | 6 |
| **Thai Udon & Peanut (Vegan),** 1 cup | 6 |
| **Traditional Spinach Salad with Bacon,** 1 cup | 5 |
| **Won Ton Chicken Happiness,** 1 cup | 4 |

| ▲ Power Foods | *PointsPlus*™ value |
|---|---|
| **SIGNATURE PREPARED SALADS** | |
| **Ambrosia with Coconut (Vegetarian),** 1/2 cup | 6 |
| **Artichoke Rice Salad (Vegetarian),** 1/2 cup | 5 |
| **Aunt Doris' Red Pepper Slaw (Fat-free, Vegan),** 1/2 cup | 2 |
| **Baja Bean & Cilantro Salad (Low-fat, Vegan),** 1/2 cup | 4 |
| **BBQ Potato Salad (Vegetarian),** 1/2 cup | 5 |
| **Carrot Raisin Salad (Low-fat, Vegetarian),** 1/2 cup | 3 |
| **Chinese Krab Salad,** 1/2 cup | 4 |
| **Citrus Noodles Salad with Snow Peas (Vegetarian),** 1/2 cup | 4 |
| **Classic Antipasto (Tossed Salad),** 1 cup | 8 |
| **Dijon Potato Salad with Garlic Dill Vinaigrette (Vegan),** 1/2 cup | 4 |
| **Field Corn & Very Wild Rice (Vegetarian),** 1/2 cup | 5 |
| **Greek Couscous Salad with Feta Cheese and Pinenuts (Vegetarian),** 1/2 cup | 5 |
| **Green Chile Ranch with Spicy Tortilla Chips (Vegetarian),** 1 cup | 7 |
| **Italian White Bean Salad (Vegan),** 1/2 cup | 4 |
| **Jalapeño Potato Salad (Vegetarian),** 1/2 cup | 5 |
| **Joan's Broccoli Madness (Non-Vegetarian),** 1/2 cup | 5 |
| **Lemon Rice with Cashews (Vegan),** 1/2 cup | 4 |
| **Mandarin Noodles Salad with Broccoli (Low-fat, Vegan),** 1/2 cup | 4 |
| **Mandarin Shells Salad with Almonds (Low-fat, Vegan),** 1/2 cup | 3 |
| **Old Fashioned Macaroni Salad with Ham,** 1/2 cup | 6 |
| **Oriental Ginger Slaw with Krab (Low-fat),** 1/2 cup | 2 |
| **Penne Pasta Salad with Chicken in a Citrus Vinaigrette (Low-fat),** 1/2 cup | 3 |
| **Pesto Pasta Salad (Vegetarian),** 1/2 cup | 5 |
| **Picnic Potato Salad (Vegetarian),** 1/2 cup | 5 |
| **Pineapple Coconut Slaw (Vegetarian),** 1/2 cup | 4 |
| **Poppyseed Coleslaw (Vegetarian),** 1/2 cup | 3 |
| **Red Potato & Tomato (Vegetarian),** 1/2 cup | 5 |
| **Roasted Potato Salad with Chipotle Chile Vinaigrette (Vegan),** 1/2 cup | 3 |
| **Shrimp & Seafood Shells Salad,** 1/2 cup | 6 |
| **Smoky Ham & Cheddar Broccoli Slaw,** 1/2 cup | 7 |
| **Southern Dill Potato Salad (Low-fat, Vegetarian),** 1/2 cup | 3 |
| **Southwestern Rice & Beans Salad (Low-fat, Vegetarian),** 1/2 cup | 2 |
| **Spicy Cajun Shells (Vegetarian),** 1/2 cup | 8 |
| **Spicy Southwestern Pasta Salad (Low-fat, Vegan),** 1/2 cup | 3 |
| **Summer Barley Salad with Black Beans (Low-fat, Vegan),** 1/2 cup | 3 |
| **Sweet & Sour Broccoli Slaw (Low-Fat, Vegan),** 1/2 cup | 4 |
| **Sweet Marinated Vegetables (Fat Free, Vegan),** 1/2 cup | 2 |
| **Tabouli (Vegan),** 1/2 cup | 5 |
| **Thai Citrus & Brown Rice (Vegan),** 1/2 cup | 6 |

*Signature Prepared Salads (cont'd)*

| ▲ Power Foods | *PointsPlus*™ value |
|---|---|
| **Thai Noodle Salad with Chicken & Peanut Sauce,** 1/2 cup | 5 |
| **Three Bean Marinade Salad (Vegan),** 1/2 cup | 5 |
| **Tomato Cucumber Marinade Salad (Vegan),** 1/2 cup | 2 |
| **Tuna Tarragon Salad,** 1/2 cup | 7 |
| **Turkey Chutney Pasta Salad,** 1/2 cup | 6 |
| **Wheat Berry & Curry (Vegetarian),** 1/2 cup | 5 |
| **Whole Grain Fiesta Couscous (Vegetarian),** 1/2 cup | 7 |
| **Wild Rice & Chicken Salad,** 1/2 cup | 8 |
| **Zesty Tortellini Salad (Vegetarian),** 1/2 cup | 6 |

## SALAD DRESSINGS & CROUTONS

| ▲ Power Foods | *PointsPlus*™ value |
|---|---|
| **Avocado Ranch Dressing,** 2 Tbsp | 4 |
| **Bacon Dressing,** 2 Tbsp | 4 |
| **Balsamic Vinaigrette (Non-Vegetarian),** 2 Tbsp | 5 |
| **Basil Vinaigrette,** 2 Tbsp | 4 |
| **BBQ Vinaigrette,** 2 Tbsp | 2 |
| **Blue Cheese Dressing,** 2 Tbsp | 4 |
| **Citrus Vinaigrette,** 2 Tbsp | 4 |
| **Cranberry Orange Vinaigrette (Low-fat),** 2 Tbsp | 2 |
| **Creamy Italian Dressing,** 2 Tbsp | 3 |
| **Cucumber Dressing (Reduced Calorie),** 2 Tbsp | 2 |
| **Fat Free Honey Mustard Dressing,** 2 Tbsp | 1 |
| **Fat Free Italian Dressing,** 2 Tbsp | 1 |
| **Garlic Parmesan Seasoned Croutons,** 5 pieces | 2 |
| **Green Chili Ranch Dressing,** 2 Tbsp | 4 |
| **Honey Lime Cilantro Vinaigrette,** 2 Tbsp | 3 |
| **Honey Mint Lemonade Dressing,** 2 Tbsp | 4 |
| **Honey Mustard Dressing,** 2 Tbsp | 4 |
| **Italian Vinaigrette with Basil & Romano Cheese,** 1 Tbsp | 4 |
| **Kahlena French Dressing,** 2 Tbsp | 3 |
| **Monterey Blue Salad Dressing,** 2 Tbsp | 3 |
| **Parmesan Pepper Cream Dressing,** 2 Tbsp | 4 |
| **Pineapple Vinaigrette,** 2 Tbsp | 3 |
| **Ranch Dressing,** 2 Tbsp | 4 |
| **Roasted Garlic Dressing,** 2 Tbsp | 3 |
| **Smoky BBQ Vinaigrette,** 2 Tbsp | 3 |
| **Spicy Buffalo Ranch Dressing,** 2 Tbsp | 4 |
| **Spicy Southwest Chipotle,** 2 Tbsp | 5 |
| **Strawberry Balsamic Vinaigrette,** 2 Tbsp | 4 |
| **Sweet Maple Dressing,** 2 Tbsp | 5 |
| **Thousand Island Dressing,** 2 Tbsp | 3 |
| **Warm Bacon Dressing,** 2 Tbsp | 3 |
| **Chow Mein Noodles,** 1/4 cup | 2 |
| **Plain Croutons,** 5 pieces | 1 |
| **Tomato Basil Croutons,** 5 pieces | 2 |

## SOUP & CHILI

| ▲ Power Foods | *PointsPlus*™ value |
|---|---|
| **8 Vegetable Chicken Stew,** 1 cup | 4 |
| **Albondigas Locas (A Meatball Soup),** 1 cup | 5 |
| **Asian Ginger Broth (Low-fat, Vegetarian),** 1 cup | 0 |
| **Beef & Barley Stew,** 1 cup | 5 |
| **Better Than Mom's Beef Stew,** 1 cup | 7 |
| **Big Chunk Chicken Noodle (Low-fat),** 1 cup | 4 |
| **Border Black Bean & Chorizo,** 1 cup | 6 |
| **Broccoli Cheese (Vegetarian),** 1 cup | 7 |

| ▲ Power Foods | *PointsPlus*™ value |
|---|---|
| **Canadian Cheese with Smoked Ham,** 1 cup | 10 |
| **Cheese Stuffed Cappelletti Soup (Non-Vegetarian),** 1 cup | 7 |
| **Chesapeake Corn Chowder (Non-Vegetarian),** 1 cup | 8 |
| **Chicken & Rice,** 1 cup | 4 |
| **Chicken Fajitas & Black Bean Soup,** 1 cup | 7 |
| **Chicken Pot Pie Stew,** 1 cup | 8 |
| **Chicken Tortilla Soup with Jalapeño Chiles & Tomatoes (Low-fat),** 1 cup | 2 |
| **Chili Cheeseburger,** 1 cup | 7 |
| **Chunky Potato Cheese Soup with Thyme (Vegetarian),** 1 cup | 6 |
| **Classical French Onion Soup (Non-Vegetarian),** 1 cup | 4 |
| **Classical Minestrone Soup (Low-fat, Vegan),** 1 cup | 3 |
| **Classical Shrimp Bisque,** 1 cup | 6 |
| **Continental Lentil & Spinach (Low-fat, Vegetarian),** 1 cup | 3 |
| **Corned Beef & Cabbage,** 1 cup | 4 |
| **Country Corn & Red Potato Chowder (Non-Vegetarian),** 1 cup | 6 |
| **Cream of Broccoli Soup (Vegetarian),** 1 cup | 7 |
| **Cream of Chicken Soup,** 1 cup | 8 |
| **Cream of Mushroom Soup (Non-Vegetarian),** 1 cup | 8 |
| **Cream of Rosemary Potato (Non-vegetarian),** 1 cup | 9 |
| **Creamy Herbed Turkey Soup,** 1 cup | 9 |
| **Creamy Vegetable Chowder (Vegetarian),** 1 cup | 7 |
| **Curried Yellow Split Pea (Low-fat, Vegetarian),** 1 cup | 5 |
| **Deep Kettle House Chili (Low-fat),** 1 cup | 4 |

| ▲ Power Foods | *PointsPlus*™ value |
|---|---|
| **Deep Kettle House Chili with 33% more meat!,** 1 cup | 6 |
| **Deep Kettle House Chili with 50% More Meat!,** 1 cup | 7 |
| **El Paso Lime & Chicken Soup,** 1 cup | 4 |
| **Field of Creams - Cauliflower with Proud to be American Cheese (Vegetarian),** 1 cup | 8 |
| **Field of Creams - Sweet Tomato Basil (Vegetarian),** 1 cup | 6 |
| **Fire Roasted Green Chile & Corn Chowder with Bacon,** 1 cup | 7 |
| **Garden Fresh Vegetable Soup (Low-fat, Vegetarian),** 1 cup | 3 |
| **Garden of Eatin' (Low-fat) (Vegetarian),** 1 cup | 3 |
| **Golden Yam Bisque (Vegetarian),** 1 cup | 5 |
| **Green Chile Stew with Pork,** 1 cup | 4 |
| **Irish Potato Leek Soup (Vegetarian),** 1 cup | 7 |
| **Lemon Chicken Orzo,** 1 cup | 6 |
| **Loaded Baked Potato & Cheese with Bacon,** 1 cup | 8 |
| **Longhorn Beef Chili,** 1 cup | 5 |
| **Marvelous Minestrone Soup with Bacon,** 1 cup | 6 |
| **Minestrone with Italian Sausage,** 1 cup | 5 |
| **Moroccan Garbanzo & Lentil Bean (Low-fat, Vegetarian),** 1 cup | 5 |
| **Mulligatawny Soup (Non-Vegetarian),** 1 cup | 6 |
| **Neighbor Joe's Gumbo (Non-Vegetarian),** 1 cup | 5 |
| **New Mexican Corn Tortilla with Chicken,** 1 cup | 5 |
| **New Orleans Jambalaya (Non-Vegetarian),** 1 cup | 6 |
| **Old Fashion Vegetable Soup (Low-fat, Vegetarian),** 1 cup | 2 |

Soup & Chili (cont'd)

| ▲ Power Foods | *PointsPlus™* value |
|---|---|
| **Pinto Bean & Basil Barley (Low-fat, Vegetarian),** 1 cup | 4 |
| **Posole Soup with Pork,** 1 cup | 3 |
| **Potato Tomato & Spinach (Low-fat, Vegetarian),** 1 cup | 4 |
| **Ratatouille Provencale (Fat-free, Vegan),** 1 cup | 3 |
| **Roasted Mushroom with Sage (Non-Vegetarian),** 1 cup | 9 |
| **Rustic Tuscan Stew (Low-fat, Non-Vegetarian),** 1 cup | 3 |
| **Santa Fe Black Bean Chili (Low-fat, Vegan),** 1 cup | 4 |
| **Savory Turkey Harvest,** 1 cup | 6 |
| **Smoky Pinto & Brown Rice (Low-fat, Vegetarian),** 1 cup | 4 |
| **Southwest Tomato Cream (Vegetarian),** 1 cup | 3 |
| **Southwest Tomato Cream Soup (Vegetarian),** 1 cup | 3 |
| **Southwest Turkey Chowder with Bacon,** 1 cup | 7 |
| **Spicy Sausage & Pasta Soup,** 1 cup | 8 |
| **Split Pea & Potato Barley (Low-fat, Vegetarian),** 1 cup | 4 |
| **Split Pea Soup with Ham,** 1 cup | 7 |
| **Sweet Tomato Onion Soup (Low-fat, Vegan),** 1 cup | 2 |
| **Texas Red Chili (Non-Vegetarian),** 1 cup | 5 |
| **Three-Bean Turkey Chili (Low-fat),** 1 cup | 4 |
| **Tomato Chipotle Bisque (Non-Vegetarian),** 1 cup | 7 |
| **Tomato Parmesan & Vegetables (Low-fat, Vegetarian),** 1 cup | 3 |
| **Turkey Cassoulet with Bacon,** 1 cup | 6 |
| **Turkey Vegetable Soup,** 1 cup | 5 |
| **U.S. Senate Bean with Smoked Ham,** 1 cup | 4 |
| **Vegetable Medley Soup (Low-fat, Vegetarian),** 1 cup | 2 |
| **Vegetarian Harvest Soup (Vegan),** 1 cup | 5 |
| **White Bean & Lime Chicken Chili,** 1 cup | 5 |
| **X-treme Spice Vegetable Chili with Energy Boost (Low-fat, Vegetarian),** 1 cup | 2 |
| **Yankee Clipper Clam Chowder with Bacon,** 1 cup | 9 |

## HOT TOSSED PASTAS/ KITCHEN FAVORITES

| ▲ Power Foods | *PointsPlus™* value |
|---|---|
| **4-Cheese Alfredo (Vegetarian),** 1 cup | 10 |
| **Arizona Marinara (Vegetarian),** 1 cup | 9 |
| **Broccoli Alfredo with Basil (Vegetarian),** 1 cup | 10 |
| **Bruschetta (Vegetarian),** 1 cup | 6 |
| **Carbonara Pasta with Bacon,** 1 cup | 8 |
| **Chicken Tetrazzini,** 1 cup | 13 |
| **Cilantro Lime Pesto (Vegetarian),** 1 cup | 10 |
| **Creamy Bruschetta (Vegetarian),** 1 cup | 10 |
| **Creamy Herb Chicken,** 1 cup | 8 |
| **Curried Pineapple & Ginger (Low-fat, Non-Vegetarian),** 1 cup | 5 |
| **Fettuccine Alfredo (Vegetarian),** 1 cup | 10 |
| **Fire-Roasted Tomato & Basil Alfredo (Vegetarian),** 1 cup | 10 |
| **Garden Vegetable with Italian Sausage,** 1 cup | 8 |
| **Garden Vegetable with Meatballs,** 1 cup | 8 |
| **Greek Mediterranean (Vegetarian),** 1 cup | 8 |
| **Hand-Crafted Mexican Beans (Low-fat, Vegetarian),** 1 cup | 6 |
| **Italian Sausage with Red Pepper Puree,** 1 cup | 7 |

| ▲ Power Foods | *PointsPlus™* value |
|---|---|
| **Italian Vegetable Beef,** 1 cup | 8 |
| **Lemon Cream with Capers (Non-Vegetarian),** 1 cup | 11 |
| **Linguini with Clam Sauce,** 1 cup | 10 |
| **Macaroni & Cheese (Vegetarian),** 1 cup | 9 |
| **Nutty Mushroom (Vegetarian),** 1 cup | 11 |
| **Oriental Green Bean & Noodle (Low-fat, Vegetarian),** 1 cup | 6 |
| **Pasta Florentine (Vegetarian),** 1 cup | 10 |
| **Penne Arrabbiatta (Vegetarian),** 1 cup | 9 |
| **Ragin Cajun with Andouille Sausage,** 1 cup | 10 |
| **Roasted Eggplant Marinara (Vegetarian),** 1 cup | 9 |
| **Roasted Mushroom Alfredo with Rosemary (Vegetarian),** 1 cup | 10 |
| ▲ **Salsa de Lupe (Fat-free, Vegan),** 1/4 cup | 0 |
| **Sauteed Balsamic Vegetables (Vegan),** 1/2 cup | 3 |
| **Smoked Salmon & Dill,** 1 cup | 10 |
| **Smoky BBQ Baked Beans (Low-fat, Non-Vegetarian),** 1 cup | 8 |
| **Spicy Italian Sausage & Peppers,** 1 cup | 9 |
| **Steamed Vegetables with Lemon Herb Butter (Vegetarian),** 1/2 cup | 3 |
| **Stuffing (Non-Vegetarian),** 1/2 cup | 6 |
| **Tomato Spinach Whole Wheat (Vegetarian),** 1 cup | 7 |
| **Tuscany Sausage with Capers & Olives,** 1 cup | 6 |
| **Vegetable Ragu (Vegetarian),** 1 cup | 7 |
| **Vegetarian Marinara with Basil (Vegetarian),** 1 cup | 6 |
| **Walnut Pesto (Vegetarian),** 1 cup | 8 |

| ▲ Power Foods | *PointsPlus™* value |
|---|---|
| **FRESH BAKED MUFFINS & BREADS** | |
| **Apple Cinnamon Bran Muffin (96% Fat-free),** 1 | 3 |
| **Apple Raisin Muffin,** 1 | 4 |
| **Banana Nut Muffin,** 1 | 4 |
| **Bruschetta Focaccia,** 1 piece | 4 |
| **Buttermilk Cornbread (Low-fat),** 1 piece | 4 |
| **Cappuccino Chip Muffin,** 1 | 5 |
| **Caribbean Key Lime Muffin,** 1 | 5 |
| **Carrot Pineapple Muffin with Oat Bran,** 1 | 4 |
| **Cherry Nut Muffin,** 1 | 4 |
| **Chipotle Lime Butter,** 1 Tbsp | 3 |
| **Chocolate Brownie Muffin,** 1 | 5 |
| **Chocolate Chip Muffin,** 1 | 5 |
| **Country Blackberry Muffin,** 1 | 5 |
| **Cranberry Orange Bran Muffin (96% Fat-free),** 1 | 3 |
| **Fruit Medley Bran Muffin (96% Fat-free),** 1 | 3 |
| **Garlic Asiago Focaccia,** 1 piece | 4 |
| **Georgia Peach Poppyseed Muffin,** 1 | 4 |
| **Indian Grain Bread (Low-fat),** 1 piece | 5 |
| **Lemon Vanilla Butter,** 1 Tbsp | 2 |
| **Maple Walnut Muffin,** 1 | 6 |
| **Old World Greek Focaccia,** 1 piece | 5 |
| **Pauline's Apple Walnut Cake,** 1 piece | 6 |
| **Pesto & Sun-dried Tomato Focaccia,** 1 piece | 5 |
| **Pumpkin Raisin Muffin,** 1 | 4 |
| **Quattro Formaggio Focaccia,** 1 piece | 4 |
| **Roasted Potato Focaccia,** 1 piece | 4 |
| **Sauteed Vegetable Focaccia,** 1 piece | 5 |
| **Sourdough Bread (Low-fat),** 1 piece | 4 |
| **Southwest Chipotle Focaccia,** 1 piece | 4 |
| **Spiced Pumpkin Muffin with Cranberries,** 1 piece | 5 |

*Fresh Baked Muffins & Breads (cont'd)*

| ▲ Power Foods | PointsPlus™ value |
|---|---|
| **Strawberry Buttermilk Muffin,** 1 | 4 |
| **Sweet Cherry Butter,** 1 Tbsp | 2 |
| **Sweet Orange & Cranberry Muffin,** 1 | 5 |
| **Sweet Strawberry Butter,** 1 Tbsp | 2 |
| **Taffy Apple Muffin,** 1 | 4 |
| **Tangy Lemon Muffin,** 1 | 4 |
| **Thai Chicken Focaccia with Peanuts,** 1 piece | 5 |
| **Wildly Blue Blueberry Muffin,** 1 piece | 4 |
| **Zucchini Nut Muffin,** 1 | 4 |

## MORNING MENU/BREAKFAST

| ▲ Power Foods | PointsPlus™ value |
|---|---|
| **Blueberry Sauce/Blueberry Stir-in,** 2 Tbsp | 2 |
| **Granola Topping,** 2 Tbsp | 3 |
| ▲ **Homemade Oatmeal (Plain),** 3/4 cup | 3 |
| **Mediterranean Sunrise Pasta,** 1 cup | 6 |
| **Potatoes O'Brien,** 1/2 cup | 4 |
| **Scrambled Eggs,** 1/2 cup | 3 |
| **Sticky Granola Clusters with Almonds,** 1/4 cup | 7 |
| **Strawberry Sauce/Strawberry Stir-in,** 2 Tbsp | 1 |
| **Tom's Country Gravy,** 2 Tbsp | 2 |
| **Warm Marion Blackberry Sauce,** 1/4 cup | 2 |

## DESSERTS

| ▲ Power Foods | PointsPlus™ value |
|---|---|
| **Apple Cobbler,** 1/2 cup | 10 |
| **Apple Medley (Fat-free),** 1/2 cup | 2 |
| **Banana Pudding,** 1/2 cup | 4 |
| **Banana Royale (Fat-free),** 1/2 cup | 2 |
| **Butterscotch Pudding (Low-fat),** 1/2 cup | 4 |
| **Candy Sprinkles (Low-fat),** 1 Tbsp | 2 |
| **Caramel Apple Cobbler,** 1/2 cup | 11 |
| **Caramel Syrup,** 2 Tbsp | 4 |
| **Cherry Apple Cobbler,** 1/2 cup | 9 |
| **Chocolate Chip Cookie,** 1 small | 2 |
| **Chocolate Frozen Yogurt (Fat-free),** 1/2 cup | 3 |
| **Chocolate Lava Cake,** 1/2 cup | 9 |
| **Chocolate Pudding (Low-fat),** 1/2 cup | 4 |
| **Chocolate Pudding (Low-fat, No Sugar Added),** 1/2 cup | 3 |
| **Chocolate Syrup,** 2 Tbsp | 3 |
| **Cranberry Apple Cobbler,** 1/2 cup | 9 |
| **Gelatin (Fat-free),** 1/2 cup | 2 |
| **Gelatin (Sugar Free, Fat-free),** 1/2 cup | 0 |
| **Granola Topping,** 2 Tbsp | 3 |
| **Green Tea Mousse,** 1/2 cup | 5 |
| **Hot Lemon Lava Cake,** 1/2 cup | 8 |
| **Nutty Waldorf Salad (Low-fat),** 1/2 cup | 2 |
| **Oatmeal Raisin Cookie,** 1 small | 3 |
| **Pineapple Gelatin (Fat-free),** 1/2 cup | 3 |
| **Pineapple Upside-down Cake,** 1/2 cup | 7 |
| **Raspberry Apple Cobbler,** 1/2 cup | 10 |
| **Rice Pudding (Low-fat),** 1/2 cup | 3 |
| **Shortcake,** 1 cake | 6 |
| **Sugar-free Cherry Chocolate Mousse,** 1/2 cup | 1 |
| **Sugar-free Chocolate Mousse,** 1/2 cup | 1 |
| **Sugar-free Lemon Mousse,** 1/2 cup | 1 |
| **Sugar-free Raspberry Mousse,** 1/2 cup | 1 |
| **Sugar-free Strawberry Mousse,** 1/2 cup | 1 |
| **Tapioca Pudding (Low-fat),** 1/2 cup | 4 |
| **Vanilla Pudding,** 1/2 cup | 4 |
| **Vanilla Soft Serve (Reduced Fat),** 1/2 cup | 4 |
| **Warm Carrot Cake with Cream Cheese Lava,** 1/2 cup | 8 |

| ▲ Power Foods | *PointsPlus*™ value |
|---|---|
| **TACOS** | |
| **Crunchy Taco Supreme®, 1** | 6 |
| **DOUBLE DECKER® Taco, 1** | 8 |
| **DOUBLE DECKER® Taco Supreme®, 1** | 9 |
| **Grilled Steak Soft Taco, 1** | 7 |
| **Ranchero Chicken Soft Taco, 1** | 7 |
| **Soft Taco Supreme® - Beef, 1** | 7 |
| **Spicy Chicken Soft Taco, 1** | 4 |
| **BURRITOS** | |
| **1/2 lb Beef & Potato Burrito, 1** | 14 |
| **1/2 lb Beef Combo Burrito, 1** | 11 |
| **7-Layer Burrito, 1** | 13 |
| **Burrito Supreme® - Beef, 1** | 11 |
| **Burrito Supreme® - Chicken, 1** | 10 |
| **Burrito Supreme® - Steak, 1** | 10 |
| **Chili Cheese Burrito, 1** | 10 |
| **Fiesta Burrito - Beef, 1** | 10 |
| **Fiesta Burrito - Chicken, 1** | 9 |
| **Fiesta Burrito - Steak, 1** | 9 |
| **Grilled Stuft Burrito - Beef, 1** | 18 |
| **Grilled Stuft Burrito - Chicken, 1** | 16 |
| **Grilled Stuft Burrito - Steak, 1** | 16 |
| **Spicy Chicken Burrito, 1** | 11 |
| **CHALUPAS** | |
| **Chalupa Baja - Beef, 1** | 11 |
| **Chalupa Baja - Chicken, 1** | 10 |
| **Chalupa Baja - Steak, 1** | 10 |
| **Chalupa Nacho Cheese - Beef, 1** | 10 |
| **Chalupa Nacho Cheese - Chicken, 1** | 9 |
| **Chalupa Nacho Cheese - Steak, 1** | 9 |
| **Chalupa Supreme - Beef, 1** | 10 |
| **Chalupa Supreme - Chicken, 1** | 10 |
| **Chalupa Supreme - Steak, 1** | 10 |

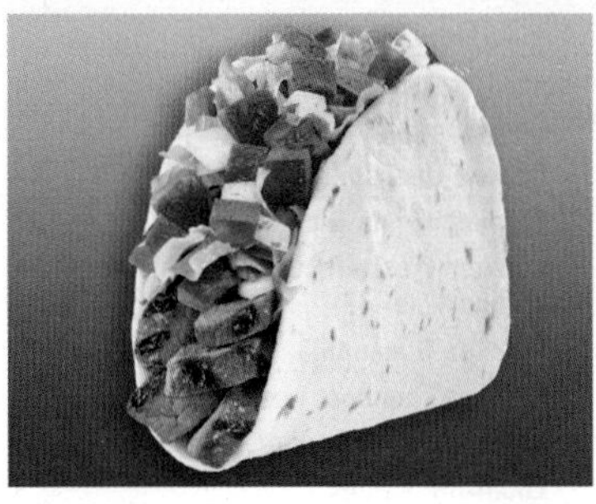

| ▲ Power Foods | *PointsPlus*™ value |
|---|---|
| **GORDITAS** | |
| **Gordita Baja® - Beef, 1** | 9 |
| **Gordita Baja® - Chicken, 1** | 8 |
| **Gordita Baja® - Steak, 1** | 8 |
| **Gordita Nacho Cheese - Beef, 1** | 8 |
| **Gordita Nacho Cheese - Chicken, 1** | 7 |
| **Gordita Nacho Cheese - Steak, 1** | 7 |
| **Gordita Supreme® - Beef, 1** | 8 |
| **Gordita Supreme® - Chicken, 1** | 8 |
| **Gordita Supreme® - Steak, 1** | 8 |
| **FRESCO STYLE BURRITOS** | |
| **Bean Burrito, 1** | 8 |
| **Burrito Supreme® - Chicken, 1** | 8 |
| **Burrito Supreme® - Steak, 1** | 8 |
| **Fiesta Burrito - Chicken, 1** | 8 |
| **FRESCO STYLE TACOS** | |
| **Crunchy Taco, 1** | 4 |
| **Grilled Steak Soft Taco, 1** | 4 |
| **Ranchero Chicken Soft Taco, 1** | 4 |
| **Soft Taco - Beef, 1** | 5 |

# TACO BELL®

| ▲ Power Foods | *PointsPlus*™ value |
|---|---|
| **SPECIALTIES** | |
| **Cheese Quesadilla,** 1 | 12 |
| **Chicken Fiesta Taco Salad,** 1 | 20 |
| **Chicken Fiesta Taco Salad without Shell,** 1 | 11 |
| **Chicken Quesadilla,** 1 | 14 |
| **Chicken Taquitos,** 1 serving | 8 |
| **Crunchwrap Supreme®,** 1 | 15 |
| **Enchirito® - Beef,** 1 | 9 |
| **Enchirito® - Chicken,** 1 | 8 |
| **Enchirito® - Steak,** 1 | 9 |
| **Express Taco Salad,** 1 | 15 |
| **Fiesta Taco Salad,** 1 | 22 |
| **Fiesta Taco Salad without Shell,** 1 | 12 |
| **Mexican Pizza,** 1 | 14 |
| **MexiMelt®,** 1 | 7 |
| **Southwest Steak BORDER BOWL®,** 1 | 15 |
| **Spicy Chicken CRUNCHWRAP SUPREME®,** 1 | 15 |
| **Steak Quesadilla,** 1 | 14 |
| **Steak Taquitos with Guacamole,** 1 | 10 |
| **Steak Taquitos with Salsa,** 1 | 8 |
| **Steak Taquitos with Sour Cream,** 1 | 10 |
| **Tostada,** 1 | 6 |
| **Zesty Chicken BORDER BOWL®,** 1 | 17 |
| **Zesty Chicken BORDER BOWL®, without dressing,** 1 | 11 |
| **NACHOS & SIDES** | |
| **Cheesy Fiesta Potatoes,** 1 serving | 8 |
| **Cinnamon Twists,** 1 serving | 5 |
| **Mexican Rice,** 1 serving | 3 |
| **Nachos,** 1 serving | 9 |
| **Nachos BellGrande®,** 1 serving | 20 |
| **Nachos Supreme,** 1 serving | 12 |
| **Pintos 'N Cheese,** 1 serving | 4 |

| ▲ Power Foods | *PointsPlus*™ value |
|---|---|
| **VALUE MENU™** | |
| **1/2 Lb. Cheesy Bean & Rice Burrito,** 1 | 12 |
| **Bean Burrito,** 1 | 9 |
| **Big Taste Taco,** 1 | 11 |
| **Caramel Apple Empanada,** 1 | 8 |
| **Cheese Roll-up,** 1 | 5 |
| **Cheesy Double Beef Burrito,** 1 | 12 |
| **Crunchy Taco,** 1 | 4 |
| **Soft Taco - Beef,** 1 | 5 |
| **Triple Layer Nachos,** 1 serving | 9 |

| ▲ Power Foods | *PointsPlus™* value |
|---|---|

## 10 GRAMS OR LESS OF FAT

| | |
|---|---|
| **Bean Burrito (without cheese),** 1 | 8 |
| **Chicken Softshell Taco,** 1 | 5 |
| **Crispy Taco,** 1 | 5 |
| **Softshell Taco,** 1 | 5 |
| **Taco Burger (without cheese),** 1 | 6 |
| **Texas Style Chili (without cheese),** 1 serving | 4 |

## TACOS

| | |
|---|---|
| **Chicken Softshell Taco with Cheese,** 1 | 4 |
| **Taco Bravo®,** 1 | 9 |
| **Taco Burger,** 1 serving | 7 |

## BURRITOS

| | |
|---|---|
| **Bean Burrito,** 1 | 9 |
| **Beef Grilled Burrito,** 1 | 16 |
| **Beefy Burrito,** 1 | 11 |
| **Chicken & Potato Burrito,** 1 | 12 |
| **Chicken Grilled Burrito,** 1 | 15 |
| **Combination Burrito,** 1 | 10 |
| **Crunchy Chicken and Potato Burrito,** 1 | 16 |
| **Meat & Potato Burrito,** 1 | 13 |
| **Super Burrito,** 1 | 12 |

## CHALUPA

| | |
|---|---|
| **Chipotle Chicken Chalupa,** 1 | 6 |

## SPECIALTIES

| | |
|---|---|
| **Cheese Quesadilla,** 1 | 12 |
| **Chicken Quesadilla,** 1 | 13 |
| **Chicken Taco Salad (without dressing),** 1 serving | 12 |

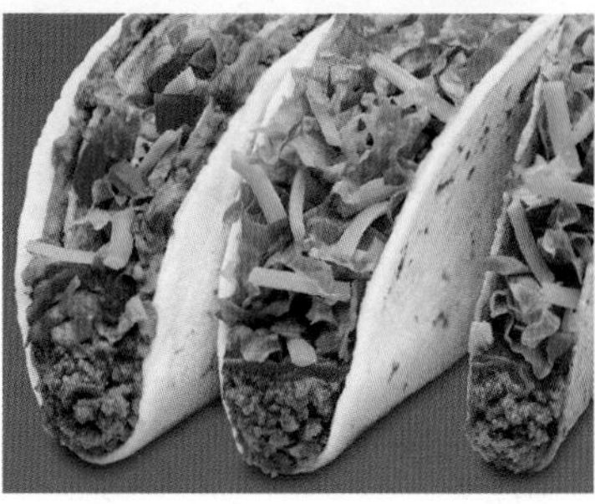

| ▲ Power Foods | *PointsPlus™* value |
|---|---|
| **Crunchy Chicken (without sauce),** 1 serving | 12 |
| **Crunchy Chicken Taco Salad (without dressing),** 1 | 18 |
| **Super Nachos,** 1 small serving | 12 |
| **Super Nachos,** 1 regular serving | 22 |
| **Super Potato Olés®,** 1 small serving | 17 |
| **Super Potato Olés®,** 1 regular serving | 27 |
| **Taco Salad (without dressing),** 1 | 14 |

## LOCAL FAVORITES
(NOT AVAILABLE AT ALL LOCATIONS)

| | |
|---|---|
| **Chili Cheese Potato Olés®,** 1 serving | 16 |
| **Chili Enchilada,** 1 | 8 |
| **Chilito,** 1 | 9 |
| **Mexi Rolls® without Nacho Cheese,** 2 | 3 |
| **Ranch Burrito - Beef,** 1 | 12 |
| **Ranch Burrito - Chicken,** 1 | 10 |
| **Smothered Burrito,** 1 | 13 |

## SIDES

| | |
|---|---|
| **Chili without Crackers,** 1 serving | 6 |
| **Chili without Crackers & Cheese,** 1 serving | 4 |
| **Mexican Rice,** 1 serving | 7 |
| **Nachos,** 1 serving | 11 |

*Sides (cont'd)*

| ▲ Power Foods | *PointsPlus™* value |
|---|---|
| **Potato Olés®,** 1 small serving | 11 |
| **Potato Olés®,** 1 large serving | 20 |
| **Potato Olés® - Kid's Meal/Breakfast Portion,** 1 serving | 8 |
| **Refried Beans,** 1 serving | 7 |
| ▲ **Refried Beans (without cheese),** 1 serving | 6 |
| **Texas Chili without Crackers,** 1 serving | 6 |
| **Texas Chili without Crackers & Cheese,** 1 serving | 4 |

## SNACKS

| | |
|---|---|
| **Buffalo Chicken Snackarito™,** 1 serving | 8 |
| **Chips & Queso,** 1 serving | 12 |
| **Cini-Sopapilla Bites®,** 1 serving | 5 |
| **Ranch Chicken Snackarito™,** 1 serving | 7 |

## CONDIMENTS

| | |
|---|---|
| **Guacamole,** 1 serving | 2 |
| **Hot Sauce,** 1 serving | 0 |
| **Mild Sauce,** 1 serving | 0 |
| **Nacho Cheese,** 1 serving | 3 |
| **Pico de Gallo,** 1 serving | 0 |
| ▲ **Salsa,** 1 serving | 0 |
| **Sour Cream,** 1 serving | 3 |
| **Super Hot Sauce,** 1 serving | 0 |
| **Bacon Ranch Dressing,** 1 serving | 4 |
| **Creamy Italian Dressing,** 1 serving | 4 |
| **House Dressing,** 1 serving | 2 |
| **Ranch Dressing,** 1 serving | 5 |

| ▲ Power Foods | *PointsPlus™* value |
|---|---|

## BREAKFAST MENU®

| | |
|---|---|
| **Breakfast Burrito - Bacon,** 1 | 14 |
| **Breakfast Burrito - Sausage,** 1 | 17 |
| **Breakfast Egg Burrito,** 1 | 11 |
| **Breakfast Egg Burrito - Bacon,** 1 | 13 |
| **Breakfast Egg Burrito - Sausage,** 1 | 16 |
| **Breakfast Taco - Bacon,** 1 | 7 |
| **Breakfast Taco - Sausage,** 1 | 8 |
| **Scrambler Burrito - Bacon,** 1 | 14 |
| **Scrambler Burrito - Sausage,** 1 | 16 |
| **Potato Olés® Scrambler - Bacon,** 1 small | 17 |
| **Potato Olés® Scrambler - Bacon,** 1 regular | 27 |
| **Potato Olés® Scrambler - Sausage,** 1 small | 19 |
| **Potato Olés® Scrambler - Sausage,** 1 regular | 31 |

## DESSERTS

| | |
|---|---|
| **Apple Grande,** 1 serving | 8 |
| **Choco Taco,** 1 | 11 |
| **Churro,** 1 serving | 3 |
| **Giant Goldfish® Grahams,** 1 bag | 2 |

| ▲ Power Foods | *PointsPlus*™ value |
|---|---|

## TACOS

| | |
|---|---|
| **Crisp Ground Beef Taco,** 1 | 7 |
| **Crisp Ground Beef w/sour cream taco,** 1 | 7 |
| **Junior Soft Taco,** 1 | 8 |
| **Soft Chicken Taco,** 1 | 9 |
| **Soft Chicken Taco,** 1 | 6 |
| **Soft Ground Beef Taco,** 1 | 10 |
| **Super Soft Chicken Taco,** 1 | 13 |
| **Super Soft Chicken Taco - wheat tortilla,** 1 serving | 13 |
| **Super Soft Ground Beef Taco,** 1 | 14 |
| **Super Soft Ground Beef Taco - wheat tortilla,** 1 | 15 |

## BURRITOS

| | |
|---|---|
| **Beef Bean & Cheese Burrito,** 1 | 12 |
| **Big Juan® Chicken Burrito,** 1 | 14 |
| **Big Juan® Ground Beef Burrito,** 1 | 16 |
| **Chicken & Black Bean Burrito,** 1 | 12 |
| **Chicken B.L.T. Burrito,** 1 | 18 |
| **Chicken Casita Burrito,** 1 | 12 |
| **Crisp Chicken Burrito,** 1 | 5 |
| **Crisp Ground Beef Burrito,** 1 | 11 |
| **Crisp Pinto Bean Burrito,** 1 | 9 |
| **Crispy Chicken Ranchero Burrito,** 1 | 16 |
| **Ground Beef Casita Burrito,** 1 | 13 |
| **Soft Meat Burrito,** 1 | 5 |
| **Soft Pinto Bean Burrito,** 1 | 9 |
| **Soft Veggie Burrito,** 1 | 13 |

## OTHER FAVORITES

| | |
|---|---|
| **Bean Tostada,** 1 | 6 |
| **Cheddar Melt,** 1 | 6 |
| **Chicken Chimichanga,** 1 | 15 |

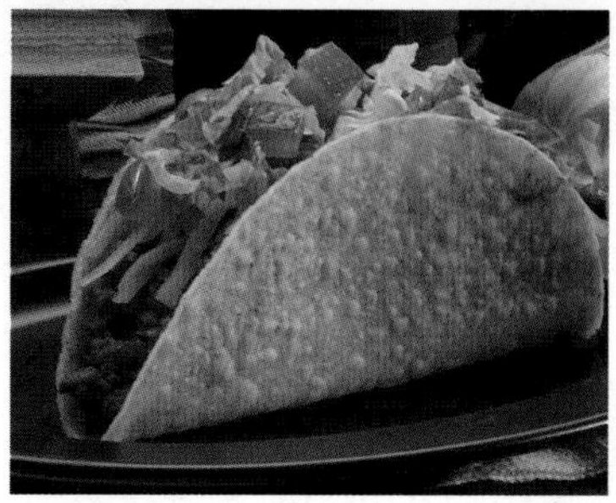

| ▲ Power Foods | *PointsPlus*™ value |
|---|---|
| **Chicken Enchilada,** 1 | 5 |
| **Chicken Tostada,** 1 | 8 |
| **Ground Beef Chimichanga,** 1 | 16 |
| **Ground Beef Enchilada,** 1 | 7 |
| **Ground Beef Tostada,** 1 | 9 |
| **Nachos,** 1 grande | 24 |
| **Taco Burger,** 1 | 12 |

## INDIVIDUAL ITEMS

| | |
|---|---|
| **10" Flour Tortilla,** 1 | 5 |
| **11" Wheat Tortilla,** 1 | 3 |
| **Cheddar Cheese,** 1 serving | 2 |
| **Chipotle Ranch,** 1 serving | 5 |
| **Filing, Crispy Chicken Strips,** 1 | 3 |
| **Filling, Fajita Chicken Strips,** 1 serving | 2 |
| **Filling, Ground Beef,** 1 | 3 |
| **Guacamole,** 1 serving | 1 |
| ▲ **Salsa Fresca,** 1 serving | 0 |
| **Salsa Verde,** 1 serving | 0 |
| **Sour Cream,** 1 serving | 1 |
| **Taco Shells,** 1 | 3 |
| **Thousand Island Dressing,** 1 serving | 4 |
| **Tortilla Salad Bowl, 10",** 1 | 7 |

# TACOTIME®

| ▲ Power Foods | *PointsPlus™* value |
|---|---|
| **SIDES** | |
| **Cheddar Fries,** 1 large serving | 19 |
| **Cheddar Fries,** 1 medium serving | 12 |
| **Cheddar Fries,** 1 small serving | 10 |
| **Mexi Fries®,** 1 large serving | 15 |
| **Mexi Fries®,** 1 small | 7 |
| **Mexi Fries®,** 1 medium serving | 11 |
| **Mexi-Rice,** 1 serving | 2 |
| **Refritos (w/o chips),** 1 | 5 |
| **Refritos (with chips),** 1 | 6 |
| ▲ **Salsa Nuevo,** 1 | 0 |
| **Stuffed Fries,** 1 small serving | 9 |
| **Taco Chips,** 1 serving | 4 |
| **SALADS** | |
| **Chicken Taco Salad, regular,** 1 regular serving | 8 |
| **Ground Beef Taco Salad,** 1 regular serving | 9 |
| **Tostada Delight Chicken Salad,** 1 | 11 |
| **Tostada Delight Ground Beef Salad,** 1 | 12 |
| **DESSERTS** | |
| **Churro with cinnamon & sugar,** 1 | 7 |
| **Churro, plain,** 1 | 6 |
| **Crustos,** 1 | 8 |
| **Empanada (apple),** 1 | 6 |
| **Empanada (cherry),** 1 | 6 |
| **Empanada (pumpkin),** 1 | 7 |

▲ Power Foods — *PointsPlus™* value

## HAND SCOOPED FROZEN YOGURT

|  | *PointsPlus™* value |
|---|---|
| **Blueberries & Cream,** 1/2 cup | 3 |
| **Butter Pecan Frozen,** 1/2 cup | 4 |
| **Chocolate Chocolate,** 1/2 cup | 3 |
| **Chunky Chocolate Cookie Dough,** 1/2 cup | 4 |
| **Peaches & Cream,** 1/2 cup | 3 |
| **Peanut Butter Delight,** 1/2 cup | 5 |
| **Pralines & Cream,** 1/2 cup | 4 |
| **Psychedelic Sorbet,** 1/2 cup | 2 |
| **Rainbow Cream,** 1/2 cup | 3 |
| **Rocky Road,** 1/2 cup | 4 |
| **Strawberries and Cream,** 1/2 cup | 3 |
| **Vanilla Bean,** 1/2 cup | 3 |
| **Vanilla Chocolate Chip,** 1/2 cup | 4 |
| **White Chocolate Mousse,** 1/2 cup | 4 |

## SOFT SERVE FROZEN YOGURT

|  | *PointsPlus™* value |
|---|---|
| **Cake Batter,** 1/2 cup | 3 |
| **Cheesecake,** 1/2 cup | 3 |
| **Chocolate,** 1/2 cup | 3 |
| **Classic Tart,** 1/2 cup | 2 |
| **Coffee,** 1/2 cup | 3 |
| **Fat Free Dutch Chocolate,** 1/2 cup | 3 |
| **Golden Vanilla,** 1/2 cup | 3 |
| **Mango Sorbet,** 1/2 cup | 3 |
| **No Sugar Added Fat Free Chocolate,** 1/2 cup | 3 |

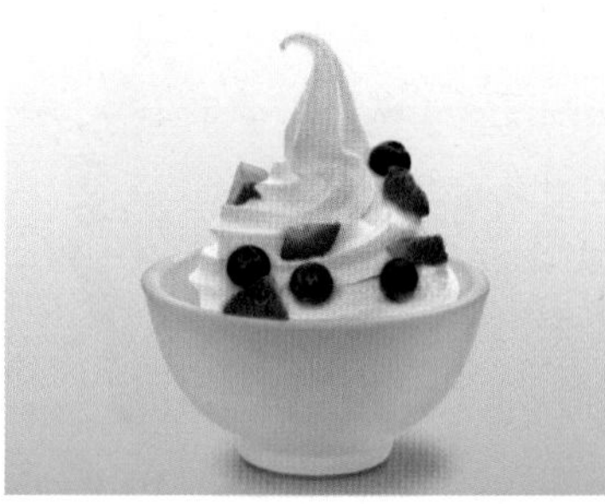

▲ Power Foods — *PointsPlus™* value

|  | *PointsPlus™* value |
|---|---|
| **No Sugar Added Fat Free Mountain Blackberry,** 1/2 cup | 3 |
| **No Sugar Added Fat Free Peach,** 1/2 cup | 3 |
| **No Sugar Added Fat Free Strawberry,** 1/2 cup | 3 |
| **No Sugar Added Fat Free Vanilla,** 1/2 cup | 3 |
| **No Sugar Added White Chocolate Macadamia,** 1/2 cup | 3 |
| **Old Fashioned Vanilla, fat free,** 1/2 cup | 3 |
| **Orange Sorbet,** 1/2 cup | 3 |
| **Peanut Butter,** 1/2 cup | 3 |
| **Raspberry Sorbet,** 1/2 cup | 3 |
| **Strawberry,** 1/2 cup | 3 |
| **Strawberry Kiwi Sorbet,** 1/2 cup | 3 |
| **White Chocolate Mousse,** 1/2 cup | 3 |

# THE EXTREME PITA®

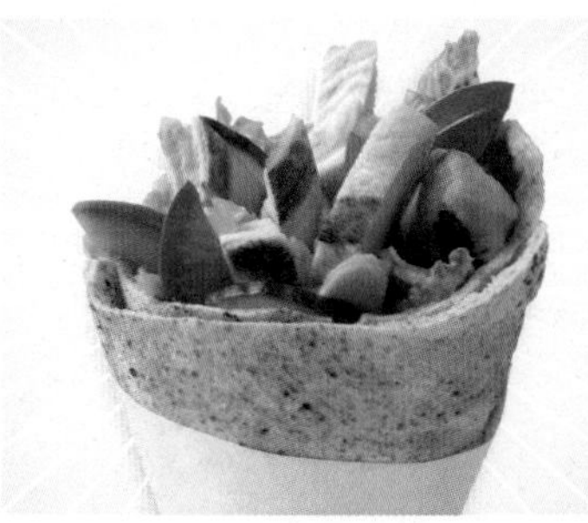

▲ Power Foods — *PointsPlus™* value

## CLASSIC PITAS

| Item | PointsPlus™ value |
|---|---|
| **Big Country (Chicken & Steak),** 1 | 13 |
| **Grilled Steak Pita,** 1 small | 7 |
| **Market Fresh Veggie,** 1 small | 4 |
| **Market Fresh Veggie,** 1 regular | 6 |
| **Meatball Pita,** 1 small | 13 |

## CHEF INSPIRED PITAS

| Item | PointsPlus™ value |
|---|---|
| **Bourbon Chipotle Chicken Pita,** 1 small | 10 |
| **Chicken Caesar,** 1 small | 8 |
| **Chicken Caesar,** 1 regular | 12 |
| **Chicken Souvlaki,** 1 small | 9 |
| **Chicken Souvlaki,** 1 regular | 15 |
| **Fiesta Mexican Pita,** 1 small | 9 |
| **Mandarin Chicken Pita,** 1 small | 9 |
| **Maple Dijon Chicken Pita,** 1 small | 6 |
| **Rustic Italian Pita,** 1 small | 9 |
| **Thai Beef Pita,** 1 small | 8 |
| **Thai Chicken Pita,** 1 small | 7 |

▲ Power Foods — *PointsPlus™* value

## FLAT BAKED PITAS

| Item | PointsPlus™ value |
|---|---|
| **Bourbon Chipotle Chicken,** 1 | 13 |
| **Buffalo Chicken,** 1 | 11 |
| **Extreme Classic,** 1 | 12 |
| **Hawaiian Luau,** 1 | 13 |
| **Mediterranean Chicken,** 1 | 12 |
| **Pepperoni Extreme,** 1 | 11 |
| **Rustic Italian,** 1 | 11 |
| **Thai Beef,** 1 | 13 |
| **Thai Chicken,** 1 | 11 |

## FREESTYLE PITAS

| Item | PointsPlus™ value |
|---|---|
| **Buffalo Chicken,** 1 | 8 |
| **Buffalo Chicken,** 1 regular | 6 |
| **Extreme Club,** 1 small | 7 |
| **Extreme Club,** 1 regular | 10 |
| **Falafel Fanatic,** 1 small | 7 |
| **Falafel Fanatic,** 1 regular | 10 |
| **Grilled Chicken,** 1 small | 6 |
| **Grilled Chicken,** 1 regular | 8 |
| **Gyro,** 1 small | 9 |
| **Gyro,** 1 regular | 14 |
| **Philly Cheese Steak,** 1 small | 7 |
| **Philly Cheese Steak,** 1 regular | 13 |

## PITA BREAD

| Item | PointsPlus™ value |
|---|---|
| **Pita Bread,** 1 small | 4 |
| **Pita Bread,** 1 regular | 5 |

## CHEESE

| Item | PointsPlus™ value |
|---|---|
| **Cheddar Cheese,** 1 regular | 3 |
| **Feta Cheese,** 1 regular | 2 |
| **Mozzarella,** 1 small serving | 1 |
| **Mozzarella,** 1 regular serving | 3 |

| ▲ Power Foods | *PointsPlus*™ value |
|---|---|
| **BREAKFAST PITAS** | |
| **BLT Pita,** 1 | 6 |
| **Ham Pita,** 1 | 5 |
| **Omelette Pita,** 1 | 9 |
| **Eggstreme Pita,** 1 | 7 |
| **Eggstreme Bacon Pita,** 1 | 9 |
| **Eggstreme Ham Pita,** 1 | 9 |
| **SIDES & APPETIZERS** | |
| **Bruschetta Pita,** 1 serving | 6 |
| **Cheesy Garlic Pita with Hummus,** 1 serving | 9 |
| **Hummus Dip,** 1 serving | 4 |
| **Pita Chips,** 1 serving | 4 |
| **Tzatziki Dip,** 1 serving | 2 |
| **SALAD** (WITH DRESSING) | |
| **Traditional Greek Salad,** 1 serving | 10 |
| **SALADS** (WITHOUT DRESSING) | |
| **Grilled Chicken Caesar Salad,** 1 serving | 7 |
| **Mandarin Chicken Salad,** 1 serving | 12 |
| **Maple-Dijon Chicken Salad,** 1 serving | 5 |
| **DRESSINGS & SAUCES** | |
| **Balsamic Vinaigrette Dressing,** 1 small serving | 1 |
| **Greek Feta and Oregano Dressing,** 1 small serving | 2 |
| **Light Caesar Dressing,** 1 small serving | 1 |
| **Light Italian Dressing,** 1 small serving | 0 |
| **Light Ranch Dressing,** 1 small serving | 1 |
| **Maple Dijon Vinaigrette Dressing,** 1 small serving | 1 |
| **Spicy Asian Sesame Dressing,** 1 small serving | 2 |
| **BBQ Sauce Regular,** 1 small serving | 1 |
| **Hot Cajun BBQ Sauce,** 1 side serving | 1 |
| **Hot Cajun BBQ Sauce,** 1 regular serving | 2 |
| **Bistro Sauce,** 1 serving | 4 |
| **Bourbon Chipotle Sauce,** 1 small serving | 1 |
| **Chipotle-Mayonnaise,** 1 small serving | 1 |
| **Chipotle-Mayonnaise,** 1 regular serving | 3 |
| **Light Mayonnaise,** 1 small serving | 1 |
| **Dijonaisse,** 1 small serving | 1 |
| **Honey Mustard,** 1 small serving | 1 |
| **Hummus,** 1 side serving | 1 |
| **Hummus,** 1 regular serving | 2 |
| **Mole Sauce,** 1 small serving | 1 |
| **Sour Cream,** 1 small serving | 1 |
| **Sweet Chili Thai Sauce,** 1 small serving | 1 |
| **Tzatziki Sauce,** 1 regular serving | 1 |
| **Tzatziki Sauce,** 1 small serving | 0 |
| **KIDS MENU** | |
| **6" Cheese Flat Baked Pita,** 1 | 10 |
| **6" Pepperoni Flat Baked Pita,** 1 | 8 |
| **Chicken Pita,** 1 | 6 |
| **Ham and Cheese Pita,** 1 | 7 |
| **Grilled Cheese Wedge,** 1 serving | 9 |
| **Ham & Cheese Wedge,** 1 serving | 8 |

# THE LOOP RESTAURANT

| ▲ Power Foods | *PointsPlus™* value |
|---|---|

## SANDWICHES, HOT DOGS & BURGERS (WITHOUT CONDIMENTS)

| | |
|---|---|
| **BBQ Grilled Chicken Sandwich,** 1 | 17 |
| **BBQ Grilled Chicken Sandwich, without bun,** 1 | 11 |
| **Cajun Grilled Chicken Sandwich,** 1 | 13 |
| **Cajun Grilled Chicken Sandwich, without bun,** 1 | 7 |
| **Cajun Grilled Fish Sandwich,** 1 | 11 |
| **Cajun Grilled Fish Sandwich, without bun,** 1 | 6 |
| **Cajun Grilled Tuna Sandwich,** 1 | 11 |
| **Cajun Grilled Tuna Sandwich, without bun,** 1 | 5 |
| **Grilled Chicken Sandwich,** 1 | 14 |
| **Grilled Chicken Sandwich, without bun,** 1 | 9 |
| **Grilled Fish Sandwich,** 1 | 11 |
| **Grilled Fish Sandwich, without bun,** 1 | 6 |
| **Grilled Teriyaki Chicken Sandwich,** 1 | 12 |
| **Grilled Teriyaki Chicken Sandwich, without Bun,** 1 | 6 |
| **Grilled Tuna Sandwich,** 1 | 11 |
| **Grilled Tuna Sandwich, without bun,** 1 | 6 |
| **Portobello Mushroom Sandwich,** 1 | 9 |
| **Portobello Mushroom Sandwich, without bun,** 1 | 3 |
| **Veggie Melt Focaccia,** 1 | 17 |
| **Sauteed Mushrooms for Sandwiches,** 1 serving | 1 |
| **Hot Dog, Chicago,** 1 | 12 |
| **Hot Dog, Chicago, without bun,** 1 | 8 |
| **Hot Dog, Chili Cheese,** 1 | 16 |
| **Hot Dog, Chili Cheese, without bun,** 1 | 12 |
| **Hot Dog, Plain,** 1 | 11 |
| **Hot Dog, Plain, without bun,** 1 | 7 |
| **Black Bean Burger,** 1 | 10 |
| **Black Bean Burger, without bun,** 1 | 4 |
| **Cheddar Bacon Burger,** 1 | 20 |
| **Cheddar Bacon Burger, without bun,** 1 | 15 |
| **Loop Burger,** 1 | 16 |
| **Loop Burger, without bun,** 1 | 10 |
| **Loop N Bleu Burger,** 1 | 18 |
| **Loop N Bleu Burger, without bun,** 1 | 13 |
| **Loop N Cheese Burger,** 1 | 18 |
| **Loop N Cheese Burger, without bun,** 1 | 12 |
| **Loop N Swiss Burger,** 1 | 18 |
| **Loop N Swiss Burger, without bun,** 1 | 12 |

## WRAPS

| | |
|---|---|
| **Cajun Chicken Wrap,** 1 | 15 |
| **Cajun Chicken Wrap, without wrap,** 1 | 7 |
| **Cajun Fish Wrap,** 1 | 8 |
| **Cajun Fish Wrap, without wrap,** 1 | 5 |
| **Chicken Caesar Wrap,** 1 | 16 |
| **Chicken Caesar Wrap, without wrap,** 1 | 8 |
| **Chicken Salad Wrap,** 1 | 15 |
| **Chicken Salad Wrap, without wrap,** 1 | 7 |

## ENTRÉES (NOT INCLUDING SIDES)

| | |
|---|---|
| **Cajun Chicken,** 1 serving | 4 |
| **Cajun Salmon,** 1 serving | 8 |
| **Cajun Tuna,** 1 serving | 5 |
| **Chicken Fingers,** 1 serving | 22 |
| ▲ **Grilled Chicken,** 1 serving | 5 |
| **Salmon,** 1 serving | 8 |
| ▲ **Tuna,** 1 serving | 5 |

| ▲ Power Foods | PointsPlus™ value |
|---|---|

## SIDES ITEMS

| Item | PointsPlus™ value |
|---|---|
| **Bleu Cheese Chips,** 1 serving | 18 |
| **Focaccia with Marinara Sauce,** 1 slice | 3 |
| **French Fries (served with sandwich),** 1 serving | 7 |
| **French Fries (side order),** 1 serving | 12 |
| **Fruit Salad,** 1 serving | 2 |
| **Onion Rings (served with sandwich),** 1 serving | 9 |
| **Onion Rings (side order),** 1 serving | 14 |
| ▲ **Steamed Veggies,** 1 serving | 1 |

## SPECIALTY PIZZAS (MEDIUM)

| Item | PointsPlus™ value |
|---|---|
| **Artichoke,** 1 slice | 7 |
| **Barbeque,** 1 slice | 8 |
| **Bianco,** 1 slice | 6 |
| **California,** 1 slice | 5 |
| **Cilantro,** 1 slice | 7 |
| **Giardino,** 1 slice | 6 |
| **Grilled Mushroom,** 1 slice | 7 |
| **Margherita,** 1 slice | 6 |
| **Mediterranean,** 1 slice | 6 |
| **Rustica,** 1 slice | 7 |
| **Sausage and Goat Cheese,** 1 slice | 7 |
| **Veggie,** 1 slice | 6 |

## CHEESE PIZZA

| Item | PointsPlus™ value |
|---|---|
| **Thin Crust Cheese Pizza, Medium,** 1 slice | 6 |
| **Thick Crust Cheese Pizza, Medium,** 1 slice | 11 |

## PIZZA TOPPINGS (FOR THIN & THICK CRUST PIZZA)

| Item | PointsPlus™ value |
|---|---|
| **Anchovies,** 1 serving | 0 |
| ▲ **Artichokes,** 1 serving | 0 |
| **Asiago Cheese,** 1 serving | 1 |
| **Bacon,** 1 serving | 1 |
| **Chicken,** 1 serving | 0 |
| **Extra Cheese,** 1 serving | 1 |
| **Extra Marinara Sauce,** 1 serving | 0 |
| **Garlic Cloves, Roasted,** 1 serving | 1 |
| **Goat Cheese,** 1 serving | 0 |
| ▲ **Green Peppers,** 1 serving | 0 |
| **Ground Beef,** 1 serving | 1 |
| **Ham,** 1 serving | 0 |
| ▲ **Jalapenos,** 1 serving | 0 |
| **Mushrooms, Portabello,** 1 serving | 0 |
| **Mushrooms, Sauteed,** 1 serving | 1 |
| **Olives, Black,** 1 serving | 0 |
| **Olives, Kalamata,** 1 serving | 0 |
| **Onions, Caramelized,** 1 serving | 1 |
| **Onions, Sauteed,** 1 serving | 1 |
| **Pepperoni,** 1 serving | 1 |
| **Pork,** 1 serving | 0 |
| ▲ **Red Peppers, Roasted,** 1 serving | 0 |
| **Ricotta Cheese,** 1 serving | 1 |
| **Sausage,** 1 serving | 1 |
| **Spinach, Sauteed,** 1 serving | 1 |
| **Tomatoes, Marinated,** 1 serving | 1 |
| ▲ **Tomatoes, Roma, Sliced,** 1 serving | 0 |
| **Tomatoes, Sun Dried,** 1 serving | 0 |
| **Vegetables, grilled,** 1 serving | 1 |

## SALADS (WITHOUT CROUTONS OR DRESSING)

| Item | PointsPlus™ value |
|---|---|
| **Caesar Salad,** 1 large | 4 |
| **Caesar Salad with Chicken,** 1 large | 7 |
| **Cajun Chicken Salad,** 1 salad | 5 |
| **Crispy Chicken Salad,** 1 salad | 13 |
| **Crunchy Broccoli Salad,** 1 salad | 9 |
| **Gorgonzola Walnut Salad,** 1 salad | 12 |
| **Greek Salad,** 1 large | 5 |
| ▲ **House Salad,** 1 large | 1 |

*Salads (cont'd)*

| ▲ Power Foods | *PointsPlus*™ value |
|---|---|
| **House Salad with Chicken,** 1 salad | 5 |
| **Walnut, Cranberry and Goat Cheese Salad,** 1 salad | 13 |

## SALAD DRESSINGS

| ▲ Power Foods | *PointsPlus*™ value |
|---|---|
| **1000 Island,** 1 serving | 7 |
| **Balsamic Vinaigrette,** 1 serving | 10 |
| **Bleu Cheese,** 1 serving | 6 |
| **Caesar,** 1 serving | 9 |
| **Honey Dijon,** 1 serving | 9 |
| **Honey Dijon, Fat Free,** 1 serving | 2 |
| **Light Italian,** 1 serving | 2 |
| **Lite Ranch,** 1 serving | 6 |
| **Lite Raspberry Vinaigrette,** 1 serving | 4 |
| **Ranch,** 1 serving | 6 |
| **Shallot Vinaigrette,** 1 serving | 9 |
| **Sweet Red Wine Vinaigrette,** 1 serving | 7 |

## SOUPS

| ▲ Power Foods | *PointsPlus*™ value |
|---|---|
| **Beef Pot Roast,** 1 bowl | 5 |
| **Black Bean,** 1 bowl | 4 |
| **Boston Clam Chowder,** 1 bowl | 7 |
| **Broccoli Cheese,** 1 bowl | 7 |
| **Chicken and Dumpling,** 1 bowl | 11 |
| **Chicken Enchilada,** 1 bowl | 8 |
| **Chicken Gumbo,** 1 cup | 2 |
| **Chicken Noodle,** 1 cup | 2 |
| **Chili,** 1 bowl | 14 |
| **French Onion,** 1 bowl | 3 |
| **Italian Style Wedding,** 1 cup | 4 |
| **Minestrone,** 1 cup | 1 |
| **Mushroom and Brie Bisque,** 1 bowl | 7 |
| **Potato with Bacon,** 1 bowl | 7 |
| **Shrimp and Black Bean,** 1 bowl | 4 |
| **Tomato Bisque,** 1 bowl | 9 |
| **Twice Stuffed Baked Potato,** 1 bowl | 11 |
| **Vegetarian Vegetable,** 1 bowl | 2 |

## CRACKERS & CONDIMENTS

| ▲ Power Foods | *PointsPlus*™ value |
|---|---|
| **Crackers, Melba Snacks,** 1 pack | 1 |
| **Crackers, Premium Gold,** 1 pack | 1 |
| **Crackers, Sesame Bread Wafers,** 1 pack | 1 |
| **Crackers, Sesame Breadsticks,** 1 pack | 1 |
| **Croutons,** 1/3 cup | 2 |
| **Croutons,** 1/2 cup | 3 |
| **Oyster Crackers,** 1 package | 2 |
| **A-1 Steak Sauce,** 1 Tbsp | 0 |
| **Cholula Hot Sauce,** 1 tsp | 0 |
| **Dipping Sauce for Onion Rings,** 1 serving | 13 |
| **Garlic Mayonnaise,** 1 serving | 9 |
| **Grey Poupon Mustard,** 1 tsp | 0 |
| **Heinz 57 Steak Sauce,** 1 Tbsp | 0 |
| **Ketchup,** 1 serving | 2 |
| **Lemon Dill Mayonnaise,** 1 serving | 8 |
| **Louisiana Hot Sauce,** 1 tsp | 0 |
| **Mayonnaise,** 1 Tbsp | 3 |
| **Mustard,** 1 tsp | 0 |
| **Tartar Sauce,** 1 serving | 6 |

## KIDS MENU (WITHOUT SIDE ITEMS)

| ▲ Power Foods | *PointsPlus*™ value |
|---|---|
| **Kids Burger,** 1 | 11 |
| **Kids Chicken Fingers,** 1 serving | 13 |
| **Kids Fries,** 1 serving | 5 |
| **Kids Grilled Cheese,** 1 sandwich | 12 |
| **Kids Hot Dog,** 1 | 11 |
| **Kids Mac N Cheese,** 1 serving | 9 |

## MILKSHAKES

| ▲ Power Foods | *PointsPlus*™ value |
|---|---|
| **Butterfinger,** 1 | 37 |
| **Chocolate,** 1 | 28 |
| **Oreo,** 1 | 36 |
| **Strawberry,** 1 | 25 |
| **Vanilla,** 1 | 23 |

| ▲ Power Foods | *PointsPlus*™ value |
|---|---|

## DESSERTS

| | |
|---|---|
| **Brownie,** 1 | 11 |
| **Carrot Cake,** 1 piece | 27 |
| **Cheesecake,** 1 piece | 14 |
| **Chocolate Cake,** 1 piece | 22 |
| **Crème Brulee Cheesecake,** 1 slice | 17 |
| **Key Lime Pie,** 1 slice | 16 |
| **Marble Cheesecake,** 1 slice | 18 |
| **Tiramisu,** 1 slice | 14 |
| **Chocolate Chip Cookie,** 1 cookie | 10 |
| **Chocolate Chunk Cookie, Regular,** 1 cookie | 10 |
| **Chocolate Chunk Cookie, Large,** 1 cookie | 17 |
| **Oatmeal Raisin Cookie,** 1 cookie | 6 |
| **Peanut Butter Cookie,** 1 cookie | 11 |
| **White Chocolate Macadamia Nut Cookie,** 1 cookie | 11 |

## BEVERAGES

| | |
|---|---|
| **Coke,** 1 serving | 5 |
| **Diet Coke,** 1 serving | 0 |
| **Light Lemonade,** 1 serving | 0 |
| **Pink Lemonade,** 1 serving | 5 |
| **Root Beer,** 1 serving | 6 |
| **Sprite,** 1 serving | 5 |

# TIM HORTONS®

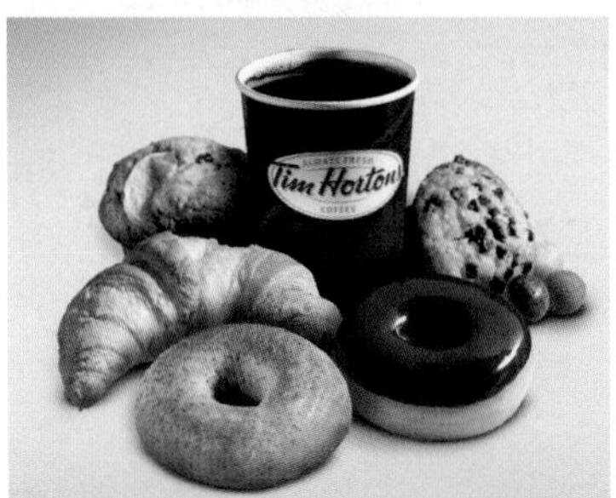


▲ Power Foods — *PointsPlus*™ value

## YEAST DONUTS

| | |
|---|---|
| **Apple Fritter Donut,** 1 | 8 |
| **Blueberry Fritter Donut,** 1 | 9 |
| **Chocolate Dip Donut,** 1 | 6 |
| **Honey Dip Donut,** 1 | 6 |
| **Maple Dip Donut,** 1 | 6 |

## CAKE DONUTS

| | |
|---|---|
| **Chocolate Glazed Donut,** 1 | 7 |
| **Old Fashion Glazed Donut,** 1 | 9 |
| **Old Fashion Plain Donut,** 1 | 7 |
| **Sour Cream Plain Donut,** 1 | 7 |

## FILLED DONUTS

| | |
|---|---|
| **Angel Cream Donut,** 1 | 9 |
| **Blueberry Donut,** 1 | 6 |
| **Boston Cream Donut,** 1 | 7 |
| **Canadian Maple Donut,** 1 | 7 |
| **Strawberry Filled Donut,** 1 | 6 |

## OTHER DONUTS

| | |
|---|---|
| **Honey Cruller,** 1 | 9 |
| **Walnut Crunch Donut,** 1 | 10 |

▲ Power Foods — *PointsPlus*™ value

## YEAST TIMBITS®

| | |
|---|---|
| **Honey Dip Timbit,** 1 | 2 |

## CAKE TIMBITS®

| | |
|---|---|
| **Chocolate Glazed Timbit,** 1 | 2 |
| **Old Fashion Plain Timbit,** 1 | 2 |
| **Sour Cream Glazed Timbit,** 1 | 3 |

## FILLED TIMBITS®

| | |
|---|---|
| **Banana Cream Timbit,** 1 | 2 |
| **Blueberry Timbit,** 1 | 2 |
| **Lemon Timbit,** 1 | 2 |
| **Strawberry Filled Timbit,** 1 | 2 |

## MUFFINS

| | |
|---|---|
| **Banana Nut,** 1 muffin | 11 |
| **Blueberry,** 1 muffin | 9 |
| **Blueberry Bran,** 1 muffin | 8 |
| **Chocolate Chip,** 1 muffin | 12 |
| **Cranberry Blueberry Bran,** 1 muffin | 8 |
| **Cranberry Fruit,** 1 muffin | 10 |
| **Fruit Explosion,** 1 muffin | 10 |
| **Low Fat Blueberry,** 1 muffin | 8 |
| **Low Fat Cranberry,** 1 muffin | 8 |
| **Raisin Bran,** 1 muffin | 10 |
| **Strawberry Sensation,** 1 muffin | 10 |
| **Wheat Carrot,** 1 muffin | 11 |
| **Whole Grain Raspberry,** 1 muffin | 11 |

## BAGELS (WITHOUT SPREAD)

| | |
|---|---|
| **Blueberry,** 1 | 7 |
| **Cinnamon Raisin,** 1 | 7 |
| **Everything,** 1 | 7 |
| **Onion,** 1 | 7 |

| ▲ Power Foods | *PointsPlus*™ value |
|---|---|
| **Plain,** 1 | 7 |
| **Poppy Seed,** 1 | 7 |
| **Sesame Seed,** 1 | 7 |
| **Twelve Grain Bagel,** 1 | 8 |
| **Wheat & Honey Bagel,** 1 | 8 |

## CREAM CHEESE

| | |
|---|---|
| **Garlic and Herb,** 1 serving | 4 |
| **Light Plain Cream Cheese,** 3 Tbsp | 2 |
| **Light Strawberry Cream Cheese,** 3 Tbsp | 3 |
| **Plain Cream Cheese,** 3 Tbsp | 3 |

## BREAKFAST

| | |
|---|---|
| **Bacon, Egg, and Cheese,** 1 sandwich | 11 |
| **Bagel BELT™,** 1 serving | 12 |
| **Egg and Cheese,** 1 sandwich | 10 |
| **Hash Brown,** 1 serving | 3 |
| **Sausage, Egg, and Cheese,** 1 sandwich | 14 |

## TIM'S OWN® SANDWICHES

| | |
|---|---|
| **BLT,** 1 sandwich | 12 |
| **Chicken Salad,** 1 sandwich | 10 |
| **Egg Salad,** 1 sandwich | 10 |
| **Ham & Swiss,** 1 sandwich | 11 |
| **Toasted Chicken Club (with lettuce, tomato, bacon & honey mustard),** 1 sandwich | 12 |
| **Turkey Bacon Club,** 1 sandwich | 11 |

## COUNTRY BUNS

| | |
|---|---|
| **White,** 1 | 6 |
| **Whole Wheat,** 1 | 6 |

| ▲ Power Foods | *PointsPlus*™ value |
|---|---|

## SOUPS, STEW & CHILI

| | |
|---|---|
| **Beef Noodle,** 1 bowl | 3 |
| **Chicken Noodle,** 1 bowl | 3 |
| **Cream of Broccoli,** 1 bowl | 5 |
| **Creamy Field Mushroom,** 1 bowl | 4 |
| **Hearty Potato Bacon,** 1 bowl | 6 |
| **Hearty Vegetable,** 1 bowl | 2 |
| **Minestrone,** 1 bowl | 4 |
| **Split Pea with Ham,** 1 bowl | 4 |
| **Turkey and Wild Rice,** 1 bowl | 3 |
| **Vegetable Beef Barley,** 1 bowl | 3 |
| **Chili,** 1 bowl | 9 |
| **Beef Stew,** 1 bowl | 6 |

## YOGURT & BERRIES

| | |
|---|---|
| **Creamy Vanilla Yogurt and Berries,** 1 serving | 4 |
| **Strawberry Yogurt and Berries,** 1 serving | 4 |

## SNACKS & BAKED GOODS

| | |
|---|---|
| **Apple Fritter,** 1 | 8 |
| **Cheese Croissant,** 1 | 6 |
| **Cherry Cheese Danish,** 1 | 6 |
| **Chocolate Danish,** 1 | 9 |
| **Cinnamon Roll - Frosted,** 1 | 13 |
| **Cinnamon Roll - Glazed,** 1 | 12 |
| **Maple Pecan Danish,** 1 | 8 |
| **Plain Croissant,** 1 | 6 |
| **Plain Tea Biscuits,** 1 | 6 |
| **Raisin Tea Biscuit,** 1 | 8 |

# TIM HORTONS®

| ▲ Power Foods | *PointsPlus*™ value |
| --- | --- |
| **COOKIES** | |
| **Caramel Chocolate Pecan,** 1 cookie | 6 |
| **Chocolate Chunk,** 1 cookie | 6 |
| **Oatmeal Raisin Spice Cookie,** 1 | 6 |
| **Peanut Butter,** 1 cookie | 7 |
| **Peanut Butter Cookie,** 1 | 7 |
| **Triple Chocolate Cookie,** 1 | 7 |
| **White Chocolate Macadamia Nut,** 1 cookie | 7 |
| **BEVERAGES** | |
| **Café Mocha,** 1 cup | 5 |
| **English Toffee,** 1 cup | 6 |
| **English Toffee Cappuccino,** 1 cup | 6 |
| **French Vanilla,** 1 cup | 6 |
| **French Vanilla Cappuccino,** 1 cup | 7 |
| **Hot Chocolate,** 1 cup | 6 |
| **Hot Smoothee,** 1 cup | 7 |
| **Iced Cappuccino,** 1 cup | 7 |
| **Iced Cappuccino with milk,** 1 cup | 4 |
| **Flavor Shot,** 1 serving | 0 |

▲ Power Foods — *PointsPlus™* value

## BURGER SUBS
(WITHOUT DRESSING & ADDITIONAL CHEESE)

|  | PointsPlus™ value |
|---|---|
| **All American Cheeseburger,** 1 small | 15 |
| **All American Cheeseburger,** 1 regular | 22 |
| **All American Cheeseburger,** 1 large | 29 |
| **Big Tub,** 1 small | 18 |
| **Big Tub,** 1 regular | 23 |
| **Big Tub,** 1 large | 42 |
| **Burger Special,** 1 small | 17 |
| **Burger Special,** 1 regular | 25 |
| **Burger Special,** 1 large | 36 |
| **Cheeseburger,** 1 small | 16 |
| **Cheeseburger,** 1 regular | 25 |
| **Cheeseburger,** 1 large | 34 |
| **Mushroom Burger,** 1 small | 17 |
| **Mushroom Burger,** 1 regular | 24 |
| **Mushroom Burger,** 1 large | 35 |
| **Pizza Burger,** 1 small | 17 |
| **Pizza Burger,** 1 regular | 25 |
| **Pizza Burger,** 1 large | 35 |
| **Taco,** 1 small | 15 |
| **Taco,** 1 regular | 23 |
| **Taco,** 1 large | 30 |

## BURGER SUB WRAPS
(WITHOUT DRESSING & ADDITIONAL CHEESE)

|  | PointsPlus™ value |
|---|---|
| **All American Cheeseburger,** 1 small | 12 |
| **All American Cheeseburger,** 1 regular | 17 |
| **All American Cheeseburger,** 1 large | 25 |
| **Big Tub,** 1 small | 15 |
| **Big Tub,** 1 regular | 20 |
| **Big Tub,** 1 large | 30 |
| **Burger Special,** 1 small | 15 |
| **Burger Special,** 1 regular | 20 |
| **Burger Special,** 1 large | 32 |
| **Cheeseburger,** 1 small | 14 |
| **Cheeseburger,** 1 regular | 26 |
| **Cheeseburger,** 1 large | 30 |

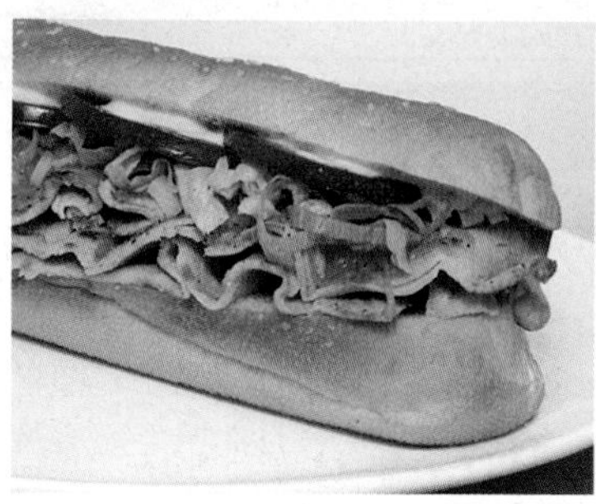

▲ Power Foods — *PointsPlus™* value

|  | PointsPlus™ value |
|---|---|
| **Mushroom Burger,** 1 small | 14 |
| **Mushroom Burger,** 1 regular | 21 |
| **Mushroom Burger,** 1 large | 30 |
| **Pizza Burger,** 1 small | 14 |
| **Pizza Burger,** 1 regular | 27 |
| **Pizza Burger,** 1 large | 31 |
| **Taco,** 1 small | 13 |
| **Taco,** 1 regular | 20 |
| **Taco,** 1 large | 26 |

## CHICKEN SUBS
(WITHOUT DRESSING & ADDITIONAL CHEESE)

|  | PointsPlus™ value |
|---|---|
| **Chicken & Broccoli,** 1 small | 12 |
| **Chicken & Broccoli,** 1 regular | 15 |
| **Chicken & Broccoli,** 1 large | 22 |
| **Chicken & Cheddar,** 1 small | 11 |
| **Chicken & Cheddar,** 1 regular | 15 |
| **Chicken & Cheddar,** 1 large | 22 |
| **Chicken Club,** 1 small | 14 |
| **Chicken Club,** 1 regular | 19 |
| **Chicken Club,** 1 large | 31 |
| **Chicken Parmesan,** 1 small | 8 |
| **Chicken Parmesan,** 1 regular | 12 |
| **Chicken Parmesan,** 1 large | 17 |
| **Grilled Chicken,** 1 small | 6 |
| **Grilled Chicken,** 1 regular | 9 |
| **Grilled Chicken,** 1 large | 11 |

# TUBBY'S® GRILLED SANDWICHES

| ▲ Power Foods | *PointsPlus*™ value |
|---|---|
| **CHICKEN SUB WRAPS** (WITHOUT DRESSING & ADDITIONAL CHEESE) | |
| **Chicken & Broccoli,** 1 small | 8 |
| **Chicken & Broccoli,** 1 large | 17 |
| **Chicken & Broccoli,** 1 regular | 15 |
| **Chicken & Cheddar,** 1 small | 8 |
| **Chicken & Cheddar,** 1 large | 16 |
| **Chicken & Cheddar,** 1 regular | 12 |
| **Chicken Club,** 1 small | 11 |
| **Chicken Club,** 1 regular | 16 |
| **Chicken Club,** 1 large | 25 |
| **Chicken Parmesan,** 1 small | 5 |
| **Chicken Parmesan,** 1 regular | 9 |
| **Chicken Parmesan,** 1 large | 12 |
| **Grilled Chicken,** 1 small | 3 |
| **Grilled Chicken,** 1 regular | 6 |
| **Grilled Chicken,** 1 large | 7 |
| **DELI SUBS** (WITHOUT DRESSING & ADDITIONAL CHEESE) | |
| **Club Sub,** 1 small | 13 |
| **Club Sub,** 1 regular | 19 |
| **Club Sub,** 1 large | 29 |
| **Famous,** 1 small | 13 |
| **Famous,** 1 regular | 18 |
| **Famous,** 1 large | 27 |
| **Ham & Cheese,** 1 small | 11 |
| **Ham & Cheese,** 1 regular | 16 |
| **Ham & Cheese,** 1 large | 24 |
| **Turkey & Cheese,** 1 small | 11 |
| **Turkey Club,** 1 small | 13 |
| **Turkey Club,** 1 regular | 18 |
| **Turkey Club,** 1 large | 28 |

| ▲ Power Foods | *PointsPlus*™ value |
|---|---|
| **DELI SUB WRAPS** (WITHOUT DRESSING & ADDITIONAL CHEESE) | |
| **Club Sub,** 1 small | 11 |
| **Club Sub,** 1 regular | 16 |
| **Club Sub,** 1 large | 25 |
| **Famous,** 1 small | 10 |
| **Famous,** 1 regular | 15 |
| **Famous,** 1 large | 23 |
| **Ham & Cheese,** 1 small | 9 |
| **Ham & Cheese,** 1 regular | 13 |
| **Ham & Cheese,** 1 large | 19 |
| **Turkey & Cheese,** 1 small | 9 |
| **Turkey & Cheese,** 1 regular | 13 |
| **Turkey & Cheese,** 1 large | 21 |
| **Turkey Club,** 1 small | 11 |
| **Turkey Club,** 1 regular | 16 |
| **Turkey Club,** 1 large | 24 |
| **STEAK SUBS** (WITHOUT DRESSING & ADDITIONAL CHEESE) | |
| **Mushroom Steak,** 1 small | 16 |
| **Mushroom Steak,** 1 regular | 13 |
| **Mushroom Steak,** 1 large | 33 |
| **Pepper Steak,** 1 small | 16 |
| **Pepper Steak,** 1 regular | 20 |
| **Pepper Steak,** 1 large | 33 |
| **Philly Cheesesteak,** 1 small | 13 |
| **Philly Cheesesteak,** 1 regular | 19 |
| **Philly Cheesesteak,** 1 large | 24 |
| **Pizza Steak,** 1 small | 16 |
| **Pizza Steak,** 1 regular | 27 |
| **Pizza Steak,** 1 large | 34 |
| **Portabella Mushroom,** 1 small | 14 |

| ▲ Power Foods | *PointsPlus™* value |
|---|---|
| **Portabella Mushroom,** 1 regular | 22 |
| **Portabella Mushroom,** 1 large | 30 |
| **Steak & Cheddar,** 1 small | 16 |
| **Steak & Cheddar,** 1 large | 46 |
| **Steak Cheddar,** 1 regular | 23 |
| **Steak Special,** 1 small | 17 |
| **Steak Special,** 1 regular | 20 |
| **Steak Special,** 1 large | 35 |

## STEAK SUB WRAPS
(WITHOUT DRESSING & ADDITIONAL CHEESE)

| | |
|---|---|
| **Mushroom Steak,** 1 small | 14 |
| **Mushroom Steak,** 1 regular | 20 |
| **Mushroom Steak,** 1 large | 29 |
| **Pepper Steak,** 1 small | 13 |
| **Pepper Steak,** 1 regular | 17 |
| **Pepper Steak,** 1 large | 29 |
| **Philly Cheesesteak,** 1 small | 10 |
| **Philly Cheesesteak,** 1 regular | 16 |
| **Philly Cheesesteak,** 1 large | 19 |
| **Pizza Steak,** 1 small | 13 |
| **Pizza Steak,** 1 large | 30 |
| **Pizza Steak,** 1 regular | 20 |
| **Portabella Mushroom,** 1 small | 16 |
| **Portabella Mushroom,** 1 regular | 18 |
| **Portabella Mushroom,** 1 large | 25 |
| **Steak & Cheddar,** 1 small | 13 |
| **Steak & Cheddar,** 1 regular | 20 |
| **Steak & Cheddar,** 1 large | 42 |
| **Steak & Cheese,** 1 small | 13 |
| **Steak & Cheese,** 1 regular | 20 |
| **Steak & Cheese,** 1 large | 29 |
| **Steak Special,** 1 small | 14 |
| **Steak Special,** 1 regular | 17 |
| **Steak Special,** 1 large | 31 |

| ▲ Power Foods | *PointsPlus™* value |
|---|---|

## SPECIALTY SUBS
(WITHOUT DRESSING & ADDITIONAL CHEESE)

| | |
|---|---|
| **BLT,** 1 small | 13 |
| **BLT,** 1 regular | 18 |
| **BLT,** 1 large | 32 |
| **Cold Veggie,** 1 regular | 12 |
| **Cold Veggie,** 1 large | 16 |
| **Italian Sausage,** 1 small | 14 |
| **Italian Sausage,** 1 regular | 20 |
| **Italian Sausage,** 1 large | 30 |
| **Tuna,** 1 small | 9 |
| **Tuna,** 1 regular | 13 |
| **Tuna,** 1 large | 17 |
| **Veggie Stir Fry,** 1 small | 10 |
| **Veggie Stir Fry,** 1 regular | 18 |
| **Veggie Stir Fry,** 1 large | 26 |

## SPECIALTY SUB WRAPS
(WITHOUT DRESSING & ADDITIONAL CHEESE)

| | |
|---|---|
| **BLT,** 1 small | 10 |
| **BLT,** 1 regular | 15 |
| **BLT,** 1 large | 24 |
| **Cold Veggie,** 1 small | 4 |
| **Cold Veggie,** 1 regular | 9 |
| **Cold Veggie,** 1 large | 12 |
| **Italian Sausage,** 1 small | 12 |
| **Italian Sausage,** 1 regular | 17 |
| **Italian Sausage,** 1 large | 25 |
| **Tuna,** 1 small | 7 |
| **Tuna,** 1 regular | 10 |
| **Tuna,** 1 large | 13 |
| **Veggie Stir Fry,** 1 small | 7 |
| **Veggie Stir Fry,** 1 regular | 11 |
| **Veggie Stir Fry,** 1 large | 17 |

# UNO® CHICAGO GRILL

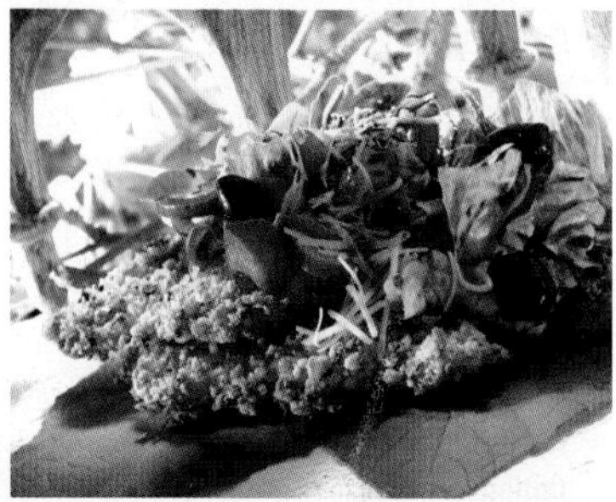

| ▲ Power Foods | *PointsPlus*™ value |
|---|---|
| **APPS** | |
| **Buffalo Bites (without sauce),** 1/3 order | 9 |
| **Buffalo Chicken Quesadilla,** 1/3 order | 10 |
| **Buffalo Wings,** 1/3 order | 12 |
| **Chi-Town Tasting Plate,** 1/4 order | 14 |
| **Crispy Cheese Dippers,** 1/3 order | 8 |
| **Muchos Nachos,** 1/3 order | 12 |
| **Onion Strings,** 1/3 order | 16 |
| **Pizza Skins,** 1/5 order | 13 |
| **Roasted Veggie Quesadilla,** 1/3 order | 8 |
| **Shrimp & Crab Fondue,** 1/5 order | 6 |
| **Steak Quesadilla,** 1/3 order | 10 |
| **SANDWICHES & BURGERS** (WITHOUT SIDES) | |
| **Firecracker Chicken Sandwich,** 1 serving (order serves 1 1/2) | 12 |
| **Grilled Chicken Sandwich,** 1 serving (order serves 1 1/2) | 10 |
| **Steak & Cheese Sandwich,** 1 serving (order serves 1 1/2) | 18 |
| **Turkey Bacon Swiss Sandwich,** 1 serving (order serves 1 1/2) | 16 |

| ▲ Power Foods | *PointsPlus*™ value |
|---|---|
| **Buffalo Chicken Panini,** 1 serving (order serves 1 1/2) | 17 |
| **It's All Greek to Me Panini,** 1 serving (order serves 1 1/2) | 14 |
| **Southwest Steak Panini,** 1 serving (order serves 1 1/2) | 19 |
| **Burger Sliders,** 1/2 order | 16 |
| **Philly Burger,** 1 serving (order serves 1 1/2) | 15 |
| **Uno® Burger,** 1 serving (order serves 2) | 14 |
| **Uno® Burger with Cheese,** 1 serving (order serves 2) | 16 |
| **Veggie Burger,** 1 serving (order serves 2) | 7 |
| **BIG BOWLS & LITTLE GREENS** (WITHOUT CRACKERS) | |
| **Balsamic Vinaigrette,** 1 serving | 6 |
| **Caesar Side Salad, with dressing,** 1 serving | 7 |
| **Gorgonzola Walnut Side Salad,** 1 serving | 8 |
| **House Side Salad,** 1 serving | 2 |
| **Blue Cheese Dressing,** 1 serving | 8 |
| **Blueberry Pomegranate Vinaigrette, low fat,** 1 serving | 2 |
| **Caesar Dressing,** 1 serving | 8 |
| **Classic Vinaigrette,** 1 serving | 5 |
| **Fat Free Vinaigrette,** 1 serving | 0 |
| **Honey Mustard,** 1 serving | 9 |
| **Ranch Dressing,** 1 serving | 7 |
| **French Onion Soup,** 1 serving | 6 |
| **New England Clam Chowder,** 1 serving | 8 |
| **Veggie Soup,** 1 serving (order serves 1 1/2) | 2 |
| **Windy City Chili,** 1 serving (order serves 1 1/2) | 7 |

| Power Foods | PointsPlus™ value |
|---|---|

## BIG GREENS (WITHOUT BREADSTICK)

| Item | PointsPlus™ value |
|---|---|
| **Asian Chicken Salad, with dressing,** 1 serving | 14 |
| **Caesar Salad, with dressing,** 1/2 order | 6 |
| **Chicken Caesar Salad, with dressing,** 1/2 order | 8 |
| **Chopped Mediterranean Grilled Shrimp Salad, with dressing,** 1/2 order | 9 |
| **Classic Cobb Salad, with dressing,** 1/2 order | 12 |
| **Honey Crisp Chicken Salad, with dressing,** 1/2 order | 11 |
| **House Salad with Grilled Chicken, without dressing,** 1/2 order | 3 |
| **House Salad, without dressing,** 1/2 order | 1 |
| **Spinach, Chicken and Gorgonzola, with dressing,** 1/2 order | 10 |

## CHICKEN (WITHOUT BREADSTICK OR SIDES)

| Item | PointsPlus™ value |
|---|---|
| **Baked Stuffed Chicken,** 1/2 order | 5 |
| **Chicken Milanese,** 1/2 order | 12 |
| **Chicken Parmesan,** 1/2 order | 15 |
| **Chicken Thumb Platter®,** 1/2 order | 7 |
| **Grilled Chicken with Mango Salsa,** 1/2 order | 3 |
| **Grilled Rosemary Chicken,** 1/2 order | 7 |

## PASTA (WITHOUT BREADSTICK)

| Item | PointsPlus™ value |
|---|---|
| **Chicken & Broccoli Fettuccine,** 1/2 order | 18 |
| **Chicken and Penne with Chablis White Wine,** 1/2 order | 13 |
| **Chicken Spinoccoli®,** 1/2 order | 18 |
| **Penne Bolognese,** 1/2 order | 10 |
| **Rattlesnake Pasta,** 1/2 order | 18 |
| **Shrimp Scampi,** 1/2 order | 15 |
| **Tortellaci,** 1/2 order | 13 |
| **Tuscan Chicken Penne,** 1/2 order | 16 |
| **Tuscan Roasted Vegetable Penne,** 1/2 order | 14 |

## FLATBREAD PIZZAS

| Item | PointsPlus™ value |
|---|---|
| **BBQ Chicken Flatbread,** 1/3 pizza | 9 |
| **Cheese & Tomato Flatbread,** 1/3 pizza | 7 |
| **Mediterranean Flatbread,** 1/3 pizza | 8 |
| **Pepperoni Flatbread,** 1/3 pizza | 9 |
| **Roasted Eggplant, Spinach & Feta Flatbread,** 1/3 pizza | 7 |
| **Sausage Flatbread,** 1/3 pizza | 9 |
| **Spicy Chicken Flatbread,** 1/3 pizza | 10 |
| **Spinach, Mushroom & Gorgonzola Flatbread,** 1/3 pizza | 8 |

## DEEP DISH PIZZAS

| Item | PointsPlus™ value |
|---|---|
| **Cheese & Tomato Deep Dish Pizza,** 1/3 pizza | 16 |
| **Chicago Classic Deep Dish Pizza,** 1/3 pizza | 21 |
| **Farmer's Market Vegetable Deep Dish Pizza,** 1/3 pizza | 15 |
| **Numero Uno Deep Dish Pizza,** 1/3 pizza | 18 |
| **Prima Pepperoni Deep Dish Pizza,** 1/3 pizza | 17 |
| **Spinoccoli Deep Dish Pizza,** 1/3 pizza | 17 |

## GLUTEN FREE PIZZAS

| Item | PointsPlus™ value |
|---|---|
| **Gluten Free Cheese Pizza,** 1/3 pizza | 8 |
| **Gluten Free Pepperoni Pizza,** 1/3 pizza | 9 |
| **Gluten Free Vegie Pizza,** 1/3 pizza | 9 |

# UNO® CHICAGO GRILL

| ▲ Power Foods | *PointsPlus*™ value |
|---|---|
| **SMOKE, SIZZLE & SPLASH (WITHOUT BREADSTICK OR SIDES)** | |
| ▲ **10 oz Top Sirloin,** 1 serving (order serves 2) | 6 |
| **Baked Haddock,** 1 serving (order serves 2) | 7 |
| **BBQ Shrimp, Grilled & Skewered,** 1 serving (order serves 2) | 4 |
| **Brewmasters Grill NY Sirloin,** 1 serving (order serves 2) | 7 |
| **Fish & Chips Platter,** 1 serving (order serves 2) | 12 |
| **Grilled BBQ Salmon,** 1 serving (order serves 2) | 8 |
| **Grilled Shrimp and Sirloin,** 1 serving (order serves 2) | 8 |
| **Lemon Basil Salmon,** 1 serving (order serves 2) | 6 |
| **Salmon, Shrimp and Haddock Combo,** 1 serving (order serves 2) | 20 |
| **Sirloin Steak Tips,** 1 serving (order serves 2) | 7 |
| ▲ **Sirloin, 8 oz,** 1 serving (order serves 2) | 5 |
| **SATISFYIN' SIDES** | |
| **Brown Rice with Ocean Spray Sweetened Dried Cranberries and Mango,** 1 serving | 5 |
| **French Fries,** 1 serving | 12 |
| **Mashed Potato,** 1 serving | 9 |
| **Rice Pilaf,** 1 serving | 6 |
| **Roasted Seasonal Vegetables,** 1 serving | 2 |
| **Skinless Baked Potato,** 1 serving | 13 |
| **Steamed Broccoli,** 1 serving | 2 |
| **Steamed Seasonal Vegetables,** 1 serving | 3 |
| **Uno Breadstick,** 1 serving | 6 |

| ▲ Power Foods | *PointsPlus*™ value |
|---|---|
| **FREEZERS** | |
| **Chocolate Cookie Freezer,** 1 serving | 13 |
| **Chocolate Monkey,** 1 serving | 9 |
| **Raspberry Lime Ricky,** 1 serving | 5 |
| **Strawberry Smoothie,** 1 serving | 8 |
| **Tropical Fruit,** 1 serving | 9 |
| **DESSERTS** | |
| **All American,** 1/2 order | 8 |
| **Brownie Bowl,** 1/2 order | 12 |
| **Chicago Cheesecake,** 1/2 order | 13 |
| **Mini All American Hot Apple Crumble,** 1 serving | 9 |
| **Mini Hot Chocolate Brownie Sundae,** 1 serving | 10 |
| **Mini Macadamia Nut White Chocolate Chunk Deep Dish Sundae,** 1 serving | 20 |
| **Uno Deep Dish Sundae,** 1/2 order | 19 |

| ▲ Power Foods | *PointsPlus™* value |
|---|---|
| **6" SANDWICHES** | |
| **Baked Chicken Grinder,** 1 | 14 |
| **Baked Chicken Grinder (without mayonnaise, cheese, or dressing),** 1 | 7 |
| **BLT Grinder (without mayonnaise, cheese, or dressing),** 1 | 12 |
| **Buffalo Chicken Grinder (without dressing or cheese),** 1 | 10 |
| **Cheesesteak Grinder,** 1 | 18 |
| **Chicken Cordon Bleu Grinder,** 1 | 17 |
| **Chicken Cordon Bleu Grinder (without mayonnaise, cheese, or dressing),** 1 | 13 |
| **Chicken Parmesan Grinder,** 1 | 17 |
| **Chicken Parmesan Grinder (without mayonnaise, cheese, or dressing),** 1 | 12 |
| **Chicken Salad Grinder,** 1 | 23 |
| **Chicken Salad Grinder (without dressing or cheese),** 1 | 18 |
| **Ham and Cheese Grinder,** 1 | 17 |
| **Ham and Cheese Grinder (without mayonnaise, cheese, or dressing),** 1 | 11 |
| **Ham and Turkey Grinder,** 1 | 16 |
| **Ham and Turkey Grinder (without mayonnaise, cheese, or dressing),** 1 | 10 |
| **Italian Grinder,** 1 | 19 |
| **Italian Grinder (without mayonnaise, cheese, or dressing),** 1 | 15 |
| **Light Turkey Grinder,** 1 | 10 |
| **Meatball Grinder,** 1 | 25 |
| **Meatball Grinder (without dressing or cheese),** 1 | 20 |
| **Reuben (without dressing or cheese),** 1 | 6 |
| **Reuben Grinder,** 1 | 14 |
| **Roast Beef Grinder,** 1 | 17 |

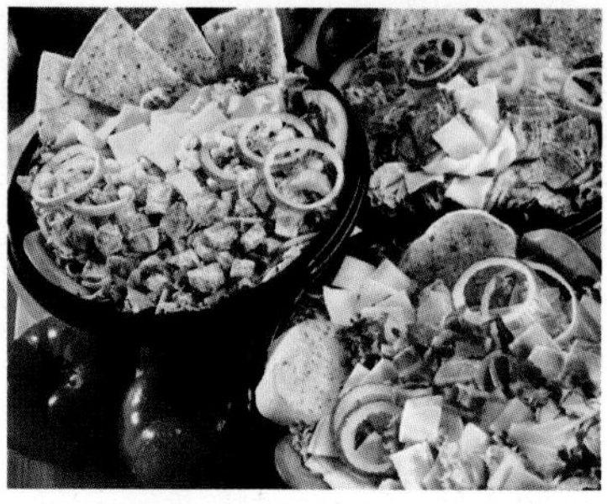

| ▲ Power Foods | *PointsPlus™* value |
|---|---|
| **Roast Beef Grinder (without mayonnaise, cheese, or dressing),** 1 | 12 |
| **Sirloin Steak Grinder,** 1 | 17 |
| **Sirloin Steak Grinder (without dressing or cheese),** 1 | 11 |
| **Spicy Chicken Grinder,** 1 | 17 |
| **Spicy Chicken Grinder (without mayonnaise, cheese, or dressing),** 1 | 10 |
| **Tuna Grinder,** 1 | 22 |
| **Tuna Grinder (without dressing or cheese),** 1 | 17 |
| **Turkey Grinder,** 1 | 15 |
| **Turkey Grinder (without mayonnaise, cheese, or dressing),** 1 | 10 |
| **Turkey Reuben Grinder,** 1 | 21 |
| **Veggie Grinder,** 1 | 12 |
| **Veggie Grinder (without dressing or cheese),** 1 | 7 |
| **SOUPS** | |
| **Chicken Noodle Soup,** 1 cup | 3 |
| **French Onion Soup (without cheese or sourdough),** 1 cup | 2 |
| **Tomato Bisque,** 1 cup | 9 |

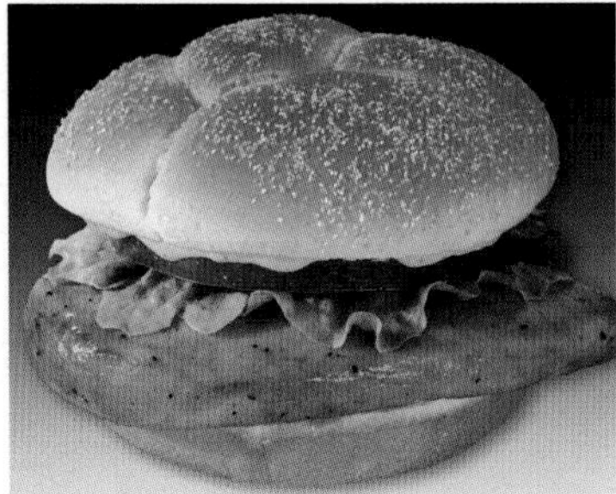

▲ Power Foods — *PointsPlus*™ value

## SANDWICHES

|  | PointsPlus™ value |
|---|---|
| **Bacon Deluxe Single,** 1 sandwich | 17 |
| **Bacon Deluxe Double,** 1 sandwich | 23 |
| **Bacon Deluxe Triple,** 1 sandwich | 30 |
| **Baconator®,** 1 sandwich | 26 |
| **Cheeseburger, Kids' Meal,** 1 burger | 7 |
| **Chicken Club Sandwich,** 1 sandwich | 17 |
| **Crispy Chicken Sandwich,** 1 sandwich | 10 |
| **Crispy Chicken Sandwich, Kids' Meal,** 1 sandwich | 9 |
| **Double Stack™,** 1 burger | 9 |
| **Double w/Everything and Cheese,** 1 sandwich | 20 |
| **Grilled Chicken Go Wrap,** 1 wrap | 7 |
| **Hamburger, Kids' Meal,** 1 burger | 6 |
| **Homestyle Chicken Fillet Sandwich,** 1 sandwich | 12 |
| **Homestyle Chicken Go Wrap,** 1 wrap | 8 |
| **Jr. Hamburger,** 1 sandwich | 6 |
| **Jr. Cheeseburger,** 1 sandwich | 7 |
| **Jr. Cheeseburger Deluxe,** 1 sandwich | 8 |
| **Jr. Bacon Cheeseburger,** 1 burger | 8 |
| **Single with Everything,** 1 | 12 |
| **Spicy Chicken Fillet Sandwich,** 1 sandwich | 12 |
| **Spicy Chicken Go Wrap,** 1 wrap | 8 |
| **Triple with Everything and Cheese,** 1 sandwich | 27 |
| **Ultimate Chicken Grill Sandwich,** 1 sandwich | 9 |

## SANDWICH COMPONENTS

|  | PointsPlus™ value |
|---|---|
| **1/4 lb. Hamburger Patty,** 1 patty | 6 |
| **American Cheese,** 1 serving | 2 |
| **American Cheese Jr.,** 1 serving | 1 |
| **Applewood Smoked Bacon,** 1 strip | 1 |
| **Bacon Jr.,** 1 strip | 0 |
| **Crispy Chicken Patty,** 1 patty | 6 |
| **Dill Pickles,** 4 pieces | 0 |
| **Homestyle Chicken Fillet,** 1 fillet | 6 |
| **Honey Mustard Sauce,** 1 serving | 1 |
| **Iceberg Lettuce Leaf,** 1 serving | 0 |
| **Jr. Hamburger Patty,** 1 patty | 2 |
| **Ketchup,** 1 serving | 0 |
| **Mayonnaise,** 1 serving | 1 |
| **Mustard,** 1 serving | 0 |
| **Natural Swiss Cheese,** 1 serving | 2 |
| **Onion,** 4 pieces | 0 |
| **Premium Bun,** 1 roll | 5 |
| **Ranch Sauce,** 1 serving | 1 |
| **Sandwich Bun,** 1 roll | 3 |
| **Spicy Chicken Fillet,** 1 fillet | 6 |
| **Tomato,** 1 slice | 0 |
| **Tortilla,** 1 | 3 |
| **Ultimate Chicken Grill Fillet,** 1 fillet | 3 |

| ▲ Power Foods | PointsPlus™ value |
|---|---|

## BONELESS WINGS & CRISPY CHICKEN NUGGETS

| Item | PointsPlus™ value |
|---|---|
| **Kids' Meal Chicken Nuggets,** 4 pieces | 5 |
| **Chicken Nuggets,** 5 pieces | 6 |
| **Chicken Nuggets,** 10 pieces | 13 |
| **Bold Buffalo Boneless Wings,** 1 serving | 14 |
| **Honey BBQ Boneless Wings,** 1 serving | 16 |
| **Sweet & Spicy Asian Boneless Wings,** 1 serving | 14 |
| **Barbecue Nugget Sauce,** 1 packet (2 Tbsp) | 1 |
| **Heartland Ranch Dipping Sauce,** 1 packet (2 Tbsp) | 4 |
| **Honey Mustard Nugget Sauce,** 1 packet (2 Tbsp) | 4 |
| **Sweet & Sour Nugget Sauce,** 1 packet (2 Tbsp) | 1 |

## SIDE SELECTIONS

| Item | PointsPlus™ value |
|---|---|
| **Buttery Best Spread,** 1 packet | 1 |
| ▲ **Side Salad,** 1 | 1 |
| **Caesar Side Salad, without dressing,** 1 | 2 |
| **Chili,** 1 small serving | 4 |
| **Chili,** 1 large serving | 7 |
| **French Fries,** 1 small serving | 9 |
| **French Fries,** 1 medium serving | 11 |
| **French Fries,** 1 large serving | 14 |
| **French Fries,** 1 kids serving | 6 |
| **Hot Chili Seasoning,** 1 packet | 0 |
| **Mandarin Orange Cup,** 1 serving | 2 |
| ▲ **Plain Baked Potato,** 1 potato | 7 |
| **Sour Cream & Chives Baked Potato,** 1 potato | 8 |
| **Saltine Crackers,** 2 | 1 |

## GARDEN SENSATIONS® SALADS

| Item | PointsPlus™ value |
|---|---|
| **Chicken BLT Salad,** 1 salad | 12 |
| **Chicken Caesar Salad,** 1 salad | 4 |
| **Mandarin Chicken® Salad,** 1 salad | 4 |
| **Southwest Taco Salad,** 1 salad | 10 |

## SALAD DRESSINGS & TOPPINGS

| Item | PointsPlus™ value |
|---|---|
| **Ancho Chipotle Ranch Dressing,** 1 packet | 2 |
| **Balsamic Vinaigrette Dressing,** 1 packet | 2 |
| **Classic Ranch Dressing,** 1 packet | 6 |
| **Fat Free French Dressing,** 1 packet | 2 |
| **Honey Dijon Dressing,** 1 packet | 7 |
| **Italian Vinaigrette Dressing,** 1 packet | 4 |
| **Light Classic Ranch Dressing,** 1 packet | 3 |
| **Light Honey Dijon Dressing,** 1 packet | 3 |
| **Oriental Sesame Dressing,** 1 packet | 5 |
| **Supreme Caesar Dressing,** 1 packet | 4 |
| **Thousand Island Dressing,** 1 packet | 8 |
| **Reduced Fat Acidified Sour Cream,** 1 packet | 1 |
| **Crispy Noodles,** 1 packet | 2 |
| **Homestyle Garlic Croutons,** 1 packet | 2 |
| **Roasted Almonds,** 1 packet | 4 |
| **Seasoned Tortilla Strips,** 1 packet | 3 |

## FROSTY™ TREATS

| Item | PointsPlus™ value |
|---|---|
| **Chocolate Frosty™,** 1 small | 9 |
| **Chocolate Frosty™,** 1 large | 14 |
| **Chocolate Fudge Frosty™ Shake,** 1 small | 11 |
| **Coffee Toffee Twisted Frosty™, Chocolate,** 1 | 15 |

*Frosty™ Treats (cont'd)*

| ▲ Power Foods | PointsPlus™ value |
|---|---|
| **Coffee Toffee Twisted Frosty™, Vanilla,** 1 | 15 |
| **Frosty™-cino,** 1 small | 10 |
| **Frosty™-cino,** 1 large | 14 |
| **M&M's® Twisted Frosty™, Chocolate,** 1 | 15 |
| **M&M's® Twisted Frosty™, Vanilla,** 1 | 15 |
| **Nestle® Toll House® Cookie Dough Twisted Frosty™, Chocolate,** 1 | 13 |
| **Nestle® Toll House® Cookie Dough Twisted Frosty™, Vanilla,** 1 | 13 |
| **Oreo® Twisted Frosty™, Chocolate,** 1 | 12 |
| **Oreo® Twisted Frosty™ Vanilla,** 1 | 12 |
| **Strawberry Frosty™ Shake,** 1 small | 11 |
| **Strawberry Frosty™ Shake,** 1 large | 14 |
| **Vanilla Frosty™,** 1 junior | 4 |
| **Vanilla Frosty™,** 1 small | 8 |
| **Vanilla Frosty™,** 1 large | 14 |
| **Vanilla Bean Frosty™ Shake,** 1 small | 11 |
| **Vanilla Bean Frosty™ Shake,** 1 large | 13 |
| **Vanilla Frosty™ Float with Coca-Cola,** 1 | 11 |

## BEVERAGES

| ▲ Power Foods | PointsPlus™ value |
|---|---|
| **Barq's® Root Beer,** 1 kids serving | 5 |
| **Coca-Cola®,** 1 kids serving | 5 |
| **Coffee,** 1 small | 0 |
| **Coffee Creamer,** 1 | 1 |
| **Coke Zero™,** 1 kids serving | 0 |
| **Dasani® Water,** 1 bottle | 0 |
| **Diet Coke®,** 1 kids serving | 0 |
| **Dr. Pepper®,** 1 kids serving | 5 |
| **Fanta® Orange,** 1 kids serving | 5 |
| **Hi-C® Flashin Fruit Punch,** 1 kids serving | 5 |
| **Minute Maid® Light Lemonade,** 1 kids serving | 0 |
| **Nesquik® Low Fat Chocolate Milk,** 1 bottle | 4 |
| **Nesquik® Low Fat White Milk,** 1 bottle | 3 |
| **Non-Nutritive Sweetener,** 1 packet | 0 |
| **Pibb Xtra®,** 1 kids serving | 5 |
| **Sprite®,** 1 kids serving | 4 |
| **Sugar,** 1 packet | 0 |
| **Sweet Tea,** 1 kids serving | 3 |

| ▲ Power Foods | *PointsPlus™* value |
|---|---|
| **ORIGINAL RECIPE BAGELS (WITHOUT SPREAD)** | |
| **Blueberry Bagel,** 1 | 6 |
| **Cinnamon Raisin Bagel,** 1 | 6 |
| **Egg Bagel,** 1 | 6 |
| **Everything Bagel,** 1 | 6 |
| **Honey Wheat Bagel,** 1 | 6 |
| **Jalapeño Bagel,** 1 | 6 |
| **Onion Bagel,** 1 | 6 |
| **Plain/Water Bagel,** 1 | 6 |
| **Pumpernickel Bagel,** 1 | 6 |
| **Rye Bagel,** 1 | 6 |
| **Sesame Bagel,** 1 | 6 |
| **SPECIALTY BAGELS** | |
| **Cheese Bagel,** 1 | 7 |
| **Everything Cheese Bagel,** 1 | 7 |
| **Jalapeño Cheese Bagel,** 1 | 8 |
| **Onion Cheese Bagel,** 1 | 7 |
| **Pizza Bagel,** 1 | 8 |
| **CREAM CHEESE** | |
| **Cucumber Onion Cream Cheese,** 1 serving | 3 |
| **Garlic Herb Cream Cheese,** 1 serving | 3 |
| **Honey Nut Raisin Cream Cheese,** 1 serving | 3 |
| **Jalapeno Green Chili,** 1 serving | 3 |
| **Low Fat Cream Cheese,** 1 serving | 2 |
| **Non-Fat Cream Cheese,** 1 serving | 1 |
| **Onion Cream Cheese,** 1 serving | 2 |
| **Regular Cream Cheese,** 1 serving | 3 |
| **Sour Cream & Onion Cream Cheese,** 1 serving | 3 |

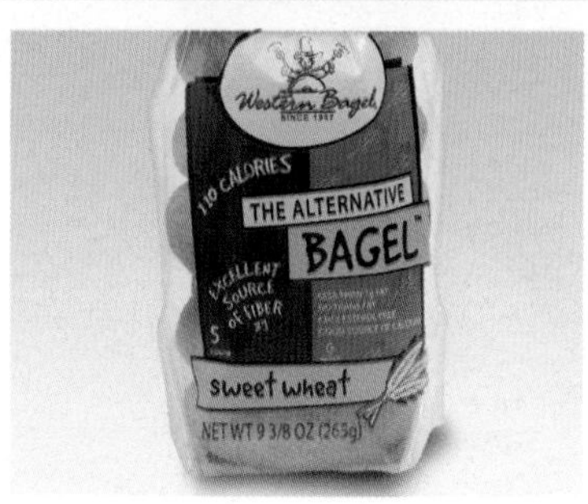


| ▲ Power Foods | *PointsPlus™* value |
|---|---|
| **Spinach Herb Cream Cheese,** 1 serving | 2 |
| **Sun Dried Tomato Cream Cheese,** 1 serving | 3 |
| **Vegetable Cream Cheese,** 1 serving | 2 |
| **THE ALTERNATIVE BAGEL** | |
| **Cinnamon Spice,** 1 | 3 |
| **Country white,** 1 | 3 |
| **Country White,** 1 | 3 |
| **Perfect 10 Bagel Healthy Grain,** 1 | 4 |
| **Roasted Onion,** 1 | 3 |
| **Sweet Wheat,** 1 | 3 |
| **Very Blueberry,** 1 | 3 |
| **THE ALTERNATIVE ENGLISH MUFFIN** | |
| **Plain,** 1 | 2 |
| **Wheat,** 1 | 2 |
| **THE ALTERNATIVE PITA** | |
| **Plain,** 1 | 3 |
| **Wheat,** 1 | 3 |

# WHATABURGER®

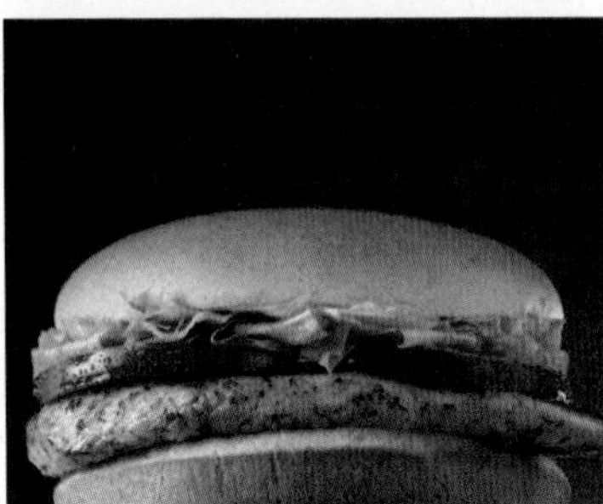

| ▲ Power Foods | *PointsPlus*™ value |
|---|---|

## BURGERS, CHICKEN & FISH

| | |
|---|---|
| **Chicken Strip,** 1 piece | 5 |
| **Chicken Strips,** 2 pieces | 10 |
| **Chicken Strips,** 3 pieces | 16 |
| **Chicken Strips (with gravy),** 4 pieces | 23 |
| **Grilled Chicken Sandwich,** 1 | 12 |
| **JUSTABURGER®,** 1 | 8 |
| **WHATABURGER®,** 1 | 16 |
| **WHATABURGER JR®,** 1 | 8 |
| **WHATACATCH® Sandwich,** 1 | 13 |
| **WHATACHICK'N® Sandwich,** 1 | 14 |

## SPECIAL REQUEST

| | |
|---|---|
| **WHATABURGER® (without bun oil),** 1 | 15 |
| **WHATACHICK'N® Sandwich (without bun oil & salad dressing),** 1 | 12 |
| **WHATACHICK'NR® Grilled Chicken Sandwich (without bun oil & salad dressing),** 1 | 11 |

## SALADS

| | |
|---|---|
| ▲ **Salad Garden, without dressing,** 1 | 1 |
| **Salad, Chicken Strips,** 1 | 15 |
| **Salad, Grilled Chicken, without dressing,** 1 | 6 |

| ▲ Power Foods | *PointsPlus*™ value |
|---|---|

## SIDE ORDERS

| | |
|---|---|
| **Cheese, American,** 1 small slice | 1 |
| **Cheese, American,** 1 large slice | 2 |
| **French Fries,** 1 small serving | 7 |
| **Gravy, White Peppered (for chicken strips),** 1 serving | 2 |
| ▲ **Jalapeno Sliced,** 1 serving | 0 |
| ▲ **Jalapeno, Whole,** 1 | 0 |
| **Onion Rings,** 1 medium serving | 11 |
| **Texas Toast,** 1 slice | 4 |

## BREAKFAST

| | |
|---|---|
| **Biscuit,** 1 | 8 |
| **Biscuit and Gravy,** 1 | 16 |
| **Honey Butter Chicken Biscuit,** 1 | 17 |
| **Biscuit Sandwich with Bacon, Egg, & Cheese,** 1 | 13 |
| **Biscuit Sandwich with Egg & Cheese,** 1 | 12 |
| **Biscuit Sandwich with Sausage, Egg, & Cheese,** 1 | 18 |
| **Biscuit with Bacon,** 1 | 9 |
| **Biscuit with Sausage,** 1 | 15 |
| **BREAKFAST-ON-A-BUN®, with Bacon,** 1 | 9 |
| **BREAKFAST-ON-A-BUN®, with Sausage,** 1 | 15 |
| **Egg Sandwich,** 1 | 8 |
| **Pancakes with Bacon, 3 pancakes, 2 slices bacon** | 17 |
| **Pancakes with Sausage, 3 pancakes, 1 sausage patty** | 22 |
| **Pancakes, plain,** 1 serving | 15 |
| **Taquito with Bacon & Egg,** 1 | 10 |
| **Taquito with Bacon, Egg & Cheese,** 1 | 11 |
| **Taquito with Potato & Egg,** 1 | 11 |
| **Taquito with Potato, Egg & Cheese,** 1 | 12 |

| ▲ Power Foods | *PointsPlus™* value |
|---|---|
| **Taquito with Sausage & Egg,** 1 | 10 |
| **Taquito with Sausage, Egg & Cheese,** 1 | 12 |
| **Hash Brown Sticks,** 4 | 5 |

## SHAKES & MALTS

| | |
|---|---|
| **Malt, Chocolate,** 1 small | 18 |
| **Malt, Chocolate,** 1 medium | 29 |
| **Malt, Chocolate,** 1 kids | 14 |
| **Malt, Strawberry,** 1 small | 18 |
| **Malt, Strawberry,** 1 medium | 28 |
| **Malt, Strawberry,** 1 kids | 14 |
| **Malt, Vanilla,** 1 small | 16 |
| **Malt, Vanilla,** 1 medium | 26 |
| **Malt, Vanilla,** 1 kids | 13 |
| **Shake, Chocolate,** 1 small | 17 |
| **Shake, Chocolate,** 1 kids | 14 |
| **Shake, Strawberry,** 1 small | 17 |
| **Shake, Strawberry,** 1 kids | 14 |
| **Shake, Vanilla,** 1 small | 15 |
| **Shake, Vanilla,** 1 kids | 12 |

## DESSERTS

| | |
|---|---|
| **Cinnamon Roll,** 1 | 11 |
| **Cookie Chocolate Chunk,** 1 | 7 |
| **Cookie White Chocolate Chunk Macadamia Nut,** 1 | 7 |
| **Hot Apple Pie,** 1 | 6 |
| **Hot Pumpkin Pie,** 1 serving | 9 |

# WHITE CASTLE®

| ▲ Power Foods | *PointsPlus*™ value |
|---|---|
| **SANDWICHES** | |
| **White Castle,** 1 | 4 |
| **Double White Castle,** 1 | 7 |
| **Cheeseburger,** 1 | 5 |
| **Double Cheeseburger,** 1 | 8 |
| **Bacon Cheeseburger,** 1 | 5 |
| **Double Bacon Cheeseburger,** 1 | 10 |
| **Jalapeno Cheeseburger,** 1 | 5 |
| **Double Jalapeno Cheeseburger,** 1 | 9 |
| **Chicken Breast Sandwich with Cheese,** 1 | 5 |
| **Chicken Ring Sandwich,** 1 | 5 |
| **Chicken Ring Sandwich with Cheese,** 1 | 5 |
| **Fish Sandwich with cheese,** 1 | 5 |
| **SIDE ORDERS** | |
| **Chicken Rings,** 6 rings | 9 |
| **Clam Strips,** 1 regular serving | 7 |
| **Fish Nibblers,** 1 regular serving | 8 |
| **French Fries,** 1 regular serving | 8 |
| **Mozzarella Cheese Sticks,** 3 sticks | 7 |
| **Onion Chips,** 1 regular serving | 13 |
| **CONDIMENTS & DIPPING SAUCES** | |
| **BBQ Sauce,** 1 packet | 0 |
| **Fat Free Honey Mustard Sauce,** 1 packet | 1 |
| **Marinara Sauce,** 1 container | 0 |
| **Seafood Sauce,** 1 container | 1 |
| **Tartar Sauce,** 1 serving | 1 |
| **White Castle Zesty Zing Sauce,** 1 container | 3 |
| **Maple Syrup,** 1 container | 3 |
| **Ranch Dressing,** 1 container | 4 |
| **Crave Cooler Coke,** 1 small | 4 |

# WINCHELL'S® DONUTS

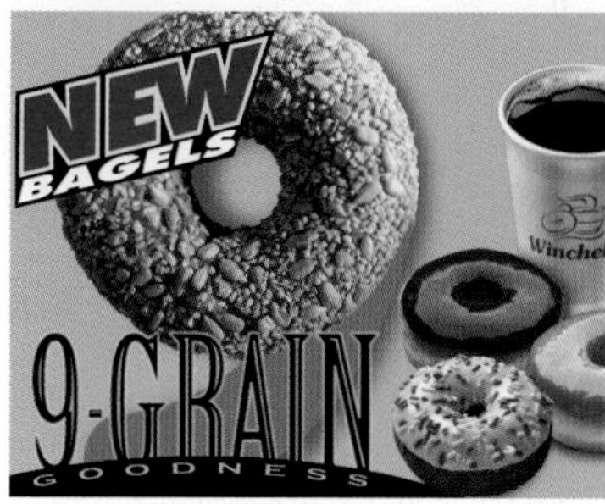


| ▲ Power Foods | *PointsPlus*™ value |
|---|---|
| **CAKE DONUTS** | |
| **Plain Cake,** 1 | 7 |
| **Iced Cake,** 1 | 9 |
| **RAISED DONUTS** | |
| **Chocolate Rounds,** 1 | 6 |
| **Chocolate Twist,** 1 | 11 |
| **Glazed Rounds,** 1 | 6 |
| **Glazed Twist,** 1 | 11 |
| **BAKED PRODUCTS** | |
| **Croissant,** 1 | 14 |

# YUM YUM® DONUTS

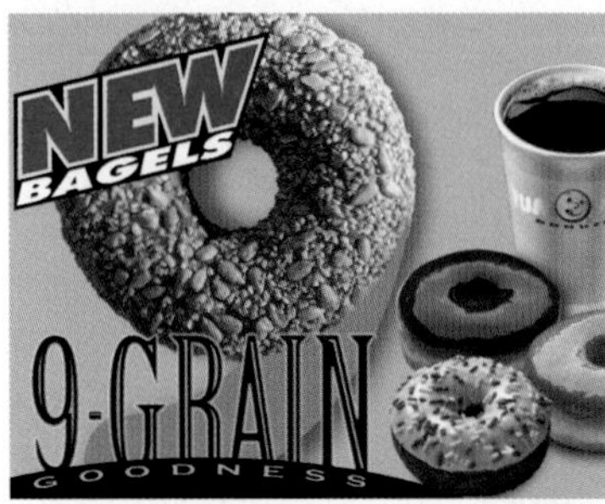


| ▲ Power Foods | *PointsPlus*™ value |
|---|---|
| **CAKE DONUTS** | |
| **Plain Cake,** 1 | 7 |
| **Iced Cake,** 1 | 9 |
| **RAISED DONUTS** | |
| **Chocolate Rounds,** 1 | 6 |
| **Chocolate Twist,** 1 | 11 |
| **Glazed Donuts,** 1 | 6 |
| **Glazed Twist,** 1 | 11 |
| **BAKED PRODUCTS** | |
| **Croissant,** 1 | 14 |

# TRADEMARK & PHOTOGRAPHY ACKNOWLEDGMENTS

Weight Watchers® gratefully acknowledges receipt of the nutrition information and photographs submitted by the participating restaurants for use in this ***Dining Out Companion*** and lists the following trademark information as supplied by the restaurants.

A & W is a registered trademark of A & W Restaurants, Inc.

Au Bon Pain is a registered trademark of ABP Corporation.

BLIMPIE is a registered trademark of Kahala Corp. and/or its subsidiaries, Scottsdale, AZ.

Bojangles' is a registered trademark of Bojangles' International, LLC.

Bruegger's is a registered trademark of Bruegger's Enterprises, Inc.

Bruster's Real Ice Cream is a registered trademark of Bruce Reed.

Burger King is a registered trademark of Burger King Brands, Inc. Other trademarks are used by Burger King with permission of the trademark's owner.

Camille's Sidewalk Café is a registered trademark of Beautiful Brands International.

Captain D's Seafood is a registered trademark of Captain D's, LLC.

Caribou Coffee is a registered trademark of Caribou Coffee Company.

Carl's Jr. is a registered trademark of Carl Karcher Enterprises, Inc.

Carvel is a registered trademark of Carvel Corporation.

Chevy's Fresh Mex is a trademark of Real Mex Restaurants, Inc.

Chick-fil-A is a registered trademark of CFA Properties, Inc.

Chili's Grill & Bar is a registered trademark of Brinker International Payroll Company, LP, a Delaware Corporation. Other trademarks, if used, are used with permission of the trademark's owner.

Chipotle Mexican Grill is a registered trademark of Chipotle Mexican Grill, Inc.

Church's Chicken is a trademark of Church's Chicken.

Cold Stone Creamery is a registered trademark of Cold Stone Creamery, Inc.

Corner Bakery Cafe is a registered trademark of CBC Restaurant Corp.

Country Kitchen Restaurant is a registered trademark of Kitchen Investment Group, Inc. Other trademarks are used by Country Kitchen Restaurant with permission of the trademark's owner.

Cousins Subs is a registered trademark of Cousins Subs.

Culver's is a registered trademark of Culver Enterprises, Inc. Other trademarks are used by Culver's with permission of the trademark's owner.

# TRADEMARK & PHOTOGRAPHY ACKNOWLEDGMENTS

DQ and the ellipse shaped logo are trademarks of Am. D.Q. Corp., Mpls., MN © 2010.

Denny's is a registered trademark of Denny's Corp. Other trademarks are used by Denny's Corp. with permission of the trademark's owner.

Dippin' Dots is a registered trademark of Dippin' Dots, Inc.

Domino's Pizza is a registered trademark of Domino's Pizza, Inc.

Donatos Pizza is a registered trademark of Donatos Pizza LLC.

Dunkin' Donuts is a registered trademark of DD IP Holder LLC. Used with permission.

Earls is a registered trademark of Earls Restaurants Ltd.

Eat'n Park is a registered trademark of Eat'n Park Restaurants.

El Pollo Loco is a registered trademark of El Pollo Loco, Inc.

Emerald City Smoothie is a registered trademark of ECS Company LLC.

Famous Dave's is a registered trademark of Famous Dave's of America, Inc.

Fazoli's is a registered trademark of Fazoli's System Management, LLC, Lexington, KY.

Fresh Choice is a registered trademark of Fresh Choice, LLC.

Freshëns is a registered trademark of Yogurt Ventures USA, Inc.

Godfather's Pizza is a registered trademark of Godfather's Pizza, Inc.

Golden Corral is a registered trademark of Golden Corral Corporation.

Golden Spoon Frozen Yogurt is a registered trademark of Golden Spoon, Inc.

Green Burrito is a registered trademark of Santa Barbara Restaurant Group, Inc.

Hardee's is a registered trademark of Hardee's Food Systems, Inc.

HuHot Mongolian Grill is a registered trademark of HuHot Mongolian Grills, LLC.

Jack in the Box is a registered trademark of Jack in the Box, Inc.

Jet's Pizza is a registered trademark of Jet's America, Inc.

Joe's Crab Shack is a registered trademark of Ignite Restaurant Group.

Jreck Subs is a registered trademark of Jreck Subs.

KFC is a registered trademark of KFC Corporation, Louisville, KY.

Kolache Factory is a registered trademark of Kolache Factory Inc.

Lee's Famous Recipe Chicken is a registered trademark of Lee's Famous Recipes Inc.

# TRADEMARK & PHOTOGRAPHY ACKNOWLEDGMENTS

Long John Silver's is a registered trademark of Long John Silver's, Inc.

Maid-Rite is a registered trademark of Maid-Rite Corporation.

Maui Wowi Hawaiian Coffee & Smoothies is a registered trademark of Maui Wowi Hawaiian Inc.

McDonald's is a registered trademark of McDonald's Corporation and its affiliates.

Miami Subs Pizza & Grill is a registered trademark of Miami Subs of Delaware, Inc. Other Trademarks are used by Miami Subs Pizza & Grill with permission of the trademark's owner.

Moe's Southwest Grill is a registered trademark of Moe's Franchisor LLC.

Monical's Pizza is a registered trademark of Monical Pizza Corporation.

Mrs. Fields is a registered trademark of The Mrs. Fields' Brand, Inc.

Noodles & Company is a registered trademark of Noodles and Company, a Delaware Corporation.

Old Chicago is a registered trademark of Rock Bottom Restaurants, Inc.

Olive Garden is a registered trademark of Darden Concepts, Inc., a wholly owned subsidiary of Darden Restaurants, Inc.

On The Border Mexican Grill & Cantina is a registered trademark of Brinker International Payroll Company, LP, a Delaware Corporation. Other trademarks, if used, are used with permission of the trademark's owner.

Outback Steakhouse is a registered trademark of OS Asset, Inc.

Papa Gino's is a registered trademark of Papa Gino's Holding Corporation.

Papa Murphy's TAKE 'N' BAKE PIZZA is a registered trademark of Papa Murphy's International, Inc.

Petro's Chili & Chips is a registered trademark of Petro's Franchise Group, LLC.

Piccadilly is a registered trademark of Piccadilly Restaurants, LLC.

The Pizza Hut name, logos and related marks are trademarks of Pizza Hut, Inc. and are used with permission.

Planet Smoothie is a registered trademark of Planet Smoothie LLC.

Pollo Tropical is a registered trademark of Carrols Corporation.

Port of Subs is a registered trademark of Port of Subs, Inc.

Roly Poly Sandwiches is a registered trademark of Roly Poly Franchise Systems LLC.

# TRADEMARK & PHOTOGRAPHY ACKNOWLEDGMENTS

Romano's Macaroni Grill and Macaroni Grill are both registered trademarks of Mac Acquisition IP LLC, a Delaware limited liability company. Other trademarks, if used, are used with permission of the trademark's owner.

Rubio's Fresh Mexican Grill is a registered trademark of Rubio's Restaurants, Inc.

Sandella's is a trademark of Sandella's LLC.

Schlotzsky's is a registered trademark of Schlotzsky's Franchise LLC.

Sizzler is a registered trademark of Sizzler USA Franchise, Inc.

Smoothie King is a registered trademark of Smoothie King Franchises, Inc.

Sonic, America's Drive-In is a registered trademark of America's Drive-In Brand Properties LLC.

Souper Salad is a registered trademark of Souper Salad, Inc.

Starbucks and the Starbucks logo are registered trademarks of Starbucks U.S. Brands, LLC.

SUBWAY Restaurants is a registered trademark of DAI.

Sweet Tomatoes and Souplantation are registered trademarks of Garden Fresh Restaurant Corp.

Taco Bell is a registered trademark of Taco Bell Corp. All rights reserved.

TACO JOHN'S is a registered trademark of Taco John's Seasonings Limited Partnership.

TacoTime is a registered trademark of Kahala Franchising, L.L.C. and/or its licensors.

TCBY is a registered trademark of TCBY Systems, LLC.

The Extreme Pita is a registered trademark of Extreme Pita IP.

Tim Hortons is a registered trademark of Tim Hortons USA Inc.

Tubby's is a registered trademark of Tubby's Sub Shops

Uno Chicago Grill is a registered trademark of Pizzeria Uno Corporation.

W.g. Grinders is a registered trademark of W.g. Grinders, Inc.

Wendy's is a registered trademark of Oldemark LLC and is licensed to Wendy's International, Inc.

WHATABURGER is a registered trademark of Whataburger Restaurants L.P.

Winchell's Donuts is a registered trademark of Winchell's Franchising, LLC.

Yum Yum Donuts is a registered trademark of Yum Yum Donut Shops, Inc.

Zoopa is a registered trademark of Fresh Choice, LLC.

# NOTES

# NOTES

## NOTES